1 MONTH OF
FREE
READING

at

www.ForgottenBooks.com

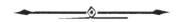

By purchasing this book you are eligible for one month membership to ForgottenBooks.com, giving you unlimited access to our entire collection of over 1,000,000 titles via our web site and mobile apps.

To claim your free month visit: www.forgottenbooks.com/free855004

ISBN 978-0-365-28381-2
PIBN 10855004

THE

PENINSULAR

JOURNAL OF MEDICINE

AND

THE COLLATERAL SCIENCES.

EDITED BY

E. ANDREWS, A.M., M.D.,

DEMONSTRATOR OF ANATOMY IN THE UNIVERSITY OF MICHIGAN.

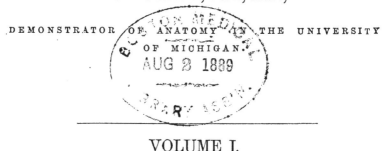

VOLUME I.

ANN ARBOR, MICHIGAN:

Printed for the Proprietors, by

GEORGE E. POMEROY & CO.

TRIBUNE OFFICE, DETROIT.

1853-4.

THE

PENINSULAR

JOURNAL OF MEDICINE

AND

THE COLLATERAL SCIENCES.

EDITED BY

E. ANDREWS, A.M., M.D.,

.DEMONSTRATOR OF ANATOMY IN THE UNIVERSITY OF MICHIGAN.

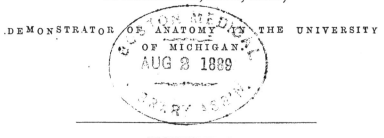

VOLUME I.

ANN ARBOR, MICHIGAN:

Printed for the Proprietors, by

GEORGE E. POMEROY & CO.

TRIBUNE OFFICE, DETROIT.

1853-4.

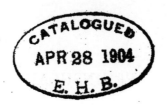

INDEX TO VOLUME I.

THE

PENINSULAR

JOURNAL OF MEDICINE

AND THE COLLATERAL SCIENCES.

| VOL. I. | JULY, 1853. | NO. I. |

ORIGINAL COMMUNICATIONS.

Art. I.—*Physiology of Spiritual Table Tipping.* By E. Andrews, M.D.

This veriest humbug that ever exhaled from the caverns of delusion, has brought to light one remarkable physiological truth, viz: *the power of other functions of the mind besides the will over the muscles.* Physicians should lose no time in investigating it, for another opportunity equally good may not occur in a century. Besides, physicians owe it to society to expose delusions which are based on physiological phenomena, since they alone are competent to do it. They should examine it, therefore, that their exposure may not be the laugh of ignorance, but the piercing sarcasm of men who understand the nature of what they speak.

The Rev. Charles Beecher, of N. J., at the request of an ecclesiastical association, has written a small work on this subject, in which he takes the ground that the "manifestations" are actually the work of evil spirits. His admission of the spirituality of the performances has had a bad effect in this region. All the tipsy tables have tipped with unwonted confidence ever since, and thousands, who held it to be mere nonsense before, are now staggered to learn that a Beecher has decided for the spirits.

We shall give this work a brief review for two reasons: one is, because many physicians who may not see the work itself will, nevertheless, have to combat the influence of its name, and the other is, because it is a fine sample of the pranks cut up by the nervous system, which, no longer content to delude hysterical girls, and superstitious old men and women, has in these last days, bestrode the pulpit, and made a learned divine, one from a family of ecclesiastical giants, think that there is actually a telegraph from the infernal regions, and that we are in the daily receipt of despatches from the devil.

The treatise in question commences, very necessarily, with a statement of the facts. Now, good reader, what kind of a statement of facts do you suppose was made by this clergyman of mighty name, this Beecher, who was appointed by the New York and Brooklyn Association to report on Spiritual Rappings. You who are accustomed to the searching, fact-sifting of scientific bodies—you possibly imagine that he commences with a careful description of the observations and experiments whereby he determined the phenomena, and with a clear statement of the tests whereby he sifted out the error, and analyzed the whole to the ultimate fact elements. Most learned doctor, you are mistaken. The whole question of facts is contained in a dozen lines. Here it is:

"The facts which constitute the pneumatic argument arrange themselves in four classes:—

"Class 1. Mysterious intelligent sounds and movements.

"Class 2. Involuntary polyglott speaking and writing.

"Class 3. Apparitions.

"Class 4. Doctrines, revelations, poems, prophecies and medical prescriptions, all delivered through the above instrumentalities."

This is all he has to say about the facts. The subsequent pages are learned and eloquent, but to what purpose? In science we are accustomed to require our authors to state item by item, all the circumstances in which their facts were observed, and all the tests to which they were subjected, because experience has shown that assertions not thus scrutinized are not worth a fig, and all arguments based on them, though they may be very logical, prove no more than a puff of nonsense.

He next proceeds to do battle with two opposing theories, which he handsomely demolishes, for he is good at the sword exercise of argument. He also brings up "*od*" or "*odyle*" with evident approbation, as the means by which evil spirits effect their communications with men, women and tables, upsetting the latter, jerking the elbows of the former, and kicking up a row generally.

This odyle is a name given to a supposed agent or force, by Baron von Reichenbach, of Vienna. It is supposed to be diffused throughout the universe, and the Baron has written a book of some 400 pages, filled with his observations and experiments upon it. At some future time we may review it for the amusement of our readers, at present suffice it to say that the majority of his phenomena were evidently nothing but the disordered sensations of the "sensitive" and "nervous" subjects upon whom he experimented. The Baron was evidently entirely ignorant of the pathology of the nerves of sensation. Whoever reads his work without understanding physiology will wonder and admire, but a physiologist will wonder and laugh.

The rest of Beecher's essay is devoted to showing that the tipping and rapping spirits are evil and not good spirits.

We have had some acquaintance with ecclesiastical bodies, and we think we can account for the production of this curious document without any disparagement to that noble profession. Clergymen, as a body, are not engaged in discovery. Their business is not so much to investigate new truths, as to enforce old ones; hence, in their associations they assign topics to each other, not so much for the investigation of facts as to develope originality of thought and fire of expression. In all probability the Congregational Association of New York and Brooklyn cared not one fig for the *investigation* of this humbug, but knowing that Mr. Beecher held some peculiar notions upon it, wished to enliven their meeting by drawing forth his ideas and his eloquence.

But laying Beecher aside, what and how much is there in these "manifestations." We have taken some pains to investigate the matter, and we affirm, as the result of our observations, that if you reject one-half of all the accounts for falsehood, and then two-thirds of the remainder for exaggeration and mistake, there will remain the following solid facts:

1st. Disordered innervation, causing delusions of the senses and spasmodic twitching of the muscles in all parts of the body.

2nd. Tables, stands, etc., by placing the medium's hands flat upon the upper surface, may be made to move about the room, get upon a sofa, dance to music, and tip out intelligent answers to questions *without any consciousness of voluntary exertion by the medium.*

3rd. The medium may write communications and answers to questions *without any voluntary directing of the hand or pencil.*

Any one who will seat half a dozen ladies of nervous temperament at a table, and cause them to hold their hands immoveably upon it for an hour, may produce the manifestations of twitching and disordered sensation, and a few repetitions will generally suffice to develope the table-moving power.

The character of many of the mediums is such as to leave no doubt that their agency is involuntary, at the same time our investigations have demonstrated the action of the muscles. They usually suppose that with the hands laid flat upon the smooth top of a table, it is impossible for muscular action to take effect, and we have often seen them raise the hand so as only to touch the table with the ends of their fingers and thumbs—a manœuvre which satisfies most observers that there is no muscular action in the case.

Our first experiment was to see whether this position of the hands was a sufficiently rigid test. To our surprise we found that with merely the tips of our fingers touching the table we could imitate all the evolutions of the spirits. We caused it to traverse the room in every direction, made it dance to music, and mount up upon the sofa, and with the tip of one finger pressed upon the top of it, we could use force enough to cause it to lie slowly down upon its side, and to rise up again. We next took a circular cherry table, four feet in diameter, and placing our hands flat upon the top, we forced it to walk up the perpendicular walls of our office, and then, top downward, to walk all about the ceiling. Being thus satisfied that muscular power was competent to the effect, we proceeded to test for its actual existence.

The mediums were confident that the table heaved and moved spontaneously beneath their hands. We placed a sheet of paper beneath their hands, when lo! the table stood still while the paper slid all over it. We next placed a book under their hands, and two round wooden pencils under the book as rollers. The book rolled about with great activity, but the indignant table would not budge an inch. We then placed our own hands under those of the medium, when we could distinctly feel the latter pushing and pulling upon our own. It was evident, therefore, that the power was exerted by the medium, not by the table. Lastly, we placed our fingers upon the tendon of the latissimus dorsi muscle where it crosses the axilla, and having ascertained that it was relaxed, requested the spirits to tip, when we could feel the tightening of the tendon as it drew the arm back. The muscular action was decided.

We next proceeded to test by questions, both vocal and mental, by which we ascertained the following facts:

1. When the question was vocal and the medium knew what the answer should be, *the spirit invariably replied correctly.*

2. When the question was such that the medium neither knew the answer, nor could have any possible chance of hitting right by coincidence, *the response was invariably wrong.*

3. When there was a chance of hitting right by coincidence, as in questions of yes and no, or questions of numbers and some others, the answers were sometimes right and sometimes wrong.

4. If the questions were mental, and no chance of guessing right existed, the answers were *always false.* If, in addition, the countenance

was so guarded as not to show *when* a mental question was asked, the answers were not only false in substance, but out of time with the question; and answers repeatedly came *when no questions had been asked.*

The following are our notes of one of these dialogues. It was a writing medium of the most unquestionable integrity. Having ascertained that the spirit could answer questions otherwise than by yes and no, we proceeded both with vocal and mental questions.

Question. (vocal) Will the spirits communicate?

Spirit. Yes.

Q. (vocal,) Whose spirit is writing now?

S. William Bassett's.

Q. (mental,) William, how many brothers has J——?

S. Yes.

Q. (mental,) Where does the oldest one live?

S. No.

Q. (mental,) Are they both married?

S. Yes. (This was incorrect.)

Q. (mental,) How many sisters has he?

S. Yes.

Q. (mental,) Who married his sister?

S. Yes.

Q. (vocal,) Will the table tip?

S. Yes.

Q. (vocal,) In how many minutes?

S. 10. (The spirit used figures.)

Q. (vocal,) Will the spirit write it in letters?

S. Ten. (Here the company went to the table and sat half an hour, but it would not tip.)

Q. (vocal,) What has been performing here to-night? (Here the pencil wrote something which was probably meant for "spirits," but it was nearly illegible and looked more like the word "infernal."

Medium to the Spirit. That isn't good; can't you write a little plainer? ·

The pencil then wrote after the former word very distinctly, S-p-i-r-t-s, "Spirts;" whereupon we took the slate and read the communication to the company, "Infernal Spirts." It was obvious to those present that the "infernal spirts" did not stand very rigid testing.

Putting together these with other facts, therefore it was clear that the knowledge of the medium and the chances of conjecture, had some connection with the correctness or incorrectness of the answers; in short, that the communication came from living souls in this world, not from "infernal spirts" of the other. And yet the high and irreproachable character of the mediums compelled us to believe that their actions were not vol--untary. The question then remained, Can the mental states express themselves in muscular actions *without* the intervention of the will?

The table-tippers and spirit-writers have developed one great truth, which, though previously known in special applications, has only recently seemed to receive a full general acknowledgment, and that is this: Not only the will, but every other function of the mind is a natural stimulant to the muscles, competent, when acting with the will, to give it double effect, but also able to act without it and produce *intelligent involuntary actions.*

Undoubtedly the clearest development of this principle is seen in the muscles of the countenance. These are handed over almost entirely to the involuntary class, and almost all their action is in response to the stimulus of thought and emotion; there is no volition, no consciousness of their action. It is certain, therefore, that thought and emotion, as well as volition, have control over muscular power.

We hold that every muscle in the body is subject to the same influence, and that the reason why we do not notice it, is because the superior power of volition masks the effects of the other mental functions. If this is true, then we should expect that by giving these functions a relative preponderance over the will, they would re-assert their motor power and bring the muscles under their control. This may be done by giving the emotions unusual power, as in terror or in pain, the involuntary writhing and recoiling of which are too familiar; or it may be done by concentrating the thoughts on a particular action and withholding the will. This is the method of the mediums, and by it they secure action which corresponds to thought without volition.

Normally, however, this power acts in conjunction with the will. This is the triple strength which nerves the limbs of men under intense excitement—the superadded force which renders them competent to meet great emergencies. We often see at a fire instances where men, with a very slight *voluntary* effort, will pick up and carry off a piece of furniture which they could not lift in their cooler moments. A striking instance of the tremendous energy of this superadded force occurred in one of the old Scottish wars. A soldier struck a horseman with a battle-axe with such violence, that the weapon at one blow clove down through the rider and his horse, killing both, and then broke a paving-stone beneath.

The common experiment of a few persons lifting another on the tips of their fore-fingers is another instance. Standing around, they all take breath together, and at a given signal they blow under the person to be raised, when he rises like a cork. So striking is the result, and so little is the consciousness of exertion, that the operators often imagine that the person is raised by the breath they blow under him, and not by their fingers. It is obvious, however, that the sole use of the breath is to be a signal, and by the formality of the preparation, to concentrate their thoughts intently on the desired action.

Here, then, we have the power for producing the spiritual manifestations, viz: muscular power without volition, and without distinct consciousness. It now remains to show how involuntary power can produce intelligent actions, which is quickly done.

The most striking law of this involuntary force is its tendency to execute whatever motions the mind dwells upon, even contrary to the will. Who has not felt the irresistible disposition to move his head when sitting for a daguerreotype, simply from fixing it so strongly in mind that that motion must not be made. So in the above cases of excitement, the superadded force comes in to execute the movements upon which the mind is intent: hence it coincides with volition. The case is the same in a thousand instances in life where a vivid conception of an action causes an unconscious imitation of it. It is seen also in skilled musicians, in whom the mere desire to have a certain note prompts the requisite motion of the fingers without any consciousness of volition, and it is remarkable that this involuntary style of action gives a more delicate and perfect execution than acts of mere will.

Now the Spiritualists have the merit of having demonstrated that this involuntary power may be separated from the voluntary, and made to act alone; and also that the thought or wish of any motion is as efficient as willing the motion. This is the whole mystery of involuntary writing and tipping. Any sensitive person may try the experiment for himself. Take a pencil in the hand, and without any support for the arm, hold the point lightly on a sheet of paper until the hand begins to twitch and tremble with nervousness and fatigue—a little superstitious awe will help— then looking earnestly at the pencil, picture in your fancy vividly the letters you wish to produce. If you are of a nervous temperament, you will now feel an involuntary impulse of the hand in the requisite directions, and by perseverance and repetition, you may in a little time become a writing medium, a telegraph operator for the devil, as Beecher would say, but really, one over whose muscles fancy has usurped the place of will.

We have proved this by actual experiment, and have been able ourselves to write involuntary communications. Table tipping is still easier.

Since writing the above we see by the journals that Dr. Carpenter, of England, has put forth an essay in which he proves that other acts of mind than the will may control the muscles. We have also just received a letter from Dr. John C. Norton, a highly intelligent physician of Ill., in which he says: " In regard to the writing, I have probed the matter to the very bottom. I have been a writing medium, and can demonstrate by an analysis of my own mind while engaged in receiving communications, that the spirits of the dead are not at all concerned in it. I do not take the ground that it is all imposture; in fact I know better. *The will has nothing to do with the actions performed, and yet they are all the work of the mind.*"

We are perfectly aware that most unexplainable stories are every day told, but be wary of two things, first, of phenomena not rigidly tested, and secondly of second-hand statements. We have in our investigations detected eye-witnesses of the very highest integrity, in egregious false statements in consequence of their excitement.

In conclusion, we give it as our own impression, that the claim of " spirituality " for the " manifestations " is an unmitigated humbug, and we are willing to test it with any decent medium that dare try it. We will ask twenty plain and fair questions, and we defy any medium in or out of Michigan to answer them all correctly, either by writing, rapping or tipping; and we will set a suitable table in the middle of our room, and after we have taken the proper measures to prevent the application of muscular action and mechanical force, we defy all the spirits out of Pandemonium to move it a single foot.

Art. II.—*Epilepsy, Treated by Ligation of the Common Carotid Artery.* Case reported by Z. Pitcher, M.D.

In the summer of 1849, a young woman of fine physical developments and more than ordinary cerebral activity, called at my office for professional advice. From the statement then made, it appeared that she was subject, at irregular intervals, to attacks of Epilepsy. The attacks also varied in form, or force, and in the number that might occur in any given day or night, having relation to the intensity of the exciting circumstances concerned in their production. Ordinarily, the paroxysms which occurred in the day time, were such as M. Esquirol terms *Petit Mal*, whilst the nocturnal ones were usually of the violent convulsive character, called in the French schools, the *Grand Mal*. Of these two varieties, she states that she has had as many as twenty-four in twenty-four hours. At other times, a week or two would elapse without a return of either.

This person was, at the time of this conversation, twenty-two years old, and had been subject to this form of disease, since the seventeenth year of her age, prior to which time, the menstrual function had been fully established.

Miss ———— first felt, what she now regards the premonitory indications of her disease, when about thirteen years old. This was a strange and indescribable sensation in the right arm. For some time the sensation was confined to the forearm. At length it passed above the elbow, and, finally, its place of appearing became fixed at the point where the Omo-hyoideus muscle emerges from under the Trapezius. From this time, it could be recognised as the aura epileptica, being peculiar in this respect, that the patient was always impressed with the idea that a warm liquid was issuing from the place affected.

During this interview, I became impressed with the analogies in this case, as to age, sex, mental and physical endowments, to one which terminated fatally a few years before, in which I was permitted to make an autopsic examination, where the pons varolii and medulla oblongata were found very much indurated. At the same time, I learned that she had been under the treatment of intelligent physicians, both at Geneva and Buffalo; from which, I came to the conclusion, that I had nothing to hope from ordinary medication. These circumstances led me, after trying the effects of Conium and Stramonium, to form the resolution of cutting off from the brain, by applying a ligature to the carotid artery, one half of the blood distributed to that organ.

It may be well to state, that I had taken pains to assure myself that there was no disease of the medulla spinalis, no effusion into the theca vertebralis, no caries of the spinal column, no disease of the heart or respiratory organs, no disorder of the stomach or collatitious viscera, no impediments to the performance of the functions of the uterus or ovaria; in fine, no evidence of complication, either by mental disorder, physical derangement, or habits of body, exterior to the cerebral centre, to which the seizures could, with any degree of certainty, be referred.

The ligature was applied below the omo-hyoideus, whilst the patient was under the influence of chloroform. No unfavorable symptom occurred. Since the operation, the *aura* has never returned, neither have the grave and convulsive forms of the disease. For more than two years, there was no seizure of any kind. But, within the past year, when exercise is omitted, and any unpleasant mental disturbance takes place at the same time, very slight returns of the *Petit Mal* occur, but never to occasion loss of consciousness. The health of the young woman is now perfect. Her temper, which had been rendered irritable, by the disease of her nervous centre, is very much improved, and her appreciation of existence greatly enhanced.

The space alloted to this case will admit of no remarks.

NOTE:—Having, at the time of the operation, no friend accustomed to administer anaesthetics, I availed myself of the services of Dr. J. B. Brown, now of the U. S. Army, by whom the artery was tied.

Detroit, 1853.

ARTICLE III.—*Report of Cases, by* PROFESSOR PALMER, *of Chicago.* *Combination of Chloroform and Opium.*

JANUARY 14TH, 1853.—Was called to Wm. Roselle, American, aged 62, strong and muscular, but of somewhat intemperate habits.

The history of the case, as given by himself, was that thirty-eight days before, he received a fall, striking his left shoulder against a fence. This was followed by pain, tumefaction, and inability to move the arm. He had been under the care, and been visited some eight or ten times, by a Homœopathic practitioner, who appends an M. D. to his name, and had taken various pillets, as he thought, with but little effect upon his shoulder, though he insisted they operated as a cathartic upon his bowels! He said his shoulder had been repeatedly examined, but what his attendant considered the nature of the difficulty he did not know. On examination of the shoulder, a dislocation of the head of the humerus, downwards and forwards under the margin of the pectoral muscle, was found.

Considering an attempt at reduction justifiable, although between five and six weeks had passed since the occurrence of the displacement, Drs. De Laskie Miller and H. A. Johnson, and Mr. A. Young present and assisting. "Jarvis' Adjustor" was applied, and the patient put under the influence of chloroform, though not to the extent of complete insensibility. Gradual extension was made in the direction of the axis of the limb, it being at the same time gently rotated backwards and forwards until the head of the bone was felt superficially in the axilla, below and a little interior to its natural situation. When by means of a strap passed under the arm of the patient and over the shoulder of the operator, the head of the bone was lifted obliquely upwards and backwards into its proper cavity. The head of the bone slipped into its place, not with the usual abrupt snap or shock, as in a recent case, but as if the smooth, hard surfaces were covered with some semi-solid substance, as they doubtless were. The extending cords were immediately relaxed,—the arm carried to the side when the joint was found in place,—the shoulder presenting its usual rotundity. Proper dressings were applied, and the progress of the case was gradual, but satisfactory, as long as observed.

The time employed in the reduction did not exceed fourteen minutes from the commencement of extension, and the suffering of the patient during the whole operation, was very inconsiderable

Jarvis' Adjustor, though by no means an indispensable article in the reduction of dislocations, yet in the facility with which the requisite force can be applied and regulated, and in the freedom allowed for the necessary manipulations, possesses advantages over all ordinary apparatus. While the chloroform is invaluable, not only in preventing suffering, but also by producing muscular relaxation, and thereby greatly faciliating the process. By the adoption of these modern *American* improvements, ordinary uncomplicated dislocations need not be a dread to the Surgeon.

TUESDAY, FEBRUARY 1ST, 4 O'CLOCK, A. M.—Called to Bridget, Jordan, Irish, aged 28, exceedingly small, height as afterwards taken, four feet six inches; in labor with her sixth child, all five having been still-born from severity of labor, caused by disproportionate size of mother and child. History, as obtained from midwife in attendance, and from the patient, was, that she was taken in labor on Sunday morning, two days before, and that about noon of the same day "the waters broke and a hand came down." Pains had recurred frequently ever since, and were most of the time severe. The patient, though so small, appeared to have much firmness of constitution, and had been in good health. There was considerable feverish excitement and tenderness of the abdomen and parts, the pulse full and firm. On examination, the right hand and arm of a full sized fœtus, at term, was found presenting externally, the palm upward as the mother lay upon her back, and the thumb was towards her right thigh, showing the back of the child to the back of the mother, and the head towards the right side. From the long continuance and severity of the pains, the shoulder was pressed down deep into the pelvis, and this result was further increased by the tractive efforts of the midwife upon the arm, and who expressed the hope that the labor would soon be over. No motion of the child was felt, and no sound of the fœtal heart was heard on auscultation. The great disproportion between the size of the woman and child, the great length of time (nearly forty hours) since the discharge of the waters, the firm contraction of the uterus from the severity of the pains about the child, and its impaction in the pelvis rendered the case one of unusual difficulty and embarrassment. Of course, in all cases of this kind turning is the remedy if practicable, and evisceration, a tedious

and dangerous dissection, the only alternative, and in this case it was
evident that if turning was to be attempted, the use of all the means
possible tending to facilitate the operation and diminish the shock
and other injurious consequences to the system would be required.—
An attempt at turning was decided upon. The indications clearly
were to produce general and especially uterine relaxations, to prevent
the terrible suffering during the process, and to guard against inflammation. Keeping these indications in view, the following course
was pursued. A large dose (about one grain) of Morphine was
administered, and as its effects began to be fully realized, the patient
was placed in a proper position for turning, a vein was opened and
blood taken until the pulse was decidedly softened; the administration
of Chloroform was then commenced, and cautiously persevered in,
until its full anæsthetic effect was produced. The operation then commenced, and although it was somewhat difficult, the hand being almost
paralyzed by the firmness of the pressure, a foot was brought down and
filleted, the arm gradually receded, and in half an hour the patient was
delivered of a dead male child, weighing nearly nine pounds. Under the
use of anodynes, fomentations and laxatives, the woman did well and speedily
" got up. " I have been somewhat minute in the details of this case,
because, to me at least, it possesses more than ordinary interest, not only
from the difficulties it presented, but likewise from the combination of
remedies which were used to overcome them. The bleeding and opium
are old remedies of established reputation. The philosophy of their use
is well understood. Latterly, however, chloroform or ether has taken the
place of opium. In all ordinary cases, the full effect of either of these
anæsthetic articles, fulfills the necessary indications, and is all that is
required. Nearly five years ago, and without any known precedent as a
guide, I used chloroform with the most gratifying results where turning
was performed in a first labor, and where the waters had been drained off
for twelve hours. I considered that the administration of a large opiate,
the usual treatment, would have been more effectual in producing uterine
relaxations, and that cases would occur requiring the use of that remedy;
but where turning could be effected *without* too much violence under the
use of chloroform, it was the preferable agent, as no dose of the opiate
compatable with the safety of the patient could prevent severe suffering,
and the completion of the safe delivery of the child, after the turning,
would be likely to be protracted by the continued absence of uterine
contractions for a considerable length of time; and although the combined administration of an opiate and chloroform suggested itself, I did
not venture upon it, fearing for the immediate safety of the patient from
the combined influence of those powerful agents. Up to the time of the

occurrence of the case of Bridget Jordan, I have been detailing, I had had no experience, and have yet seen no account of their full and united effects, but the necessity for a greater amount of *uterine* relaxation than chloroform would produce, and for a greater degree of insensibility than a safe dose of opium would accomplish, induced me to run the hazard of combining their effects, and the result was all that could be desired. The anæsthesic was complete, but in no respect unpleasant. Neither the pulse, the respiration or the countenance was materially affected. In the flushed, heated and sensitive condition of the patient, the bleeding certainly aided the relaxation; and I apprehend rendered the other means less dangerous, as well as guarded against what we have in such cases so much to dread as a sequel, severe inflammation.

Chicago, April, 1853.

Art. IV.—*Description of a new plant discovered by* John C. Norton, M. D., *Ill.*

I send you a description of a species of Nasturtium, which I find here growing upon the springy side hills, and which I have taken the liberty to name " pinnatifida."

Description.—Pod somewhat flattened, turned upwards; flowers small, light yellow, in a terminal corymb; petals of the length of the calyx; stem upright sub-pubescent; leaves doubly and triply pinnatifid; lower leaves, segments ovate or rounded; upper leaves, segments linear oblong, involute. Pubescence on stem and leaves appearing glutinous under a lens. One to two feet high: moist side hills bordering on Rock River, Illinois. May 14, 1852.

Art. V.—*Strangulated Inguinal Hernia, from imperfect descent of the Testicle of the right side, Orchitis. By* Wm. Brodie, M. D.

On the evening of the 2d November, 1852, I was called into the country some 30 miles distant, to operate upon David G——, a farmer, for Strangulated Hernia. Upon my arrival, I found him lying upon his back, on the bed, with his limbs drawn up. Cold, clammy perspiration, pulse weak and small, countenance anxious, at times suffering extreme pain, followed with vomiting. Poultices of pulverized charcoal had been applied for sometime to the part.

Upon examination, I found a large tumor in the right groin, irregular upon its convexity, the superior portion hard, the inferior tense but elastic, the whole exquisitely sensitive. The upper portion of the tumor lay directly over the external abdominal ring.

The lower portion of the swelling gave the usual impulse upon coughing, satisfying me that this was the Hernial protrusion.

Upon examination of the scrotum, I found therein but one testicle. He informed me that from a boy there had always been a small swelling in the upper portion of the groin, which upon pressure, gave a sensation like that produced by squeezing the testicle in the scrotum.

Having placed him in a position favorable to the reduction of the Hernia, I raised up the lower border of the testicle with the left hand, and with the right grasped the sac, making pressure in the axis of descent for a few minutes, when the gut returned with its significant gurgle. Immediate relief was felt. The patient being somewhat exhausted, I ordered him some stimulus, and gave him an opiate.

The testicle was, in this case, the cause of the strangulation, having in its passage downwards into the scrotum, (from some cause,) stopped upon its exit through the external abdominal ring.

The Hernia, which was of some years standing, he had always been able to reduce himself, until this occasion, his manipulations to reduce it gave rise to inflammation of the testicle, which from its increased size, closed up the ring, and pressing upon the neck of the sac, prevented its return. It was, in fact, the stricture.

The case is interesting in two points; first in its rarity, and second in its diagnosis. The attending physician had tried in vain to reduce the mass, and as a dernier resort, said an operation must be performed.

Two interesting cases are detailed in the London Lancet, pages 358, 359 and 360, of vol. 2, 1852; however in neither of these did orchitis exist.

Before leaving, I gave directions for treating the orchitis, and placed him again in the hands of his former physician. I have since heard from him, and learned that he has recovered.

Detroit, Michigan, April 6th, 1853.

ART. VI.—*Cancerous Growths.* *Experiments of* DR. H. A. JOHNSON. *Artificial Tissues.* *By* E. ANDREWS, M. D.

Cancer growths have long defied the investigations of knife and microscope, of retort and crucible, to disclose the conditions of their malignancy. Probably bolder sweeps must be made by the wing of Science, before we shall see the unlocking of this mystery. The scope of investigation, however, at present leads us to hope that we may yet succeed in forming artificial tissues, and learn from them the conditions of their growth and means of their extermination.

Dr. Johnson, one of the enterprising editors of the N. W. Medical Journal, has given this subject an examination He remarks (vol. 1,¶ 1, new series,) that the anatomical cause of the malignancy of cancer is the continual and irrepressible growth and reproduction of cells. He next shows, by chemical analysis, that there is in these growths a remarkable predominance of inorganic salts, and also remarks upon the fact that malignant growths are most frequently found where cell growths predominate, as in glands and mucous membranes, but most frequently of all in those glands to which there is a special determination of these salts, as the testes and the mammae. The experiments of Beneke and others have even shown that these salts, particularly those of lime, soda and potash, may actually be made to generate bodies resembling cells, out of the body. Dr. Johnson repeated and varied these experiments, with a view to ascertain whether these salts might not have such a cell producing power as to account for the inordinate cell growth of cancer. His notes are as follows:

"Exp. No. 1. Albumen, fat and water intimately mingled together. Exposed to a uniform temperature of 104° F. Examined after nine hours—contains oil globules, granules, and a few imperfect celluloid bodies. After twenty-two hours no perceptible change noticed.

Exp. No. 2. Albumen, oil, water and phosphate of lime. At the expiration of ten hours, contains granules and bodies resembling the cells found in pus and mucus. After twenty-two hours, granules previously noticed very abundant—bodies resembling pus or mucus globules, with masses of matter very similar to those sometimes found in the urine, and composed of epithelial scales. After seventy hours fewer of the granules and a large number of the celluloid bodies. Upon the addition of acetic acid, dark spots are seen having all the appearance of nuclei; each globule seems to have a perfect cell wall.

Exp. Nos. 3, 4, 5 and 6 were variations of Nos. 1 and 2, by subjecting to pressure during the process, and by adding to the preparation a small quantity of super carb. soda in solution. The results were similar to those previously noticed.

Exp. No. 7. Oil, phosphorus and water enclosed in a piece of bladder, and placed in a cup containing albumen. After thirty-six hours, the albumen in the cup contains granules and celluloid bodies as in previous experiments—the bladder is nearly empty with the exception of gas with which it is distended. In the drop of fluid remaining there is found an abundance of the phos. lime, oil globules and the celluloid bodies. Acetic acid affects them precisely as it does organic cells. Ether renders the walls more opaque.

Exp. No. 8. Repetition of No. 7, with like results.

Exp. No. 9. Albumen, water, and super carb. soda in a glass tube, closed by clean, fresh membrane, and immersed in a cup containing oil, water and phos. lime held in solution by acetic acid. After twenty hours the fluid in the cup contains granules, celluloid bodies, and triangular prismatic crystals, almost exactly like those of the triple phosphate found in the urine. In the tube are granules and a few celluloid bodies.

Exp. No. 10. Albumen, water, phosphate of lime, slightly acidulated with acetic acid, in a tube closed by membrane, and placed in a cup containing oil, super carb. soda, and water. After twenty hours the fluid has all passed out of the tube into the cup, which contains bodies like those already described, and others of greater size, more irregular outline, and containing large distinct nuclei.

Exp. No. 13. Oil, phos. lime, and water slightly acidulated, in a tube closed by membrane and placed in a cup containing albumen, water and carb. potass. After twenty-four hours the cup and tube both contained celluloid bodies of small size and very regular outline."

From these experiments he concludes that the inorganic salts favor cell development, and that the presence of these salts in excess is the cause of that ungovernable growth and reproduction of cells which is the element of destruction in every cancer.

He derives from these facts two indications of treatment. First, to prevent the receiving of the salts into the system. This he would accomplish by making the diet as purely vegetable as the patient will bear, vegetable food containing less of the obnoxious substances than animal. The second indication is to remove from the system as much as may be the salts that accumulate in it. To this end he would make free use of the organic acids, particularly the lactic, because these acids readily dissolve the calcareous and other salts, and these keep them in a condition to be eliminated by the proper excretory organs. This subject of the formation of artificial tissues is still under investigation in Europe. The British and Foreign Medico-Chirurgical Review for April speaks of artificial cells formed by M. Panum, from the serum of blood, resembling milk corpuscles. He first obtained from the serum a substance resembling the caseine of common cheese; this substance he dissolved by adding phosphate of soda, and then added butter and sugar in the proper proportions for milk. The whole being shaken up and then allowed to cool, had the white color and very much the taste of real milk. Under the microscope, corpuscles like milk corpuscles were observed, and also bodies like nuclei of cells with nucleoli in them. Animals readily drank and digested this artificial milk, but it differed from the natural product in not being capable of perfect coagulation.

M. Melsens has been experimenting with artificial fibrous tissue and membrane. He makes a saturated solution of albumen and some salt, and then exposes it to a violent shaking. In consequence of the agitation the clear solution becomes turbid with fibres, which, when allowed to come to rest and settle in one stratum, form a sort of membrane. These fibres, under the microscope, have a clean outline and look like perfectly organized bodies, resembling the yellow fibrous tissue. These experiments are interesting, as tending to bring all the resources of science to settle the question whether art can originate organized tissues. The above experiments, plausible as they seem, are not perfectly satisfactory; for, although we can understand that a globule of oil floating in a saline albuminous solution, might, by chemical action, form a solid covering or sack around itself, it is not clear that it would be any thing more than a chemical precipitate on the surface of the oil. It is not fairly proved yet whether these artificial cells can or cannot perform the vital functions of secretion, reproduction and nutrition. A similar remark may be made of the fibres spoken of. The form resembles that of known organized fibre, but whether they are possessed of any property of life is not known. The fibrous form is not decisive as to vitality, because we can easily conceive that the curling eddies in the agitated fluid might draw the forming albuminous precipitate into fibres and shreds without a particle of living tissue being in existence. Yet it is gratifying to find that investigators are going on in the attempt to form living tissue, for if they succeed they will shed a flood of light on obscure diseases, and if they ultimately fail, it will be almost as valuable as a negative result, as success would be for a positive one. It will be a great point gained when we know whether organic synthesis is or is not possible to the chemist.

SELECTIONS.

From the Boston Medical and Surgical Journal.

Hygienics of Temperance.   *By* Samuel A. Cartwright, M.D., *New Orleans, late of Natchez.*

Whether water or alcohol be the better health-preserving agent, is a question to be determined by observation. Some account of the effects of each on a number of the Æsculapii themselves, is herewith respectfully presented to that profession whose office it is to keep in tune the curious harp of man's body, and to take cognizance of everything which preserves or disturbs its harmony. Nothing tends more to preserve or disturb its harmony than water and alcohol. Hence the members of the medical profession, who may take sides in the temperance controversy, now agitating the people of every State in the Union, are not to be regarded as out of their province, but in a field properly belonging to them, where instead of being viewed as intruders or intermeddlers, they are, by virtue of their calling, entitled to rank as chiefs.

The writer is one of three physicians, who located in Natchez thirty years ago. The new comers found only *one* practitioner in the city belonging to the same temperance school with themselves. The country and villages within fifteen miles around afforded only *three* more. All the rest believed in the hygienic virtues of alcoholic drinks, and taught that doctrine by precept and example. Besides the practising physicians, there were ten others in the city and adjacent country who had retired from the profession. They were all temperate. Thus, including the new comers, the total number of temperance physicians, in and near Natchez, thirty years ago, consisted of seventeen. Of these, five have died:—Dr. Henry Tooley, aged about 75 years; Dr. Andrew M'Creary, aged 70; Dr. J. Ker, 60; Dr. Wm. Dunbar, 60; Dr. James A. McPheeters, 49. In 1823, the average ages of the seventeen was about 34 years. According to the Carlisle tables of mortality, and those of the Equitable Insurance Company of London, seven insteal of five would have been the ratio of mortality in England. Those at present living are Drs. D. Lattimore, W. Wren, Stephen Duncan, James Metcalf, W. N. Mercer, G. W. Grant, J. Saunderson, Benj. F. Young, T. G. Elliott, —— Phœnix, Prof. A. P. Merrill, and the writer.

On the other hand, every physician of Natchez and its vicinity, thirty years ago, whether practising or retired, who was in the habit of *tippling*, as the practice of drinking alcoholic beverages is called, has long since been numbered with the dead! Only two of them, who were comparatively temperate, lived to be gray. Their average term of life did not exceed 35 years, and the average term of life of those who were in the habit of taking alcoholic drinks frequently between meals, on an empty stomach, did not reach thirty years. In less than ten years after they commenced the practice, the most of them died, and the whole of them have subsequently fallen, leaving not one behind in the city, country or village, within twenty miles around.

To fill the places of those who died or retired from the profession, sixty-two medical men settled in Natchez and its vicinity between the years 1824 and 1835, embracing a period of ten years; not counting those of 1823 already mentioned. Of the sixty-two new comers, thirty-seven were temperate, and twenty-five used alcoholic beverages between meals, though not often to the extent of producing intoxication. Of the thirty-seven who trusted to the hygienic virtues of nature's beverage—plain unadulterated water—nine have died, and twenty-eight are living. Of the twenty-five who trusted to the supposed hygienic virtues of ardent spirits, all are dead, except three! and they have removed to distant parts of the country. Peace be to their ashes! though mostly noble fellows, misled by the deceitful syren, singing the praises of alcoholic drinks, to live too fast and to be cut off in the outset of useful manhood, it is to be hoped they have not lived in vain; as by their sacrifice, science has gained additional and important proof of the fallacy of the theory, which attributes health-preserving properties, in a southern climate, to alcoholic beverages in any shape or form.

While referred to in the mass, to correct a popular delusion, it would be unnecessary and improper to drag their names before the public. Not so, however, with those who owe life, fortune and reputation to avoiding the shoals on which their brethren were wrecked. The public have a right to know who they are, and the cause of temperance is justly entitled to all the influence attached to their names. According to the Carlisle tables, and those of the Equitable Insurance Company, of London, thirty-seven individuals, at the average age of twenty-five years, (which was about the average age of the new-comers who settled in Natchez), would, in a quarter of a century, lose nine of their number; whereas, of the thirty-seven temperance doctors, only nine have died in twenty-eight years. Of these, Drs. Wm. P. Foster, Cornell and Ferguson fell by the yellow fever of 1825; Dr. John Bell came to the south with phthisis pulmonalis, from New Hampshire, and was the son of the Governor; Dr. H. Perrine, of quinine notoriety, was killed by the Indians in the Florida war; Dr. E. Johnson returned to Kentucky and died; Dr. Ogden fell a victim to some chronic ailment; Dr. J. W. Monette, always a dyspeptic, died after he had finished his history of the Valley of the Mississippi, and had made a handsome fortune by his practice; and Dr. Thomas Davis was cut off by the yellow fever of 1839—making nine in all. The remaining twenty-eight are still living, or were when last heard from. Dr. Campbell removed to London, where he was practising medicine at last advices. Dr. J. Thistle, a year ago, removed to Davenport, Iowa. Dr. Wm. M. Guin is at present a United States Senator from California. Drs. Stewart, Walker, Pollard, French, Hubbard, Page, Sydney Smith and E. C. Hyde, removed to Louisiana, and are all engaged in the planting business, except the three last. Drs. Freiott and Weston returned to New York, Dr. Holt to

Kentucky, Dr. James Young removed to Memphis, and Dr. Woodworth to Illinois. The remainder are still in Natchez and its neighborhood. They are Drs. F. A. W. Davis, Harpour, the two Leggetts, Asa Metcalf, J. Foster, Atchison, Wood, Chamberlain, Ward, Calhoun and Abercrombie.

If the property of all the temperate doctors of Natchez and its vicinity, dead and living, including those who have moved away, and including those who have retired from the profession, embracing those of 1823, and all who came in up to 1835—fifty-four in number—were equally divided, each would have upwards of a hundred thousand dollars for his share. Temperance, in that portion of the South, at least, is not only hygienic, but auriferous. They all began life poor, with nothing but their profession for a livelihood. Some of them are in the possession of millions, and have long since retired from the duties of their profession. They nevertheless belong to the medical public, and have no right to object to their names being brought before that public for the scientific purpose of proving to the physicians, at the north, the hygienic virtues of temperance in the south. Many northern temperance men are so weak in the faith, as to be led to believe, on their coming south, that rain and river water (the only kind to be had in Natchez, New Orleans, and some other parts of the South) actually requires the addition of some stimulating liquid to make it healthful. This weakness or distrust of temperance principles is owing to the want of well-authenticated facts from the south, bearing on the question. Facts are better than theory to enable not only physicians, but the people generally, to form rules of conduct on a subject of such importance. To have their proper weight, they should be authenticated, and the important truth made known, that of the whole number of temperance doctors of 1823 (thirty years ago), in Natchez and its vicinity, more than two-thirds are still living in the year 1853, at ages varying from 55 to 85 years; that of the whole number of the intemperate, of the same period, not one remains, in town or country; that of thirty-seven temperate and twenty-five intemperate physicians, who came in afterwards, between the years 1824 and 1835, all of the former are living except nine, and all of the latter are dead except three. Hence it was necessary to mention the names of the temperance physicians, many of whom are known abroad as well as at home, as living proofs of the important truth, that a temperate and upright life is the surest, safest and best road to health, wealth, longevity and respectability.

Many young medical men, as well as others, on coming South, mistake the noise of bar-rooms and grog-shops for the public sentiment of the country. Hence they are too apt to plunge into dissipation, under the delusion that water is unwholesome unless mixed with stimulants ; and that it is, moreover, essential to popularity and a good introduction to business, "when in Rome to do as Rome does." The error lies in mistaking the purlieus for the true Rome of the South, and in the erroneous theory which attributes to alcoholic beverages the hygienic properties that pure, unadulterated water alone possesses. It was not by dram-drinking that the above-named medical men preserved their health. Their names being known, they can be interrogated and answer for themselves. It was not by grog-shops, or the influence or agency of the inmates of such places, that they succeeded in business, and came into the inheritance of the fat of the land.

It is to be deplored that there should be any discrepancy of council among medical men in regard to the use of alcoholic drinks. While physicians, in perfect health, make use of such beverages, and attribute to them hygienic virtues, the public will be slow to regard them as poisonous to the blood of a healthy man. Much of the evil lies in the inattention bestowed on the subject in our systems of medical education, since the voice of the American Hippocrates, Benj. Rush, ceased to echo in the lecture-room. "Man, who is the servant and interpreter of nature, can act and understand no farther than he has, either in operation or contemplation, observed of the method and order of nature." Those who can master this first principle of the Novum Organum, found in its first sentence, will at once perceive why physicians, even the most skilful and experienced, are as liable as other men to fall into error and to be unsafe guides on any subject they have not studied or only superficially examined. They have studied arsenic thoroughly, and they know what effects it produces in large doses and small, in sickness and in health, and can even detect the minutest portion of it in the tissues; but very few of them have thus studied alcohol, and become aware of the truth, that if it be a little slower, it is nevertheless as sure a poison.

Canal St., New Orleans, May 23, 1853.

Tabular Statement of (Thirty-three) Deaths from Inhalation of Chloroform during Surgical Operations.

The New York Journal of Medicine gives a very valuable article on Chloroform, with a tabular view of all the known deaths from it in this country and Europe. We copy the article, omiting the table on account of its length.—Ed.

We have been at no little pains to collect and arrange in the second table, an account of all the cases of deaths from chloroform, &c., which have occurred in this country. But in so doing we have not included those imperfectly reported, or those in which the persons have taken it without the advice and aid of a professional person—these latter are manifestly cases of death by accident or suicidal, and therefore ought not to be included in an estimate of the dangers of a judicious administration of anæsthetics. That there have occurred cases which will not be found included in these tables we have no doubt; for in the search which we have instituted into our periodical literature we have found occasional allusions to cases, of which we could gain no particulars of sufficient importance to demand a place in the table which we have here constructed. As it regards the physiology, pathology and treatment of the accident, we commend the remarks which precede and follow these tables, from the able pens of 'Dr. Cormack, the talented editor of the *Associa-tion Medical Journal,* Dr. Snow, and Mr. Nunnelly, to the careful perusal of our numerous readers.—*Eds. N. Y. Journal of Medicine.*

Among the now innumerable cases in which chloroform has been administered with the object of procuring insensibility to pain during surgical operations, (about thirty-three, *Eds. N. Y. Jour. Med.*) cases have been recorded, in Europe and America, in which death was the immediate result of 'its inhalation. We cannot suppose that all the deaths which have occurred have been made public; yet, even allowing the number to be doubled, the small proportion which they must bear to the total number of cases, shows that they supply no argument against the judicious use of chloroform; at the same time they teach us the advisability of using at least moderate precautions when we employ so potent an agent.

We propose to exhibit the cases in a tabular form; and in so doing, we shall avail ourselves of the elaborate paper published by Dr. Snow, in the *London Journal of Medicine* for April, May and June, 1852, adding such cases as we have met with in other journals since that date. We may also refer to Mr. Nunnelly's numerous experiments and obser-vations, published in the *Transactions of the Provincial Medical and Surgical Associations* for 1849.

Several points present themselves for consideration, principally with regard to the cause of death.

1. Dr. Snow lays much stress on the necessity of sufficiently diluting the chloroform; and, as is well known, is much opposed to the plan of using a handkerchief or napkin, which appears to have been the only apparatus used in most of the fatal cases.

In the *London Journal of Medicine,* April 1853, p. 322, he says: "There is no reason to believe that any of the accidents from chloroform have arisen from the continued exhibition of the vapor, well diluted with air. On the contrary, the sudden manner in which the alarming symp-toms came on in every case, shows that they were produced by the res-piration of air containing not less than eight or ten per cent. of the vapor; and, from the history of the cases, it is most probable that the heart was disabled, in most instances, by the direct action of the chloroform. No systematic means were taken for properly diluting the vapor with air, in any case in which death has happened. The chloroform was exhibited on a handkerchief or towel, or piece of lint, in all the cases but three; and, in two of these, it was not applied by a medical man. In order to show how easy accidents may happen with chloroform, I must beg atten-tion to a few circumstances connected with its physical as well as physi-ological properties. On a former occasion, I showed (*Medical Gazette,* vol. xliii. p. 414), both from experiments on animals, and the amount of chloroform consumed in inhalation, that the average quantity of it in the blood of an adult patient, when insensible to the surgeon's knife, is about eighteen minims, and that, if twice that amount were present in the blood, it would suffice to cause death, even if it were uniformly distribu-ted. Now, thirty-six minims of chloroform, when in the form of vapor, only occupy thirty-seven and a half cubic inches, or very little more than a pint. It is true that the vapor of chloroform does not exist in a separate state at the ordinary temperature and pressure of the atmosphere; but air, when saturated at sixty degrees, contains rather more than twelve per cent. of the vapor; and, supposing the air to contain ten per cent., which it does when the chloroform dew point is at 55 deg., the thirty-six minims would be contained in 375 cubic inches of air, more than half of which might possibly be in the lungs at one time." To prevent this result, he recommends and uses a special apparatus fitted with valves; and would also have the chloroform diluted with an equal part of rectified spirit, when—as must often occur when an inhaler cannot be conveniently procured—a handkerchief or sponge must be used. The effects of chloroform, administered in this way, are slower in being produced; but then the chance of a fatal result is much diminished. This is a valuable suggestion; and an equally important point to be attended to, in our opinion, is that, during operations, it should be the *special business of a competent person to watch carefully the effects of the chloroform on the patient from the commencement of inhalation.* Of course, no medical man—and no one else should attempt to give chloroform—would think of at once closing up the nostrils and mouth of the patient with a saturated handkerchief, sponge or lint, to the exclusion of atmospheric air.

2. The symptoms and post-mortem appearances recorded, point to the arrest of the heart's action as the cause of death; and in the majority of the autopsies, this organ is mentioned as having been soft and flabby. Yet, according to Dr. Snow, it has not in any case been extensively diseased: while he has "several times given chloroform during surgical operations, when very marked disease of the organ existed, and to a great number of old people, in whom the arcus senilis in the cornea might lead to ·suspicion of its being affected with fatty degeneration." While, then, heart-disease is scarcely a contra-indication to the use of chloroform, it should make us exceedingly careful to administer it slowly, and to watch its effects; and with these precautions we may adopt Dr. Snow's view, that it will then be even beneficial. "The action of chloroform on the circulation, when sufficiently diluted with air, is that of a stimulant. It has a very marked effect in preventing syncope during surgical operations; and, as syncope is attended with danger in diseases of the heart, there is reason to believe that the careful administration of chloroform is a means of safety to patients who, notwithstanding the heart-disease, have to undergo an operation. Moreover, the pain of even a slight operation has generally the effect of accelerating the pulse to about twice its natural frequency; and it is well known that mental excitement, muscular exertion, or any other cause which has such an influence on the circulation, may occasion sudden death where there is disease of the heart; but, as the pulse usually remains of its natural frequency and force during an operation under the effects of chloroform, this circumstance further confirms the conclusion, that the careful use of this agent is a source of safety, and not of danger, to the patient with heart-disease. In these patients, however, I think it desirable to conduct the inhalation in such a manner that excitement and struggling may be avoided, and not to prolong the use of chloroform longer than is absolutely necessary, for protracted insensi-

bility is sometimes followed by depression. I am happy to be able to quote the opinion of Dr. Sibson, who has paid great attention to the subject of chloroform, in favor of its employment under certain circumstances where there is disease of the heart. He says: 'persons, the subjects of heart-disease, when the dread of a severe operation is great, may sometimes be peculiarly benefitted by the careful and short production of anæsthesia during the cutting part of an operation.'"— *Medical Gazette*, vol. xlii. p. 111.

Is the action of chloroform on the heart local, or does the paralysis of this organ take place through the influence of chloroform on the excitomotor system? This is a question open to investigation.

3. With regard to the treatment in cases where chloroform appears to be inducing a fatal effect, we know but little. Mr. Nunnelly suggests sudden dashing of cold water on the face and chest, or producing a moderate stream of air by means of a fan—moderate interrupted pressure on the chest and abdomen being at the same time employed. Dr. Snow places great reliance on the performance of artificial respiration, which, he believes, "would restore the patient in most instances, if it were put in force within half a minute after the breathing had ceased." He also advises that blood should be taken from the jugular vein, if the patient does not very quickly begin to show signs of returning animation.—*Association Med. Jour.*

From the Buffalo Medical Journal.

Opium. The opinions thereon of SHRAPPENKUTTEL SMELFUNGIS, M.D.

"I acknowledge no procrustean creed, decapitating nonconformity!"

All is blue in the office of Smelfungus. He is blowing a cloud, and the room is filled with the aroma of tobacco, about the paternity of which there can be no doubt—it is genuine Connecticut and no mistake.

"Longevity," he says, "cannot be considered a characteristic of the materia medica. From the earliest days of medicine, emphemeræ have arisen; fluttered out their existence, and disappeared from the view. But other articles there are which possess inherent vitality, which have been for ages the main pillars of therapeutics; and which still stand firm in their stately proportions. And stateliest, with firmest shaft of these, is opium.

"Opium! mysterous drug, whose potency is felt not only in the body, but in the recesses of the mind: where is the link that connects the sleepy poppy with the grandest powers of our nature? By what deep-hidden agency does it lull the racked nerve to quiet, and steal upon the mind with gorgeous dreams, extending time and space beyond conception? No man has yet returned from these close penetralia with power to tell their secrets. Used daily and hourly for many centuries, it is still unknown, misunderstood, abused, and underrated. De Quincy, wrapped in Elysian dreams by its still influence, quaffing by imperial pints his ' happiness in bottles,' with powers of utterance never equaled, 'speaking as never man spake,' has lifted the silver vail, only to reveal behind it the blackness of darkness. He has called from out the depths: but his voice is choked by sorrow, and we hear sighs only—*suspira de profundis.* Oh, mighty agent! instrument by which the soul dips down to Acheron, and gazes through he portals of Tartarus; no power can interpret or destroy thee!"

" Now Smelfungus,' I venture to insinuate, "you are on stilts as long as that euphonious baptismal name of yours, and allow me to suggest, you are gyrating rather awkwardly. How are you going to get down?"

Smelfungus looked grieved, holds silence for a moment, and then abruptly changes his style of address.

"Have you noticed, my friend, how all things work together for good to them that love physic? Have you seen how, out of this expectant humbug, have come goodly things—figs from thistles, grapes from thorns? Our otherwise Expectant must needs do something. His lazy theory was to wait for positive indications; and, very naturally, one externally recurring indication was the relief of pain. So our friend, Expectant, follows it out, and when you come to examine his treatment, you find here, there, everywhere, opium, and opium alone, prescribed in all the ills that flesh is heir to, from Abscess to Unknown. Of course, this was nonsense and error. Better and more scientific was old Dr. G.'s prescription for a 'singing in the head, viz., a poultice of old music books applied to the coccygeal region, with the luminous idea of ' drawing the music down!' There's revulsive treatment for you! But after all, good cometh from every new thing. Some of expectant's patients get well, and that without regard to old time depurative theories. And some of these were cases whereof Dame Nature had not the handling. Dame Nature is a blotch! To relieve a pleuratic inflammation, she fills one side of the chest with water; a remedy from which the patient might well pray to be delivered. But Expectant coming to a case of incipient pleuritis, makes a homœpathic diagnosis, called it ' pain in the side,' and gives it three or four grains of opium therefor. Patient gets well instanter. Well, Expectant comes to another patient, finds her with low-typhoid symptoms, and abdominal tenderness, but not much else to complain of. In the absence of any decided indications, Expectant prescribes his eternal opium. By-and-by this patient, too, recovers, and Mr. Observer, standing by, beholds a case of puerperal peritonitis cured by opium.

"From all this, I, sir, sitting in philosophic judgment, derive the great fact that we know nothing about opium. Tell us, old Monument, who have for forty years dealt out your opinion, what know you about it? Did you ever dream that it was a *curative* you were handling, and not 'a palliative merely? Man of the Microscope and testing tube read for us this deep, this Sphynx-like riddle. Are we yet—we staunch old regulars—to yield the field in this matter? Is opium the curative means, the efficient drug in our mixed prescriptions of calomel et opii. aa.grs.iij.? For look you, country practitioner dealing Schieffelin's best powdered from the blunt point of your old jack-knife, you old Clyster-pipe, who have not weighèd a prescription these half-score years, your small doses of opium weigh three stout grains!

"*Rest!* That is the word. Here, in rest and sleep, 'tired nature's sweet restorer' lies the secret. One sensible thing that Dame Nature does, is to put her patients to bed—to so prostrate their lusty muscles, that the sturdy knees give way, and the recumbent posture becomes necessary. Here, then, is the great curative, and opium is a means thereto. 'Old functional Harmony' used to tell us with extremest unction, that 'uterine contraction was the remedy for uterine hæmorrhage.' Not lead, nor ergot, not cold water, not compression, not the tampon, but any one, or all of these, which could bring on uterine contraction. So here in inflammation. Rest is our remedy—not calomel, nor antimony, not blood-letting, not opium, but any one or all, or none of these, so that you secure rest.

"There is a vague idea, derived from some exploded theories, that calomel has, *jure divino*, a certain control over inflammation—that the presence of calomel in the stomach, simultaneously with inflammation in the viscera, is incompatible. Now, good Sir Hunker! you know that I —Smelfungus—have the highest respect for you of the conservative school. You know that on every occasion I have ranked myself among you—have bowed to the existence of a liver—and scouted at the pretensions of these new comers, who bear that flaunting 'banner with the strange device,' *Young Physic.* But, my dear sir, we must compromise or surrender. Let us come down a peg or two and we shall still be men of note. Let us use a little Twigg's hair dye, and rejuvenate ourselves— gray hairs are at a discount now-a-days. Look you! only a day or two since a certain divine declared a decided preference for young physicians over old. He had the hardihood to intimate that one good theory, round and well established, was worth ten years' experience. He was a Scotchman, and I said to him, that 'it behoveth a Scotchman to be right, for if he be wrong he be forever, and eternally wrong.' Between you and I, my aged friend, it is about time to cave. Now I have a talent for compromises, and I can propose a satisfactory arrangement which shall govern this vexed question of Calomel *vs.* Opium. Let us hereafter say nothing about being 'bilious.' That's all well enough at the bed-side, but it is ruled out of professional intercourse. Let us give our calomel as we did of old to all patients of firm fibrinous habits, whose blood has a tendency to plastic exudation. So much we claim for our side of the house. Now, we may as well (needs must when the devil drives,) concede to Young Physic, that calomel shall be withheld in cases where this condition does not obtain, viz., in those manifold diseases where the blood has a tendency to fluidity. I fear that this will narrow down the amount of the drug used, but we must come to it. Don't you recollect feeding calomel, for a fortnight on a stretch, to that strumous little girl with dysentery, last year? How fast she did gain, didn't she? And how nicely you could trace the curative influence of the calomel, couldn't you?" And Smelfungus puts his tongue to his cheek, and makes a mysterious gesture with his thumb over the left shoulder. And I can imagine Editor Flint perusing this backsliding confession of Smelfungus with a quiet smile and a chuckle, which means 'I told you so!' But Smelfungus loves freedom of action; he cannot bear to be fattened by the green withes of tradition. Witness the motto at the head of this article.

But touch him gently, Dr. Flint! or you may yet see Smelfungus astride his old bilious Rosinate, charging the windmills of natural medicine with the stern voiced war cry:—"*Floret Colomelas—ruat cœlum!*"

> "Salts, sir, in all his steps—manna in his eye—
> In every gesture, calomel and rhubarb."

Smelfungus loves fun, and from no recent occurrence has he derived so many good horse-laughs as from the developments at Bellevue *in re* of opium in puerperal peritonitis.

"Dr. Clark would have made no great stir with his interesting experiments in peritonitis, had he not been so severely criticised. Not but that Dr. Clark's treatment was a goodly instance of *a priori* reasoning applied to therapeutics—brilliant in its conception, and triumphant in its success. But the fun of the matter lies in the criticism of the New York Medical Gazette. 'This,' he says, 'comes of making hospital doctors of mere theorists.' He tells us that we must look in the dead-house records for the results of such treatment. *Of course* the patients are dead. He stops not to enquire about it—they are dead *de necessitate;* and he sheds his tears over them as freely as a child in the measles. Smelfungus can see him; leading a lachrymose group of anxious inquirers beside the green shores and still waters of the East River. With solemn step and slow, he conducts them down the gravel walks of Bellevue, 'twixt cabbages and onion beds, and sadly points to the little dead-house, as filled with the mementoes of Dr. Clark's recklessness.

"But they look in vain—these women are not yet defunct, but still live to bend as best they may, with abdomen probulgent over their wash tubs, the spared monuments of human folly."

> "Oh, that mine enemy had written a book!"

If I were to tell you, gentle reader, all that Smelfungus says about the matter, I should detract from that solemnity, which becomes the pages of a medical journal. A pompous dignity is the main-stay of our profession, and by a parity of reasoning a medical monthly should indulge in no unseemly cachinnations. VALE.

From " Ranking's Abstract," Art. 114.—Medical Times and Gazette, June 19.

Treatment of Croup by Warm Vapor and Emetics. By W. BUDD, M. D., Bristol.

"The subjoined extract is taken from a clinical lecture upon six cases of croup. The author first directed attention to the general pathological phenomena; after which he remarked as follows on the microscopic appearances of the exudation:"—

"The histological and other characters of the exudation itself are very important. If you examine a portion of the false membrane under the microscope, you will see that it is essentially made up of cells or corpuscles lying in a granular blastema. These cells bear, as you will remark, a very close resemblance to the common pus-corpuscle. Pus-corpuscles are, in fact, as I have endeavored to show you at greater length elsewhere, none other than these same cells, dead—most probably in a higher state of oxidation, and otherwise chemically altered. Here and there, however, a stray cell is seen, making, by its fusiform shape, a tendency to rudimentary but abortive development.

"The most important character of the blastema in which the corpuscles are imbedded, is the large number of fat-granules it contains.

"The presence of this large quantity of fat in the morbid product, besides presenting another point in common with pus, is probably connected in some way with its low capacity for organization. These characteristics are constant in the false membrane of croup. They are also occasionally met with in inflammatory exudation from other surfaces; especially in such as occur under direct exposure to air, or as the effect of malignant poisons—or, in weak and cachectic persons, whatever the cause of the inflammation. Such exudations have, in fact, received the epithet *croupal*, in testimony of this likeness to the croupal type.

"As a croup, they are especially characterised by a proneness to degenerate into pus, and other kindred fluid products, with a tendency to the development of corrosive, and, in some cases, of still more noxious qualities. This close affinity of the exudation to pus, is, in croup, a character of great moment; since, in virtue of it, a product which was, at first, solid and adherent, and firmly choking up the air-channel, may, by a slight change of conditions, give place to a fluid secretion, offering no serious mechanical obstacle to the ingress of air, or to its own expulsion. In cases of recovery, some such secretion always supersedes the croupal, and is, in fact, the chief instrument of that separation from the surface beneath, which prepares the way for its ejection.

"The condition of the mucous membrane itself varies much in different cases and in different stages of the disease. As a general rule, it presents less vascular redness than is seen in other forms of inflammation of the same degree.

"Of this, two different explanations have been offered. One, that the gorged capillaries are relieved from their distension by the outpouring of the effused lymph; the other, that they are choked up with white products of the same nature as the exudation itself. Which of these explanations is the true one, or whether either adequately represents the fact, I will not pretend to decide.

"Besides being inflamed, the larynx and under surface of the epiglottis are generally found fretted and ulcerated, and a similar but still more extensive destruction of substance often effects the tonsils also. These alterations are, in great part, the result of the corrosive action of the morbid product. The material of the false membrane is no sooner poured out than it becomes the seat of catalytic changes, which, being communicated to the living membrane, (whose power of resistance is lowered by disease, and whose elements are already prone to dissolution,) lead to its disintegration. Direct exposure to air, the presence of sufficient moisture, and the heat of the underlying, diseased surface, all concur to give activity to these chemical changes in the morbid product."

"Having disposed of the local changes in croup, the author next alludes to the mode of death, which is by apnœa, or the privation of oxygen; he also speaks at length on the pathology of the disease, concluding with the following remarks on the treatment, to which he accords the preference:"

"This, it is scarcely necessary to say, embraces two principles and fundamental objects;—the first, to promote the separation and expulsion of such false membrane as may be already formed—the second, to prevent the formation of new false membrane, by means calculated to moderate or to alter the character of the inflammation to which the morbid product owes its origin. Now, long before adopting the precise method of treatment applied to the cases I shall presently have to relate, many considerations had led me to suppose, (in common, I doubt not, with many others,) that the most direct as well as most effectual means of securing both objects would probably be found in suitable modification of the atmosphere breathed by the patient.

"On the other hand, it had appeared to me equally clear, on the same grounds, that the great obstacle to the cure of the local disease of the windpipe, is the direct chemical action of the double current of air passing over the inflamed surface. There is, indeed, much reason to believe, that the effect of air, and specially of the oxygen it contains, in keeping up inflammation, (itself a process of rapid oxidation,) in already diseased parts, as well as in exciting inflammation in parts whose power of resistance to common chemical agency is, through some cause, lowered, is only beginning to be appreciated.

"Yet there would seem to be little doubt, not only that this agency of the air is most large and influential, but that a knowledge of it furnishes a principle fertile in application as well to the cure as to the prevention of disease. The reality of such an agency as that here assumed, may be made evident in many ways. In the first place, the consuming and destructive power of the active principle of the air we breathe on living tissue, generally, is universally known.

"Every day as much of the substance of the living body as is represented by the flesh, and other nitrogenous constituents, we appropriate in the shape of food, is reduced from the living state to that of dead chemical compounds by this consuming agent. Here the oxygen of the air is, it is true, in solution in the blood, and in dynamic and physiological relation with the tissue with which it unites, but in the gaseous form also, and on the surface of the body—acting not physiologically now, but pathologically—its effects under certain conditions are scarcely less marked.

"Thus, for instance, to certain forms of serous membrane, especially if to its own power the depressing effect of cold be added, air is most deadly. Admitted into the pleura, the peritoneum, or arachnoid, (as I once saw in a person in whom the trephine was used for the removal of a piece of scull, which was supposed, through irregularity of form, to be the cause of inveterate epilepsy in the patient,) cold air often excites the most intense inflammation — a result which there is no reason to doubt is mainly due to the chemical action of the oxygen it contains on the delicate membrane which lines these cavities.

"It may, indeed, be objected, that this offers no analogy to the case before us, since the epithelium, which covers the air-tubes, is, not only like that of the surface of the body generally, proof against any injurious action from the air, but is actually destined to protect the underlying tissues from its corroding influence. This is undeniably true. But, on the other hand, the susceptibility which this structure does not possess by nature, it may readily, and from various causes, acquire, and to almost as high a degree as that of the serous membranes themselves.

"In the state of health it remains unharmed; but let its natural power of resistance be weakened, either along with that of the rest of the body, as in general debility, however occasioned, or through some defect in its own nutrition, and cold air becomes almost as injurious to it as to the peritoneum or pleura. I have already often had occasion to show you that the bronchitis of the weak, of the aged, of the emphysematous, is, for the most part, the result of the direct chemical action of the air, on a mucous membrane whose power of resistance is lowered, either by general debility or by some defect, permanent or transient, in its own nutrition; or, what is more common still, by both. Excluding specific and epidemical influences, the records of bronchitis in the Reports of the Registrar-General, may be read as an illustration, on the broad scale, of this position.

"The power of air, under certain conditions, to set up the most intense inflammation of the mucous membrane of the air-tubes, was very distinctly shown in a case which fell under my notice some years ago. It was a case in which it became necessary to perform tracheotomy, to rescue a boy from impending suffocation, produced by rapid swelling in the structures about the larynx, caused by his having accidentally swallowed boiling water. The difficulty of breathing had existed but a short time; there was little or no secondary congestion of the lung; the boy was previously in good health, and the operation was skilfully performed. Barring the intervention of some new element, therefore, there appeared to be no assignable cause for the particular mischief which followed. But the air which the boy breathed, instead of passing through a long and tortuous channel, and becoming warmed on the way, as in the state of nature, entered now by a short and direct cut into the bronchi. At the same time, the weather was cold; and, as no sufficient precautions were taken to give the air of the apartment a suitable temperature, the result was the most intense and diffuse bronchitis, which well nigh marred the success of the operation.

"That common air may have a very damaging effect on this mucous tract, is, therefore, a fact beyond dispute. It would be easy to extend much further, if need were, the proof of its operation. But perhaps, after all, it was scarcely necessary to illustrate at such length a position which you might have found no difficulty in conceding at once.

"The fact itself, however otherwise viewed or described, is not only a part of familiar knowledge, but precautions founded on the perception of it are so universal as to have the force and character of a common instinct. If, then, the air we breathe have power to set up inflammation on a surface not before diseased, how much more damaging is it likely to be to a surface already inflamed. The inflamed trachea in croup is sheathed, it is true, from the direct influence of this element by the intervening false membrane.

"This is seldom, however, the case throughout the disease. For, besides that in its early stage, there is always a time when false membrane is not yet formed, the instances are rare in which even after its formation the larynx is not partially or completely denuded of its adventitious covering, once at least during the course of the complaint. In almost every case, if narrowly watched, it will be found that distinct flakes of false membrane are, at some time or other, coughed up with great temporary relief to the sufferer.

"So that it is precisely at the moment when the best hopes are excited by the occurrence of this incident, that the prejudicial action of the raw air in keeping alive the inflammation in the now bare and diseased surface, steps in to disappoint them.

"As the air is more injurious the colder it is, it naturally occurred to me, that the first object in the treatment would be to raise the temperature of the air breathed by the patient to a suitable point. The second was to saturate the air thus warmed with watery vapor. On many grounds, indeed, it seemed to me not improbable, that — whether by modifying the physical constitution of the false membrane itself, or, perchance, by promoting a more serous secretion beneath it, or in both ways at once — the moisture thus generated might specially aid in the separation and expulsion of the morbid product, and possibly also prevent its being formed anew.

"It is for more enlarged experience to say to what degree these important objects are likely to be realized by these simple means. The result we have as yet obtained are perhaps too few to build upon securely. Nevertheless, as far as they go, they surpass the best expectations that could have been formed of this method of treatment. If they warrant nothing more, they at least encourage to a further trial of it.

"The mode of proceeding is simple enough. The sick child is placed in a bed, closed on all its sides with a double curtain. Into this bed is introduced a large earthenware pan nearly filled with all but boiling water, and into the water is plunged, from time to time, a heated brick, for the purpose of disengaging steam, care being taken to have the brick completely submerged.

"By this means the atmosphere within the curtain is constantly kept at a temperature of from 75° to 80° Fahr., and surcharged with vapor. Where it is practicable, the mother is placed in the bed with the child, in order to reconcile it to the strangeness of its situation. As convalescence approached, this was on several occasions found to be a useful precaution.

"The only other measure adopted, was to give an emetic from time to time, whenever the struggle for breath seemed more than commonly urgent. Not, however, for the sake of the antiphlogistic effect of the antimony or other agent employed, but to help, by that mechanical succussion which the act of vomiting causes, and which daily experience shows to be so effectual for this end, in the expulsion of the morbid product. This is the great and paramount use of emetics in the treatment of croup, and it is one the more to be valued *since there is no substitute for it.*"

From the London Lancet.

ST. MARY'S HOSPITAL.—*Performance of Tracheotomy in a case of Uterine Epilepsy.* Under the care of DR. TYLER SMITH.

Dr. Marshall Hall has advanced the opinion that spasmodic closure of the glottis, and consequent partial suffocation, is the cause of the most distressing symptoms, as well as the most injurious consequences in the severer forms of epilepsy. Hence he proposes tracheotomy as a means of reducing the severer forms to a milder type.—*Ed.*

We need not remind the readers of The Lancet of Dr. Marshall Hall's views respecting the operation of tracheotomy in epilepsy; they have had ample opportunity of becoming acquainted, in the pages of this journal, with Dr. Hall's reasons for recommending this operation, and the facts which have from time to time been published in support of this mode of treatment. There can be no doubt respecting the benefit which has, in several cases of epilepsy, been obtained by tracheotomy, as laryngismus is one of the symptoms especially calling for relief, and we have much pleasure in offering an account of the following case, lately treated by Dr. Tyler Smith, which presents the peculiarity of the convulsive disease being in its origin dependent on uterine derangement.

Sarah B——, the wife of a gamekeeper, at Debden, in Essex, was admitted into this hospital on the 13th of January, 1853. The patient has had four children, and has been the subject of epilepsy of the most severe character, from the appearance of puberty. At this time she acted as nurse to a child who suffered severely from fits, and it was supposed that this circumstance had some influence in causing the first fits which occurred to the present patient. For some years the fits occurred with great regularity at each catamenial period, as many as twenty seizures frequently occurring before and during the menstrual flow. Of late she has menstruated scantily, and at irregular intervals, but the fits have pretty generally attended the periodical discharge. The attacks of convulsion were preceded by screaming, after which she would be violently thrown down, and the respiration so arrested by laryngismus, as to produce frightful lividity of the head and face. This poor woman had been reduced, by the long continuance of her malady, to such a state of fatuity as to be quite unable to attend to her domestic affairs, and, in several instances, violent mania had followed and preceded the seizures. On two occasions she has been confined as a lunatic. Her head and face bear the marks of many wounds produced by falls at the onset of fits. In 1850, she suddenly fell in a fit across a bed in which her child, an infant of seventeen months old, was laid, and killed it on the spot. Her husband was absent half an hour, and when he returned found his wife nearly insensible by the side of the dead infant.

There could be no question, therefore, that this was one of the gravest instances which could occur of this terrible disease. The patient was not considered a fit subject for permanent abode in an asylum, but in her own cottage she was a source of constant danger to herself or others. We proceed to give a detail of her case from the date of her admission to the present time.

Jan. 19th, or sixth day after admission.—The catamenia were present, and she had one fit, but not of a very severe character.

Twelfth and thirteenth days.—After the catamenia had ceased, she had a fit each day. These fits were severe, and she was thrown violently to the ground, but they were not of long duration. She had a a fourth fit eight days afterwards, and on the following she had two others. Single fits followed on every third day after this, so that during the month which she passed in the hospital before the operation, nine seizures occurred.

After the patient had passed one month in the hospital, Feb. 13th, tracheotomy was performed by Mr. Lane. An instrument was used on this occasion which we believe had not before been tried upon the living subject, contrived by Mr. Thomson, late of University College. It is a modification of an instrument, which some of our readers may remember seeing at the Great Exhibition, and opens the trachea by a double lancet, piercing the tube horizontally between the tracheal rings. In ordinary cases this instrument would have the advantage of opening the trachea by one incision, without dividing the rings, but in this case the integuments were first divided, as the woman suffered from an enlarged thyroid gland. The puncture of the windpipe immediately produced tracheal cough, and whistling respiration began at once through the aperture. Very little blood was lost, and that which passed down the trachea was readily coughed out through the tube. Chloroform was used, and during the early part of the anæsthesia the limbs were rigid and convulsed, but the spasm passed away after the puncture of the trachea, and she did not have a perfect fit. The patient was now placed in a warm situation in her ward, and a gauze cravat put round her neck. No inflammation of the trachea, or other ill consequence followed upon the operation.

Two days after the opening the windpipe she became restless and disturbed in the night. Heat of skin, raised pulse, and furred tongue were present on the next day, and she was very unruly. In the evening she threw the medicine-glass at the sister of the ward. Dr. Tyler Smith prescribed a febrifuge and an active aperient, and on the subsequent evening the catamenia appeared. During two whole days previously, she had been so incoherent as to require constant watching. On several occasions she pulled the inner tube out of its place; but during this time she had nothing like a fully-formed convulsion. After the appearance of the catamenia, the cerebral disturbance subsided, and she has since remained collected and rational. The last fit was that which occurred the day before the operation.

We shall watch the result of Dr. Tyler Smith's case with great interest, and shall not fail to place the particulars before the readers of the " Mirror." It is hoped that as long as the tracheal tube is worn, she will not suffer from a fully-formed attack. If such should be the happy event, it would remain to be seen what effect the abortive seizures, minus the convulsions, would have upon the nervous system ; and how far the partial abeyance of the disorder would favor the action of medicine and regimen, and allow of the restoration of the intellect from the blows dealt by the hundreds of convulsions of which this poor creature has, in a long course of years, been the victim. Dr. Tyler Smith will do a great service if he can help us to a solution of these important points. We should state that in his remarks upon the case, he observed that, sixteen or seventeen years ago, he had at Bristol, assisted his then senior fellow-pupil, Mr. W. P. H. Eales, now practising at Plymouth, to perform tracheotomy in a case in which a man had fallen into the water, in a fit, while crossing a plank from the quay to his barge. The man did not recover, but Mr. Eales thus performed, under almost identical circumstance, an operation precisely similar to the successful one of Mr. Lane, of Uxbridge, which has deservedly excited so much attention.

From the Boston Medical and Surgical Journal.

Dr. King's Address on Quackery—Its Causes and Effects.

There are some medical societies in New England, whose by-laws declare that it shall be deemed disreputable and unlawful for any fellow of such society to consult, directly or indirectly, with any person who is not a fellow—such offences being punishable with fine or expulsion. In some of the States no one is allowed to practice medicine or prescribe for the sick until he has a diploma recorded on the books of the town in which he is located. In France, every new scheme that is rejected by the regular faculty is instantly suppressed. All these are salutary provisions, and tend to guard the public against imposition. The importance of medical societies has been too much overlooked. Besides State societies, district and village societies, with their quarterly or monthly meetings, should be everywhere established. These are schools in which every member may learn something, and by comparing himself with others, keep regulated and posted up, and become an abler and better practitioner. Here a healthy emulation is encouraged, private animosities are dismissed, jealousies and heart-burnings are cured. Here the passions are hushed, the feelings chastened and the tongue curbed. Some poet says, "Mountains interposed make enemies of nations, which else, like kindred drops, had mingled into one." Scripture, reason and all experience, assure us that a house divided against itself cannot stand. When any class of men wish to accomplish an object for the good of the whole, they find it necessary to form associations and act in concert. By such means, men who could do nothing as individuals, form powerful associations and accomplish important purposes with perfect ease. Political parties are always wide awake upon this subject; when an election is pending, the cry is organize, organize! Religious and moral associations act upon the same principle, and acquire power by similar means. Mechanics and laborers, without capital and without influence as individuals, by forming associations and acting in unison, acquire immense power. They can almost change the time of the sun's rising; they have already shortened the day from about fourteen to ten hours. When they think proper, they raise their wages. Nothing is wanted to accomplish anything they wish, but perfect and unflinching concert of action.

The art of healing, as our profession is sometimes called, has always been too much shrouded in mystery. Its origin is probably nearly coeval with the human race, although very little is known of its early history. More than two thousand years ago we find her in Egypt, the bantling of a superstitious priesthood, having darkness for her mantle, and mystery for her swaddling clothes; and from that day to the present, this same evil genius has clung to her skirts and prowled around her temples, polluting her sanctuaries and dishonoring her disciples. Under its shadow quackery reposes. It is the ambrosia and nectar which sustains it, the banner under which its disciples rally, and the tower of refuge to which they fly. Science seeks to banish mystery from the world, and expose to open day every important truth; to strip medicine of every unhallowed covering, and show, not merely to physicians, but to the public as far as it may be understood, every physiological, pathological and therapeutic process. The patient and his friends should be allowed to know all that they can correctly understand of the nature and treatment of his case. The more genuine knowledge an individual possesses the less is he liable to be imposed upon by false pretenders; but a knowledge of one science or art is no sure protection against fraud or imposition connected with some other science. There are men who are learned in everything else but medicine, and who become the unaccountable dupes of new and false medical schemes, and thereby do much mischief; for the public erroneously suppose that because a man understands the languages, mathematics, &c., he must of course know everything else. In general, the man who has the most plain common sense, who is accustomed to reason at every step he treads, is least liable to be suddenly carried away by new schemes. Those who are sound to the core, whose minds are thoroughly disciplined and trained to correctness of thought, are not easily led astray by phantoms.

Such men were Jefferson and Adams, Calhoun and Clay, Story and Webster. Neither of these men ever swallowed a Brandreth's pill, or tasted Swain's Panacea, or drank Townsend's Sarsaparilla, or bathed in Davis's Pain Killer. No irregular practitioner ever entered their doors, or prescribed for their families. Their medical advisers were among the most learned and accomplished of the profession. No Botanic, Thomsonian, Hydropath, Homœopath or Eclectic, was ever summoned to their sick chamber, or wanted beside their beds. In their most trying moments they took advice only of regular physicians, and obeyed them implicitly. No others were allowed to moisten their burning lips, or wipe the cold damp from their brows. Every one of these men has added his dying seal to the testimony of his whole life, against quackery of every kind, and in favor of regular scientific medicine. This is testimony of a high order, and it behooves the world to heed it. It stands out in bold relief, which no finesse can hide, or sophistry destroy.

The followers and supporters of new schemes in medicine have always supposed that some mighty revolution was taking place, and that the old practice, as they have always called the only true system, was destined soon to be forgotten. So thought the followers of Serapion, Empiricus, Paracelsus, and a host of other pseudo-reformers of previous times; and so think now the friends and followers of each of the phantom schemes of the present day. But this is a grand mistake. All the baseless visions of ancient times have long since passed away as a dream of the night, and those which have cast their phosphorescent glimmerings upon the present age, are fast passing into twilight. In those wild fields no century plants have yet been found; all belong to the cryptogamic class and mushroom genus.

From a review of the past, and a contemplation of the future, I see no cause of alarm or discouragement, if the profession will only be faithful to its high vocation. Some of the ancients believed that the art of healing was a direct gift from heaven. This sentiment, although fabulous in its origin, should nevertheless be held in everlasting remembrance. It accords with the just dignity and importance of the office of the art. If physicians will do all their duty, no lasting ills can betide them. An immutable law declares that all that is false must pass away. The empty ravings of fanatic quackery must lash themselves into repose, and everything that is erroneous in our own system should be cast off without regret, whilst all that is true and valuable will stand firm and unimpaired by time. Occasional whirlwinds and hurricanes must be encountered; but even these help to purify the atmosphere and make it more serene. And if some darker hour shall come, when errors and mistakes, and falsehood and fraud, in one confused mass, threaten society with an universal deluge; when reason seems to have left her throne to folly and madness; when imposters have multiplied like clouds of locusts, and the whole horizon becomes filled with the coruscations of strange stars, even then every honest and true man may look around with unconcern, and say with the poet, "Truth crushed to earth, shall rise again." Volcanoes may demolish mountains and bury cities in their dust and lava; pyramids may crumble to atoms, ocean waves dissolve the continents, and time place his desolating hand upon all material objects; but truth is eternal, and can never be overthrown.

*Review of an Address to the graduates of the Medical Department of
the University of Michigan, on the Romance and Reality of Ancient
Medicine. Delivered by DR. M. A. PATTERSON, of Tecumseh, Mich.,
Regent of the University from the First District.*

This address opens with an allusion to the imposing and romantic ceremony through which a student passed, in receiving the honors of the
School of Medicine of Salernum, the first to obtain celebrity in Europe,
and which was established in the eleventh century. It then proceeds as
in the following extracts, which give a specimen of the style of the author,
as well as to state several matters regarding the University which we
wish all our readers to know:

" Although our simple customs allow of no imposing ceremonies—although
we may not, with the spirit of ancient romance, place the gilded volume in
your hands, to remind you, when far from the scene of your present associations, that the true Physician must be a student through life—although we
may not present you with the talismanic ring, designed to wed you to your
profession, and to protect you from future evil, as the bride of the olden time
was wedded to her lover and protected by the precious amulet with which her
finger was adorned—although we may not crown you with laurel, as an em-
blem of your present triumph, and dismiss you with the kiss of affection, as a
parent would part with a beloved son—we may, without fear of violating the
cold formalities of society, which too frequently arrest upon the lips the warm
emotions of the heart, congratulate you in this your hour of triumph, and rejoice with you in this your hour of joy. Your aim has been high and honorable, and you have faithfully earned the reward of years of patient study. In
place of the fading laurel wreath, you are crowned with the approbation of
your teachers, and with the approving smiles of your friends, whose expectations you have answered, whose hopes you have fulfilled.
Hitherto your minds have been severely tasked with prolonged efforts to obtain a thorough knowledge of the facts and principles which constitute the
foundation and superstructure of Medical Science. That you have diligently
improved your time, and have profited by the instruction afforded in this admirable and humane department of our University is evident, from the recent
close and scrutinizing examination of your attainments, sustained with credit
to yourselves, and which has entitled you to the highest honors your Professors could bestow upon you—honors which, under the wise regulations of the
University, can be awarded only to those who by long and diligent study have
earned them. No favoritism can gain admission here, no exclusive privileges
darken these halls. The people of our state have founded this Institution for
the sole purpose of enabling our talented and energetic young men to acquire
a superior medical education, that they may become efficient agents, under
God, to spread the blessings of this education throughout the land. And, that
there shall be no undue influence of station or of wealth springing up here,
no aristocracy of feeling to cast its blighting shadows over this temple, devoted to a purely benevolent object, they invite students to come here, as the
ancient prophet invited those who thirsted after spiritual knowledge, " without money and without price."
Our people have an abiding faith in the generous principle that literary and
professional education should be placed within the reach of all their children;
and should the time ever come, which we trust is far distant, when the departments of the University cannot be sustained on this principle, they will close
its doors, and wait for the further development of the resources of that fund
which has ever been regarded, even amid the most trying financial embarrassments of the *speculative era*, as a sacred deposit for sacred purposes.
To Michigan belongs the honor of being the first State in the Union, perhaps

in the world, to establish literary, scientific, and professional education upon a purely republican model, a model which, while it lowers not in the slightest degree the highest standard of study approved by the oldest and proudest Universities of our land, is one step in advance of all of them in the march of human progress : as it practically teaches that so great a blessing as education, from the lowest up to the topmost rounds of its most elevated departments shall be free. On this righteous principle, this noble conception of man's duty to his fellow man, our educational system will grow with our growth and strengthen with our strength, developing and polishing the gems of mind as they are gathered from our intellectual treasures, until our literary and professional men shall be as much admired for their learning and skill, as are the natural treasures, so liberally scattered by the hand of Providence over our Peninsulas, for their beauty and usefulness.

After the severe course of study which for a long period has taxed your mental powers, you are entitled to a season of repose, of relaxation of mind, before entering upon the still more arduous duties of your profession. We will not disturb this hour of rest, which you have earned by the toil of many days, with an ambitious effort to force upon your attention an elaborate essay ; neither will we interrupt the happy current of your present thoughts, by assuming the privilege of a patriarch in medicine, and presenting you with the customary, and often formidable, budget of " good advice." Such things have become so common and cheap that you can purchase in the shops for a shilling, more, we trust, than your necessities will ever require. We believe that we are addressing gentlemen who know what is due to others as well as to themselves, who acknowledge the influence of christian principles upon their understandings and their hearts, who have been early instructed in the rules which experience has sanctioned for the government of society; and these few things embrace the substance of man's duty to his neighbor and to his God. If any are destitute of this knowledge, they will soon discover its importance in the bitter school of experience, where they will learn the value of the precept inscribed by the poet on the Temple of Apollo, " KNOW THYSELF."

The author now approaches the proper subject of the address, "the romance and reality of ancient medicine," in the following paragraph, which briefly gives its scope and object:

"We design to carry your minds back to the periods of remote antiquity, when our present science, with its brilliant departments of real and practical knowledge, supported by a proud array of learning, talent and skill, was, in the minds of the ancient physicians of Greece, like the faith of the Christian, ' The substance of things hoped for, the evidence of things not seen.' And, in our transit from the present to the past, we will endeavor to catch a glimpse, a mere glimpse, of ancient medicine, with its Romance and Reality."

He speaks of the popular superstitions and scholastic dogmas, which, even down to a comparatively modern period, retarded the growth and development of medical science, covering the jewels of truth in heaps of the rubbish of error, leaving the difficult task to the moderns of separating the real from the ideal, the useful from the worthless, and of sweeping the latter into holes and corners.

We are then informed that the records of Greece furnish the first notice of a physician, in the account of Chirou, the Centaur, who, probably, from being seen frequently on horseback visiting his patients, came to be considered by the imaginative Greeks, as " half man and half horse."

The second physician on record was the far-famed Aesculapius—represented as the son of Apollo, and the pupil of Chirou, and who, after being dispatched with the thunderbolt of Jupiter, hurled by the hand of the jealous Pluto, who feared from the skill of the great physician, the depopulation of the infernal region, was worshipped as the god of medicine, and had temples erected to him in various parts of Greece, and later, in Rome also. The sick were treated in these temples by incantations, by poetry and music, and in some instances by the administration of drugs, and the use of other less fanciful means—but the whole art was "dragged down on one hand to the lowest depths of superstition and credulity by a dishonest and crafty priesthood, and mystified on the other, apparently beyond extrication, by the dreamy speculations of a false philosophy."

This state of things continued until Hippocrates, the physician of Cos, arose, separated religion from medicine, and taught that "diseases are produced by the influences of the ever-changing external elements, and by the war of passions within the body; and that to the experienced observer of natural causes, under the guidance of a sound and discriminating judgment, is delegated the power of restoring health by the use of natural remedies, which, if not seasonably applied, the sufferer might in vain look for relief to the ministers of the gods."

By the philosophical spirit breathed in his writings, by his cautiously following nature in the treatment of disease, and by his unbending integrity and active humanity, he has well earned the title of the "Father of Medicine," and the grateful regard of mankind.

The address then refers to the Egyptian Herophilus, the *first human Anatomist*, and paints in strong colors the emotions he must have experienced, in prosecuting his investigations, and the indispensible necessity to any true science of medicine, of such knowledge. On the duty of affording facilities for anatomical examinations, our author uses the following language, which we specially commend to the notice of our readers:

"While we sacredly regard the feelings of friends and relatives, and would indignantly frown upon all illegal attempts to disturb the depositories of the dead, we have a right to ask of community, in the name of suffering humanity, to regard with friendly feelings the researches of the Anatomist—for the sake of the living, in all cases of obscurity to afford him an opportunity of discovering the cause of death, and to encourage in every laudable way the labors of those whose work, emphatically, is ' a labor of love.' "

We have not space to follow the author, with any particularity, in his account of the different schools of dogmatists, empirics, methodics, or eclectics, and pneumatics, and their learned (!) disputes—of the vain pretenders to superior wisdom, or of the practices of the priests of the temples* who often undertook to restore those "given up by the regular

---

* "We learn something of their practice from a record found among the ruins of an Esculapian temple on an island in the Tiber, which, from the name of Antonius being mentioned, was probably recorded in the first century of the Christian era. As it belongs to the romance of our subject, we here present you with a translation of the precious document:

'In these days a certain Caius being blind, the Oracle directed that he should approach the holy altar from the right to the left, and bend the knee, and placing five fingers upon the altar, should then raise his hand and place it upon his own eyes, and he saw clearly; the people being present and rejoicing that such a great miracle was performed under our Emperor Antonios.

"Lucius being affected with a pain in his side, and having been despaired

doctors "—and must even pass over the interesting account of the celebrated Galen, the greatest and the last of the ancient medical school founders, and his far-famed system of humoral pathology, which held almost undisputed sway for thirteen hundred years, and which, in its subtle web of philosophical fiction, contained the elements of much important truth.

We must also forego to dwell upon the account of the wonderful Paracelsus, who may be styled the father of quacks, and who startled the physicians of the dark ages with the announcement, "that the very down on his bald pate had more knowledge than all their writers, the buckles of his shoes more learning than Galen and Avicennes, and his beard more experience than all their universities," and who, like many of his successors, died of intemperance, "though he professed to have discovered a marvelous elixer which would preserve health and beauty, and prolong life to infinity."

In this view of ancient medicine, in the address, only some of the more important parts of which we have briefly alluded, the author has shown much of romance with its reality; but we must bear in mind that it was not medicine alone, that at this period was involved in darkness. Philosophy and religion no less, were in this condition. But the time soon came when, as in the language of the address,

"The Creator again said, 'Let there be light, and there was light'—when the human mind awoke from the sleep of ages, and asserted the dignity of its nature by shaking off the fetters of a delusive form of religion, and the trammels of an equally delusive philosophy—when Luther battled the corruptions of the church and Bacon exposed the fictions of Aristotle—when the art of printing disseminated the doctrines of the reformers of divinity, philosophy and medicine, and the bold cheered on the good work, whilst the timid trembled, as they beheld one after another of the strongholds of credulity and superstition tottering under the sturdy blows of the men of the new era, until the human mind was set free; and man, in the redeemed places of his earthly heritage, was permitted to doubt the infallibility of priest-craft, philosopher-craft, and doctor-craft.

"If, under the ministrations of Luther, man was born again spiritually, under the teachings of Bacon he was born again intellectually, And thus the age of knowledge was renewed with increased splendor and usefulness—not by the mere revival of ancient literature, with its web of romance and reality, but by the influence of Luther's Bible on the conscience, and of Bacon's Organon on the understanding."

* * * * * * * * *

"Our medical fathers proved themselves worthy of the new era, for the light of their minds illuminated every department of medicine. In their hands the crude art of the middle ages was elevated, and assumed the form and dignity of a real science; and in the hands of their successors it h s been

---

of by all men, the God returned the Oracle that he should come, and taking ashes from the altar, should mingle them with wine and place it upon his side; and he recovered, and returned thanks to the God, and the people congratulated him.

"Julian vomiting blood, having been despaired of by all men, the God responded from the Oracle that he should approach and take from the altar the fruit of the pine, and eat it with honey for three days; and he recovered, and returning gave thanks publicly in the presence of the people.

"Valerius Aprus, a soldier, being blind, the God returned the Oracle that he should come and mingle the blood of a white cock with honey, and use it as an eye-salve for three days—and he saw, and came back and returned thanks publicly to the God."

still further improved, until, when compared with other departments of human knowledge, it has become a reliable science—the hope of the diseased, and the admiration of the intelligent in every part of the world."

This able address, manifesting a great amount of research, written in a style, and we have no doubt, delivered in a manner worthy of the subject and the occasion, closes with the following remarks, which, as they bear upon the subject of medical education, and medical practice in our State, we think cannot fail to interest:

"The credit of our State, which is now connected with the advancement of medical science, induced the regents to establish in this department of the University, the elevated standard of study recommended by the National Medical Association. You have cheerfully submitted yourselves to this searching ordeal, and have literally complied with its requirements; and you now stand *on a level* with the graduates of those institutions which have adopted this standard, and *above those* whose standard is lower than this.

"If such elevated attainments are considered necessary to qualify students of our University to practice their profession, we would ask of those having authority in our legislative councils, whether the time has not arrived for the application of the same rule to physicians from abroad, who may hereafter desire to establish themselves within our borders as practitioners of medicine.

"When the settlements of Michigan were in their infancy, and the labors of the few physicians who were scattered over the Territory were infinitely greater, and far less remunerative than the labors of the physicians of the present time; no one was allowed to practice medicine in the Territory unless his testimonials of respectable qualifications were approved by the established Board of Medical Censors. Population was scarce at that period, and the health and life of every human being was a matter of public concern. When Michigan became a State, and population more abundant, the annual destruction of individual health, and the loss of a few lives by mal-practice, may have been considered of minor importance, if thought of at all, compared with the establishment of the great principle of *free competition.* But there is a just limit to competition, and that limit regards the traffic in life and health   Those who engage in trade without capital or knowledge of the business, are almost certain to fail: their failure merely results in mortified vanity and the loss of property. The latter may be regained by industry, and the former removed by common sense. But when a physician fails from ignorance of his duties, his failure involves the loss of health, and frequently of life. The former may be restored by skillful treatment, after weeks or years of suffering; but we have no Promethean fire with which to enkindle the light of life thus rudely extinguished."

We are aware that we have extended this notice, and presented quotations, perhaps, beyond the limits which are usual in an article upon similar occasions; but the intrinsic interest of the subject, the able manner in which it is treated, and the personal acquaintance of many of our readers with the author, will abundantly serve as our apology.

EDITORIAL.

Meeting of the National Medical Association.

The sixth annual meeting of the American Medical Association commenced in the City of New York, May the 3d, and was the largest and one of the most important yet held. Some seven or eight hundred delegates were in attendance, and every State in the Union, with possibly one or two exceptions, was represented by some of the ablest men in the profession. We have space only for the most meagre sketch of the proceedings, and any report, however complete, would very far fail in giving a full and correct impression of the interest excited, and the effect produced upon those present, and through them upon others, of the meeting together of such a body of men to consult upon the improvement, the honor, and the usefulness of the profession.

After the chair was taken by the President, Dr. B. R. Welford of Va., and a few remarks made by him, congratulating the members upon the return of the anniversary, the thronged attendance of delegates, and the flattering prospects and advancement of the profession generally, Dr. F. C. Stewart, Chairman of the Committee of Arrangements and Reception, came forward, and in a congratulatory address, referring to the origin of the Association in that State, the mighty object it has in view, the labors already performed, and the achievements accomplished, as evinced in the five published volumes of " Transactions," and the awakened spirit of improvement throughout the ranks of the profession, cordially welcomed the members of the Association in the name of the united profession of New York, to the city and its hospitalities.

After the calling of the rolls of delegates a recess was taken to allow the representatives from each State to appoint one of their number to constitute a committee for the nomination of officers and committee of the Association for the ensuing year, and propose a place for the next meeting of the body.

After the recess an invitation was presented from the Medical Society of Mo., and the members of the profession in St. Louis, to make that city the place of the next meeting. After discussion, a motion unanimously prevailed instructing the nomination committee to report in favor of St. Louis.

Dr. Condie of Pa., Chairman of the Committee of Publication, reported upon the disposal of the volumes of " Transactions," defended the committee from censure, in consequence of the tardy issue of the books from the press, alleging that the great quantity of matter, the maps and plates accompanying some of the articles, and the scarcity of means, was a sufficient excuse for such delay. He recommended the assessment of the present year to be raised from three to five dollars, and that the committee be authorised to determine upon what terms the printed record of transactions be furnished to members and others, which was adopted.

Treasurer's Report showed—

Cash received from all sources during year - -	$1,905
Cash paid during year - - - - - -	2,015
Balance due Treasurer - - - - -	$110

A resolution passed, authorising the Committee of Publication to furnish Chairman of Committees on Epidemics with volumes of published Transactions.

A large number of communications were received from various public institutions in New York and vicinity, inviting members to visit them.

The President proceeded to read the Annual Address. This was a lengthy document, written in an elaborate and elegant style, and containing many useful and important suggestions, and breathing a mingled spirit of judicious conservatism and enlightened reform.

Among the many subjects dwelt upon in the address were the evils arising from a low standard of acquirements for entrance into the profession, produced by the injudicious chartering of schools and the competition for members and money among them ; strongly advising a proper Board of Medical Examiners in each State, having nothing to do with the schools, and therefore raised above pecuniary and other temptations, who should decide who were qualified for entering the profession. Another prominent subject was the adulteration of drugs, as proved by the reports of Inspectors appointed under the law of Congress on the subject—the part which this Association had in procuring the enactment of that law—and the importance of having similar State laws for covering the whole ground, and preventing domestic, as we now had prevented foreign, adulterations. The importance of the enactment of laws for the securing of a uniform system of registration of Marriages, Births, and Deaths, considered professionally and in relation to all the other interests of the country, was strongly urged, and a reference made to the Legislature of his own State (Virginia) as having set the example. The importance of local and State organizations of the profession for accomplishing all the purposes of this body, and elevating the profession, was illustrated, and the address closed by strongly appealing to the members to unite with ardor for the honor and dignity of the noble profession.

A discussion occurred upon the propriety of employing an able chemist to analyse the various prominent nostrums of the day, and publishing the results in public papers, but no definite action was taken.

The Nominating Committee reported the following names as officers for the year, who were unanimously elected by the Association :—

President—Dr. JONATHAN KNIGHT, Ct.
Vice Presidents—Dr. USHER PARSONS, R. I.
LEWIS CONDIT, N. J.
H. R. FROST, S. C.
H. L. HOWARD, O.
Secretaries—Dr. E. BEADLE, N. Y.
Dr. E. L. LAMOINE, Mo.
Treasurer—Dr. FRANCIS CONDIE, Pa.

The Chairman of Committee of Arrangements presented a programme of proceedings from the 3rd to the 6th inclusive, embracing the time of meeting and adjournment, the entertainments at the residences of several prominent citizens and physicians during the evenings, and excursions to public institutions, &c.

Arrangements were made by which members were allowed free admission to various galleries of art, scientific curiosities, &c.

SECOND DAY—MAY 4th.

Many new delegates arrived, and were announced. A resolution was carried that " Representatives of the Army and Navy shall be admitted as delegates to this body when appointed by the chiefs of their respective bureaus."

Reports of Standing Committees being in order, Prof. Meigs of Philadelphia presented an extended report on diseases of the Cervix Uteri, which, with all other reports of Standing Committee when completed, went to the Committee on Publication.

Dr. Condie, Chairman of Committee on Tubercular Diseases, stated that he had not had time to complete his report on that subject, although he had given it much attention, and had collected many materials. He would, he hoped, be able to report fully at the next annual meeting. Committee continued.

Dr. Emerson, of Pa., presented a report on " The Agency of Refrigeration produced by Upward Radiation of Heat as an exciting cause of Disease." An abstract of the report was read, dwelling principally upon the sudden reduction of temperature produced by radiation of heat in the night, when the body is not protected from the open sky. Many illustrations given of persons so exposed in malarious districts, and the effect in developing fever, &c. The whole tendency of the report was to show how an acquaintance with a single law of nature may, by following out its relations, be made to shed a new light upon obscure subjects, and to lead to the correction of errors. The sanatory lesson designed to be inculcated was the great importance of guarding against the refrigerating effects of *nocturnal radiations*, especially in sickly places, and during epidemic periods.

Dr. Campbell, of Ga., presented a report on " Typhoid Fever," of which he gave a verbal synopsis, tracing the cause to a lesion of the ganglionic system of nerves.

Dr. Atlee, of Lancaster, Pa., Chairmon of the Committee on the Epidemics of New Jersey, Delaware, and Pennsylvania, said he could not report for the reason that he had not been furnished with materials by a history of the diseases which had prevailed in his district. It was impossible for any man to learn by observation of the prevalence of all the epidemics in the three States included within his territory. He regretted that so much apathy existed with the profession generally upon a subject of so much importance.

After some discussion, Dr. Palmer, of Chicago, proposed a resolution,— "That this Association earnestly recommend to the local societies, in all' portions of the country, to appoint committees, whose duties it shall be to record the prevalence of epidemic or other diseases, and the general state of health in their respective localities, and transmit the said reports to the Chairman of the Committee of this body on Epidemics, belonging to such locality. Such local report to be sent through a similar Committee of the State Societies, where they exist."

This, together with another resolution, instructing the Secretaries to circulate the above resolution through every State in the Union, in such a manner as to give it the widest publicity, were adopted.

Dr. Sutton, of Tennessee, presented an abstract report on the Epidemics of that State.

Dr. Pitcher, of Detroit, Chairman of the Committee on Medical Education, presented a report which was read at length, and listened to with much attention, and with decided expressions of approbation. The report deprecated the low standard of Medical Education in this country, though regarding it as having been somewhat elevated since the establishment of this Association. It dwelt upon the importance of a thorough preliminary education, and of a protracted and systematic drilling in schools of medicine, giving the greatest prominence to elementary medical subjects—as Astronomy, Physiology, Pathology, Chemistry, Materia Medical, Toxicology, &c., before taking the student into an hospital or clinique, and confusing him with cases which he cannot understand.

The report regarded that system of Medical Education the best which embraced two grades of medical schools—the one Elementary or Preparatory, the other Practical or Clinical. The one is best located more or less remote from the destructive allurements of a great city; the other, where hospital advantages systematized and rendered practical and practicable, can be had, and made a principal means of instruction. The absurdity of taking a young student into the wards of an hospital, with scores of others, where but a momentary and imperfect glance can be obtained of the patient, and but a few fragmentary sentences can be heard from the teachers, as they together hurry on from one bed to another, was forcibly stated—and in view of the difficulties that must ever attend the giving of hospital instruction to the great mass of students, the report dwelt with just emphasis on what must, after all, be considered the best kind of clinical instruction—that of the intelligent private preceptor, the student watching by the bed-side of patients, and observing carefully cases in their different stages as they occur in ordinary practice.

The sentiments of the report were illustrated by a reference to the Medical Department of the University of Michigan—its leading features were given, and the fact pointed out that it had complied in general with the recommendations of this Association.

The report concluded with the following resolutions, which were unanimously passed :—

Resolved—That the Association re-affirm its formerly-expressed opinions, on the value and importance of general education to the student and practitioner of medicine, and that it would gladly enlarge its rule on the subject, so as to include the Humanities of the schools, and the Natural Sciences.

Resolved—That in the opinion of this Association, a familiar knowledge of the elements of Medical Science should precede clinical instruction.

Resolved—That in order to accomplish the latter, the hospitals, when elevated to the ranks of schools of practice, and the intelligent private preceptor, are the most efficient instrumentalities to be used for that purpose.

Dr. J. M. Smith, of New York, Chairman of the Committee on Voluntary Essays rewarding of prizes, reported fifteen received—and the awarding of prizes to the two following :—First, "On the Cells, its Pathology," &c. On opening the accompanying sealed envelope, the author was found to be Dr. Waldo G. Burnet of Boston. The second prize was awarded to the author of "Fibrous Diseases of the Uterus, hitherto considered incurable,"—Dr. Washington L. Atlee of Philadelphia.

Dr. Marsh of Albany, then presented a lengthy paper on "Morbus Coxarius," or hip disease. He gave a short abstract of its contents, and afterwards, during a recess of the Association, dwelt more at length on the subject in the Crosby-street Medical College. His position was, that "Dislocation" seldom or never took place in this disease—that deformity arose from absorption of acetabulum and of the head of the femur, and that the principal indication of treatment is to prevent the pressure of the diseased surfaces together which causes such absorption and the continuance of the disease ; and this is to be affected by permanent extension.

AFTERNOON SESSION.

Dr. Chas. A. Lee offered a resolution severely censuring those Medical Schools which gave two courses of lectures annually. Though the spirit of the resolution was approved, it was regarded by some as premature, and laid on the table.

Dr. Buck of New York, read a paper on Morbid Growths in the Larynx. A case of deep interest was detailed, with the various operations for relief, but finally proving unsuccessful. The morbid specimen was shown as well as a wax model of the same.

A resolution was passed appointing a committee to procure the passage of a law by Congress, conferring assimilated rank upon the Medical Officers of the Navy ; also, one appointing agents in the different States for the sale of the volumes of Transactions of the Association.

Funds were guaranteed for the payment of any premiums the Association might see fit to award.

Dr. Bolton of Richmond Va., offered a resolution highly commendatory of the course taken by the authorities of the Medical Department of the University of Michigan, in requiring due preparatory education from their students, and extending their course of lectures as recommended by this Association.

The resolution was opposed by Dr. Cox of Maryland, and Dr. Davis of Chicago, on the ground that the Association had not sufficient information as to how far the University had complied with their recommendations, to justify so marked a distinction being made, and such an implied censure upon all other schools.

It was further objected, that as it was a State institution—the tuition free, and the professors paid from the public fund, they were not entitled to such special credit as the resolution implied.

Dr. Palmer explained, stating the position of the University on the various points in question, and referring to the report of Committee on Education, read in the morning, as containing a correct and impartial statement.

Dr. Bolton said he had no interest in the University of Michigan, and had learned of its peculiarities only from the report of the committee. But it seemed reasonable that when this body had recommended certain reforms on the part of the schools, and one school had come forward and adopted those reforms, that that school should be commended for so doing. This he understood to be the case in the present instance.

Dr. Warthington Hooker said he had for some time been observing the University of Michigan. He regarded it as being placed upon a high vantage ground—that it had an important mission to fulfil among the schools, in relation to the subject of Medical Education in this country—a mission which it could fulfil as well without the special endorsement of this body—that, indeed, it was above the need of any such favor. After some more conversation, at the request of a friend of the University, the motion was withdrawn.

Dr. Thos. G. Simons, Chairman of a Committee appointed at a previous meeting of the Association, for the purpose of memorialising Congress for the passage of a law requiring all emigrant vessels to have a regular Surgeon on board, reported that the subject was presented to the Senate—had gone to a committee of that body, but had not been reported upon.

A discussion arose respecting the withholding of diplomas from such medical stduents as intended to practice irregularly ; but no definite action was taken. The sentiment seemed to prevail that the hope against quackery in every form was in encouraging none but educated and morally elevated persons to enter the profession.

Third Day.

We regret our space will not allow us to follow regularly the proceedings of this day, even to the imperfect manner, and to the limited extent, we have the two preceding days, and especially as they do not abate in interest.

Dr. W. Hooker offered a resolution, which passed, that a committee be appointed to consider the recommendations in the President's address for the organization of local Societies throughout the country.

Dr. Zeigler presented a series of resolutions on the same subject, which were referred to the committee.

Dr. Davis of Ill., from the Committee on Medical Education, read at length a very elaborate report. It evinced patient research, and was marked by its author's usual directness of thought and expression.

Dr. Yandell of Ky., in the absence of Dr. Gross, the Chairman of the Committee on Malignant Diseases, read an abstract of Dr. Gross's report, the substance of which was, that from an extensive examination into the results of operations for genuine cancer, it was advised that the knife be more sparingly used in the management of this disease.

The rest of the day was principally consumed in considering subjects of general interest to the profession, such as Medical Education, Literature, and Reform Quackery, Legal Enactments for its Suppression, &c.

After the customary resolutions of thanks to officers, to the gentlemen and institutions of New York, which had received them so hospitably, and to the Press, for its reports of their proceedings, the Association adjourned *sine die.*

In the evening a splendid banquet, got up with great expense, was served at the Metropolitan Hall, about 1,000 persons being present.

Professor W. Parker presided with great propriety, as he does everything ; but as this has but little direct bearing upon the cause of Science, and in its details was very much like other things of the kind, we omit any special account of it, not regarding this as the part of the proceedings most worthy of being held in remembrance.

The next day a large number of the delegates made an excursion about New York Harbor, and visited the institutions on Blackwell's Wards and Randall's Islands, while others left for their homes, some never to reach them.   A. B. P.

ADDRESS TO THE READER.

We come before our readers with the first number of the Peninsular Journal of Medicine and the Collateral Sciences. This enterprise has long been contemplated by the profession of Michigan, and the want of it has been severely felt. What the medical men of this region need is to concentrate their power, and organize their strength. There is intellect enough, and learning enough among them to command the highest honor and respect from community, and there is power enough to blow the breath of annihilation upon their enemies, and sweep out quackery as in a whirlwind from their path. But that intellect has never been set before the public, and their power has not been exercised. It has been an honorable, but disastrous fault of our profession, that it has been so absorbed in the business of investigation and discovery, and so occupied in the practical application of these discoveries to the relief of human misery, that it has neglected its own defence, and forgotten those arts of communication upon which depend the impressiveness of its appearance before the world. There is a justice due to ourselves as well as to the community—and to obtain it we must centralize and organize, we must meet, discuss, plan, execute. It is remarkable that every great and general movement seems to originate in many minds at once, as though a common spirit pervaded every individual. So it has been in this case. There is a spontaneous uprising of voices from every quarter, insisting that the profession of this region *must be one*, and that its actions must come forth with the irresistible force of unity. To this end it is absolutely necessary to have a sound Journal, both to be the organ of communication of the profession, and the weapon of its warfare. The State Society, which met in March, held this matter in serious consideration, and urged the establishment of such an organ, and great numbers of physicians from every part of this and adjoining States have expressed their wish for it. We are before the profession, therefore, *at their call*, and for the execution of the general design. We call, therefore, upon the medical men of Michigan to sustain us. The movement with which we are identified requires that there be a general arousing to the common interest, and though the existence of the Journal is already safe, yet the successful carrying on of the great common enterprise demands that the professional organ circulate to every medical man. This must be done by individual effort, and we feel authorized to ask for that effort. Let every one, then, who receives this number, procure us at least one new subscriber, and that part of the work is done.

On our part we shall spare no effort to render the Journal worthy of universal confidence. Its contents will consist,

1st, Of original articles, reports of interesting cases, etc.

2d, Selections from Medical Journals, and other scientific works.

3d, Editorials, including notices of proceedings of societies, and a general survey of the current scientific literature. Suitable prominence will be given to notices and reviews of new works.

The whole will constitute yearly a volume of nearly six hundred pages of medical reading. For the terms and other particulars we refer to the prospectus on the cover.

Finally, we call upon all who favor the great cause in which we are engaged to stand by us, and assist us to set a trumpet to the lips of the profession, whose sound shall be heard, to the rejoicing of the friends and the dismay of the enemies of truth and progress in science. E. A.

FORMATION OF THE STATE MEDICAL SOCIETY.

Pursuant to a call made by a large number of physicians in various parts of the State, a meeting was held at the Medical College of the University, March 30, for the purpose of organizing a State Medical Association. H. Taylor, M. D., of Mt. Clemens, was called to the chair. On motion, Drs. Andrews, Shank and Brownell were appointed a committee to report a constitution, whereupon the meeting adjourned until 2 P. M.

At 2 P. M. the meeting was called to order, Dr. Taylor in the chair. The committee then reported a constitution for the adoption of the meeting, whereupon the house proceeded to adopt it article by article.

It was moved and carried that a committee of five be appointed by the chair to nominate officers. The chair appointed Drs. Pitcher, Shank, Brodie, Andrews, of Paw Paw, and Arnold, of Monroe, as the committee.

The committee reported the names of Geo. Landon, M. D., of Monroe, for President; J. Paddack, M. D., of Pontiac, for Vice President; E. Andrews, M. D, of Ann Arbor, for Secretary; and S. H. Douglass, M. D., of Ann Arbor for Treasurer. These officers were then ballotted for and declared unanimously elected.

The President then appointed Drs. Stebbins, of Detroit, Arnold, of Monroe, and Shank, of Lansing, as the Censors of the Society. Dr. Brodie offered the following resolution, which was adopted:

Resolved, That this Society call the attention of the profession to the necessity of maintaining a Journal within this State, and that it recommends its members to use their best efforts to sustain and support the one about to be published under the title of the "Peninsular Journal of Medicine and the Collateral Sciences."

Drs. Leland, of Detroit, Paddack, of Pontiac, Andrews, of Paw Paw, Taylor, of Mt. Clemens, and Beach, of Coldwater, were chosen delegates to attend the meeting of the National Association at N. Y.

It was moved and carried that any one of the delegates may obtain a substitute, provided he be a member of this Society, and that the officers shall furnish him with the proper credentials.

Dr. Taylor, of Brooklyn, was then appointed a committee to investigate the subject of Meteorology, and to report at the next annual meeting.

Dr. Patterson, of Tecumseh, was appointed to report on the epidemics of this State.

Dr. Taylor, of Mt. Clemens, was appointed to report on the geographical distribution of diseases in this region.

It was moved and adopted that during the coming year any regular physician recommended by a member of this Society may become a member by paying the initiation fee and subscribing to the other regulations.

It was also moved and carried that the Medical Ethics of the National Medical Association be adopted by this Society. The following resolution was then offered and adopted:

Resolved, That the proceedings of this meeting be published in the first number of the Peninsular Journal, and that a copy be sent to every regular physician in the State, and that the sum of fifty dollars be appropriated to the Journal for the said purpose.

The Society then adjourned. L. S. STEVENS, M. D., *Sec'y pro. tem.*

THE

PENINSULAR

JOURNAL OF MEDICINE

AND THE COLLATERAL SCIENCES.

VOL. I.   AUGUST, 1853.   NO. II.

ORIGINAL COMMUNICATIONS.

ARTICLE I.—*Method of conducting post mortem examinations in cases of suspected poisoning.* By S. H. DOUGLASS, A.M., M.D., Prof. of Chemistry, Phar. and Med. Jur. in the University of Michigan.

Considering the extent of ignorance that prevails in the medical profession upon the proper mode of conducting post mortem examinations in cases of suspected poisoning, in which legal investigations are to follow, a few plain instructions may not be amiss to our readers.

The laboratory of the University of Michigan is the natural centre for the State, to which packages for analysis in such cases would be directed. Several years' experience in connection with this laboratory shows the fact that scarcely one in ten of these packages come to hand in such form and through such channels, as that the chain of medical evidence would be complete in a case of criminal prosecution. This ignorance of the profession is in some measure excusable, upon the ground that the books are comparatively silent upon the points to which we refer. The evil arises out of a want of attention to what might appear to most persons, upon first thought, as simple and unimportant particulars. It should, however, always be distinctly borne in mind, that in all criminal prosecutions where doubts can be thrown around a case, (and the counsel are not usually slow in the introduction of these doubts,) the prisoner is to have the benefit of them.

When called to make an examination in a case of suspected poisoning, we should first inquire whether it is to be made under the direction of the proper authorities, *i. e.* a Coroner's Jury or Prosecuting Attorney. If the body has been already buried, and is to be exhumed, the examination is best made in the open field. It is only necessary to remove the lid of the coffin without removing the remains. But before this is done all persons not officially present, or who are not to be used as witnesses, should be removed at such distance as that by no possibility they can clandestinely introduce any substance that may afterwards embarrass the analysis, or lead to false conclusions. This accomplished, we may safely remove the lid and proceed to the examination. We should first carefully inspect the exterior of the body. Every unusual appearance should be noted, such as the expression of the countenance, appearance of the skin, state of decomposition, &c. These exterior appearances may furnish but slight evidence, if any, of death by poisoning; they must, nevertheless, be noted, for in the judicial investigation they will most certainly be subjects of inquiry. The jury and counsel are, unfortunately, not usually versed in Toxicological science, and hence are prone to place undue importance upon these exterior appearances. For this reason, or perhaps in part from a morbid curiosity, they not unfrequently form the great body of the medical evidence. The witness who has not carefully examined the case in this respect, acquits himself but poorly. The counsel in the cross-examination, always ready to take advantage of his apparent ignorance, press him with vexatious questions, the jury lose their confidence in him, and he retires from the witness stand with little credit to himself or the profession he represents, even though he may have acquitted himself honorably in the judgment of that profession.

The exterior of the body having been carefully inspected, we proceed to lay open the abdomen and secure, *first*, the stomach and its contents. This is effected by passing a ligature around either extremity and removing it entire. In as much as the mucous surface cannot be examined without a sacrifice of its contents, it is better to defer such examination until such time as the analysis shall be made. *Second*, portions of the small and large intestines. These should be secured in the same manner, that is, by ligature, before removal. *Third*, portions of the liver, spleen and kidneys.

Having removed these articles, the question arises as to what disposition shall be made of them. This is an important consideration in which the profession are very liable to err. A specie jar should be procured, and its cleanliness secured by washing in pure water. The *material* introduced, the top may be secured by a piece of wet bladder or clean oil silk firmly stretched and tied. The ordinary tin cover may be placed over all. In doing all this the contact of the *material* with any substance not known to be clean should be carefully avoided. Thus we should particularly avoid allowing it to come in contact with the lid of the coffin or the coffin itself, for the brass or German silver nails with which it is made contain arsenic, and sometimes other poisonous elements. The nails have been placed in circumstances the most favorable for rapid corrosion, and mere contact of the wet material might communicate sufficient arsenic to give an arsenical reaction. If the jar is designed to be conveyed to a distance for the analysis of its contents, the cover should be secured by the private seal of the person making the examination, and placed in the custody of the proper officer, who should deliver it *in person* to the chemist. After securing the above articles for chemical analysis, Mr. Taylor gives the following general instructions for extending the examination: "1st. Examine all the important organs for marks of natural disease; and, 2d, To note down any unusual pathological appearances or abnormal deviations; although they may at the time appear to have no bearing on the question of poisoning. It is useful to bear in mind, on these occasions, that the body is inspected, not merely to show that the individual died from poison, but to prove that he has not died from any natural cause of disease. Medical practitioners commonly direct their attention exclusively to the first point; while lawyers, who defend accused parties, very properly direct a most searching examination to the last mentioned point, *i. e.* the healthy or unhealthy state of those organs which are essential to life, and with which the poison has probably not come in contact."

When all these precautions are taken the chain of medical evidence in most cases may be said to be complete. It is much to be regretted that the course we have indicated is not often followed. Thus, the examination is usually made in the presence of an indiscriminate crowd of idle spectators; the exterior appearance of the body is not observed; the stomach is laid open and the contents lost; for the purpose of removing the stench (or possibly to embarrass the analysis) some chloride of lime is added; instead of the clean jar to secure the material, it is wrapped in several newspapers, thus allowing the printer's ink to impart a fair share of its antimony, zinc, lead, and arsenic; no means are taken to preserve the identity of the material. Being too foul to be taken into the interior of a house, it is left in a tin pan or old platter in the open field for hours together, in the keeping of the crowd. It is not sent to the chemist by special messenger, but by express or by some chance person who may be passing that way on his route to California, or some distant or unknown point. He leaves it at the depot or in the hands of the runner for the hotel, who after having satisfied his curiosity as to the contents of the "newspaper," conveys it to the chemist. The chemist makes his analysis, and in the judicial investigation all these facts are made to appear—a multitude of doubts and uncertainties are thrown around the case. The prisoner is to have the benefit of these doubts. The strongest circumstantial evidence has satisfied the public of the guilt of the accused, and yet he is suffered to go at large, for the evidence of the chemist and professional man proves utterly worthless against such an array of doubts, arising from a want of attention to a few *apparently* unimportant particulars in the first examination.

We cannot close this article without alluding to one other circumstance. The medical profession are a truth-loving profession, never neglecting or refusing to make post mortem examinations when it is requested without remuneration, and in all doubtful cases being the first to request the privilege, provided death has not resulted from violence. This laudable love of truth often leads them to make examinations of the kind we have described, without considering that the examination once made, they may be compelled to expend their time and money in attendance upon the courts as witnesses, without compensation. Now, this is all wrong. Dr. Smith, in his "Analysis of Medical Evidence," makes the following very proper remarks: "For my own part, I have no delicacy as to the expression of my persuasion, that the power which assigns us over to the public prosecutor, whenever he may please to want us, from a notion that he has a right to the unrequited exercise of our best energies; and that under circumstances the most repugnant to our feelings as men, the most perplexing to our resources, the most hazardous to our reputation, and often the most dangerous (in various ways) to our personal safety—that the power is oppressive." The profession, in the cases we described, have the remedy in their own hands, to some extent at least. Let them apply it before the post-mortem examination is commenced. Our gentlemanly Emeritus Professor once gave the following advice to a graduating class: "When called upon by courts of law or juries of inquest, where questions relating to insanity, legitimacy, and murder by poison are involved, you should, in consequence of the skill required and the time employed, demand an adequate honorarium."

ART. II.—*The Batttle with Quackery—Tactics of our Warfare— The Plan of the Campaign.* By CORPORAL BULLHEAD, *of the Army of Quack-Killers.*

It is a fact at once laughable and lamentable, that with learning and truth to sustain, a common cause to defend, and a common interest at stake, the medical army has no concentration to its forces, no plan for its defence, no tactics in its warfare. It has the faintest possible shadow of an *esprit du corps*, and the loosest possible budget of an organization. We are, like "Nick Bottom's" company, "spread out into a clump, every man conjunctively by himself." While we sleep lazily around our guns, quacks of all names and colors, some in breeches, and some in petticoats, are crawling through our port-holes, and scrambling over our parapets. They eat up our rations and steal the very cartridges out of our boxes; yet not a sentinel fires his gun—there are no sentinels. Not an officer gives a command—there are no officers. I, Bullhead, self-constituted Corporal, take my rounds every morning in vain, to find some commissioned officer to give me orders.

Now look, ye few that be awake, at the mighty medical army, every man snoozing at his post. Now and then one of them getting his nose tweaked with uncommon vigor, wakes up a little to yelp an oath at the quacks, and another, hearing the disturbance, swears at the credulity of the people that patronize them, and then both turn over and sleep again. Wake up, fellow soldiers, and man your big guns! Let us have one good round at the enemy, if it is only by way of refreshment. I, Corporal Bullhead, have no serious objection to your being killed in battle, provided you be broad awake, and the enemy be positively the strongest; but I desire that that fact be clearly demonstrated by experiment, lest some historian of the wars write in his book, that the great American army of Quack-Killers, stacked its arms and went to sleep, and the Quacks came and stacked them in their graves.

Too much trouble, eh?—takes us out of the line of our profession,— diverts us from the pursuits of medicine. Well, I see that I must turn preacher and reason with ye a little, which I am the more willing to do, as I see no immediate chance of doing military duty.

Know then, fellow soldiers, that it is the opinion of Corporal Bullhead, that there never was, and never will be, a body of men banded together to accomplish any particular object, who will not have to spend a certain amount of time, money and thought, in defending their interests, and making their position respected before the world, and that too, by efforts outside of their particular line of business. Therefore, every enterprise involves two systems of action: one to do the business in hand, and the other to beat off its enemies, win the co-operation of friends and clear a field of action. Our railroad companies spend thousands of dollars to rescue their interests from attack in the legislature, and tens of thousands more to concentrate the patronage of different sections of the country upon their lines of travel. They understand that they must ground their business firmly and systematically, or they are ruined, though it do require efforts out of the line of freight and passenger-carrying.

Our brothers, the Clergy, are also perfectly aware of the same two-fold principle. They not only have seminaries to educate the new preachers, and libraries, journals, synods, conferences, associations and assemblies to keep the old ones in good preaching trim, but they devote their doughtiest warriors to protect them from external enemies. They publish books and periodicals for popular reading, they open religious departments even in secular papers, they battle their foes in open controversy on the field, and baffle them with silent influences by the fireside. They tinge the hearts of the nation on its hearth-stones.

Therefore it is that Anglo-Saxons of the mightiest intellect are dictating religion to the world, while Indians and silly old women in pantaloons, dictate its medicine.

Exactly in the same manner, we, the medical army, have got to have two parts to the plan of our campaign. The first part will be to look to the quality of the profession, and to make it a sound, learned, active and energetic body of men. A body strong in its organization, and irresistible therefore in its action. The second part will be to establish a complete system of operations to control the opinions of the people. *These two things can be done,* and when they are well done our victory is already accomplished—Quackery is wiped away.

As to the profession in itself considered, fellow soldiers, allow the Corporal to state its wants and the plan for supplying them. First then, and foremost, now and forever, we want an *organization,* an organization strong and compact, and reaching to every physician in the state and nation. This is to be accomplished first by garrisoned posts, or local medical societies, as you call them. Not county societies strictly, but societies embracing such sections of country as are most conveniently situated for meeting, irrespective of county limits. This part of the work is already moving bravely on. We have at least five local societies in active operation. One embracing Grand River Valley, one in Kalamazoo Co., one called the Serapion, consisting of medical students in the University, one in Detroit, and one in Macomb Co. Bravo! so far, fellow soldiers, we have here a number of garrisons able to take care of themselves, each competent to defend their own posts, and to live by their own intrinsic vitality. This is the true grit, the right stuff to make an army of Quack-Killers of; now let us join forces and have a State Society.— This is the way to find the men that will stand fire, and this also has been done. Late in February last, a number of physicians conceived the idea of once more trying a state organization, now that local societies were coming spontaneously into existence. The idea was contagious; other physicians were written to and replied with a hearty approval. A circular was hastily drawn up and sent out, calling a meeting for the purpose. Notwithstanding the suddenness of the movement, about fifty physicians met together at Ann Arbor, the appointed place, and organized the Peninsular Medical and Scientific Association, and although on account of the short notice there was neither show nor ceremony, there was what was still better, enthusiasm and full determination to overturn all obstacles, and compel success. Next year will see a statelier and more powerful gathering still.

So far we have done well, but, gentlemen Quack-Killers, let me show you how much better other professions do. There are about six-hundred regular physicians in the state of Michigan, and of these about fifty were present at the meeting, whereat we became enthusiastic and glorified ourselves exceedingly, to think there was so much organizable material in the Peninsular body. A few weeks afterwards, the Michigan Congregational Association, met in the same place. Now there are sixty-eight Congregational Clergymen in this State, and nearly two-thirds of the entire number were present at their annual meeting. Had our physicians come out in like proportion to our annual meeting, instead of fifty we should have had four hundred men present, and then we should have only barely equalled the zeal of our clerical friends. It must be admitted, however, that it is more difficult for a physician to leave home, than for a clergyman, yet the necessity for meeting, for organization, for combined thought, and combined action, is imperative. I propose, therefore, the following measure to remedy the evil. Its oddity may obtain for it a poor reception, yet I believe it would be very efficient:—Let every member who cannot attend, select from his acquaintances some intelligent layman, instruct him what measures he wishes to have carried, and what defeated, in the Society, pay his expenses and send him with proper credentials, as his substitute; and I propose that such delegates shall be admitted to act *pro tempore* as regular members. The physician would naturally select a man favorable to the interests of the profession, and he, feeling interested and honored, would return a stout champion for our rights among the people. Besides it would not hurt us to hear a voice from the people occasionally on our floors, to let us know how things sound and look in popular ears and eyes, and to assist us in planning measures to secure popular influence on our side. *We are too far removed from the people.* Nevertheless this would be a very imperfect substitute for the personal attendance of the physician himself, and ought not to be resorted to, except in cases where the physician absolutely *cannot* leave his patients.

The reasons why the army of Quack-Killers in this State, has not been sooner and better organized, is not for want of effort. The veterans of the profession have been struggling for it for years, against adverse influences too strong for them.

Our State was new, and the practitioners, coming from the four winds, were isolated, and intent, each on his own field of labor, as a matter of course they knew little, and cared less, for the body corporate. A wild forest region, where the Doctor, brawny with exposure to the weather and the smoke of log cabins, steered his stout sulkey dubiously among stumps and corduroy roads, or astride of his French pony, forded streams and swamps where he had to carry his saddle-bags on his shoulder to keep them above water, afforded physicians little chance to meet and communicate with each other, and rendered a journey of fifty miles to attend a meeting of the State Society, an impossibility. Besides, the necessity of combined defence was not then so pressing. Your little lily-fingered homœopathist, with his little rosewood box of little delicate sugar-plums, will not straddle his dandy legs over a forest-trained horse, to push his way through thickets, ride over pole bridges, and bivouac in the woods at night, with a sap-trough turned over for a pillow and a fire burning to keep off the wolves. But now when the forests are cut through, and wealth and population are increased, and railroads bind all parts of the Peninsula together, communication is become easy and an organization of our forces can be accomplished with facility. It must be done, for while we delay, quacks by hosts come swarming to a land where there is wealth and legal protection for them, where toil and danger are over and where there is no firmly united energetic body of physicians to assault them.

I have dwelt so long on the necessity of organization of the army because Corporal Bullhead deems that, before we can fight, we must be in existence, and he is of the opinion that a disorganized army is out of existence—it has no right to be called an army. But let no soldier suppose that organization is *all* we have to do. To train and discipline forces is not to *do* anything,—it is only getting ready to do something. After all is complete, then we are to lay a plan and execute it—we are to engage the enemy and overthrow him. I am firmly persuaded that it is in our power to destroy quacks, root and branch, from the State; but we must make good preparation, and go to the assault with union and system, before we shall accomplish it. The sum total of our preparations thus far are five living, local societies, a State Society, a flourishing Medical College, and a Medical Journal. Bravely done, so far: give but these elements their full development—make them reach every physician in the State, and we are organized: our task is then but to advance upon the enemy.

This brings us to the second part of our tactics, which is to organize a complete system of measures for controlling the popular opinions on medical subjects. In this part of our tactics we have done nothing—absolutely nothing. In France they have a medical department in the columns of the ordinary journals and papers, and at some future time we must do the same here; but at present it is not practicable, and there is nothing else substituted for it. Now, fellow-soldiers, I know you differ from me, some of you, in the measures to be adopted on this point, nevertheless let the Corporal give his opinion. If there is no popular medical literature, how is a plain, common man to decide whether he shall send for Dr. Lobelia, Dr. Hydropath, Dr. Little-pill, Dr. Big-pill, Dr. Urine-squinter, or Dr. Spirit-rapper?—for they all prefix Dr. to their titles, and that is all he can learn about them. Which of them knows any medical truth, or indeed whether any of them do, is altogether a doubtful point in his mind—he does not know what to decide—how can he? Yet medical advice must be had, the circumstances of the case compel a decision, and besides, from its very nature, the popular mind will not rest long in uncertainty. I have seen scores of men in this predicament gasping for truth as dying men gasp for breath. Consequently they betake themselves to reading anything which they can find on the subject. One man receives a copy of the Water Cure Journal, and it settles his opinion; another picks up a medical almanac or a patent medicine pamphlet, and settles his faith upon that; and a third, not lighting upon anything else, pins his faith to the advertisements in the newspapers. Here then is an imperative demand for a certain amount of medical literature, for there is a certain amount of medical thinking and reading which must be done—*which will be done*, by the people. But we, instead of coming up to the necessity of the times, and preoccupying the minds of the masses with enough correct reading and material of correct thought to fill up what time and attention they are disposed to give to medical topics, have stood haughtily aloof, saying that we would not condescend to submit our sanctified thoughts to their profane gaze, lest they trample on the pearls of truth, and turn again and rend our prescriptions. " Ignorance is the mother of devotion," said the priest of the dark ages; " Ignorance is the mother of obedience to my orders," still echoes the doctor of the nineteenth century; thus he purposed that this vacuum in the public mind should remain a vacuum. Never was there a more ludicrous blunder—a more preposterous absurdity. It was not a question *whether* the people should read, but *what* they should read. The demand was for a certain definite amount of popular medical literature—we neglected to furnish it, and as a matter of course Hydropathists, Homœopathists, Spiritualists, and the agents of patent medicines stepped in and supplied the demand. The Hydropathists publish their Water-Cure Journal *for popular reading*; their Water-Cure Manual is also for the people. The Homœopathists of Detroit publish a periodical *expressly for popular reading*, and so industrious are they in its circulation that they fling it

into the doors even of those who do not desire to see it.   Other quacks
produce a whole arsenal of advertisements, family medical almanacs, and
pamphlets for gratuitous distribution, and to cap the pyramid, there are
the handsomely bound volumes for parlor tables, discoursing on Hydropathy and Homœopathy, and filled with bugbear accounts about the terrible and "murderous Allopathists."   What have we produced to remedy the evil ?   A few popular lectures, and three miserable little school-
books on Physiology and Hygeine.   There is but one efficient remedy
needed in this branch of our tactics, and that is to satisfy the popular
craving with a sound medical literature, agreeable enough in form to attract the reader, and abundant enough in quantity to occupy all the attention the people are disposed to give the subject.

I propose, then, first, that in addition to our Peninsular Journal, which
is intended especially for scientific men, we establish a periodical of popular medical reading, to be strictly under the control of the State Society,
to be kept up in an elegant, pleasing and racy style, and filled with sound
matter suited to interest the popular mind.   Those who are opposed to
attempting to enlighten the public, must recollect that there is a craving
among the masses which *will* satisfy itself, if not with truth, then with
Hydropathy, Homœopathy, or whatever other thing happens first to offer
itself under the semblance of truth.   The popular mind always will have
a certain limited amount of medical reading, and nine cases out of ten
they will adopt the opinions of the reading which accident throws often-
est in their way.   All we have to do, therefore, is to preoccupy their attention with something more attractive and more widely circulated than
the missives of our enemies.

Now we, the profession of Michigan, are six hundred strong, and by a
contribution of fifty cents apiece, we could establish a cheap monthly,
which would drown out the Hydropathic and Homœopathic squibs, and
patent medicine pamphlets, and add ten thousand dollars a year to the
revenues of the profession.   Such a periodical, properly edited, would
even now support itself and yield a handsome income to any one who
should undertake it; but in order that it might be furnished at the cheap-
est possible rate, and obtain the widest possible circulation, it should receive a liberal donation annually from the profession.

Even the indirect benefits of such an organ would be immense; for
shallow book-makers, itinerant lecturers, and other dabblers on the outskirts of the science must then produce better wares, and pay more
respect to the profession, or receive a scourging which they would feel in
their pockets.   But the greatest benefit would be its power as a weapon
against quackery.   Our present mode of fighting consists of single com-
bats and individual broils with empirics, a kind of warfare which makes

each individual quack a distinguished character in his own neighbor-hood, and of course helps him. He is supposed to be a great man when a regular physician deems it worth while to buckle on his armor against him : but a widely spread periodical would come like a mildew on the very sources of his existence. It would destroy quackery with-out disturbing its insignificance, and slaughter quacks in their obscu-rity without dragging them into eminence, it would sweep the field like grape shot, and he that was hit by it could not boast of being the spe-cial and distinguished mark fired at. There are other items which should come in as parts of the system of action, but I have no time to detail them all. I have laid down the principles, let the particulars be worked out according to circumstances. If this plan does not suit the majority, let others be proposed. I am not tenacious of my own ideas, only give us some plan—a plan for the state, and a plan for the nation. We have had enough of inactivity, and enough of this skirmishing, now we want a grand Napoleonic system of operations. Let us have the pleasure of at least one general engagement, with the forces trained and disciplined, and the onset made in style. I, for one, want to see it tried—I want to see the battle.

Art. III.—*Amputation at the Hip Joint.* By E. M. Clark, M.D., Detroit. Reported by L. G. Robinson, M.D.

Dr. Clark was consulted, in January last, by Philip Lewis, a colored man, aged 49, on account of extensive sloughing of the left foot, and ulcers of the leg.

The latter of these had been troublesome for about eighteen months, and originated from a slight injury received near the heel. On exami-nation, the patient was found considerably emaciated, pulse about 100, with some cough, and suffering from deep-seated pain throughout the limb, which was considerably enlarged, particularly along the middle and upper third of the femur. Fluctuation was not distinct at any point, but upon introducing the exploring-needle at different places, along the upper third, bloody serum escaped freely. The disease was pronounced "Fungus Hæmatodes," and amputation regarded as the only means that could give a hope of prolonging life. Accordingly, the operation was performed on the 28th of January. The patient, being first placed fully under the influence of chloroform, the nates resting on the edge of the table, and the limb supported by an assistant; then, having placed my index finger as the compress for the Femoral Artery, the operator proceeded to make the incisions, according to Lisfranc's method, except that the entire flap was formed from the outer side of the limb, the disease having extended so high as to render it impossible to form a flap from the inner side. The vessels were promptly secured by five ligatures, and the loss of blood no more than in ordinary amputations of the femur.

The anaesthetic effects of the chloroform soon passed off, and reaction was fully established, leaving the strength of the patient not much diminished by the operation. Considerable cough and expectoration continued for several days, but finally subsided.

The pulse averaged about 110 during the first ten days subsequent to the operation, and then its frequency gradually diminished to 80.

Three-fourths of the flap united by the first intention, and gave a fair promise of a prompt and complete union of the whole, until the latter part of the third week. About this time, a *bed sore* made its appearance, over the region of the sacrum, which, on account of its situation, proved most troublesome, and served to retard the process of granulation.

The fortune of the patient was such as to deny him of almost every comfort. Living in the dismal apartments of a poverty-stricken tenement, subject to exposure from cold, and, of necessity, breathing a confined and impure atmosphere. Notwithstanding this unfavorable condition, the vital powers of the system were sustained, to a remarkable degree, and the incisions continued to granulate, until the early part of the fifth week, when, from a sudden cold, an unfavorable change took place, and, sinking rapidly, he died on the 9th of March, forty-one days after the operation.

On dissection of the amputated limb, the characteristic appearance of the disease was most distinctly exhibited.

Detroit, July 18th, 1853.

ART. IV.—*Review of an Article on Diaphragmatic Hernia.* By HENRY J. BOWDITCH, Member of the Boston Society of Medical Observation.

The Buffalo Journal for June, contains a long and interesting article on diaphragmatic hernia, by Henry J. Bowditch. The communication opens with a detail of a case of which the following is a condensed account:—

"It appears that when a child, he was surprised, on comparing his chest with those of his schoolfellows, to find that his heart did not beat as theirs' did, but to the right of the sternum. He had been troubled all his lifetime with palpitations of the heart, and by frequent "stitches" in the left side, and often had attacks of total unconsciousness, by which he was for some time wholly disabled. Sept. 25.—While resting from his work of raising a piece of timber, the derrick he had been using, broke and fell, striking him about the middle of the back, and fracturing the spine. On the fourth day he was brought to the hospital on a litter.

On examination.—Intellect unaffected; skin hot; pulse 132. A protuberance on the back, occasioned by the spinous processes of the three lower dorsal and first lumbar vertebræ. Complete paralysis of lower extremities, with slight degree of insensibility; fullness and dullness on percussion of hypogastrium.

Pulsation of heart natural, but entirely to the right of median line.— Respiration thoracic. Right chest laboring more than the left; left chest more prominent than right, both in front and at sides. On percussion, left front chest highly resonant as far as a line dropped from anterior boundary of axilla. Beyond that, dull, even on the back as far as median line; right chest natural.

On auscultation.—No respiration over whole of left chest, except from the clavicle down to the space between the second and third ribs. In its place a mixture of gurgling, whistling and blowing sounds was heard, like those heard over the abdomen, and produced by flatus and intestinal motion. These were not generally affected by cough or inspiratory effort, though sometimes excited by either. No bronchial or amphoric sound; metallic tinkling occasionally; voice natural; impulse and sounds of heart most distinct at right of sternum.

Diagnosis.—Probably rupture of diaphragm and intestines in left chest. Catheter was passed, elixir opii, gtt. p. p. p. given, and patient left for the night."

The patient lingered about three weeks and then sunk.

"The patient died October 20. The post-mortem examination was made very hurriedly, owing to circumstances beyond our control. The trunk presented no unusual appearance in front. Abdomen moderate in size, certainly not distended. On raising the sternum, the stomach, the major part of the colon, and several folds of the small intestines, with the omentum, were found in the left chest. These organs were much distended with flatus, but appeared perfectly healthy. No trace of recent lymph or injection about them on the pleura. The lung was compressed to the greatest degree, and looked like a lung that had been confined by a pleuritic effusion, save that it had not the usual *sodden* aspect observed in pleurisy. The heart was pressed to the right side, but that, with the right lung, was healthy. The liver resting upon the right side of the diaphragm, was normal. The spleen was healthy, and in its usual situation under the left ribs. The bladder was seen above the pubes, and contained about half a pint of purulent, flaky-looking, very offensive urine. A fold of small intestine was adherent to its fundus, by soft adhesions, and extended from there to the umbilicus, and was much distended with air. The diaphragm was perfectly healthy at the right side, but was almost wholly wanting at the left. It consisted,—1st, of a triangular piece, extending from front backward, This was five-and-a-half inches long from sternum to spine, and only two-and-a-half inches broad at its base, which was attached to the sternum and cartilages of ribs. Towards the spine is presented an opaque whitish rounded, somewhat cord-like aspect. On examination it was found composed of a muscle, and on each side was serous membrane, viz., pleura and peritonœum. Near the sternum aud vertebræ, for the space of about an inch, these two membranes were united, and smoothly so, the line of demarkation in the part near the spine being invisible, while in that toward the sternum they were joined by a cellular structure. The intervening space showed the muscle about one-fourth of an inch thick and the two membranes firmly attached to it.— 2nd.—There was a small semilunar portion only of the diaphragm near the spleen, lying by the side and a little underneath the intestines, that had passed into the thorax. But over the whole of the breast and a good part of the side, the peritonœum and pleura seemed continuous, forming one large smooth cavity."

Becoming interested in the subject, the author set himself to search out the history of diapragmatic hernia. He finds the first two cases in the works of Ambrose Pare, written about two-hundred and fifty years ago. Following the records down to the present time, he collects, in all, eighty-eight cases, which he makes the foundation of his article, and from which, by classification, he obtains some curious statistics. He finds that of the cases recorded, the rupture was on the left side of the diapragm forty-one times, and in the right side eighteen times. In the remaining cases it was not recorded which side was subjected to the accident. The small number of cases occurring on the right side, he accounts for by the presence of the liver on that side, which acts as a shield, protecting the diapragm, while the left side is without any such protection, and is further predisposed to the injury, by being hollowed into two sacculi by the spleen and greater extremity of the stomach. Of the hernia that occurs on the left side, a very large majority were ruptures, directly through from the peritonœal into the pleural cavities, and consequently there was no hernial sac. On the right side, however, the protrusions were usually sacculated, being covered, either with peritonœum or pleura, or both. The predominance of sacs on the right side, is owing to the following structure: Behind the ensiform cartilage. the diaphragm is imperfect; a triangular opening exists in the musculo-tendinous layer, which opening is divided into two, by a slip of fascia running forward to be attached to the posterior surface of the ensiform cartilage. These two openings are only closed by a serous membrane of the chest on one side, and of the abdomen on the other, consequently this is a favorite point for the protrusion of hernia upward into the chest, and of course a hernia at this point would carry gradually the peritonœum before it, and have a regular sac; whereas, in the other parts of the diaphragm, the hernia is more likely to be a violent rupture, rending an opening at once from the peritonœal to the pleural cavity. If, now, the position of the heart and the two lungs be taken into consideration, it will be readily perceived, that in as much as the right lung comes nearer to the mesial line than the left, at this point, the hernia will nearly always go to the right cavity of the chest. This mechanism explains beautifully the predominance of the saculated form on the right side.

TO BE CONTINUED.

Art. V.—*Meteorology.*

The subject of Meteorology is one so obviously connected both with Pathology and Hygiene, that the Peninsular Medical and Scientific Society, which was organized in March last, deemed it necessary to take immediate measures to have the Meteorology of the State investigated, recorded, and reported upon. Dr. M. K. Taylor, of Brooklyn, Michigan, was therefore appointed a committee to establish over the State a system of observations for this purpose, and to collect and report the results. No one man can accomplish such an enterprise. He must unite with him many observers in different localities. All those persons, physcians or not, who are willing to assist in making and recording such observations, are earnestly requested to communicate with Dr. Taylor, Brooklyn, Mich. The following memoranda, partly on the same subject, having been omitted in our previous number, for want of room, we subjoin them here.—Ed.

Notes of the Thermometer during the winter of 1852–3.   *By* J. C.
NORTON, M.D.

TO THE EDITOR OF THE PEN. JOUR. OF MED: *Dear Sir*—I herewith
send you some average results made from my notes of observations on
the thermometer during the past winter, which you are at liberty to publish if you see fit.

Rockford, Ill., Lat. 42 *deg.* 12 *min.* N., *Long.* 12 *deg.* W.

	Average tem. at Sunrise.	Noon.	Sunset.	Av. of Month.
November,	26.13	37.5	32.3	31.977
December,	20.41	31.9	26.12	26.14
January,	19.064	36.193	29.161	28.139
February,	16.893	32.392	25.	24.761

My botanical observations are too numerous to be profitable for publication.   I send you, however, a list of plants growing here which I
have never seen in those parts of Michigan where I have been.

LIST OF PLANTS.

Pulsatilla patens,
Ranunculus rhomboideus,
Corydalis aurea,
Nasturtium pinnatifida, (mihi,)
Arabis dentata,
Barbaria vulgaris,
Draba caroliniana,
Silene stellata,
Oxalis violacea,
Negundo aceroides,
Amorpha fruticora,
Petalosteum violaceum,
     "   candidum,
Baptisia Cucophora,
Cassia camæchrista,
Celtis occidentalis,
Morus rubra,
Pinus banksiana.

Gaura filipes,
Echinocystis lobata,
Lonicera flava,
Silphium perfoliatum,
Echinacea purpurea.
Dodecatheon media,
Collinsia verna,
Synthiris Houghtoniana,
Castillija sessiliflora,
Verbena stricta,
     "   angustifolia,
Lithospermum latifolium,
Mertusia virginica,
Polemonium reptans,
Fraxinus quadrangulata,
Populus grandidentata,
     "   balsamifera,
Cypripedium candidum.

   Rockford, Ill., May 28, 1853.

SELECTIONS.

From the Boston Medical and Surgical Journal.

Motive Power of the Blood proved by experiments on four Crocodiles. One brought to life. By SAMUEL A. CARTWRIGHT, M. D., *New Orleans, late of Natchez.*

Four crocodiles were subjected to vivisection in the court-yard of my office, on the 1st and 6th of the present month. One was nearly ten feet long, another about six and a half feet, and the other two of smaller size.

June 1st, at half past 9 o'clock, I tied the trachea of one of the smaller sized saurians, and turned it loose. At twelve minutes before 10 o'clock, I tied the trachea of another one, and proceeded at once to open the thorax and abdomen, exposing the viscera, even the heart, to view, by opening the pericardium. It was then taken from the table and placed on the floor. The largest crocodile was surrendered to Dr. Dowler, to perform any experiment he might see proper. By this time a number of medical gentlemen had assembled to witness the experiments; viz., Drs. Copes, Nutt, Hale, Wharton, Weatherly, Chaillie, Chappellier, Greenleaf, Prof. Riddell and his brother, and also Messrs. Brenan and Gordon. While the large crocodile was being secured and made fast to the table, the two others, whose tracheæ had been ligated, were moving about as actively as before the operation. Some doubted whether the ligation would kill them at all; and others were of the opinion that the exposure of the viscera and serous membranes of one of them to the action of the air, would prevent the ligation from proving fatal, as oxygen would be absorbed and carbonic acid expelled by the tissues thus exposed. The experiment reported at page 394 of the 46th volume of this Journal, June 16, 1852, where an alligator, nearly dead, revived under the scalpel of the dissector, while the ligature was still around the trachea, had given rise to that opinion; although it was subsequently demonstrated, by attempts at insufflation, that the lungs had been cut by the operator, thus giving egress to the poisonous carbonic acid and ingress to the vivifying oxygen—still the erroneous impression was left on the minds of Dr. Dowler and others, that it was the exposure of the membranes to the air by the dissection which revived the animal. In the present case the viscera and membranes were as extensively exposed to the air as in that instance. I particularly guarded against cutting the lungs or any branches of the bronchial tubes. Both animals, in less than an hour after the ligation of the trachea, were dead. The one whose viscera had been exposed, died as soon as the other. When pinching, burning and piercing the most sensitive parts of the body ceased to cause motion or to produce sensation, the first one operated on was re-placed on the table, and the viscera of the thorax and abdomen exposed by dissection. An artery was accidentally cut, and a profuse hemorrhage was the consequence. The temperature of the room was 83 deg. The inflating process was then commenced, and some faint evidences of returning vitality manifested themselves; but as the reptile had lost the greater portion of the blood in its body, the very substance I wished to vivify and set in motion by the introduction of fresh air into the lungs, I abandoned the experiment and removed the subject from the table, without regret, intending to make it answer the purposes of another experiment, to prove the error of certain reviewers, who had taken the position, "that alligators were curious animals, and might come to life themselves if let alone." Hence the determination to let this one alone, to prove to sceptics that nothing short of the admission of fresh air into the lungs can restore life in cases of asphyxia or suspended animation. It never came to, or responded to the irritants applied to its nerves, but quickly lost every remaining vestige of life after the insufflation was suspended. Even the irritability of the muscles was destroyed; thus confirming the experiment reported at page 79 of the 47th volume of this Journal, Aug. 26, 1852, where simple ligation of the trachea not only destroyed life, but muscular irritability, by poisoning the blood by the retention of carbonic acid.

The other crocodile, above mentioned, whose trachea had been tied at a quarter before 10 o'clock, and the viscera immediately exposed, was found to be dead, and at 25 minutes before 11 o'clock was replaced upon the table. Various means were used, as pinching, piercing, and burning the most sensitive parts of the body, to extort symptoms of life; and when they failed to have any effect, the inflating process was commenced. After continuing the insufflation of the lungs for some fifteen or twenty minutes, the animal came to life, snapped its jaws, opened its eyes, moved its limbs, and twisted and worked itself when pinched or cut. In the language of a by-stander *"it lived again."* It continued to live for several hours afterwards. It was brought to life at 11 o'clock. At 3 o'clock, when the company left for dinner, it was still alive, and would dodge the finger when thrust at its eyes, although not touched. Several gentlemen, before leaving, convinced themselves by that and other measures, that the reptile was not only alive, but had its sight, hearing, intelligence and the power of motion restored to it. When the company left, it was the only live crocodile in the room. Both the others had been dead for some time. The first one operated upon had been dead more than four hours—and the one which Dr. Dowler had been experimenting on was also dead, although it was the last one brought on the table.

On the 6th of June I tied the trachea of a female crocodile, about six and a half feet long, and as large around as a common sized man—Drs. Dowler, Copes, Wharton, Chappellier, Reynolds, Greenleaf and Backee being present. When animation became nearly suspended, the viscera were exposed by dissection. On opening the pericardium, the auricle of the heart happened to be pierced. The hemorrhage was profuse. A ligature was put around the slit in the auricle, but before the hemorrhage could be arrested the most of the blood in the body had escaped. Insufflation was tried, but it had very little ostensive effect. It excited the heart into action, and restored some degree of motion and sensibility; but it restored and preserved an amount of vitality sufficient to enable Dr. Dowler, to whom I resigned the half-dead female saurian, to re-produce those astonishing phenomena of the nervous system, which he has heretofore made known to the scientific world. They are of a nature to make a Nilotic ruin, a perfect chaos, of the main foundation of physiology and pshychology since the days of Moses. In the report of the experiment on the battle-ground crocodile, published Aug. 25, 1852, in the 47th volume of this Journal, it is stated that after tying the trachea, the animal died, and that Dr. Dowler, with fire, hooks and forceps, failed to produce a single nervous phenomenon he had been accustomed to show. But in this instance, a sufficient quantum of vitality remained and was kept up by the inflation, to enable him to verify to the bystanders nearly the whole of those remarkable facts he has heretofore reported in his "Contributions to Physiology." He proved with the half-dead reptile, as also with the ten foot crocodile on the 1st of June, what he had frequently proved before, viz., that sensibility, motion, the will and intelligence, continue to be manifested in the body after it has been cut off from the brain and spinal marrow; that pinching the distal portion of any divided nerve will cause motion and sensation in the part to which it is distributed; and that the same phenomena will continue to occur as the nerve is followed downward toward the part to which it is distributed. These experiments with the crocodile prove the fallacy of those dogmas, which have so long made physiology and psychology the most hypothetical, changeable and non-progressive of all the sciences. Until cut loose from the unsound learning of the dark ages, those noble sciences cannot be made to perform their proper part on the arena of practical utility. The hypotheses to which they are chained, make the cerebral system the *subjective or the me*, and the blood the *objective or the not me*. To reach the brain, the supposed seat of the subjectivity, recourse has been had to the supposition, that impressions from without are conveyed by a subtle fluid, oscillations or other means, through the nerves to the brain—the supposed exclusive residence of the mind. The latter is supposed to give its commands, which are conveyed by the same or another set of nerves to the muscles and to the different organs of the body, ordering muscular motions to be performed and pain or pleasure to be felt. Another hypothesis pre-supposes that the chief motive power of the blood is derived from the mechanical propulsion effected by the contraction of a muscle, called the heart. There are more than three millions of species of animals destitute of such an organ, and even in mammals the heart and arteries are of subsequent formation to some other structures of the body abundantly furnished with nutritive fluids. While such unsound doctrines (which need only be stated to carry their refutation upon their face,) are received as fundamental truths in physiology and psychology, it will be vain to expect that these sciences can make any progress in the field of utility and practical operations. While such errors prevail, the phenomena attributed to mesmerism, table-moving and spirit rapping, will continue to confound the wisdom of the learned, and to lead the ignorant and credulous into every species of ridiculous extravagance. Such is the natural tendency of the popular mind, when men of science are driven to the subterfuge of denying phenomena clearly demonstrable—not for the want of evidence of their existence, but for the want of something in their philosophy to explain them. Back to Moses, then, let young America, not too old or full of prejudice to learn new truths, go to take a fresh start in physiology and psychology. Physiologists and psychologists will there learn, what the experiments on the crocodile prove, that the blood is the *subjective or the me,* and that all other parts of the body are the *objective or the not me;* or, in the language of Moses, the blood is the life of the flesh, and the air is the life of the blood. Life, in the proper Hebrew sense of the term—life, consisting of motion, sensation, will, consciousness and intelligence; these are all implied by the Hebrew word translated life. Neither physicians nor theologians have fully believed in the physiological doctrines taught by Moses. Some of the former and all the latter profess to believe in the prophet, but not in the prophet's doctrines when applied to physiology. It is not as a prophet I quote him, but as a man and a learned physiologist. My experiments on the crocodile, as well as those of Dr. Dowler, show most clearly and positively, that. as far as regards the fundamental principles of the science of physiology, Moses is a great way ahead of either Carpenter or Dunglison. Dowler proves that the blood is the life of the flesh when he irritates a nerve, dissevered from the brain and spine, and produces the phenomena of life and motion in the part to which it is distributed. When the blood was previously poisoned by carbonic acid gas, as in the experiment with the battle-ground crocodile. recorded in this Journal, (page 79, vol. 47,) not a single symptom of life followed the irritation of the nerves or any other part. Muscular irritability had been destroyed by the carbonic acid destroying the life of the blood. Whereas, in other experiments, where the blood had not thus been previously poisoned, or if poisoned, its vitality had been restored by insufflation, then the irritation of any nerve, after it had been divided or after the spine and brain had been destroyed, produced the phenomena of life in the parts to which it was distributed. The brain and nerves, therefore, instead of being the primary seat and type of life, are subordinate agents, or mere conductors of vitality from the fountain of life, the blood, to the flesh and solid structure of the body.

My experiments prove that the life of the blood is derived from the atmospheric air: and that air alone, without any aid from the heart at all, is its main and principal motive power. In other words, the oxidation of the blood in the lungs is the chief motive power; or, in the language of Mrs. Willard, "the chief motive power of the blood is derived from respiration." Whether caloric, as Mrs. Willard contends, or caloric and electricity combined, be the *Phaetonitis equi* of those cars of life, called blood corpuscles, is another question, lying in hypothetical regions I have no desire to explore. It is not the occult cause of things, but the existence of the things themselves, I seek to prove. That there is such a thing as a *haematokinetic* or blood-moving power, derived from respiration is abundantly proved by artificial respiration restoring motion to the blood and bringing to life dead crocodiles. That this haematokinetic or bloodmoving power can act beyond the periphery of the animal body, is sufficiently proved by those beautiful habitations which the mollusks build, paint and polish for themselves, without the aid of head or hands. Shells are nothing more than the thing called mesmerism in the solid form.

Their frame-work consists of fibrin thrown off from the body of the ani-, mal, chinked or filled in with solid matter thrown out like the fibrin. The stumbling-block, to those educated in the doctrines of solidism and mechanical agencies, is that their philosophy will not admit them to attach ideas of life, motion, sensibility and intelligence, to any substances not provided with an apparatus to move by mechanical means, with nerves, brain, and organs especially designed for hearing, seeing, tasting, smelling and feeling. Yet the beaver and the snail have an additional sense, which has been called the *hygrometic,* enabling them to foretell changes in the weather. No organ has ever been discovered by which such knowledge is communicated. There are millions and myriads of living creatures in the ocean possessing one or more of the above-mentioned senses, and some of them sufficient intelligence to be expert navigators; yet they are liquid masses having less consistency than the blood, being mere bubbles of jelly inflated with atmospheric air, and without any solid organization whatever. Even the membrane enclosing the radiaries is as foreign to their gelatinous bodies as the shell is to the crustacea. The light, seen in the ocean near the arctic circle and the equator, is emitted by myriads of animals, not only possessing life, sensation and intelligence, but motions as *rapid as meteors.* They are of less consistence than the blood; the slightest touch resolves them into thin air and an unctious liquid. They prove that life, with all its essential attributes, does and can exist in the liquid and even in the aeriform state.

The difficulty of believing the Mosaic physiology, that the blood is the life, and air the fountain of life to the blood, is not for the want of facts proving that substances less dense possess life, but is owing to the prejudices of education founded on too narrow a platform. The platform of Harvey that the chief motive power of the blood is derived from a muscular organ, excludes the larger half of the animal creation. Fishes have no aortic heart to circulate the blood. They have a small, weak muscular organ to assist in propelling the blood into the gills, but they have no heart to propel it through the systemetic circulation. The oxygenation of the blood in the gills is a sufficient motive power. In the sturgeon the arteries are cartilaginous tubes, and can give the hæmatokinetic power, derived from the oxygenation of the blood in the gills, no assistance. The heart of the fœtus in utero does not beat time with that of the mother, nor are the blood corpuscles of the same size in the mother and her unborn child; proving that it is not the same blood, and is not circulated by the same forces, as the theory of Harvey supposes. The law, which gives the motive power to the blood of fishes—the oxidation of the blood in the gills—gives the motive power to the fœtal blood; the placenta performing for the fœtus the same office that the gills do for fishes. The fœtus in utero is, physiologically speaking, *a tadpole,* the placenta being its branchiæ or gills. When comparative anatomy is more studied, the radical error of the received doctrines of the circulation will become more apparent.

Dowler and the mesmerizers (I fear he will never pardon me for the association) have done much to expose the errors of the schools on the nervous system. The former has demonstrated repeatedly that the phenomena of sensation, voluntary motions, the will, the passions, and some degree of intelligence, can be re-produced in animals deprived of the brain and spinal marrow. Both have proved that the mind is not a prisoner in the bone called the cranium, as the learned world believe. My experiments prove that the blood, instead of being a lifeless mass, moved only as it is moved by physical forces, is highly vital, and derives from the oxygen of the air, not only its life, but a hæmatokinetic or motive power more active than that which the needle derives from the loadstone; that the motive power thus generated, is not dependent on vascular organization or any organization at all for its manifestations, as is proved by the Articulata and Radiata, and that it can carry the vital blood beyond the immediate periphery of the vascular system, as is proved by the fibrous frame-work in the shells of the Mollusca.

Canal Street, New Orleans, June 11th, 1853.

From the St. Louis Medical and Surgical Journal.

Hints for the Treatment of Hydrophobia. By Dr. MARSHALL HALL.

Many years ago I had the opportunity of watching the course of a case of hydrophobia. It occurred in a little boy: and I scarcely left the room during the eight-and-forty hours that he survived. But I need not detail the series of symptoms which occurred, and which I have described elsewhere, on the present occasion.

It has appeared to me that there are *three* modes of death in this disease:—1st. Sudden death from asphyxia. 2nd. Sudden death from secondary asphyxia. 3rd. Sudden death (for in all the cases I think the death is sudden and unexpected at the precise moment at which it occurs) from nervous exhaustion.

Either of these modes of dissolution would be averted by the timely institution of tracheotomy. Indeed, if this measure were adopted, the frightful seizures which occur from trying to take liquids would be obviated. These seizures consist in fearful attacks of laryngismus, and of convulsions of the neck and pharynx, but chiefly of laryngismus, with threatening of instant suffocation. These seizures would be disarmed of their force and terror by tracheotomy.

Tracheotomy thus obviating the *effects of laryngismus* — 1st. The sudden death from asphyxia, the immediate result of asphyxia, could not occur; and 2nd. The sudden death from secondary asphyxia, the more remote result of many attacks of laryngismus, could not occur!

There remains the sudden death from exhaustion. It is a question whether this would occur necessarily from the poison of hydrophobia. Why should it occur *necessarily* from this poison? No reason can be given for this; and we are not to be misled into a conclusion unsupported by facts, since, though all cases of hydrophobia have proved fatal, they have proved fatal by a mode by which they would not occur if tracheotomy were performed.

Could any measures be adopted to check the violence of the spasm,

—laryngismus and its effects being obviated, — such as the hydrocyanic acid, and so to prevent the subsequent exhaustion? Or could any remedies be adopted to remove this exhaustion more directly, as wine or cinchona?

These hints I throw out for the consideration of my professional brethren, in the hope of good.—*Lancet*

From the Western Lancet.

A Clinical Lecture on Epilepsy, delivered at the Commercial Hospital, Cincinnati, April 9th, 1853. By MARSHALL HALL, M.D., F.R.S., &c. Reported by L. M. LAWSON, M.D.

Dr. Marshall Hall having been invited to examine several cases of Epilepsy at the Commercial Hospital, complied with the request, and in the presence of a considerable number of physicians and students, very carefully and satisfactorily investigated three cases.

The first case was a young man, aged 25, who had been affected with Epileptic fits, at irregular intervals, for a period of nine months. They usually recurred, without any obvious exciting cause, about once in three weeks. The patient had formerly been a dairyman, and attributed the disease to the frequent draughts of new milk which he was in the habit of taking at different periods through the day, to the extent of a pint at a time. His previous health had been good. The fit lasts from ten to thirty minutes, after which he revives, but appears exhausted and imbecile for some hours. He makes some noise during the attack, does not froth at the mouth nor bite his tongue, nor is there any great lividity of countenance.

This was regarded as a comparatively mild form of the disease.

The second case was a female, aged 25, who attributes the disease to mental excitement consequent upon the birth of an illegitimate child. The disease seems to have arisen from mental causes, and the attacks are liable to recur whenever she becomes angry or otherwise agitated in mind. The fits are extremely irregular, both as it regards recurrence and intensity. At times she escapes for two or three months, and again is liable to an attack whenever she becomes mentally excited. In some instances they are very severe; but there is not complete closure of the glottis at any time. After the severe attacks, she remains more or less manical for several days. The general health is impaired, with a weak action of the heart, but no organic disease of that organ. Her physical powers are much impaired, and the mind evidently greatly weakened.

The third case was more aggravated than the first. The patient was a German, aged 21, who had suffered for about four years. His mind seemed much impaired, and no accurate history of the origin and progress of the disease could be obtained. His fits recur once in three or four weeks, or oftener if he becomes constipated. The fits are very violent, but it appears that laryngismus is not completely developed; he froths at the mouth, has stertorous breathing, and remains insensible after the convulsion ceases, for a period varying from a half to five or six hours. He does not bite his tongue.

Dr. Hall directed his attention particularly to the existence of *laryngismus*, and, after a careful examination, he reached the conclusion that the spasm of the glottis was not complete in either case. In relation to the above cases, and epilepsy in general, Dr. Hall submitted, in substance, the following remarks:—

GENTLEMEN:—I always feel confident of the result when I can have the opportunity, which I enjoy this day, of *examining* a patient or patients afflicted with epilepsy, in the very presence of my auditory. It is then not *I* who gives the lecture but the *patient*, whose very expressions are worthy of notice. *My* interrogations will be, not of a *leading* character, but merely suggestive, and yours will be the office of judge.

The first patient being introduced, I shall ask him:— How long is it since your first attack of epilepsy? This question gives us a measure of the inveteracy of the malady. I need scarcely remark that the difficulty in the cure, or rather the treatment, is proportional to the previous duration. If the cause be of hereditary origin, if it have followed convulsions in infancy, if it have already subsisted many years, a long and systematic course of treatment must be required to mitigate its symptoms. I next ask:— What do you think was the first exciting cause of your malady, or the exciting causes of subsequent attacks? Has it arisen from any affliction of mind? Or excess of any kind, especially sexual? Does it come on especially during sleep? Or has it been induced by errors in diet, or by disorder of the bowels? Or does it return at catamenial periods.

In the first patient examined, it seems that *milk* had been an exciting cause of attack, and I need scarcely say that a *pint* of milk, (the quantity drank at a time by the patient) swallowed nearly at a draught would prove a very solid meal in the stomach, unmasticated, and unmingled with the saliva, and with the bubbles of atmospheric air which are usually swallowed with solid food. We must take the fact or facts as we find them, listening to the patient's statement without bias.

I next ask — What warning sign of an approaching attack do you experience? And if there be such a warning voice, I propose energetic modes of treatment as preventives of the threatened attack. An ample dose, as 1 scruple or drachm of bicarbonate of potass, with or without an ample dose of ipecacuanha, or rhubarb, is, I think, among the most efficacious of our preventive remedies.

I next enquire, not of the patient, but of those who have been bystanders:—What are the appearances of the patient as the attack comes on and proceeds to its climax? Usually the eyes and head are fixed.— So it appears, it is in our first patient. The head is sometimes not only fixed but turned rigidly to one side; there is *torticollis*. This fixed or controlled state of the head is effected by the action of the muscles of the neck, hence I have designated the affection *trachelismus*. It is merely the expression of an obvious fact. With this state of the muscles of the neck there is compression of the large veins of the part, whence flushings and tumefaction of the face and neck, the latter of which is sometimes augmented an inch to an inch and a half in circumference. With this augmented *external* congestion of the face and neck, there is, of course, augmented *internal* congestion of the cerebrum, of the medulla oblongata, etc. These, too, are obvious facts. But from these facts, stupor and convulsions proceed, and, indeed, all the phenomena of this form of epilepsy, that is, of *Epilepsia trachelea.*

But now I ask another question:— Is there any *struggle for breath in the throat ?* any closure of the larynx? any laryngismus?

In our first patient, the case seems not to involve laryngismus. These are the symptoms which I have noticed,— the bitten tongue, insensibility, etc., but the *direst* form of Epilepsy is not yet.

When there is laryngismus, with, as is usual, violent respiratory, or rather expiratory, efforts, then are also the *direst* forms of purpurescence and tumefaction of the face, neck, tongue; of stupor, of convulsions; and, following these, coma, delirium, or perhaps mania, loss of memory or intellect, etc.

Our second patient refers her attack to mental emotion attendant on her bearing an illegitimate child. Since that time she has suffered from epileptic seizures, which have obviously obscured her faculties, and shattered her frame!

The attacks are attended by laryngismus and its effects, and are followed by stupor, temporary mania, and a tendency to suicide.

Now, gentlemen, it is obvious that laryngismus is disarmed, as it were, of its terrors, by the operation of tracheotomy. I strongly urge the trial, therefore, of this measure, not in epilepsy in general terms, but of that form of epilepsy which I designate as *Epilepsia laryngea.*

The epilepsia laryngea is the most formidable form of the disease, and is followed by the most formidable effects. Under the influence of tracheotomy, it ceases to be the epilepsia laryngea; it is reduced to another or abortive form; and its formidable effects are obviated!

I beg you, gentlemen, to reflect well on these *facts,* for facts they are! Shall we not when we see intellect, limb, life even, in danger, endeavor to arrest such calamities, even admitting that we can do no more? But this is not all, that can be accomplished, even with the direst forms.— Epilepsy may be removed altogether, wearing away the susceptibility to attacks; or at least we obtain time for other remedies.

I do not recommend trachetomy in any of these cases we have seen to day, but there arises a question whether it should not be adopted in the last case. The mind is going. Institute tracheotomy, administer the strychnia, improve and regulate the diet and bowels, and this poor creature may happily be saved from idiocy and imbecility!

I fear, gentlemen, to weary your patience, but I must add one remark: Epilepsy sometimes occurs in "hidden" seizures; its effects are then misunderstood; mania may occur, which may be homicidal or infanticidal; crime may be committed; and the poor patient may suffer the extreme penalty of the law, *because* there has been a *hidden* fit of epilepsy!

But this event is most apt to occur as a *puerperal* case; and especially in the event of giving birth to an illegitimate child, with all the affliction and torture attendant on such an event. The pueperal mania may be short, too short indeed for detection; and the miserable creature is found guilty of infanticide and pays the penalty of the law by the sacrifice of her life. Surely such an event will henceforth be rendered impossible by the speedy abrogation of a law, the relic of a dark age!

But I must conclude. Read and study this *Table*, every word of which is full of fact and of important truth. Let it remain in your library for consultation. And when the seas again divide us, let it be as a remembrancer of one who has long been attached in a peculiar manner to our profession, its scientific character, and its pure and benevolent objects. Amidst much malignant calumny I have pursued my laborious career in another country. But I have my ample reward in the warm greeting and welcome which have attended me since I have arrived in yours. Every good attend you and your noble and liberal institutions!

Excuse me, gentlemen, if I have unconsciously spoken with ardor and enthusiasm of my recent labors. I do trust that an important step is being taken in regard to our knowledge of epilepsy and certain congeneric maladies, infantile and puerperal convulsion, apoplexy, paralysis, mania, dementia, etc.; for our view of these great subjects ought to be expansive; and I have spoken with the enthusiasm which I have felt. Besides, I perceived that I was addressing the kind and generous hearted, and I could use no reserve.

[Since the departure of Dr. Hall from Cincinnati, we have received from him the following statement, which may very properly form an appendix to the preceding lecture. It will be seen that it relates to an epileptic patient who had been subjected to tracheotomy. The seizure detailed was doubtless rendered brief, or interrupted, by the tracheal tube.—REPORTER.]

"I saw Poole on Saturday last, and was fortunate enough to *witness* a fit from its beginning to its close. It was very interesting. The tube was quite patent. The fit commenced by torticollis and turning of the eyes, with general *tonic* spasm, marked in the arms and neck. He was insensible and fell; the face became very dark, and no respiratory movement was either visible or audible for nearly a minute. The muscles then became slightly relaxed, passing into a state of *clonic* spasm; and there was immediately the sound of catching respiration through the tracheal tube. In three minutes he stood up and spoke, and in two or three more he was cleaning the tube! It was an interesting exhibition of what tracheotomy can do; the moment there was an attempt at respiratory movement, the air not coming in contact with a closed larynx; *no coma*. This is one of the severest attacks since the operation, and this is a man whose life was a succession of fits before, the coma of one lasting till another supervened."—*Extract from a letter from Dr. J. Russel Reynolds, London.*

From the Buffalo Journal.

Use of Anæsthetics in Rigidity of Perinæum in First Labor. By J. H. BEECH, M.D., of Coldwater, Mich.

Holding the opinion that the small experience of the general practitioner may be rendered doubly useful to himself, and of some small avail, perhaps, to others, if placed in some reservoir whence many draw mental refreshment, I beg leave to submit the following to your consideration, and that of the profession, if you deem it worthy of a place in the Buffalo Medical Journal:

Having a desire to exercise great caution in the employment of new remedies, I began the use of anæsthetics in obstetric practice, only in cases of unusual severity, where pain seemed rather a dangerous than a warning symptom.

At first I was extremely reluctant in admitting them in first labors, desiring to give Dame Nature a fair chance with new apparatus. A case like the following, not the first which had come under my observation, and I believe not unheard of in the practice of most physicians, suggested the use of anæsthetics for a definite object, under certain circumstances. A young woman in first labor, had proceeded in about the usual manner, (except that there was excessive firmness of the os externum) until the head distended the perinæum to its utmost capacity. Venesection and tartarized antimony, etc., had lent their aid; and the perinæum had been many minutes carefully supported by the hand covered by a napkin, the reluctant *os* was slowly yielding, and time seemed the only additional remedy necessary. The pain, however, was most intolerable, and my patient, although perfectly confiding, and obedient as possible to every word of caution, hitherto, suddenly threw all her energy into one effort, which tossed her from her position, and almost from the hands of her attendants. The result was, a rupture, extending from the *fourchette* backward about two inches; the posterior commissure being about eight lines from the *raphe.* Reflection brought resolution in regard to future trials of this kind. The course of human events brought cases unlike, and at last a similar one in nearly all respects. The extreme pain appeared to be the only bar to my prospect of success.

Ether was accordingly administered by inhalation, and to my infinite gratification, the rigid parts yielded like warmed India rubber, and the head passed almost as soon as the subtle fluid had banished the cognizance of pain. The etherization had nearly subsided before the hips escaped.

Again, a similar patient came to my charge, but the whole process of dilatation, both internal and external, had been tardy and unusually painful, although nausea and vomiting were almost constant. The usual methods had been resorted to with that success which patience bestows, until the head bore hard upon the center of the perinæum.

Several strong and uterine abdominal contractions had exhibited a force sufficient to have made an independent passage, but for the support of the hand. With each effort the perinæum seemed to yield a little, and then contract with all its power, and carry all nearly back to the starting point of the last pain. The patient had nearly exhausted self-control, and although there was evidently an enlargement of the *vulva* steadily progressing, delay was dangerous, as there was a strong disposition of the parts to become dry and tender, requiring frequent artificial lubrication.

I knew the patient to be very susceptible to the influence of chloroform, and it was accordingly administered. Its effect was as soon discovered at the seat of difficulty, as by the attendant who gave it, and three or four natural contractions, in quick succession, completed the labor, with slight perception of pain.

I have exhibited both chloroform and ether, to females not primiparous, and have often thought that the external organs relaxed more readily; whereas, formerly, I had feared injury from the withdrawal of consciousness in the last stage of labor in cases like the above.   But agony as effectually destroys self-command as " Morpheus " himself, and I argue thus: the sentient nerves being quieted, Dame Nature has the more perfect control.

If the experience of others agrees with my own thus far, anæsthetics are useful adjuvants in labor with rigidity of the soft parts, especially where it possesses the character of clonic spasm.

April 18, 1853.

From the Boston Medical and Surgical Journal.

Treatment of Spermatorrhœa.

With the difficulties connected with the treatment of obstinate cases of this malady, most practitioners are familiar.   Books without number have been written on the subject; and almost every system of medicine proposes remedies, many of which on trial are found of no value whatever. It is hopeless to undertake to interrupt by medication the repetitions of the misfortune.   There are but two methods, we believe, decidedly reliable; one of them is mechanical, the other is left to the ingenuity of the reader to ascertain.   For several years past some of the very worst forms in which the disease presents itself, have been terminated in a short time, and the sufferer restored to permanent health, by a mechanical contrivance which originated, it is believed, in Boston.   The way to proceed is this: Take a piece of firm harness leather one inch wide, and make a ring or ferrule, which shall be one eighth of an inch greater in diameter than the penis.   Thrust the points of four pins, equi-distant from each other, through the walls of the ring, so that they will project through a little way on the inside, and then cut off the projecting part of the pins on the outside.   On retiring for the night, slip the ring on the organ midway, and insert cotton wool between the two, to keep the pins from pricking the flesh.   An emission seldom occurs without a full distention of the penis.   The theory of a cure, as well as the facts, are simply these.   When an erection takes place, and even before, the uniform enlargement presses the cotton, which yields, causing the points of the pins to enter the flesh, and thus the patient is instantly awakened.   This occurs as frequently as distension comes on, and the semen is therefore retained.   This, we repeat, is superior to any and all other prescriptions made use of.   Last week an instrument was left on sale at Dr. Cheever's, under the Tremont Temple, in this city, that acts precisely like the leather ring.   It is made of steel, however, clasping like a dog's collar, according to the size required, and having on its inner edge a row of sharp points.   Within this steel ring is another, extremely delicate, which opens to receive the penis, and retains it exactly in the middle.   When it begins to distend, the small ring allows the member to enlarge till it strikes the sharp points, and then the individual is awake and safe. After interrupting the emission a few times in this way, the morbid tendency in many cases is removed, and the sickly, feeble youth rallies and regains his health. Other cases may require a more constant use of the remedy, until maturer age and different circumstances render it no longer necessary.

From the New York Journal of Medicine.

A Treatise on the Epidemic Erysipelatous Fever of the United States. By H. N. BENNETT, M.D., of Bridgeport, Conn.

A disease of a peculiar character, and which has displayed a great uniformity in its general symptoms, those referable to the vital sources and centres, but at the same time presenting an extended diversity of local lesions, developed under the direction and impress of the genius of the disease, has prevailed during a period of ten or twelve years past, over a large extent of territory in the United States, extending from Vermont and New Hampshire on the north, to Virginia, Indiana, Illinois, Missouri, and Mississippi on the south and west. This disease has been described by different authors who have witnessed it, under the various appellations of "Epidemic Erysipelas," "Epidemic Erysipelatous Fever" "Black Tongue," &c.; the latter being a popular and most absurd name, derived from a rare symptom of the malady.

I have given the preference to the name of *Erysipelatous Fever,* since this malady evidently belongs to that class of diseases, which manifest notable general disorders previous to the appearance of any local symptoms or lesions. Chills, rigors, disturbances of the functions of the first passages, diminution of the urinary excretion, a quickened circulation, &c., are the premonitory symptoms of this as of other febrile diseases which appear to have their origin in a specific cause impressed upon the organism in a manner unknown to us in the present state of science.

Notwithstanding the numerous historical accounts of this epidemic in different localities, I believe no author has yet undertaken the task of producing a methodical paper, describing the disease as a distinct and well-characterized affection, and drawn up from an aggregation of all the information which can be obtained upon the subject. That Erysipelatous Fever is a disease having fixed characters, and displaying sufficient uniformity in its symptoms to impress upon it the seal of a specific malady, even when subjected to the eccentric tendencies of the epidemic impulse, I think will not be questioned by any one who has traced its history in this country. In composing the present treatise, the author will draw from all the sources of information within his reach, as well as largely from his own experience in the disease.

The first account of importance, given of this disease in this country, is that of Dr. George Sutton of Aurora, Indiana, published in the *Western Lancet,* for November, 1843. According to this writer, the disease commenced in the latter part of November, 1842, in Ripley Co., near Ripley Creek, and from thence extended in a southeasterly direction over a section of country, varying from ten to fifteen miles in width, and about thirty in length, following the course of some small streams which empty into the Ohio. A few cases occurred in the adjoining county upon the opposite side of the river. Dr. Sutton observes, that it is remarkable that it did not spread towards the west, but adds, that at about the same period, an epidemic of a similar character did prevail a little to the northwest of the locality above mentioned.

The next account in order, is that of Drs. C. Hall and G. Dexter, in the *American Journal of the Medical Sciences*, January, 1844, who adopt the name of "Erysipelatous Fever." These gentlemen give a history of the disease as it prevailed in various portions of the State of Vermont, and state, that "as far as the inquiry has been extended, the answer has corroborated the statement, that in the spring of 1842, it was noticed as an epidemic," and that "there is no satisfactory evidence that it observed any particular line of progress; on the contrary, the proof is conclusive that its course has been irregular and erratic." According to their own account, however, those sections of country bordering upon the Connecticut River, and the shores of Lake Champlain, suffered most severely from this fearful scourge. From these lines it occasionally diverged in various directions, to localities of different points of the compass, and different geological formations. The period of duration of this epidemic, according to the best sources of information, was about two years, dating from the fall of 1841, or the spring of 1842.

Another account of the same epidemic, is given by Dr. J. A. Allen, in the *Boston Medical and Surgical Journal*, January, 1844, as it manifested itself in Middlebury, Vt., a town lying upon Otter Creek, a considerable stream emptying into Lake Champlain. The disease was also prevailing at the same time in several towns in New York, also lying upon the borders of Lake Champlain and Lake George.

In the *Illinois Medical and Surgical Journal*, June, 1844, Dr. D. Meeker makes a report of this epidemic, which made its appearance at Michigan City, Ia., in December, 1843. This town lies on the southeast shore of Lake Michigan. Dr. Shipman describes the same epidemic in the same vicinity, in the *New York Journal of Medicine*, for January, 1846. He observes, that from Michigan City, it spread to St. Joseph's Co., and during the summer and autumn over a wide section of country in Northern Indiana and Southern Michigan. Dr. Shipman witnessed the disease himself at Laporte, in December, 1844, and January, 1845. According to the best information which I can obtain, this epidemic continued without any marked interruption, for a period of nearly three years, during which time it was attended by a fearful mortality in those sections of the country above mentioned.

In the same article, Dr. Shipman describes the disease as it prevailed in Central New-York, in Cortland, and the adjoining counties, where it continued its ravages for a period of over three years in different localities, commencing in the autumn of 1842. I may here observe that the streams of water in this section of New-York, generally have a southern inclination, and empty into the Susquehanna River, near the Pennsylvania line, and that the epidemic extended in this direction.

We hear from other sources, of the prevalence of the disease in Pennsylvania in 1844, described by Dr. Jesse Young; in Mississippi in 1844, described by Dr. Lovelace; in Michigan, in the vicinity of Livingston, about the same period or a little later, a brief notice of which is given in a letter to the editor of the *New York Journal of Medicine*, July, 1847, by Dr. S. Glisson.

In the fall of 1847, this epidemic appeared in our own town, dropping down upon us, as if from Pandora's box, and for a time scourging us with a severity which almost precluded Hope itself. A general history of it has been given in the *New-York Journal of Medicine*, for May, 1848, which does not extend, however, over the whole period of its duration, which was nearly one year. During this time I witnessed about 150 cases of the disease in all its forms, varying from a simple anginose affection, terminating in speedy recovery, to a most malignant case of cutaneous and areolar erysipelatous inflammation, terminating in gangrene and death.

From all that can be gathered of the history of this malady in the various sections of the country to which allusion has been made, I am able to obtain little of importance referring to the geological character of the regions invaded; and it would seem from the numerous and distant points which were attacked almost simultaneously, that no uniformity can exist in this respect in the different localities. One conclusion, however, I think may be fairly drawn, in regard to the progress of the epidemic from its points of departure. It has very uniformly followed the course of small streams, rivers, and lakes generally from the sources of rivers towards their mouths; and this fact would seem to indicate a preference for secondary and tertiary formations. This, however, if true, is not peculiar to the epidemic under consideration; it simply indicates an analogy between it and other diseases which at different periods assume the higher form of development.

These epidemics have been preceded by no unusual phenomena in the ordinary diseases incident to the seasons at which they occured, with the exception in some instances of the unusual prevalence of anginose affections. The seasons themselves have presented nothing unnatural, no atmospheric phenomena, and no tangible evidences of morbific effluvia. As the whole subject of the cause of epidemics is shrouded in mystery, I shall offer no new hypothetical views upon this point; and no positive information can be gathered, connected with the rise, progress and decline of the disease now under consideration, which throws any light upon this occult subject, with the exception, perhaps, of a bearing upon the question of contagion, to be hereafter considered.

Special Symptomatology.—Of the premonitory symptoms of this disease there is a considerable diversity. In some instances it is ushered in by the ordinary pyrexial symptoms, accompanied by sore throat more or less severe; enlarged tonsils and swelling and tenderness of the lymphatic glands of the neck; difficult deglutition; sometimes painful respiration, attended with lassitude, pain in the back and limbs, more especially of the knee joint; and frequently nausea and retchings; the breath uncommonly offensive; the tongue covered with a grayish white slime, through which the mucous membrane may be seen of a deep red color. The bowels are more or less constipated, sometimes insensible to the action of cathartics, but generally easily moved. The pulse frequent and depressed, the hands and feet cold and clammy, the skin contracted, and the general expression shrunken and haggard.

These symptoms are ordinarily succeeded, generally in twenty-four hours, by a chill, sometimes a severe rigor followed by general reaction, with frequent and bounding pulse. The chills, however, instead of subsiding, as in the accession of the hot stage of other fevers, are more persistent in their duration, and are frequently protracted through the continuance, and indeed through all the stages of the paroxysm; in some instances, also, through the remissions, even embracing the whole twenty-four hours; and although the chill sometimes continues during the period mentioned, even when the body is preternaturally warm, the skin is at the same time bathed with a copious acrid perspiration.

Another mode of attack differs very much from that just described.— The patient is suddenly overtaken in the midst of apparent health, with a sense of coldness painful in the extreme, soon followed by severe rigors. These symptoms are succeeded by pain in the head, abdomen, back and joints, or some or all of these at the same time, and in the course of twenty-four or thirty-six hours, succeeds the angina above mentioned.

The anginose affection has been observed by all authors who have described the disease. In the milder forms there is but little tumefaction of the tonsils or adjoining mucous tissues; the throat is of a bright rose color, the mucous follicles enlarged; in rare instances the mucous membrane of the posterior fauces is paler than natural, and appears as if œdematous. As the disease progresses, this membrane is often covered by a layer of mucus mingled with pus, which entirely obscures the color which the part presents at this time.

In the more malignant form, the pharynx assumes a dark purple color, which spreads gradually over the palate, tongue and sides of the cheeks, the tongue becoming very much swollen, and finally taking on a dark brown appearance. Ash-colored sloughs are frequently seen upon different portions of the mucous membrane, especially upon the roof of the mouth and vellum, which fall out leaving ulcerations of considerable depth and very unhealthy cast. In this state the exhalations from the mouth are horribly fetid, the sense of taste is abolished, and deglutition difficult and painful.

This inflammation of the throat sometimes passes down the trachea, with symptoms resembling croup; sometimes it passes up into the nostrils, and from them to the frontal sinuses, and even into the antrum maxillare. Sometimes this mucous inflammation appears to *commence* in frontal sinuses and antrum; large quantities of water are discharged from the nose, a violent pain is felt over the eyebrows or one of the malar bones, the face becoming so much swollen as to close the eyes; and these symptoms generally continue till a cutaneous erysipelas makes its appearance, or a copious discharge of bloody mucus is poured out from the nose.

The anginose affection, I believe to be a universal accompaniment of epidemic Erysipelatous Fever, and I find no authority which militates against this view. This local lesion is as common to the malady under consideration, as it is to Scarlatina, and forms a striking analogy between the two diseases. A peculiarity which occurs frequently in this angina, but not according to my experience universally, is the relaxation and elongation of the uvula, which is observed to have suspended from its extremity a pellicle of viscid limpid mucus, sometimes resting on the tongue, which is very soon reproduced after being removed by the efforts of the patient, or by a sponge introduced for this purpose, evidently owing to a constant exudation going on from the part. Dr. Peebles, of Virginia, was the first to make this observation, and he states that it occurred in all the cases which he witnessed.

Accompanying the angina, it is almost universal that the lymphatic glands of one or more regions of the neck, are inflamed and swollen.— They are readily felt by the finger in the early stages of the disease, and red lines may be often traced upon the skin passing from one to the other. In a few cases I have seen these glands enormously swollen, pass on to suppuration, or remain a long time indurated after convalescence has been established.

Neuralgic pains about the temples and in the occipital region are almost as frequent as the lesions just described, and in my opinion are mere reflections of the irritation produced by the mucous and glandular inflammations.

At a period varying from one to fifteen days after the development of the prodromi above described, various other inflammatory lesions commence, all however, bearing the impress of a specific origin, and pursuing a course under the direction of the peculiar genius of the malady. One of the most common is that of cutaneous erysipelas, which according to my experience occurs in about one-sixth of the cases. This proportion is not, however, well determined, since the disease in various localities has produced different results in regard to this point. If this efflorvescence is about to appear on any part of the cutaneous surface, the patient experiences a sense of tension, heat, pungent pains, itching, and tenderness upon pressure, with diffused redness and swelling of the skin, the swelling sometimes limited by the redness of the surface, but more often extending beyond it. The degree of tumefaction varies very much according to the depth to which the inflammatory process extends, and to the part affected. If it is quite superficial, apparently only affecting the *rete mucosum*, the tumefaction is slight and well defined, forming a perceptible line or ridge beyond which the skin is healthy. If, however, the true skin is implicated, and the subjacent layer of areolar tissue, the swelling is much greater, and is not bounded by the superficial redness. The parts for some distance beyond the red line are slightly tumefied, and many times exquisitely tender upon pressure.

TO BE CONTINUED.

From the Boston Medical and Surgical Journal.

Trephining in Apoplexy and Inflammation of the Brain.

To the Editor. Sir: From some experiments upon the gallinaceous tribe, this week, in cerebral hemorrhage and inflammation of the brain,.

.we are inclined to think the trephine worthy of a suggestion in similar diseases in man, and we will give you the reasons for our faith, and leave yourself and readers to your own deductions. In this region of country we have a disease among our fowls, well known to the old matrons of the land as distemper, but it is really nothing more nor less than a disease of the brain, of an apoplectic or inflammatory character, which is proved by dissection as well as the symptoms. We have had it among our fowls for several years, and as we appreciate our poultry very highly, we tried a variety of means, upon the old woman's plan and our own, for the cure of it, and with passing mortality. This season it attacked our fowls again, and we determined to pursue a more rational plan. In our slight cases we gave oil, and applied the cold douche with some success; in cases of a worse grade we gave oil, applied the douche, and introduced a seton in the back of the neck; and in several of our malignant cases, we *trephined the skull,* with decided success. While we write, we have a fine female fowl speedily recovering from a severe and protracted attack, which we attribute to the use of the *trephine.*

Now if the *trephine,* with a simple knife, will relieve the apoplectic condition of the chicken, a very tender animal when compared to man, will it not relieve man of the same affection? All of the great experiments to elucidate the functions of the nervous and other systems, have been performed upon inferior animals, and why should not this be equally legitimate? We performed the operation in several cases, with decided success when we least expected it, for it was a dernier resort with us. Some of the cases operated upon did succumb, and we attribute it to the late hour of the operation. The matter was entirely an accidental occurrence in our hands; but the analogy is so strong, that we cannot resist the inclination to place it before the profession, for further discussion. Some may object to it on account of its harshness. We reply, nothing is too harsh to protect human life, if no other means will succeed. If arsenic will cure gastritis, and we know it, we will adopt it; and so with everything else. We are an eclectic; and if farther experiments will confirm the position we assume that trephining will relieve or cure apoplexy and inflammation of the brain, we shall be one of the first to adopt it, whenever a proper case presents itself. We extract calculi from the bladder to keep men from dying; we cut off thighs to protect life; we excise the maxillary bones to prevent death; and the operation of *trephining* is not more dangerous than either of them. If tracheotomy will cure epilepsy, as we doubt not it will, we see no good reason why trephining should not cure *apoplexy.* We merely throw out these views to our brethren, as we are no " *wild enthusiast;*" and we hope every man in the brotherhood will give them a calm and candid reflection; remembering they are only suggestive upon facts observed in the *chicken* tribe. We shall continue to operate, as cases present themselves to us, and if we find our opinions further corroborated, or not, we will inform the fraternity of it, for we report our cases without regard to success or fatality.

Respectfully,   H. A. RAMSAY.

Thompson, Geo., April 18, 1853.

From the Boston Medical and Surgical Journal.
Boring the Cranium.

To THE EDITOR. SIR: In support of the conclusions arrived at, from experiments upon the "gallinaceous tribe," by your correspondent, Dr. H. A. Ramsay, with reference to the operation of trephining in apoplexy and inflammation of the brain, I offer the following remarks upon the subject, from an ancient and forgotten work. After bringing forward, in long and formidable array, the remedies of the time—as issues, ligatures, frictions, suppositories, and scarifications—the author continues, " 'Tis not amiss to bore the skull and let out the fuliginous vapours, because this humour hardly yields to other physic, and the head bored in two or three places avails much to the exhalation of vapours. I saw a man with brain disease at Rome, that by no remedies could be healed, but when by chance he was wounded in the head and his skull broken, he was excellently cured. Another, breaking his head with a fall from on high, was instantly recovered of his disease."

The matter is at least worthy of the serious consideration of the brotherhood, which I trust it will receive. Yours, J. STRADLEY.

Frederica, Del., May 1853.

From the Boston Medical and Surgical Journal.
Hydropathy in California.

By the following report of a Committee of the House of Representatives in California, it will be perceived that the Chairman was a sensible man, and also that hydropathy is bold in its pretensions there as well as here. There is a vein of wit running through it, which gives it a zest, and the whole tone of it very clearly shows that old birds are not to be caught with chaff. It is taken from the Alta Californian:

The Committee on State Hospitals, to whom was referred a remonstrance, by G. M. Bourne, hydriatic physician of San Francisco, would beg leave respectfully to report,

That they have carefully weighed the propositions contained in said remonstrance, and found them wanting, as follows:

1st, Because it assumes that a man has a right to place himself before the public as a practitioner of a science, of the principles of which he is entirely ignorant. He says he is in possession of no other warrant for practising the healing art than that conferred upon him by the great source of his being, or in other words, he was born with a sheep's skin, *ergo*, he has, without preparation, the natural right to practise medicine and surgery. Your Committee believe in no such logic.

2d, In the opinion of your Committee, it is not inimical to the spirit of our free institutions that the flights of erratic genius should be restrained within proper limits. The laws of every State protect its citizens from frauds practised upon them by false pretenders. If, then, the protection of property is deemed so essential, how much more carefully should health and life be protected from the impositions of ignorant pretenders and charlatans.

3d, That the medical profession has not realized the world's expectation, is lamentably true; but that it has approached any nearer so desirable a consummation since the advent of Priessnitz and hydropathy, your Committee has not been advised.

The order of Pretender, with whom your remonstrant fraternizes, has no legal existence, and, as your Committee believe, should have none.

The assertion of your remonstrant, that an immense number of astonishing and miraculous cures have been effected by means of cold water, requires confirmation; and your Committee, all of whom are medical practitioners, cannot conceive in what manner it has been made subservient to the successful management of difficult cases of parturition, and require the testimony of more than one interested witness to establish the fact. Your Committee have searched all the records within their reach, and can find no such statistics: but if, as your remonstrant asserts, a man totally ignorant of medicine and surgery did accomplish so much good, another man equally ignorant might accomplish as much evil.

Your Committee believe that no system of medicine should receive the protection of the laws of the State, to the exclusion of others. At the same time they believe that every practitioner, whether of allopathy, homœopathy, hydropathy, eclectic, botanic, uriscopic, root, herb, Indian or corn doctor, should possess some evidence of his proficiency in such science other than the ear-marks with which he was born. Your Committee are not aware that any legislative enactments are in contemplation, which will have the effect of retarding the progress of medical knowledge, as your remonstrant asserts.

, Those fathers of medicine whom your remonstrant has had the temerty to press into the service of hydropathy, never dreamed of the employment of water as a curative agent, to the exclusion of all other remedies, the advent of Priessnitz having been many centuries subsequent to this time.

" Literary celebrities " are not, in the opinion of your Committee, the proper persons to decide upon the merits of any system of medicine.

Sir John Ross and other navigators have recorded their opinion of water, no doubt verifying it as absolutely necessary to the success of navigation.

Lie-big's experiment of the chemical effects of cold water upon the animal economy, your Committee have not seen; but they can readily conceive, as your remonstrant asserts, that great changes, (if not entire dissolution) of the human body would occur under six weeks of active water treatment.

Notwithstanding " the great fiscal embarrassment of the State," your Committee believe it would be more than folly to substitute simple cold water for medicines of known and of proven utility, and discharge from our State Hospitals men of tried ability, and substitute a natural-born doctor on account of cheapness. Your Committee have heard of men who were born kings, and of others who were born fools, but no well attested case of a *born* doctor.

Your Committee would recognize the right of a female to practise medicine and surgery, if her education qualified her to perform its arduous duties. Her nature peculiarly fits her for ministering to the wants of the sick and afflicted.

In conclusion, your Committee would recommend that a copy of this report, together with a copy of your remonstrant's manifest, be transmitted to that " bourne " from whose " home for the sick " no patient will be likely ever to return, and ask to be dischared from a further consideration of the subject. J. H. ESTEP, *Chairman.*

From the Boston Medical and Surgical Journal.

Faults of Medical Writers.

[In the discourse by Dr. Samuel Jackson before the Philadelphia County Medical Society at its last annual meeting, we find the following remarks on a subject which deserves the attention of the profession generally—especially those who are in the habit, as all should be, of writing occasionally for the press.—ED.]

Let the young doctor do his very utmost in acquiring a habit of writing with *perspicuity, propriety and precision.* Let him seek no other ornament, for medical language is, like Thompson's loveliness, when "unadorned, adorned the most." No merit will make amends for the want of perspicuity. I can show whole paragraphs in our American books which have no meaning whatever, being similar in this respect to those verbose letters that Queen Elizabeth used to write when she had pre-determined to say nothing. Medical diction ought to use as few words as possible, thus going the shortest way to the end of a thought. An English writer on morbid poisons, wishing to describe the daily progress of the variolous pustule, uses the following verbosity : " You receive from a long distance, from Dublin or from Edinburgh, a lancet, on the point of which there is a little dry animal matter. This lancet has pricked the pustule of a patient suffering with smallpox, and the contents of the pustule have been suffered to dry on the lancet. Now with this lancet you make a single puncture in the arm of a healthy person, not previously defended by vaccination or otherwise, and what results ?"

Now suppose this author, Dr. Simon,"had wished to describe, also, the effect of a rattlesnake's bite, he might have begun thus : You receive from a long distance, from Utah or California, a rattlesnake, which Linnæus calls *crotalus,* it may be the species *horridus* or *durissus;* this dreadful animal has a sacculus of poison at the root of each fang, and when he bites, these sacculi pour forth their deadly contents along a groove in each fang. Now you permit this animal to bite a horse, for an experiment, or perhaps it bites one of you, and what results ? In this multiplication of useless verbiage, a great amount of time is wasted without any compensation.

In a celebrated medical journal, we have this circuitous way of saying that a certain medicine was probably useful in rheumatism : the disease was cured in eleven days; "and lemon juice, if it was not the principal remedy, certainly exerted an important influence toward the production of that end." What think you, gentlemen, of *producing* or *leading forward* an end or a cure ? One might suppose that the writer was a cobbler, and that he was talking about the *producing* or the *pulling forward* of his waxed-end. And then he has lemon-juice *making an exertion, and exerting an influence.*

Why should a writer say, "I had recourse to a medicine," if he had not previously used it in the same disease ? This word means a running backward. The simple English word *to give,* is often supplanted by the Latin word *to exhibit*; that is, to make a show of the medicine. A shopkeeper *exhibits* his goods, a physician *gives* or *orders* his medicine. Celsus took nearly all his ideas from the Greeks, but he did not copy their words. I believe he never uses the word *exhibere*, but *dare et utí*. Sometimes he says *adhibere*, but this does not mean *to make a show;* moreover, it is pure Latin. His own language was sufficient for him, except in the mere naming of diseases; and hence one reason that his style and manner are universally approved.

It is of no little importance that our young author should not practise the coining of words. A new idea may require a new word, but old ideas will always be most intelligibly introduced by known terms; hence the great English lexicographer, whose head might well be fancied as swarming with words, introduced only four in all his writings. His rule was, "to admit only such as may supply real déficiences, such as are readily adopted by the genius of our tongue, and incorporate easily with our native idiom." If a little license be granted, how will you define its limits? How will you definitely measure the old vulgar phrase *too much*? A little liberty will prove like moderate drinking, and lead to intemperance. If every writer of the present times should coin words at his pleasure, and the next generation should adopt them and add to them, what odious gibberish would then fill the air! It is told of Sir John Mandeville that, when far in northern Asia, with his retinue, their words were all frozen before they could be heard, and that, on coming south, they were suddenly thawed, and filled the air with their liberated voices. I can hardly credit this fact, as the amiable author does not relate it himself, and yet something similar may happen to the jargon of the present generation; while confined to books it may pass without much notice, but our successors may find the accumulated vocabulary to become a clattering of unmeaning voices, the mere echoes of our vanity, and as unintelligible as Sir John's thawed vocables.

In the Transactions of the American Medical Association you may find some animating specimens of these important additions to our deficient language. *Numerism, socialism, sensationalism, subjectivity, progressionist, therapeutication, truths eliminated, annexes of the heart.* A writer in vol. iv., p. 59, calls impressions "*intuitively-felt relations,*" and then inquires, "Are not all the felt relations based on immediacy and intuition, and not on representational and transmitted impressions." Truly, if men in high places continue to pour forth such floods of impurity, men in low places may well complain; hence I have ventured to notice the subject; it pertains to *self-education*, which is our present topic.

From the Boston Medical and Surgical Journal.

Therapeutic value of Veratrum Viride. By W. C. NORWOOD, M.D., of Abbeville, S. C.

We know of no agent so peculiarly adapted and so universally applicable to the treatment of febrile and inflammatory affections as the American Hellebore. With limited exceptions, it fulfils the therapeutical indications in these diseases unaided and alone; and, withal, its results are so invariable that we may expect to realize its effects, when properly administered, with the same certainty with which the husbandman anticipates an abundant harvest from the proper culture of his field.

However numerous or diversified may be the causes of febrile and inflammatory diseases, certain uniform effects or events are sure to follow them, and to correct or modify these effects is the grand aim of the practitioner. To do this successfully, a practical and experimental knowledge of the therapeutical properties of the agents calculated to modify the actions excited by these causes, is necessary; and this is the reason of my pressing so earnestly on every one the importance of thoroughly testing, and closely watching for himself, the therapeutical effects of veratrum viride; for I believe that he who fully understands its powers and applications, is in possession of the key which opens the door to triumphant success in the treatment of many diseases hitherto considered the opprobria of medicine.

I have been charged with enthusiasm, extravagance and fancy, in estimating the value of this remedy, and in urging its claims upon the profession; but years of close observation and experience have convinced me that, far from exaggerating, I have failed to do justice to the subject. Who can overrate the value of an agent capable of controlling the actions of the heart with demonstrative certainty? When it was announced, by the Italian physicians, that digitalis possessed the property of subduing and controlling morbid vascular action, medical men ardently anticipated the benefits that were about to be realized. But it proved not to possess the powers ascribed to it, and the field was again open for research and inquiry. After long observation and repeated experiment we are able to affirm, in the most positive manner, that *veratrum viride* entirely fulfils this indication. In less than twenty-four hours it will reduce a pulse of 100 or 160, to between 35 and 85 beats in the minute

But this drug possesses other important remedial powers. It is a certain and efficacious emetic; it possesses expectorant and diaphoretic properties in an eminent degree; its adanagic power is considerable, and it acts as a nervine in allaying morbid irritability.

We trust that these statements, based upon careful clinical observation and mature reflection, will induce the profession to use this remedy, and we believe that the benefits resulting to the sick from its judicious employment will be incalculable.— *Virginia Med. and Surg. Journal.*

From the Boston Medical and Surgical Journal.

Medical Vases.

Among other evidences of the labors accomplished by that indefatigable physician, Dr. Simpson, of Edinburgh, we have received within a few days a pamphlet by him upon the discovery of certain little vases, about an inch high and two-thirds of an inch in diameter, labelled in Greek, *lykion.* They are found in Greece, and occasionally in Italy, particularly in those places where there were Greek settlements in early times. The *lykion* was held by the ancients in the greatest estimation, and from the slight history of its use by practitioners of a remote age, it must have been very costly. Dr. Simpson's notes are full of interest. With praiseworthy enterprise, he has ascertained where the article was procured, and shows that it is still in repute in India, where it has always been prepared. For diseases of the eyes this *lykion* has been celebrated from the times of Dioscorides, Galen, and others equally well known for their attainments in medicine, and was considered far superior to all other remedies for certain affections of the optic apparatus. *Lykion* is in reality known as *ruswut* in Hindostan, and may be purchased at shops in most of the great towns over all India; and we therefore suggest to medical gentlemen living in ports in the United States from whence vessels are frequently sailing to Calcutta, to send an order for a few ounces. At all events, the oculists might find it to their special advantage to prescribe it. The *ruswut* is an inspissated extract from the wood and roots of several species of *berberis*, growing on the mountains principally of Upper India, and especially near Lahore. Dr. Simpson has a faculty of imparting a peculiar interest to any and every subject upon which he finds leisure to write.

From the Boston Medical and Surgical Journal.

Poisonous Dropsical Innoculation.

An accident of a singular and dangerous nature recently befel the celebrated surgeon, Prof. Langenbeck, in Berlin. Having been called in to attend a lady of high rank, in a most advanced and perilous stage of dropsy, Dr. L. deemed it necessary to proceed without delay, to puncturation, and this without waiting for other assistance. The operation was, therefore, instantly and successfully performed, and the patient, previously at death's door, relieved and saved. During the operation, however, some of the acrid discharge fell upon his hand, and was of course washed off when the work was completed; but, ere long, the hand, arm, throat and neighbouring regions began to swell, and all the febrile and inflammatory symptoms of animal poison ensued. Vigorous remedies were forthwith employed, and the danger averted, but the Professor is not yet so entirely recovered as to enjoy the full use of the side affected, whilst the venom has shown its lurking agency by causing eruptions on other parts of the body.

From the London Lancet.

Mesmerism. Good news for the Rheumatic !

Archbishop Whately, at a recent meeting of the Dublin Mesmeric Association, over which he presided, stated that he had been cured, by a week's mesmerising, of an inveterate rheumatism that had baffled the doctors. This beats all hollow Pulvermacher and his electric chains, " wherewith we are darkly bound." By the way, the Archbishop should have mentioned that the doctors under whose care he had been were homœopaths.

EDITORIAL.

The Obstetric Catechism, containing two thousand three hundred and forty-seven questions and answers on Obstetrics proper. By JOSEPH WARRINGTON, M.D. *One hundred and fifty illustrations: 12mo., pp. 445. Philadelphia: Barrington & Hoswell.* 1853.

The object of the author of this new candidate for public favor is stated, in the introductory address, to be, to furnish a convenient aid to the student during the prosecution of his preparatory labors, to be employed rather as a *text book* of knowledge already acquired by the diligent study of the more elaborate treatises with which this department of our profession is already enriched, than as a substitute for them. To the busy practitioner, also, who has little leisure for the careful perusal of elaborate monographs, especially in cases of emergency, it may prove a convenient and timely remembrancer. Employed in its appropriate sphere, we doubt whether a more appropriate form could have been assumed, as it enables the author to convey instruction with much of the vivacity and directness of oral communication. The scope of the work is even more comprehensive than most of the text books in this department, comprising beside the usual range of topics, most of the diseases and accidents of the female generative system in the impregnated condition, and not connected with their functional activity. It may, therefore, be regarded as a catechetical manual of the reproductive system of the female in its physiological as well as in its pathological conditions; and, taken as a whole, the design of the author is ably executed. More especially, however, in the practical portion is this commendation merited. In common with some other writers of the metropolitan schools, the author's views respecting the physical relation of the uterus and the ovum can scarcely, we apprehend, be said to be on a level with the high water mark of our science. We do not, however, regard it as a serious defect in a work designed especially as a practical manual of the Obstetric art. As a scientific as well as literary production, one feature of the work particularly impressed us, to wit, its purely *American character.* In the physiological, no less than in the practical portions of the work, we find American authorities cited, almost to the exclusion of transatlantic writers. This disposition to cultivate an independent nationality in matters of science as well as of civil polity, we hail with pleasure as the dawn of a new era in our scientific culture. When not transformed into mere local or sectional assumption, this feature will always constitute an additional recommendation to American students. Throughout the work the text is amply illustrated with good wood cuts, and the typographical execution of the work is altogether respectable.

Thankful for the present contribution to our medical literature, we hope at no distant day to see the mature experience of the author in a form that shall place it in the rank of standard works on Obstetric science.   A. S.

CHLORÓFORM.

The introduction of anæsthetic agents to alleviate the sufferings attendant upon surgical operations and child-birth, was hailed as a discovery which not only robbed the knife of its terror, but also so far thwarted the operation of the primitive curse, as to cause certain clerical grandmas to enter their protest against its heaven-defying use. Experience, however, has proved that the rapture of the surgeon, and the pious fear of his clerical brother, are alike premature; that the use of the most popular as well as powerful of the several anæsthetic agents is calculated to awaken no little anxiety on the part of the cautious physician, and fear on the part of his patient; and while our profession must feel that their hopes and expectations are not yet fully realized, our clerical brethren may rest assured that their wives will continue to bring forth in sorrow, for though the pangs attendant may be relieved, the chances of a sudden exit will serve to keep in force the spirit of the original penalty of mother Eve's transgression.

By the use of chloroform, we are occasionally reminded that Death's advent may most emphatically be like a thief in the night, when least anticipated. The officers of one of the London hospitals boasted of having exhibited it in over nine thousand cases, without a single death; and, as if in mockery, the grim messenger claimed its own in almost their next attempt at its exhibition.

The mode of death, too, is almost as diverse as the cases are numerous, hardly any two presenting exactly similar symptoms. This observation will be corroborated by consulting the table contained in the May No. of the New-York Journal of Medicine and Collateral Sciences for the present year. At times death is instantaneous, at others, as in Dr. Warren's case, in the Massachusetts General Hospital, it occurred after a lapse of three hours. Sometimes the respiratory movements continue after the heart has ceased to pulsate, and at others, we observe as one of its earliest manifestations, a paralyzing of the muscles of respiration. We once gave it to a parturient woman who strikingly verified this observation. The use of the agent was suspended; the patient revived, and again upon its renewal the same symptoms appeared. Several unavailing attempts were thus made in this case, and its use finally abandoned. In another case, one of amputation of the thigh, its exhibition was attended with the same result; here we persisted in our efforts for an hour, without avail, till at last, our knife acting as a stimulus to the respiratory motions, the chloroform was freely given and its full and happy effect obtained.

The amount, too, required to produce death varies; sometimes drachms, at others drops only. Twenty-five drops have proved fatal. (See table above alluded to.) One of our colleagues (Professor Denton) was about giving it to a nervous patient previous to laying open a felon on one of her fingers. To accustom her to the odor, a very few drops were put upon a handkerchief and handed her to smell of; he had hardly turned around, when he looked at her again and saw that her face was blanched, her eyes set, her muscles rigid, and respiration ceased. This case would undoubtedly have proved fatal, had not the Dr.'s admirable coolness prompted the application of a powerful stimulus. A scalpel, by no means distinguished for the keenness of its edge, was drawn slowly and firmly over the inflamed finger, cutting its way down to the bone. Just as the incision was completed the patient screamed, respiration was thus restored, and the patient and her friends considered it a beautiful exhibition of the agent in question ; and should this patient ever have occasion to have a pustule picked, she will probably insist upon taking chloroform.

We do not indulge in this train of thought from any ill effects we have ever experienced ; on the contrary, no accident has ever occurred with us.   G.

CODE OF MEDICAL ETHICS.

Adopted by the National Medical Convention, May, 1847.

The State Society, whose proceedings we published in our first number, adopted the Code of Ethics of the National Convention. As this Code is not in every Physician's Library, though it ought to be in every one's heart, we copy it for the benefit of those who have it not. To those who are familiar with it, we say that a reperusal of its lofty principles will do them no harm. —E. A.

CHAPTER I.—OF THE DUTIES OF PHYSICIANS TO THEIR PATIENTS, AND OF THE OBLIGATIONS OF PATIENTS TO THEIR PHYSICIANS.

ART. I.—*Duties of Physicians to their Patients.*

SEC. 1. A physician should not only be ever ready to obey the calls of the sick, but his mind ought to be imbued with the greatness of his mission, and the responsibility he habitually incurs in its discharge. These obligations are the more deep and enduring, because there is no tribunal other than his own conscience, to ajudge penalties for carelessness or neglect. Physicians should, therefore, minister to the sick with due impressions of the importance of their office ; reflecting that the ease, the health, and the lives of those committed to their charge, depend on their skill, attention and fidelity. They should study, also, in their deportment, so to unite *tenderness* with *firmness*, and *condescension* with *authority*, as to inspire the minds of their patients with gratitude, respect and confidence.

SEC. 2. Every case committed to the charge of a physician should be treated with attention, steadiness and humanity. Reasonable indulgence should be granted to the mental imbecility and caprices of the sick. Secrecy and delicacy, when required by peculiar circumstances, should be strictly observed ; and the familiar and confidential intercourse to which physicians are admitted in their professional visits, should be used with discretion, and with the most scrupulous regard to fidelity and honor. The obligation of secresy extends beyond the period of professional services—none of the privacies of personal and domestic life, no infirmity of disposition or flaw of character observed during professional attendance, should ever be divulged by him except when he is imperatively required to do so. The force and necessity of this obligation are indeed so great, that professional men have, under certain circumstances, been protected in their observance of secresy, by courts of justice.

Sec. 3. Frequent visits to the sick are in general requisite, since they enable the physician to arrive at a more perfect knowledge of the disease—to meet promptly every change which may occur, and also tend to preserve the confidence of the patient. But unnecessary visits are to be avoided, as they give useless anxiety to the patient, tend to diminish the authority of the physician, and render him liable to be suspected of interested motives.

Sec. 4. A physician should not be forward to make gloomy prognostications, because they savor of empiricism, by magnifying the importance of his services in the treatment or cure of the disease. But he should not fail, on proper occasions, to give to the friends of the patient timely notice of danger, when it really occurs; and even to the patient himself, if absolutely necessary. This office, however, is so peculiarly alarming when executed by him, that it ought to be declined whenever it can be assigned to any person of sufficient judgment and delicacy, For, the physician should be the minister of hope and comfort to the sick; that, by such cordials to the drooping spirit, he may smooth the bed of death, revive expiring life, and counteract the depressing influence of those maladies which often disturb the tranquility of the most resigned, in their last moments. The life of a sick person can be shortened not only by the acts, but also by the words or the manner of a physician. It is, therefore, a sacred duty to guard himself carefully in this respect, and to avoid all things which have a tendency to discourage the patient and to depress his spirits.

Sec. 5. A physician ought not to abandon a patient because the case is deemed incurable; for his attendance may continue to be highly useful to the patient, and comforting to the relatives around him, even in the last period of a fatal malady, by alleviating pain and other symptoms, and by soothing mental anguish. To decline attendance, under such circumstances, would be sacrificing to a fanciful delicacy and mistaken liberality, that moral duty, which is independent of and far superior to, all pecuniary considerations.

Sec. 6. Consultations should be promoted in difficult or protracted cases, as they give rise to confidence, energy, and more enlarged views in practice.

Sec. 7. The opportunity which a physician not unfrequently enjoys of promoting and strengthening the good resolutions of his patients, suffering under the consequence of vicious conduct, ought never to be neglected. His counsels, or even remonstrances, will give satisfaction, not offence, if they be proffered with politeness, and evince a genuine love of virtue, accompanied by a sincere interest in the welfare of the person to whom they are addressed.

Art. II.—*Obligations of Patients to their Physicians.*

Sec. 1. The members of the medical profession, upon whom are enjoined the performance of so many important and arduous duties towards the community, and who are required to make so many sacrifices to comfort, ease and health, for the welfare of those who avail themselves of their services, certainly have a right to expect and require, that their patients should entertain a just sense of the duties which they owe to their medical attendants.

Sec. 2. The first duty of the patient is, to select as his medical adviser, one who has received a regular profesional education. In no trade or occupation do mankind rely on the skill of an untaught artist; and in medicine, confessedly the most difficult and intricate of the sciences, the world ought not to suppose that knowledge is intuitive.

Sec. 3. Patients should prefer a physician whose habits of life are regular, and who is not devoted to company, pleasure, or to any pursuit, incompatible with his professional obligations. A patient should, also, confide the care of himself and family, as much as possible, to one physician—for a medical man who has become acquainted with the peculiarities of constitution, habits and pre-dispositions of those he attends, is more likely to be successful in his treatment, than one who does not possess that knowledge.

A patient who has thus selected his physician, should always apply for advice in what may appear to him trival cases, for the most fatal results often surpervene on the slightest accidents. It is of still more importance that he should apply for assistance in the forming stage of violent diseases; it is to a neglect of this precept that medicine owes much of the uncertainty and imperfection with which it has been reproached.

Sec. 4. Patients should faithfully and unreservedly communicate to their physician the supposed cause of their disease. This is the more important, as many diseases of a mental origin simulate those depending on external causes, and yet are only to be cured by ministering to the mind diseased. A patient should never be afraid of thus making his physician his friend and adviser ; he should always bear in mind that a medical man is under the strongest obligations of secrecy. Even the female sex should never allow feelings of shame or delicacy to prevent their disclosing the seat, symptoms and causes of complaints peculiar to them. However commendable a modest reserve may be in the common occurrences of life, its strict observance in medicine is often attended with the most serious consequences, and a patient may sink under a painful and loathsome disease, which might have been readily prevented had timely intimation been given to the physician.

Sec. 5. A patient should never weary his physician with a tedious detail of events or matters not appertaining to his disease. Even as relates to his actual symptoms, he will convey much more real information by giving clear answers to interrogatories, than by the most minute account of his own framing. Neither should he obtrude the details of his business nor the history of his family concerns.

Sec. 6. The obedience of a patient to the prescriptions of his physician should be prompt and implicit. He should never permit his own crude opinions, as to their fitness, to influence his attention to them. A failure in one particular may render an otherwise judicious treatment dangerous, and even fatal. This remark is equally applicable to diet, drink, and exercise. As patients become convalescent, they are very apt to suppose that the rules prescribed for them may be disregarded, and the consequences but too often, is a relapse. Patients should never allow themselves to be persuaded to take any medicine whatever that may be recommended to them by the self-constituted doctors and doctresses, who are so frequently met with, and who pretend to possess infallible remedies for the cure of every disease. However simple some of their prescriptions may appear to be, it often happens that they are productive of much mischief, and in all cases they are injurious, by contravening the plan of treatment adopted by the physician.

Sec. 7. A patient should, if possible, avoid even the *friendly visits of a physician* who is not attending him ; and when he does receive them, he should never converse on the subject of his disease, as an observation may be made, without any intention of interference, which may destroy confidence in the course he is pursuing, and induce him to neglect the directions prescribed to him. A patient should never send for a consulting physician without the express consent of his own medical attendant. It is of great importance that physicians should act in concert; for although their modes of treatment may be attended with equal success, when employed singly, yet conjointly they are very likely to be productive of disastrous results.

Sec. 8. When a patient wishes to dismiss his physician, justice and common courtesy require that he should declare his reasons for so doing.

Sec. 9. Patients should always, when practicable, send for their physician in the morning before his usual hour for going out; for by being early aware of the visits he has to pay during the day, the physician is able to apportion his time in such a manner as to prevent an interference of engagements. Patients should also avoid calling on their medical adviser unnecessarily during the hours devoted to meals or sleep. They should always be in readiness to receive the visits of their physician, as the detention of a few minutes is often of serious inconvenience to him.

Sec. 10. A patient should, after his recovery entertain a just and enduring sense of the value of the services rendered him by his physician; for these are of such a character, that no mere pecuniary acknowledgment can repay or cancel them.

CHAPTER II.—OF THE DUTIES OF PHYSICIANS TO EACH OTHER, AND TO THE PROFESSION AT LARGE.

ART. 1.—*Duties for the support of professional characters.*

Sec. 1. Every individual, on entering the profession, as he becomes thereby entitled to all its privileges and immunities, incurs an obligation to exert his best abilities to maintain its dignity and honor, to exalt its standing, and to extend the bounds of its usefulness. He should therefore observe strictly such laws as are instituted for the government of its members—should avoid all contumelious and sarcastic remarks relative to the faculty, as a body; and while, by unwearied diligence, he resorts to every honorable means of enriching the science, he should entertain a due respect for his seniors, who have, by their labors, brought it to the elevated condition in which he finds it.

Sec. 2. There is no profession, from the members of which greater purity of character, and a higher standard of moral excellence are required, than the medical; and to attain such eminence, is a duty every physician owes alike to his profession, and to his patients. It is due to the latter, as without it he cannot command their respect and confidence, and to both, because no scientific attainments can compensate for the want of correct moral principles. It is also incumbent upon the faculty to be temperate in all things, for the practice of physic requires the unremitting exercise of a clear and vigorous understanding; and, on emergencies for which no professional man should be unprepared, a steady hand, an acute eye, and an unclouded head may be essential to the well-being, and even to the life, of a fellow creature.

Sec. 3. It is derogatory to the dignity of the profession, to resort to public advertisements or private cards or handbills, inviting the attention of individuals affected with particular diseases—publicly offering advice and medicine to the poor gratis, or promising radical cures; or to publish cases and operations in the daily prints or to suffer such publications to be made—to invite laymen to be present at operations—to boast of cures and remedies—to adduce certificates of skill and success, or to perform any other similar acts. These are the ordinary practices of empirics, and are highly reprehensible in a regular physician.

Sec. 4. Equally derogatory to professional character is it for a physician to hold a patent for any surgical instrument or medicine; or to dispense a secret *nostrum*, whether it be the composition or exclsive property of himself or of others. For, if such nostrum be of real efficacy, any concealment regarding it is inconsistent with beneficence and professional liberality; and, if mystery alone give it value and importance, such craft implies either disgraceful ignorance, or fraudulent avarice. It is also reprehensible for physicians to give certificates attesting the efficacy of patent or secret medicines, or in any way to promote the use of them.

ART. II.—*Professional services of Physicians to each other.*

Sec. 1. All practitioners of medicine, their wives and their children while under the paternal care, are entitled to the gratuitous services of any one or more of the faculty residing near them, whose assistance may be desired. A physician afflicted with disease is usually incompetent to judge of his own case; and the natural anxiety and solicitude which he experiences at the sickness of a wife, a child, or any one who by the ties of consanguinity is rendered peculiarly dear to him, tend to obscure his judgment, and produce timidity and irresolution in his practice. Under such circumstances, medical men are peculiarly dependent on each other, and kind offices and professional aid should always be cheerfully and gratuitously afforded. Visits ought not, however, to be obtruded officiously; as such unasked civility may give rise to embarrassment, or interfere with that choice, on which confidence depends. But, if a distant member of the faculty, whose circumstances are affluent, request attendance, and an honorarium be offered, it should not be declined; for no pecuniary obligation ought to be imposed, which the party receiving it would not wish to incur.

ART. III.—*Of the duties of Physicians as respects vicarious offices.*

Sec. 1. The affairs of life, the pursuit of health, and the various accidents and contingencies to which a medical man is peculiarly exposed, sometimes require him temporarily to withdraw from his duties to his patients, and to request some of his professional brethren to officiate for him. Compliance with this request is an act of courtesy, which should always be performed with the utmost consideration for the interest and character of the family physician, and when exercised for a short period, all the pecuniary obligations for such service should be awarded to him. But if a member of the profession neglects his business in quest of pleasure and amusement, he cannot be considered as entitled to the advantages of the frequent and long-continued exercise of this fraternal courtesy, without awarding to the physician who officiates, the fees arising from the discharge of his professional duties.

In obstetrical and important surgical cases, which give rise to unusual fatigue, anxiety and responsibility, it is just that the fees accruing therefrom should be awarded to the physician who officiates.

ART. IV.—*Of the duties of Physicians in regard to Consultations.*

Sec. 1. A regular medical education furnishes the only presumptive evidence of professional abilities and acquirements, and ought to be the only acknowledged right of an individual to the exercise and honors of his profession. Nevertheless, as in consultations the good of the patient is the sole object in view, and this is often dependent on personal confidence, no intelligent regular practitioner, who has a license to practice from some medical board of known and acknowledged respectability, recognized by this association, and who is in good moral and professional standing in the place in which he resides, should be fastidiously excluded from fellowship, or his aid refused in consultation, when it is requested by the patient. But no one can be considered a regular practitioner, or a fit associate in consultation, whose practice is based on an exclusive dogma, to the rejection of the accumulated experience of the profession, and the aids actually furnished by anatomy, physiology, pathology, and organic chemistry.

Sec. 2. In consultations no rivalship or jealousy should be indulged; candor, probity, and all due respect should be exercised towards the physician having charge of the case.

Sec. 3. In consultations the attending physician should be the first to propose the necessary questions to the sick; after which the consulting physician should have the opportunity to make such further inquiries of the patient as may be necessary to satisfy him of the true character of the case. Both physicians should then retire to a private place for deliberation ; and the one first in attendance should communicate the directions agreed upon to the patient or his friends, as well as any opinions which it may be thought proper to express. But no statement or discussion of it should take place before the patient or his friends, except in the presence of all the faculty attending, and by their common consent; and no *opinions* or *prognostications* should be delivered, which are not the result of previous deliberation and concurrence.

Sec. 4. In consultation, the physician in attendance should deliver his opinion first; and when there are several consulting, they should deliver their opinions in the order in which they have been called in. No decision, however, should restrain the attending physician from making such variations in the mode of treatment, as any subsequent unexpected change in the character of the case may demand. But such variation and the reason for it ought to be carefully detailed at the next meeting in consultation. The same privilege belongs also to the consulting physician if he is sent for in an emergency, when the regular attendant is out of the way, and similar explanations must be made by him, at the next consultation.

Sec. 5. The utmost punctuality should be observed in the visits of physicians when they are to hold consultations together, and this is generally practicable, for society has been considerate enough to allow the plea of a professional engagement to take precedence of all others, and to be an ample reason for the relinquishment of any present occupation, But as professional engagements may sometimes interfere, and delay one of the parties, the physician who first arrives should wait for his associate a reasonable period, after which the consultation should be considered as postponed to a new appointment. If it be the attending physician who is present, he will of course see the patient and prescribe ; but if it be the consulting one, he should retire, except in case of emergency, or when he has been called from a considerable distance, in which latter case he may examine the patient, and give his opinion in *writing* and *under seal*, to be delivered to his associate.

TO BE CONCLUDED IN OUR NEXT.

THE

PENINSULAR

JOURNAL OF MEDICINE

AND THE COLLATERAL SCIENCES.

| VOL. I. | SEPTEMBER, 1853. | NO. III. |

ORIGINAL COMMUNICATIONS.

ART. I. — *Philosophy of certain Dislocations of the Hip and Shoulder, and their Reduction.* Read before the Detroit Medical Society. By M. GUNN, M.D., Prof. of Surgery in the University of Mich.

The views here advanced I have taught for the past two years to the gentlemen composing the Medical Class in the University; and I shall offer no apology for calling the attention of the Society for a few moments this evening to the subject of Dislocations of the Hip and Shoulder, and more particularly to that form of the accident, which, from the anatomical peculiarities of the joint, is one exceedingly difficult to reduce; and for the reduction of which Dr. Reid has but recently proposed a novel and efficient mode.

It is not my intention to discuss the question of priority which has been raised in reference to this subject, for there can be no doubt that Dr. Reid arrived at his conclusions by a course of reasoning and experiment; and that those conclusions were most essentially novel to a large majority of the profession. I propose rather, briefly to consider the prominent peculiarities of the joint, and the relation of the parts in a state of dislocation; the structures which oppose the return of the head of the femur to the acetabulum; the manner in which Dr. Reid's manipulations overcome this opposition; and lastly, the application of the principle involved, to the reduction of some other dislocations.

The encircling ridge which gives depth to the cotyloid cavity, presents upon its outer slope a plane, the inclination of which varies in different parts. At its posterior portion this inclination is very great, and it would seem in dislocation in this direction impossible to return the head of the bone to the cavity without lifting it completely over the ridge; upwards and backwards it is more gradual, and would seem to afford a much more easily surmountable obstacle; yet when we examine the relation of the parts in a dislocation in this direction, we find that applied to this surface, we have the anterior and inferior surface of the head and neck of the femur, the rotundity of the head corresponding with the curvature of the slope, while the edge of the acetabulum corresponds with the curvature described by the anterior and inferior surface of the neck. Although thus seemingly locked together, comparatively slight extension in the line of dislocation would cause the head to ride over the edge of the cavity, were it not bound down in this position by the surrounding tissues. Which particular tissue constitutes these bands is an important question to him who seeks to relax them. Dr. Reid, in common with the profession generally, considers the muscles the agents which thus oppose our efforts at reduction, and his manipulations are conducted with a view to relax them, while the femur acting as a lever, the head of the bone is raised clear of the edge of the cavity. With this same view we have the directions of the books and public teachers to apply extension and counter-extension *slowly* and *uniformly* in order to *tire out* the rebellious muscles. Bloodletting, antimony, and the hot bath are also called in to aid in this laudable crusade against these wicked organs.

In this view, I would respectfully differ with Dr. Reid, the teachers, books and profession, and state my honest belief that the muscles oppose our efforts very little more than they do the progress of our earth in its orbit. This belief I have repeatedly verified by experiments upon the dead subject, and the members of the medical class of 1851–2 in the University will remember those conducted before them. A subject was placed upon the table, the lower border of the gluteus maximus was raised, and a scalpel carried through the subjacent muscles, and an opening made in the posterior and superior portion of the capsular ligament. The round ligament was then divided, and the head of the femur luxated upon the dorsum of the ilium. The usual indications of this dislocation were present. The subject was placed in the proper position, a counter-extending band applied to the perinæum and fixed; the strength of two men exerted now upon the extending band, while endeavor was made to raise the head of the bone clear of the acetabulum with a jack towel, was insufficient to reduce the luxation. Reid's method of manipulation readily replaced the bone. This experiment was repeated many times, and

uniformly with the same result.   As *muscular action* could not have opposed our efforts and prevented success in this case, the question naturally
presents itself, what structure stood between effort and success ?   I answer,
the untorn portion of the capsular ligament.   In support of this view,
let us consider for a moment the position of the limb at the instant of
escape of the head from the socket during the process of dislocation.   To
do this we must bear in mind that force applied to the knee or foot while
the limb is in a state of adduction, constitutes the most frequent cause of
this dislocation.   Force thus applied adducts the limb still more powerfully before dislocation takes place, and at the moment of the escape of the
head of the bone from the socket the limb is in a direction which crosses
the thigh of the opposite side.   Immediately that the head of the bone has
cleared the edge of the acetabulum it settles into its position upon the
dorsum of the ilium, and the limb assumes the position and direction indicative of the accident.   During the dislodgement of the bone, the superior and posterior portion of the capsular ligament is ruptured, through
which the head protrudes; while from the position of the limb at the instant of protrusion, the anterior and inferior portion is very much relaxed,
thus allowing the head to ride easily over the acetabulum.   As soon as
the head settles into its position upon the dorsum of the ilium, the direction of the limb is changed, and the untorn portion of the ligament becomes more tense, and for this reason the head of the bone cannot be
readily returned to its place, till the limb is again placed in a position to
relax it.   Dr. Reid's method does this most effectually, and I conceive
that any other plan which does not accomplish this, as for instance extension and counter-extension by the pully, or Jarvis' apparatus, in the usual
direction, succeeds only by lacerating much more extensively, if not by
actually tearing the ligament completely asunder, before the head of the
bone will ride over the edge of the cavity.

The principle, then, I would seek to establish is this — *that in luxations of the hip and shoulder the untorn portion of the capsular ligament, by binding down the head of the dislocated bone, prevents its ready
return over the edge of the cavity to its place in the socket; and that
this return can be easily effected by putting the limb in such a position
as will effectually approximate the two points of attachment of that
portion of the ligament which remains untorn.*

This principle can be successfully applied to the reduction of the backward luxation of the femur into the ischictic notch, and also to the several luxations of the shoulder.   It has several times been my guide in
the reduction of the downward dislocation of the humerus into the axilla.
The patient is seated upon the floor, an assistant slowly raises the arm to
an angle of forty-five degrees to the plane upon which the patient is sitting;

and now while the assistant makes extension in this direction, the surgeon makes pressure with the hand upon the top of the shoulder, the bone readily returns to its place, and the arm is dropped to the side and secured in a sling.

White's method of reducing this luxation, which is figured in Druitt, is essentially the same, the only difference being in the position of the patient. According to his plan the patient lies upon his back, the scapule is fixed by a counter-extending band applied to the top of the shoulder, or by the hand of an assistant, while " the arm is raised from the side, and drawn straight up by the head, till the bone is thus elevated into the socket." In either method it will be seen that the upper and untorn portion of the capsular ligament, by the elevation of the arm is very much relaxed, thus giving a latitude of motion to the head which greatly facilitates its return, and which could not be obtained by any manipulation in which this relaxation was less perfect. Nine-tenths of the force spent in extension and counter-extention may be spared, in the reduction of all those dislocations in which, by alteration of the position of the limb, such relaxation is effected; and in the several luxations above specified this end is undoubtedly attainable.

Detroit, Aug. 11, 1853.

Art. II. — *Grand River Medical Association.* Communicated by J. H. Hollister, M.D., Cor. Sec'y.

Reference was made in the last Journal to this Association, and I may be permitted perhaps to occupy a brief space in your columns, in noticing its organization and present position. Not from a desire for notoriety, but that in other localities yet destitute of medical organizations, a similar effort may be made, I am induced to lay before your readers the plan of our organization, and our present anticipations.

It owed its origin to the necessity, very generally expressed, for a cultivated medical acquaintance and co-operation of the physicians of Grand River Valley. A variety of medical institutions are here represented by their graduates, engaged in the practice of medicine, and a very general desire had been felt for some time, that an organization which should promote a full and free interchange of thought and the discussion of questions relating to medicine and the collateral sciences, would be at once interesting and highly profitable.

In answer to a call by the physicians of Grand Rapids, a meeting was held at that place on the 1st Thursday of June, 1851, which resulted in the organization of the present Association.

Locally, it is represented by physicians from the counties of Ionia, Montcalm, Ottawa, Kent and Muskegan. Its constitution provides for the eligibility of those to membership, who, though not graduates of any medical school, from the time of their practice and correct medical deportment, are justly entitled to professional respect and etiquette. It also provides for the expulsion of those guilty of medical misdemeanors. Its officers are elected annually, and the retiring President, upon the closing of his term, is required to prepare a written address. An annual meeting is held on the 1st Thursday of January of each year, and an address presented, by a member appointed by the President at the last meeting. Engaging the attention of these meetings, are reports from Committees on various medical subjects, and clinical reports of general interest from the various members.

The society is now in the third year of its existence, harmonious and fully meeting the anticipations of its founders. Its 1st presiding officer was Chas. Shepard, M.D., of Grand Rapids, 2d, Alanson Cornell, M.D., of Ionia, and the present incumbent Alonzo Platt, M.D., of Grand Rapids.

Among the subjects claiming the attention of this Association is the infection, very prevalent in this vicinity, and not unfrequently fatal, known as Stomatitis Materin, or Nursing Sore Mouth. And as this subject is still referred to a Committee of Investigation, I may here divert from the subject of this article, and earnestly solicit communications from any of our professional brethren who have directed their attention to the pathology and treatment of this disease.

Each meeting brings new accessions to our numbers, and our desire is to embrace within our society every regular practitioner of Medicine in the Valley.

As a society, it will give us pleasure to co-operate with others for the promotion of medical improvement throughout the State, and we suggest the propriety of rendering ours, in common with others, auxiliary to the State Medical Society.

It seems an absolute necessity that a thorough organization, not of *drones*, but of efficient *workers*, should be effected throughout the entire State. Societies should be so located as to call out the latent energies of every genuine practitioner. The present is an age marked by a spirit of investigation. Men seek the *reason* of things, and the truth of assertions, whether in Theology, Medicine, the Natural Sciences or the Arts. Turning to the ailments incident to our present existence, they desire the *rationale* of that treatment which baffles disease and restores the invalid to health. And, in justice, they should be informed that the principles of medicines will lose nothing by investigation, and an enlightened community alone may enjoy an immunity from the barefaced and truthless assertion of arrogant, boasting quacks. A correct medical literature, and a higher standard of medical attainments by the profession, is needed; and a faithfulness on their part to impart correct views of medicine and its principles to those whose confidence they enjoy, is also needed. The people seek to be informed. We dream on, withholding from them the truth, and turning from us they devour the trash of medicated almanacs and astounding puffing advertisements. We curse a people bound to be humbugged, and are ourselves more than half to blame. That man who assumes the responsibilities of Medical practice, is in a measure responsible for the views of the community with which he mingles. Is he superficial, doubting, changing, dabbling, *sceptical*, he may look for a like regard on the part of his patrons. Is he prompt, *stable, educated, mastering* his profession, and evincing his love for it by his devotion to it, the result is unquestionable. *He must succeed!* His worth will be appreciated and his profession will be honored. Let us, then, by our devotion and energy — by the thorough training of our students, and our hearty co-operation with our fellow-laborers in our respective associations — dispel forever the idea that ours is a profession of inglorious ease. But I must cease this digression from my original purpose, which may only be explained from its expressing the predominant idea of my mind as I commenced this article, viz: The hope that in every convenient and healthy locality of the State a thorough medical organization should be made during the present year, and that at the next meeting of the State Society every auxiliary shall be *fully represented.*

Receive this, gentlemen, as the ardent desire of our Association, with the hope that it may meet a hearty response.

ART. III. — *Congenital Contraction of the Intestinal Canal.* By S. L. ANDREWS, M.D.

In a private letter from my friend, Dr. Baldwin, of Lahaina, Sandwich Islands, I have an interesting account of a case of congenital contraction of the intestinal canal. As Dr. B. has given me the case more in detail than is needful for your Journal, I have abridged it for your use. The child, a fine looking, plump female, and weighing $8\frac{3}{4}$ lbs., was born Dec. 5th, 1838. The first indication of anything abnormal was the rejection of a little sweetened water given a few hours after birth. On the following morning castor oil was rejected with bilious vomiting. A judicious use of cathartics, including suppository and enematic, the latter sometimes administered through a gum elastic catheter introduced several inches into the rectum, failed to produce any adequate evacuation of the bowels. Castor oil and other cathartics, and sometimes enematics, only excited vomiting, usually bilious. At length the contents of the intestines, in a very offensive state, were thrown off by vomiting. All that was passed, per anum, was fragments of hardened meconium, shaped to the intestines, and amounting to several inches in length. The last fragment tapered to a point at its upper extremity. Death on the 13th.

Diagnosis, contraction of the intestine, which was confirmed by the autopsy.

The rectum and colon were about half the natural size, or perhaps a little more, except a portion in the middle of the arch, where it was reduced to about half the diameter of that on each side of it. The cœcum was natural, but for twelve inches above it the small intestine was small indeed, not larger than the narrowest tape, and the canal too narrow to admit anything solid; the next six inches, proceeding towards the stomach, was very narrow, but contained a few small pieces of hardened meconium. Eighteen inches above this was larger, but crowded with viscid meconium. The remainder of the intestine to the stomach was twice the natural size. The gall bladder was large and full. The stomach and upper part of the intestine was filled with a liquid appearing like a mixture of bile and milk. The child had nursed until the last day.

The father of the child, an efficient and devoted missionary under the American Board, has disproportionately short limbs, both upper and lower. He is also afflicted with exostosis. A sister is afflicted in the same manner, and some of the children of both brother and sister have the same morbid state of the bones.

ART. IV.

EDITOR PENINSULAR JOURNAL OF MEDICINE: *Dear Sir* — I see in your Journal for the present month, a case reported by L. C. Robinson, M.D., of an amputation of the hip joint, for Fungus Hæmatodes, by E. M. Clark, M.D.

The object of calling attention to this operation for the above named disease, is to put the younger portion of the profession on their guard; for past experience has shown that to remove a Fungus Hæmatodes tumor, or to amputate a limb for that disease, not only proves unsuccessful, but hastens the time for the patient's dissolution. Professor Mott, in his lectures of the winter of 1842, states, while dwelling on Fungus Hæmatodes of the eye-ball, that it has been extirpated again and again, but the disease returns in all its force, and bids defiance to all our skill, and destroys the patient. Professor Parker states that he has not seen this disease removed either by extirpation or amputation. Although the wound may heal, yet the disease will attack in a short time the original location, on the stump, after amputation. Dr. Gibon, in his Surgery, after giving a long detailed account of cases of this disease, closes by stating, (in reference to a tumor that he had just removed,) "The only further remark I deem it necessary to make in relation to this case is, that could I have known the tumor to have been of the nature of fungus hæmatodes, I should certainly not have undertaken to remove it, upon the ground that there is not a single well-attested case on record in which this inveterate malady has been successfully removed by extirpation, and very few where the patient has recovered after amputation.

I will cite a case in my own practice, in which Judge Brink, of Milford, Pa., consulted me with reference to a fungus hæmatodes that involved his hand and wrist. He had been told that it was a cancer. I informed him that it was not, but told him what the disease was, and that he need not expect to live very long. He was anxious to have the arm amputated. I told him if it was, there was no doubt but the disease would attack the stump. He chose to be well for a short time, that he might settle his Judicial and other business, for he could not as he then was. Having a full understanding with the parties, I amputated above the elbow. The stump healed kindly, and in fourteen days he returned home, to all appearance well. But in seven months the fungus reappeared, and in two months from that time he died.

These cases, out of many, are cited to prove the folly of attempting to remove fungus hæmatodes, either by extirpation or amputation. I should not have amputated in any case if it were not for the reasons stated above. Except this disease, all other matters were favorable.

Was there any hope of recovery in the case reported by Dr. Robinson? — the pulse 100, the patient emaciated, having a cough, and poorly provided with the necessaries of life. And was it prudent under such circumstances to amputate? Experience tells us, *No!*

Detroit, August 15, 1853. ISAAC S. SMITH, M.D.

Art. V.—*Spiritual Functions of Tables.* By John C. Norton, M.D., of Rockford, Illinois.

Dr. Andrews:—I have just received the first number of your Medical Journal, in which I was pleased to see an article explaining some of the mysteries of Spirit Rapping. Having myself spent some time in investigating this subject, I was naturally curious to see whether both of us had arrived at the same conclusions; and, what was my gratification at finding, that we had not only arrived at the same end, but had reached it by precisely the same route. I tried the same experiments which you have mentioned, with exactly the same results. I thought I had brought out something new in regard to the principle of muscular action, but I find there is nothing new under the sun, for others have been bringing out the same views. I believe you said nothing of *placing weight upon a table.* It is claimed that spirits are able to hold a table down so that it can scarcely be lifted from the floor, and I have seen people make strong efforts to lift a stand upon which the spirits had been told to place weight, without succeeding. If I were to attempt to explain this, I should refer to kindred phenomena connected with Mesmerism, and ask, How is it that a person is fastened to the floor, or to a chair, by the influence of the operator? No one, I believe, pretends that the subject of mesmeric influence is moved upon by the spirits of the dead to act as he does. If, then, there are natural forces of sufficient power to thus hold a man down, why should we assume that there is no natural force capable of fastening a table to the floor? But, let us see what that force is which renders such material assistance to the force of gravitation. I recollect once asking a *subject* of mesmerism the following question—"Do you suppose you had the power to do differently from what you were told by the operator you would do?" The answer was—"I suppose I had the power, but my attention was so fixed upon the operator that I was incapable of making an effort at resistance." The answer is similiar to the one given to the question—"Can a bird forsake its young?" "Yes, if she wants to, but she can't want to." The power of the will is so overcome by emotions that we are incapable of forming a correct estimate of weight or of our own physical strength. To a person who has been for a long time sick, a light body appears heavy, and so to a very strong man, heavy objects appear very light. It is obvious then, that our ideas of weight depend as much upon our bodily and mental states as upon real specific gravity, and are solely the result of comparison. The spirits influence the *mind* and not the table. The *force* that holds men and tables down, is a *want of force.* Of this any one may satisfy himself by a simple experiment: Place a table upon the platform of a scale, and weigh it accurately with the persons who are to take their position by it. Now command the spirits to place weight upon it. It is clear that if weight is actually placed upon the table the balances will quickly show it; but what is the fact? Awful to relate, the spirits are "weighed in the balances and found wanting!"

But how can we be so deceived as to think the table heavier than it really is? Why, my friend, it is the easiest thing in the world. I will tell you how I have seen people deceived, and how others may be.— They form in their minds an estimate of what the table ought to weigh, and in nine cases out of ten never think to lift it before the spiritual weight is placed upon it. They are then told to lift, gently at first, and afterwards with more force, to be careful not to make any sudden effort, lest they should break the connection of the circuit. By lifting thus gently, at first, and gradually increasing the effort, the muscles are tired and the mental processes are interfered with, so that we are led to make an incorrect estimate. Our imagination helps to make up the weight, and in accordance with a well known law of physiology, the mere direction of the attention to the sensation of resistance in the table, makes that sensation more acute, so that here is another cause of deception. I do not wish, Mr. Editor, to occupy too much of the valuable space of your journal, with matters which may be interesting to none but myself, otherwise I might write a great deal upon the subject of *Spiritual Communications.* I only wished to show to the spiritual enthusiast " *how plain a tale would put them down.*"

ART. VI.—*Review of an Article on Diaphragmatic Hernia.* Written by HENRY J. BOWDITCH, Member of the Boston Society of Medical Observation. Concluded from page 63.

THE writer next proceeds with a long and somewhat tedious analysis of the symptoms, and accompanying circumstances mentioned in the recorded cases of this accident; but as many of them are mere accidental complications, many others such plain results as must necessarily accompany any such case, and as few important deductions are made from them, we hasten on, concentrating for the reader only what is of practical value.

The displacement of the viscera consisted in the passage of the liver, spleen, stomach, colon, or small intestines, or several of these together, into the pleural cavity. This, of course, compressed the lungs more or less, and generally pushed the heart to one side. From this position of the viscera, the diagnosis may be often clearly made out. The displacement of the heart will cause its pulsations to be felt and heard in a new position, as for instance on the right side. The compression of the lungs will cause the respiratory murmurs to be heard only in the upper part of the chest, while below there will be dulness on percussion if the liver or spleen alone have passed up, or resonance accompanied with the usual gurgling intestinal sounds, if the stomach or colon, distended with flatus, has ascended. There will also be more or less dyspnæa in consequence of the pulmonary compression.

He proceeds to show that this disease may continue for years, — yes, even from birth, without any very marked symptoms. The displacements and dyspnæa may be so slight as to occasion but little inconvenience, until some fall or accident either rends through the whole diaphragm, cutting off at once the power of respiration, or changes the position of the intestine, so as to strangulate it. In the latter case, the physician who is called, finds all the symptoms of strangulation without any visible hernia, and the accompanying dyspnæa assists to produce a case so obscure that few dare to diagnose it. The great danger is that of confounding it with colic, and therefore treating it most erroneously.

In a case where this disease exists, it is obvious that the patient is in constant danger. He is liable at any moment to strangulation of the hernia, without the possibility of reducing it by taxis. Writers have recorded the immediate cause of the fatal attack in thirty-four cases, which the author has condensed into a table, as follows:

TABLE.

"By a Fall,	-	-	-	-	-	in 9	cases.
" Violent emetic	-	-	-	-	" 3	"
" Laxative medicine	-	-	-	" 1	"
" Drunkenness -	-	-	-	-	" 5	"
" Irritating ingesta	-	-	" 2	"
" Excess at a ball	-	-	-	" 1
" Bullet wound	-	-	-	" 1	"
' Stab,	-	-	-	-	" 3	"
" Blow,	-	-	-	-	-	" 1	"
" Violent and sudden strain,	-	-	-	" 1	"
" Being run over, -	-	-	-	" 3	"
" Violent crying,	-	-	-	" 1
" Labor pains,	-	-	-	-	" 2	"
" A long walk,	-	-	-	-	" 1	"

34

From these facts it is inferred that the patient suffering under this hernia, ought to discontinue all employments and exercises that subject him to great strain upon the abdominal muscles, or render him liable to shocks and falls, and select some quiet occupation. He should be instructed also to abstain rigidly from debauchery and excess in eating and drinking, and never indulge in food calculated to stimulate inordinate intestinal motions.

In case the disease proceeds to strangulation, the only ordinary remedies which the writer recommends are the bath, ether, and sometimes opium. As this, however, is but indirect treatment, he proposes as a dernier resort, to lay open the abdomen, find the stricture and divide it.

"Sacs," he says, "commence about the lower and front part of the mediastinum, therefore near this is a proper place to commence the incision. Passing along the edge of the ribs for the space of three or four inches, we should divide the muscles and come upon the peritonæum covering the lower part of the diaphragm, and reflected thence upon the inner side of the abdominal muscles. It would be possible, I think, to push aside this membrane and not enter the cavity of the peritoneal sac, until we might be able to make out the exact place of stricture, and there a very slight incision only would be necessary. But in this operation there is at present so much of difficulty owing to the proximity of important organs, and to the distension and alteration of position of the abdominal organs, that it will probably have few to perform it, especially as the disease is so rare that no person would be likely to have more than one or two opportunities for operating during his whole life time."

Art. VII. — *Observations on Dropsy, with cases; as read before the Detroit Medical Society, by* Wm. Brodie, M.D.

There is perhaps no one disease or set of symptoms of disease, that so baffles the best intentions and well-directed skill of the medical profession as that of dropsy. I am aware that dropsy is considered by many as only a symptom of disease, while by others as the disease itself.

1st. Says Watson's Med. Lect., "It is often uncertain while the patient is yet alive what or where the primary disease may be; and even after death we sometimes cannot discover any organic change that would account for the effusion. Practically speaking, in such cases the Dropsy is the disease and the sole object of our treatment.

2d. "Dropsy is in fact, to a medical eye, in all cases, something more than an effect or symptom of disease. The imprisoned liquid is often a cause of other symptoms, embarrassing by its pressure important functions and even extinguishing life.

. "The removal of the dropsy (although the original cause, of which it was a symptom, may remain untouched,) will often restore a patient to comparative comfort, and in his belief, for the time to a state of health."

We see, then, that when dropsy depends upon organic disease, we have two sets of symptoms to be distinguished, viz: those depending upon the primary disease, and those upon the collected fluid. "The latter," says

Watson, "often the most grievous, are often to be got rid of, while the former, frequently permanent, are also seldom complained of or felt, except when effusion is the result."

Several cases of interest have occurred of late in St. Mary's Hospital, in which the truths above related have a particular bearing, of which I will relate two, and at the same time have the pleasure of shewing to you the Pathological specimens producing the dropsies above referred to.

John Smith, laborer, aged about 40 years, was admitted into the Hospital, March 22, 1853, complaining of great abdominal distension, and sense of pressure upon the stomach. Upon examination we found the abdomen distended with fluid pressing the intestines and stomach upon the diaphragm. The liver, owing to the effusion, was indefinable in its limits; he was emaciated, and at times had a short hacking cough, which troubled him most at night. The bowels were irregular in their action, and the discharges were frequently of a dysenteric character, and attended in their passage with some pain and tenesmus. Urine was rather scanty. Auscultation shewed embarrassed action of the lungs, more particularly upon the left side. The patient was placed under treatment, and for a time improved considerably, so that he was able to leave his bed and walk about. The abdomen became soft, and the effusion nearly gone. However, he soon again became restless, with the loss of sleep, a short hacking cough, hiccup, the effusion returned to the abdomen, his feet began to swell, and on June 3d he died.

On the following day I made the autopsy, assisted by Dr. Davenport. We found the cavity of the abdomen filled with a serous yellow fluid, quite clear, of which we removed a water-pail full. The Peritoneum was quite healthy, the spleen nearly double the common size and firm in its texture, the bladder firmly contracted, and the liver larger than natural and Cirrhosea.

The appearance of the liver as seen in health was destroyed, and its color changed to yellow, its texture was firm and not easily torn. The kidneys were natural and healthy. The right lung was healthy, and also the pleura surrounding and covering the same. The left was pressed up close to the clavicle by a serous effusion, in which were flakes of Lymph. The lung texture itself was healthy, as also the pleura costales and pulmonary; but the pleura covering the inferior portion of the diaphragm, was thickened and inflamed, and from this proceeded the effusion embarrassing the action of the lung and heart, and producing the hiccup and short cough which hastened his death. The heart was healthy in all its parts.

In regard to the liver, as being the primary cause of the dropsy in this case, we found it enlarged. It may be asked how could this condition produce dropsy? Says Watson, "There is one special form of liver dis-

.ease which, though not the sole, is *the grand* cause of passive and simple
ascites.   It has long been noticed that mere enlargement is not the most
common condition of the liver met with in Hepatic dropsy, but rather the
small, hard contracted viscus. Mere increase in the size of the organ may interfere but little with the portal circulation, whereas a shrinking and diminution of bulk must needs do so.   In point of fact, that particular state
of the liver which the French have termed Cirrhosis, and which is familiarly known to Anatomists as hobnailed, is the great source of passive
ascites.

That the dropsy in this case depended upon the liver, I have not the
slightest doubt.   A purely cirrhosed liver need not necessarily to be diminished in size; for, as I understand the term, it is applicable to the
color of the organ, and that the condition called hobnailed is the same
organ in a much more advanced condition of the disease.   Thus a morbid
process is set up in the liver — a chronic inflammation — the capsule of
Glisson becomes thickened and presses upon the nutrient arteries of the
lobules, causing an absorption of the same.   The coloring matter of the
bile is diffused throughout the liver, and produces, 1st, the cirrhosis, or
yellow appearance.   At this stage the effusion doubtless commences, and
should this be not too rapid, nor any other morbid process be set up to
hasten death, the liver will begin to contract, that is the capsular portion,
the areolar tissue begins also to shrink, and the spaces in which it rami-
fies on the surface of the liver are pulled inwards, the surface becomes
irregular and knobby, and studded with little rounded eminences like the
heads of nails, and then we have a hobnailed liver.   Had there been no
other cause to hasten the death of Smith, I have no doubt but that the
dropsy could have been so controlled that in the end he could have been
said to have died of hobnailed liver.

Peter Lopan was admitted into the Hospital with the following symptoms. A small pustular eruption upon the lower extremities, and some
at the base of the neck anteriorly, which soon yielded to treatment. Also,
with difficult respiration, a general fulness of the chest, neck, head, and abdomen.   And soon the extremities, both upper and lower, became anasarcous.   Bowels were confined, but easily acted upon.   Urine scanty, and
high colored.   Respiration difficult from the first, which difficulty increased.   The effusion became more general and he died.

On the following day I made the autopsy, assisted by Dr. Davenport.
The areolar tissue was distended with fluid — the cavity of the abdomen
was partly filled with the same.   All the abdominal viscera was healthy
with the exception of the kidneys, which organs were enlarged and congested, but no degeneration of the texture could be seen with the naked
eye.   The thorax contained some fluid, also the pecardium was dis-

tended. Lungs healthy in texture, but effused with the serous fluid, like
a sponge, and pressed into the upper portion of the thorax. No obstruction could be found to retard the return of the venous blood to the
heart except the serous effusion in the lungs. Heart in situ but slightly
Hypertrophied. Right auricle and verticle distended with blood and
dilated. Left side normal.

I have cited these two cases as having the same termination, viz:
dropsy, but arising from different causes. The primary disease in Smith
was cirrhosis, in that of Lapan passive dilitation of the right heart.

The first symptoms in each were the serous effusion or dropsy; the
first in the abdomen, the second in the lungs, head and extremities. In
neither case was there organic Lesion sufficient to account for death so
soon. What caused their death? 1st, The organic Lesion producing
the dropsy, and 2d, the dropsy, by its mechanical pressure impeding the
action and functions of other organs, upon the perfect action of which
vitality depends.

The Pathology of dropsies is of great interest to the profession, a
correct knowledge of which not only materially aids us in its treatment,
but, in fact, correct treatment can only be based upon it, and altogether
upon it must depend our prognosis of the disease.

ART. VIII.—*Letter from*.CORPORAL BULLHEAD, *of the Army of Quack
Killers, to the Editor.*

DEAR DOCTOR: After I had harangued the army, some of them raised
up and buckled on their armor, some said the Corporal was a fool, and
some didn't wake up at all. So I saw that it was necessary that yet
more should be done before we could go to battle in good hope of victory. Therefore I set out to reconnoitre the field.

In the first place I went down to the land of the Buckeyes, where
there was a great national assembly of scientific men in session, to see
what medical men of strength we had among them. Pierce, the mathematician, was Commander in Chief. Then the Chaplain prayed, and
after him the Commander made a speech, and the whole army of naturalists shouted applause, and addressed themselves to the work of advancing the cause of science. I found here that the medical men of the
nation ranked high among the lovers of all science and the destroyers of
all error. St. John, Kirtland, Ridell, Burnett, and large numbers of other
distinguished men were there from the medical corps, and shone among
the most brilliant of the assemblage.

I discovered, too, that quacks in medicine are quacks in everything else, and a laughing stock in all things; for a certain professor of homœopathy made a speech on the pebbles of Ohio, in particular, and the stratified rocks of the earth in general, wherein he maintained that these rocks were not the mud and gravel of ancient oceans, but with their coal sandstones, and pebbly conglomerates, were chemical precipitates from solution. After much laughter and some loss of time, the Association succeeded in getting rid of the subject, but not without difficulty, for the homœopathic Professor, not content with two discussions upon it was bent upon thrusting his pebble theory before them a third time.

During my stay in the Forest City I went to view the U. S. Marine Hospital. This is a fine building of hewn stone, about one hundred feet in length, and presenting a fine appearance. It is only partly finished, and contains but nine or ten patients. Rather extensive quarters I thought for so few men. However, the government builds for coming centuries, and when these great lakes shall swarm with the vessels carrying produce for a dense population settled on all their shores, the wisdom of these ample accommodations will be manifest. Should war occur, they may even be found too small. Turning down the street, I saw a conveyance marked the "Water Cure Omnibus," which plies three times a day between the docks and a Hydropathic institution in the suburbs. Thither I bent my way, for, thought I, all these fortresses of the enemy should be reconnoitered, for over their walls some day our forces are bound to go, if the Corporal has his way. Arriving at the place, I found a good sized two story building pleasantly located in a nook on the edge of a piece of forest. The woods around were laid out into walks, and seats were built under the trees. A carriage road descended into a deep ravine in the rear, which had been dammed up, thus producing a small pond of cold spring water at the bottom. Here was a boat and a bath house, and also a water ram that forced a stream up to the main building above. Returning up the hill, I found a gymnasium for exercise, containing a bowling alley, ropes, ladders, swings, etc. In front of the institution a small, badly contrived fountain was playing — eight or ten small streams about as large as would flow through a crow quill. Nevertheless moving water is always beautiful, and the effect was very pleasing. After some delay a servant came to the door to admit myself and the friend who was with me. We asked if we could have an opportunity to view the establishment. She said she guessed not, but she would go in and inquire. After some further delay a young man came and offered to show us the bath. This proved to be a large room about fifteen feet by thirty. The water tank stood above it. One end was partitioned off for the plunge bath. It consisted of a large vat four feet and a half deep, and about fifteen feet square, and was supplied by a pipe constantly discharging into it. The rest of the room was vacant. In one corner was a closet for the douche bath. The apparatus consisted of a pipe of about three quarters of an inch bore, which pointed perpendicularly down from the ceiling, and a rope outside which the operator pulled to bring down the blessing. The young man pulled it for our edification, and it shot down a stream with such force as must certainly make a patient jump, if it did not cure him. Opening into the hall adjoining, was a series of rooms used in the operation of packing, as we were informed.

I have no more time just now, Doctor, but I assure you I have been "spying out the nakedness of the land" of humbug, and you shall hear from me soon.

SELECTIONS.

From the London Lancet.

Creasote Inhalation in Phthisis, Bronchitis.

SIR: Will you permit me to call the attention of the profession to a plan of treatment which I have found of great benefit in many diseases of the chest. I believe that it has been tried before, but I cannot at present lay my hand upon any account respecting it. I allude to the inhalation of the vapor of creasote combined with steam.

The first case in which I employed it was one of phthisis, in which the cough was peculiarly distressing, in consequence of the presence of necrosis and suppuration in both ears, which were attended with severe and constant throbbing pain. A host of opiates were tried, one after another, but had to be given up, from the sickness and headache they produced. I tried creasote inhalation on speculation; and it answered so remarkably well, that its use was continued to within a few days of death. The patient always expressed himself as very grateful for the relief it gave to the cough.

Encouraged by the success attending this, I determined to try it in other cases, some of chronic bronchitis, the majority of phthisis. In all I have found it most useful in allaying cough, and checking secretion and expectoration. By allaying the cough, and thus increasing the comfort of the patient, it seems in some degree to increase the strength; at any rate, it saves its diminution. It does not of itself appear to possess any curative power. As a palliative, it is useful in all cases; and I have heard it spoken of most gratefully by a patient who only lived to use it for three or four days.

The mode of using it is very simple. I direct from four to ten drops of creasote to be placed in an old teapot, and a small quantity of boiling water to be poured over it. The spout is to be protected by a piece of flannel, and the steam inhaled through that until it begins to feel cool. Care must be taken, of course, not to put too much water in. This answers well enough in poor practice. In hospital and private practice more elegant apparatus may be used. An inhaler made by Weiss answers remarkably well. It consists of a closed tin can, holding about three pints; at the top are two large tubes which communicate with the interior; one is furnished with an ivory mouth-piece, to prevent the lips being burned by the hot metal; the other is turned upwards, and through this the creasote and water are readily introduced. The size of the tubes makes the inhalation of the steam peculiarly easy. When this is employed I find that the temperature of the water should not exceed 150 degrees. The immediate effects are a feeling of warmth about the throat, and a sensation " as if you had lungs under your ribs," followed by reduced irritability of the mucous membrane, and subsequently by evidence of the creasote having entered the blood.

It would take up too much space were I to detail all the cases in which I have employed it in hospital and private practice; one will suffice, and will serve to indicate the routine treatment I have adopted in phthisis.

A. B., seaman, aged 30, was admitted into the Northern Hospital with severe cough, dyspnœa, and profuse expectoration. He had been ill for three months, during which he had emaciated considerably. The pulse was 130, and there were copious night sweats. On examining the chest, I found solidification of the apex of the left lung, and coarse mucous rales all over the same side, both anteriorly and posteriorly. At the apex of the right lung there was tubular breathing in one spot, and prolonged expiration in another. The expectoration was of thick, semi-transparent mucus, free from air bubbles, and mixed here and there with grey tubercular patches. He was ordered to have creasote inhalation three or four times, and to take internally half an ounce of cod-liver oil, with twenty-five minims of tincture of iron, three times daily. The severity of the symptoms abated in the course of the week, and in six weeks the man was convalescent. The right lung now seems perfectly healthy; all traces of solidification have disappeared from the apex of the left; the respiration there, and over the whole of that lung, has become natural. The pulse has come steadily down to 72. The man has gained flesh, and the capacity of the chest, as evidenced by the power to take in a deep inspiration, has signally increased.

I may mention, that the use of iron has been adopted in consequence of the effect it had on a little girl, who had been previously employing creasote inhalation and cod-liver oil for some weeks without any indication of improvement. In her case, the whole of the left, and the upper part of the right lung were implicated: but I could not detect any cavities. The case seemed hopeless, when she began with the tincture of the sesquichloride, in addition to her other medicine. In two days an improvement was seen; in four it was confirmed; and, in less than six weeks after, she was running about the wards rosy and well, and has continued so up to the present time — about two months more.

I am, &c.,   THOMAS INMAN, M.D.

Liverpool.

From the London Lancet.

On the treatment of Thecal Abscess. By WILLIAM CUMMING, Esq., M.R.C.S.

Inflammation and suppuration in the thecæ of the fingers are of great importance in practice. In these cases it is necessary to know what to do, and the proper time for interference. The need of early opening, in cases of thecal abscess, is an axiom in surgery, neglect of this involving the loss of the use of the finger. The difficulty is not in the use of the remedy, but in recognizing the case which requires it. While on the one hand it is desirable to leave no cure to the risk of the result of unrelieved thecal abscess, and on the other not to adopt a severe measure without real necessity, I have often made a deep incision, thinking that the theca was affected, when after-observation has made me think that this need not have been done, or suppuration at the back or side of the finger has shown that the theca was not the part affected.

I remember a case some years ago of a woman who showed me the extreme phalanx of the finger severely inflamed, which she would not consent to have incised. I saw the finger a day or two after, quite well. These and similar cases have made me look with some attention to those marks, which might more clearly show that the theca was the part inflamed, and suppurating inflammation of the superficial cellular tissue of the finger may be left to its own progress, or advantageously be allowed to point before the lancet is used. Thecal abscess must never be left to itself, as it will certainly damage or completely destroy the finger.

It is said by many that inflammation of the theca alone calls for an incision into it. I do not know that the signs of this would be sufficiently clear or urgent to lead us to do this, while I am certain that as soon as the theca is distended with pus the signs are positive, and admit of no delay.

When there is suppuration in the theca, the finger is swollen, tense, throbbing, and perhaps red; in addition to these characters, which may occur in superficial inflammation, there are others more distinctive—great pain on pressing over the course of the tendon. If the finger, which is generally slightly flexed, be bent backwards, the tension and stretching of the tendon and theca give great pain; this can generally be done without pain if the theca is not involved. The pain is so urgent as to prevent the patient sleeping. There is fluctuation deep in the finger felt from one side of the tendon to the other. These characters I have found in thecal abscess, and to indicate almost certainly its presence, and calling at once for an incision into the theca. I will mention a few of the cases on which these remarks are founded.

A. B——, aged thirty. A few weeks after her confinement the forefinger of the right hand became very painful. No incision was made. When I first saw her, three weeks afterwards, there was an opening in the palm, and one at the back of the finger, which discharged freely. All power of flexing the finger was lost.

A middle-aged man showed me his thumb, which had been swollen, and in great pain, for more than a week. A small opening had formed at its anterior surface, from which pus was just beginning to flow. An incision into the theca was made, allowing pus to escape, and giving relief, but the tendon sloughed, and a large piece of dead bone came away.

These cases show the result of thecal abscess unrelieved by incision.

A young man had great pain in the thumb, with swelling. The first time I saw him there was distinct fluctuation from one side of the tendon to the other; great pain, which prevented sleep. An incision was at once made into the theca; pus escaped freely and the case did perfectly well.

A German, working in a sugar-house, had swelling, tension, and pain in the extreme phalanx of the middle finger. The finger began to be painful four days before I was sent for; so much so last night as to keep him from sleeping. There was superficial swelling and redness at the back of the finger, but distinct fluctuation from one side of the tendon to the other, and pain on stretching the finger back. An incision was followed by a free escape of pus, which gave immediate relief, and, in a few days the finger was well.

A lad, aged sixteen, had had pain in the finger five days, which prevented him sleeping at night. Extreme phalanx of right fore-finger, tense, swollen, red, and throbbing; fluctuation distinct, and pain on pressing over the course of the tendon. On incision, pus gushed out freely, followed by immediate relief.

In three cases these were the characters presented on first seeing them, and the incision was made at once, with a scalpel, into the theca. An attention to these characters of thecal abscess will guide us to their relief and cure, and save us, in many instances, from the mortification of making a deep and painful incision without any benefit.

The tension and pain deep in the situation of the finger, the deep fluctuation, and the severe pain preventing sleep, are the distinctive marks of thecal abscess.

May, 1853.

From the Southern Journal of Medical and Physical Sciences.

Different Modes of arresting Hemorrhage from the Extraction of Teeth. By BENJAMIN WOOD, M.D., Nashville, Tenn.

Dr. A. Saltonstall, of Columbus, Ohio, Miss., reports a case (American Jour. Dental Science, Oct. 1852) of hemorrhage from the extraction of a tooth, which, having resisted the usual means — astringents, escharotics and compression — was arrested by an artificial fixture acting both as compress and actual cautery. He "took a piece of pure silver plate, and cut it in shape to fit between the teeth and cover the lips of the orfice about the eighth of an inch on each side. This was bent to fit the parts, and heated to a white heat, and suddenly applied to the place, where it remained several days. When it was removed the coagulum came away with it. The orfice was examined, and a very delicate covering, resembling tissue paper, had formed over it."

Dr. Levison, of England, in an article published about a year ago, says, that in cases of excessive hemorrhage, where the ordinary styptics cannot be depended upon, " we may arrest the dangerous hemorrhagic flow with certainty by destroying the vessels with the bi-chloride of zinc," and gives cases where this agent, as a last resort, had been successful in his hands. In alveolar hemorrhage, pieces of cotton dipped into the bi-chloride were forced down to the alveolar cavities. It was attended, however, with great pain.

It may be remarked that in some cases where success is ascribed to the last remedy employed, the result may have been owing to a natural stasis of blood from exhaustion of the patient; such hemorrhages sometimes continuing for hours, until after fainting, and then ceasing altogether without any intervention. An interesting case of the kind was related to us a few years ago by a reliable lady who was herself the subject. The bleeding had continued with but occasional and partial intermissions for three days. On the night of the third it ceased, and she retired, but about midnight she was awakened by a renewed flow of blood. Exhausted by the loss of blood and sleep, she merely arranged a wash-bowl upon a chair so as to receive the blood as it flowed from her mouth, and with her head supported by a pillow, she soon fell asleep.— In this position she was found early the next morning, in a state of unconsciousness. The bleeding had effectually ceased.

It is fortunate these cases rarely occur. We have had but few that were troublesome. Besides the use of nitrate of silver (which as a styptic we have found more reliable than anything else that we have used), and the application of pressure, we have in two or three instances resorted to a partial *torsion of the bloodvessels* at the bottom of the aveolar cells, This depends upon the principle that the mouths of the vessels contract more readily when lacerated than when divided with a smooth cut or broken short off, as may happen in extracting a tooth, and that mechanical irritation has a tendency to induce contraction. *The modus operandi* (as we received it while under pupilage, from our brother, Dr. J. S. Wood) consists in passing a stylet or an ordinary excavator of the proper shape, to the bottom of the socket, until a twinge of pain is felt, and then giving the instrument a sudden turn, so as to twist or lacerate the artery — its situation being indicated by the impression made upon the nerve which it accompanies.

We know of but one instance in this vicinity, of death having occurred in consequence of the kind of hemorrhage under notice. This was in Russellville, Ky., about two years ago. The patient's tooth was broken in extracting, leaving a portion of the fang which could not be gotten out. Pressure, as well as styptics, &c., was tried, but without arresting the hemorrhage, the man dying, according to the recollection of our informant, in about fifteen hours after the operation. We would like very much to be favored with a report of the case in full.

In case a tooth is broken and the bleeding proceeds from the pulp, cavity or nerve canal, the obvious means of arresting it would be to plug the orifice with a metalic or wood stopping. A hickory peg or sliver would perhaps be as good as anything. If the orifice be too small to receive a stopping, it should be enlarged by means of a drill.

Pressure applied directly to the bleeding vessels and retained in its place is reliable in such cases of hemorrhage; but there is sometimes considerable difficulty experienced in its application. A ready and effectual means is to roll up pellets of cotton firmly in the fingers, of a size to suit the alveolar cells, and introduce them with considerable force, notwithstanding it be attended with considerable pain, as it always is, we believe when the hemorrhage has continued for some time. They may be wet with some styptic solution, or coated with powdered lunar caustic. After the first pellett has been introduced, we usually fill the remainder of the cavity with one of a larger size, and if it be a molar tooth with two or three bi-furcations, cover the whole with a third, sufficiently large for the purpose but no larger, crowding the edges under the margins of the gums, which in ordinary conditions, where the blood possesses its due amount of fibrin, and is of a plastic character, will be found to adhere to the cotton with sufficient tenacity to retain it in its place. It will be safest to let this stopping remain until loosened by the suppurative process. If not thrown off, however, or removed in the course of a few days, the pellets thus introduced are apt to prove the source of great suffering in the sockets, bespeaking the inflammatory action preparatory to suppuration; but when this occurs we think they may be removed at once, regarding it as evidence that active reparation has commenced.

The "waxed cones" recommended by Dr. B. B. Brown, which are made by cutting a piece of linen previously coated with melted beeswax, into tapering strips and rolling these in a form to suit the sockets to which they are to be applied, may be used to great advantage in many cases.

Editorial Correspondence of the Charleston Medical Journal and Review.

Medical Teaching in Paris; Epidemic of Typhoid Fever, Treatment of; M M. Briquet, Bouilland and Louis; Post Mortem; Statistics; Suicides; Asiatic Cholera; Puerperal Fever; M. Trousseau; Treatment of Rheumatism by Quinine and Veratrine; Service of M. Guersant at Hospital for sick children; Surgical operations; Cervical Rheumatism; Erectile Tumour; Cours d'Accouchement in Paris; Sages-femmes; Recent expression of the views of M. Coste on Embryology; Honors conferred upon Americans, &c.

PARIS, MARCH 5th, 1853. }
Rue de Seine, St. Germain. }

D. J. CAIN, M.D: *Dear Sir* — As I have quite a *melange* to introduce, it is best, perhaps, to address this communication to you personally. Good reasons exist for the non-appearance of one in the March number but these shall be reserved for your private ear.

We are in the midst of a period in the year when medical science is pursued with more vigor than any other — when the Professors at the *Ecole de Medicine* are in the midst of the winter campaign, some of them with an audience of a hundred, others with upwards of a thousand. Now also there are a legion of lecturers, public and private, who occupy almost every hour of the twenty-four at the *Ecole Practique,* and in private rooms in the neighborhood. Besides, each Interne or Chief of the Chiniques of any note, has his private class of four or five at the Hospitals, who, for twenty-five to fifty francs per month, enjoy the privilege of making visits and examinations, and of studying, auscultation and percussion with him during the evening. The College of France, the Sorbonne and the Jardin des Plantes, have each also its corps of lecturers and Professors, who discourse on general subjects — Law, Theology, Ancient and Modern Literature, &c.; but among whom, nevertheless, are found M. M. Geoffroy Saint Hiliare, Flourens, Milne Edwards, Coste, and during the summer, M. M. Orfiila, Magendie and Bernard. The latter has just completed an extremely interesting private course on Experimental Physiology with vivisections, and we had intended replacing this letter with a portion of our notes taken during their delivery. A friend, however, having furnished us with some of his own, we willingly send them, possibly continuing the subject ourselves at a future time, when more leisure should be allowed us. We may add that M. Ludovic's Demonstrations at the school for Practical Anatomy have also been quite instructive. He was, you are aware, the collaborator of Bongery in the preparation of his plates, and one of the most adroit dissectors in Paris.

Among those first alluded to, M. M. Denouvilliers and Orfila attract much the largest number of followers. We have for two months been attending M. Malgaigne, at the School of Medicine, during which time he has confined himself to the Surgical treatment of maladies of the Eye; M. Denouvilliers has consumed the same period in the introductory portions of general Anatomy, having only within a few days commenced with a particular region. One may judge from this how minutely they pass over the subjects allotted to them, in my opinion consuming a disproportionate amount of the space in treating of only a fractional part of what demands consideration, and what the student will require. However, they allow him more years in which to earn his diploma here than in the United States, and can thus afford to be thorough. We are aware that it is impossible for the same condition of things, however desirable, to exist in our country, until Governments, whether State or General, shall forcibly assume the direction and expenses of certain species of educational establishments, and wrest from the hands of one set that may be unfit, the power to confer diplomas upon others equally incapable of assuming the responsible duties of the physician who *suddenly* goes out to cure a thousand various maladies, each with its own peculiar history, its characteristic phases and relations. Thus aiding the well selected power which instructs and which confers; liberating the professors from the thraldom of pecuniary competition, and leaving them to that of intellectual; thus enabling them to direct all their energies in elevating and ennobling the profession. If the reward of the professor depends upon, and is in proportion to, the number of those who enrol in his school, he must at times enter into strife with ignoble rivals, the worst of human passions mingle in the contest, underbidding and depreciation ensue, and the profession sways backward as often as it does forward, instead of moving directly and constantly upward in the path of progress.

An epidemic of Typhoid Fever is very prevalent in Paris at present, and it is seen in all the Hospitals. In these it is quite interesting to witness the variety of treatment adopted by each physician of note, as his medical tendencies incline; that pursued respectively by M. M. Boulland, Briquet and Louis, whom I have followed, presents many points of difference, and it has been difficult to determine on which side the scale of success leans. We hope, however, to be able to send a paper by a medical friend who has watched closely the service of the former, and who can furnish some testimony with respect to his mode of employing the lancet in this disease. M. Louis very generally administers Seltzer water, vinous lemonade, and adopts, to a certain extent, the expectant system. M. Briquet at La Charite pursues what appears to me rather a middle course. He abstracts blood in the early stage of some cases which seem peculiarly fitted for it. I may observe here that I have also heard M. Trousseau say, that even as late as during the second and third septenary period, he was in the habit of bleeding to prevent the increase, or destroy the congestion of the lungs which so often exhibits itself, its approach and presence being of course easily discoverable by the physical signs. M. Briquet relies with much confidence, (and my own observation in his wards can sustain him,) upon the application of cups and scarification to the mastoid region during delirium and coma of Typhoid. It completely checks the increase of these dangerous symptoms, as I have repeatedly witnessed. He does not give mercury internally, but applies plasters of mercurial ointment over the entire abdomen until the secretions become active, or the tongue and skin exhibit the desired moisture. This method of using the remedy might more easily reconcile itself to those who so much doubt respecting the advantages of its internal administration. He gives ordinary Bordeaux wine during the period of convalescence. These means, thus generally expressed, are often associated in his practice with the use of ice, administered in every possible way, and through every channel — bladders filled with it are applied to the scalp, it is dissolved in the mouth, and given with enemata. One of his Internes mentioned to me this morning that he had lost but one case within three weeks. There are between twenty and fifty sick of the disease in each service of the Hospitals, and few of these fail to present gargouillement, the characteristic rose mark and sudamia.

As the subject of typhoid fever has been much discussed of late at the South, and in the pages of this Journal, it may not be thought useless to consider the following autopsy which I witnessed at La Charite a few days since. It is instructive, as indicating the characteristic march of the disease in an individual in whose system it was not modified by medicines. The subject, a man of about 33 years of age, of good conformation when he entered the Hospital, presented every favorable condition save the existence of the endemic; this had seized upon him as it had upon most of those who had within the last year or two moved from the country to Paris, and who did not live under favorable hygienic conditions. He had been bled, but absolutely no medicines were taken, with the exception of *tisans* and mucilaginous drinks. Notwithstanding the entire lining membrane of his *stomach* was intensely red, and exhibited all the traces of severe inflammation: there was some exudation of plastic lymph, and the particles of coloring matter seemed infiltrated beneath the mucous coat; when scraped off with a sharp bistoury, the surface beneath was white. Thirty of Payer's glands were enlarged and inflamed, decreasing in size from the commencement of the colon, until they disappeared in the small intestines. The largest were about an inch and a quarter in diameter, with elevated edges, presenting, as M. Briquet re-marked, precisely the appearance of carcinoma; the surface of those situated most inferiorly exhibited the yellow summit, indicating the commencement of gangrene. No other portion of the intestinal canal was diseased, if we exclude the above enlarged mesenteric glands. The *spleen* was four times the ordinary size, though it did not appear that the deceased had suffered from intermittent fever. The cavities of the *heart* contained some fibrinous deposits, and its muscular tissues were soft. The lungs showed previous inflammation of the bronchia, and the lower lobes were still engorged; these did not compromise the life of the individual, as quite a large portion was spongy and elastic. The consistence of the *brain* was firm, no fluid was found in the ventricles, but there was venous engorgement on its surface. The *liver* and other organs remained quite natural.

. Four cases of Asiatic Cholera appeared at Hotel Dieu during the month of January— so said the journals and the physicians! I heard M. Louis observe, a few mornings since, that the diarrhœa or cholorine, which had since existed to a certain extent, had not respected any class of the patients, not excepting those with typhoid fever. Before leaving the subject of this latter affection, which is now on the decline, I append a few statistical items which I have selected and re-arranged from a mass of valuable matter contained in the *Moniteur.* It may afford data for comparative estimates in the United States.

. On the first of March there were 1,422 sick of the disease, 4,344 having been the maximum of those sick in the Hospitals. At the same time the number of the sick, generally, has descended from 6,735 to 6,618. From the 19th to 27th of February, (9 days,) 131 had died of 1,253 sick of typhoid in hospitals, or about 1 in 100 — a proportion less than has characterized any previous epidemic. The winter has been a very wet one, the Seine having been higher than for many years past, and snow having fallen frequently within the last month.

During the year 1852, there were 29,873 deaths in Paris. 29,664 had the relations of sex, age and disease indicated. Of these 16,220 were males, and 14,444 females. In 1851 there were 29,709 deaths; 15,110 males, 14,699 females. The most fatal period of life was under three months; the least, between six and eight years. Among the 29,-664 deaths, maladies of the chest, digestive apparatus, and Typhoid Fever occurred most frequently. Of Pulmonary Phthisis, there died 2,073 males, 2,038 females; of Pneumonia, 1,279 males, 1,346 females; of Pulmonary Catarrh, 849 males, 955 females; of Enteritis, 1,395 males, 1,365 females; of Typhoid Fever, 603 males, 503 females. The temperature was quite elevated during the whole year, though there were few atmospheric variations. Of the 29,873, 10,157 were in hospitals, remainder *a domicile,* a word which may well be retained to mark those sick in the city, but not in the medical establishments. In 1829, when statistical researches commenced to attract greater attention, there were 17,101 deaths *a domicile,* and 9,884 in the hospitals, the population then being 776,241. In 1832, the numbers rose to 30,843 dead *a domicile,* 15,-481 in hospitals. This increase is accounted for by the presence of Asiatic Cholera. 1814, the year of the war, was the most fatal, there being

24,197 deaths, the severest epidemic of Typhoid ever experienced in Paris, contributed to swell the number of victims. The most melancholy reminiscences are said even now to attach to this sad epoch, which elicit a great deal of generous sympathy.

We observe, from comparative observations, that the number of persons carried to the Morgue annually varies from 250 to 320 males, from 40 to 60 females, and from 15 to 25 new born — the males generally being to the females in the ratio of about five to one. From the year 1819 to 1828, there were transported to this spot 2,765 cadavers, of which 485 were female. To show the depressing effect of an epidemic, I will cite for comparison, the two years 1831 and 1832, when the population was of course nearly the same. In the former there were 232 bodies of males, and 67 females, and 5 new born. In 1832, the year of cholera, 1,007 of males, and 225 of females. It must be remembered that these include not only suicides, but those also destroyed by accidents. It is remarkable that among the suicides of the past year there were 4 boys between 8 and 15 years of age, and 6 girls; 13 boys of from 15 to 20 years, and 9 girls. There were, also, 8 men and 4 women of from 70 to 80 years of age.

On account of the severity of Peuperal Fever at the Clinique of the School of Medicine, M. Paul Dubois has had to discontinue the reception of parturient women. The epidemic was attended with considerable mortality. They have not, however, been able to practice fumigations or purification, as the *Bureau of Administration* have been forced to occupy the beds with Typhoid patients — so great is the need at present of accommodation for the sick.

Our readers are aware that M. Trousseau has been appointed in the place of M. Chomel, at Hotel Dieu, where his cliniques are very popular indeed. It is a source of extreme regret to many that he has thus been forced to leave the *Hopital des Infants Maladies*, and to discontinue his usual course of Lectures during the summer on Meteria Medica and Therapeutics. The treatment of acute rheumatism by Quinine, commenced by Briquet, and to a certain extent discontinued, on account of the doubtful character of the termination of one or two cases in which large quantities were administered, has been revived of late, and the impression respecting it gains favor daily. I have seen M. B. give it with good effect quite often. M. Valleix employs and recommends it at La Pitie, and I hope to be able to send a paper on the subject by a gentleman who attends his *Services* and Lectures. One gramme (15 grains) is administered once or twice a day, and the patient kept partly quininized. The gravity of the usual symptoms daily decrease, and it seems to be not at all hostile to cordiac complications. M. Trousseau, in commenting upon this, and expressing his favorable impression, alluded also to the expense attending the use of this agent, accompanying it at the same time with the relation of a remarkable instance of recovery from acute articular Rheumatism, which was then in his wards. It was true, he added, that it was yet an isolated case, but the repetition of the means used might give equally favorable results. It followed the employment of Veratrine after the method reccommended by M. Daniel. (?) The patient, a woman under middle age, suffered intense pain in the articulations, high fever with endo-carditis exhibiting itself by a derangement of the first sound at the base of the heart — (sigmoid valves of aorta) — with a souffle prolonged into the large vessels, and accompanied with an alteration in the left ventricle also. In 62 hours she was absolutely cured, leaving not the slightest trace of fibrile excitement, the presence of a slight souffle alone remains. One half of a millegramme (about 1-10th of a grain,) was given in the form of pill, each day increasing the quantity, and, when the pains were relieved, continuing it in the same dose every second day. Its influence on the circulation in this case was prodigious, to use M. Trousseau's expression; the pulse fell to 42, and when I heard of the patient two days after, it was still at this reduced rate. Veratrine, we are aware, is one of the active principles of colchium, and it is, therefore, not surprising that it should possess some power in acute Rheumatism, more particularly in those dependent upon the arthritic diathesis, gout, etc.

From the London Lancet.

The Table Turning Delusion.

The following letter from Professor Faraday is extracted from the *Times* of Thursday last:

To the Editor of the Times: — Sir: I have recently been engaged in the investigation of table-turning. I should be sorry that you should suppose I thought this necessary on my own account, for my conclusion respecting its nature was soon arrived at, and is not changed; but I have been so often misquoted, and applications to me for an opinion are so numerous, that I hoped, if I enabled myself by experiment to give a strong one, you would consent to convey it to all persons interested in the matter. The effect produced by table-turners has been referred to electricity, to magnetism, to attraction, to some unknown or hitherto unrecognised physical power able to effect inanimate bodies — to the revolution of the earth, and even to diabolical or supernatural agency. The natural philosopher can investigate all these supposed causes but the last; that must to him, be too much connected with credulity or superstition to require any attention on his part.

Believing that the first cause assigned — namely, a *quasi* involuntary muscular action (for the effect is with many subject to the wish or will) —was the true cause, the first point was to prevent the mind of the turner having an undue influence over the effects produced in relation to the nature of the substances employed. A bundle of plates consisting of sand-paper, mill-board, glue, glass, plastic clay, tinfoil, cardboard, gutta percha, vulcanized caoutchouc, wood, and resinous cement, was therefore made up and tied together, and being placed on a table, under the hand of a turner, did not prevent the transmission of the power; the table turned or moved exactly as if the bundle had been away, to the full satisfaction of all present. The experiment was repeated, with various substances and persons, and at various times, with constant success; and henceforth no objection could be taken to the use of these substances in the construction of apparatus. The next point was to determine the place and source of motion — *i. e.,* whether the table moved the hand or the hand moved the table; and for this purpose indicators were constructed. One of these consisted of a light lever, having its fulcrum on the table, its short arm attached to a pin fixed on a cardboard, which could slip on the surface of the table, and its long arm projecting as an index of motion. It is evident that if the experimentor willed the table to move towards the left, and it did so move *before* the hands, placed at the time on the cardboard, then the index would move to the left also, the fulcrum going with the table. If the hands involuntarily moved towards the left *without* the table, the index would go towards the right; and if neither table nor hands moved, the index would itself remain immovable. The result was that when the parties saw the index it remained very steady; when it was hidden from them, or they looked away from it, it wavered about though they believed that they always pressed directly downwards; and when the table did not move, there was still a resultant of hand force in the direction in which it was wished the table should move, which however, was exercised quite unwittingly by the party operating. This resultant it is which, in the course of the waiting time, while the fingers and hands become stiff, numb and insensible by continued pressure, grows up to an amount sufficient to move the table or the substances pressed upon. But the most valuable effect of this test-apparatus (which was afterwards made more perfect and independent of the table) is the corrective power it possesses over the mind of the table-turner. As soon as the index is placed before the most earnest, and they perceive — as in my presence they have always done — that it tells truly whether they are pressing downwards only or obliquely, then all effects of table-turning cease, even though the parties persevere, earnestly desiring motion, till they become weary and worn out. No prompting or checking of the hands is needed — *the power is gone*; and this only because the parties are made conscious of what they are really doing mechanically, and so are unable unwittingly to deceive themselves. I know that some may say that it is the card-board next the fingers which moves first, and that *it* both drags the table and also the table-turner with it. All I have to reply is, that the card-board may in practice be reduced to a thin sheet of paper weighing only a few grains, or to a piece of goldbeaters' skin, or even the end of the lever, and (in principle) to the very cuticle of the fingers itself. Then the results that follow are too absurd to be admitted: the table becomes an incumbrance, and a person holding out the fingers in the air, either naked or tipped with goldbeaters' skin or cardboard, ought to be drawn about the room, &c.; but I refrain from considering imaginary yet consequent results which have nothing philosophical or real in them. I have been happy thus far in meeting with the most honorable and candid though most sanguine persons, and I believe the mental check which I propose will be available in the hands of all who desire truly to investigate the philosophy of the subject, and, being content to resign expectation, wish only to be led by the facts and the truth of nature. As I am unable, even at present, to answer all the letters that come to me regarding this matter, perhaps you will allow me to prevent any increase by saying that my apparatus may be seen at the shop of the philosophical instrument maker—Newman, 122, Regent Street.

Permit me to say, before concluding, that I have been greatly startled by the revelation which this purely physical subject has made of the condition of the public mind. No doubt there are many persons who have formed a right judgment or used a cautious reserve, for I know several such, and public communications have shown it to be so; but their number is almost as nothing to the great body who have believed and borne testimony, as I think, in the cause of error. I do not here refer to the distinction of those who agree with me and those who differ. By the great body, I mean such as reject all consideration of the equality of cause and effect; who refer the results to electricity and magnetism— yet know nothing of the laws of these forces; or to attraction — yet show no phenomena of pure attractive power; or to the rotation of the earth, as if the earth revolved round the leg of a table; or to some unrecognised physical force, without inquiring whether the known forces are not sufficient; or who even refer them to diabolical or supernatural agency, rather than suspend their judgment, or acknowledge to themselves that they are not learned enough in these matters to decide on the nature of the action. I think the system of education that could leave the mental condition of the public body in the state in which this subject has found it must have been greatly deficient in some very important principle.

I am, Sir, your very obedient servant,

M. FARADAY.

Royal Institution, June 28, 1853.

From the N. W. Medical and Surgical Journal.

Oxalate of Lime, and its relations to certain forms of Neuralgia. Read before the Cook County Medical Society. By H. A. JOHNSON, M.D.

We are indebted for what we know of this deposit mostly to Dr. Golding Bird. From his observations he was led to the conclusion, that oxalate of lime occurs in more than one-third of the cases in connection with an excess of uric acid or urate of ammonia, that in all cases there is an excess of urea, and that it is frequently accompanied by an excess of the phosphates; he also thinks it probable, that the uric and oxalic diatheses are both produced by the same morbid influences.

Uric acid, as existing in normal urine, is, without doubt, derived from the nitrogenized tissues of the body, but when found in excess, it may usually be traced either to ingesta, which the juices of the stomach have not the power to dissolve, or to a too rapid destruction of tissues under the influence of heat, &c., as in fevers and inflammations; can oxalic acid be traced to a similar source?

Dr. G. Bird has presented a very ingenious theory for the production of this acid from urea and uric acid, but there is generally an excess of one or both of these ingredients accompanying the oxalic deposits. Should we expect this to be the case, if the abnormal product was the result of a transformation of the urea and uric acid? It seems to me not. My own observations have been limited, but I have thought, from a careful study of quite a number of cases, that, while a temporary functional disease of the digestive organs or the introduction into the digestive tube of a large amount of food, difficult of perfect solution in the juices of the stomach, will generally give rise to uric acid deposits in the urine, chronic disease of the alimentary canal, whether functional or organic, will *more* generally be found to exist with the oxalic diathesis.

In quite a large number of instances in which I have observed the oxalate of lime in the urine, the patients have not only been affected with dyspepsia, but have also been subject to severe attacks of neuralgia. In the first few instances, the neuralgic pains were confined to the lower extremities, and I strongly suspected that they were produced by mechanical irritation of the vesical mucous membrane from the crystals of the oxalate with which the urine was loaded at the commencement of the attack, but which, towards the termination, were replaced by an excess of the phosphates.

I have since observed neuralgic pains in the face, superior extremities, and in the chest, co-existing with oxaluria, and, after carefully studying a number of cases, it seems to me evident, that the neuralgia and the urinary deposits sustain to each other an intimate relation through a common cause, viz: the derangement of the digestive organs.

It is perhaps probable that oxalic acid, whether produced from mal-assimilated food, as I think, or, from a metamorphosis of urea and uric acid, may exist first in combination with ammonia, as Dr. G. Bird has suggested. If so, it is possible that it may, instead of being selected by the kidneys, and combining in those organs with lime, be precipitated in the tissues. The crystals of this new salt, many of them smaller than blood globules, and presenting sharp angles and edges, may thus, by mechanical irritation, act directly upon the suffering structures, producing that intense and indescribable pain, for controlling which anodynes and narcotics have so little power.

Permit me to allude to my own personal experience. During the last few months I have been frequently annoyed by neuralgic pains, and always after eating freely of oranges. I had never been in the habit of using this fruit until during my recent visit south, but while in Natchez and New Orleans, it constituted almost my only diet. I also ate very freely of it during my return home.

It is to my mind an interesting fact, that the first neuralgic pain that I ever experienced, so far as my memory serves me, was in Natchez. Since my return I have frequently partaken of the fruit, and almost always with the same result, pains of a neuralgic character in the face, chest, knee, dorsum of the foot, &c. These facts induced me to institute the following experiment.

At 8 o'clock A. M., I breakfasted on beef steak, potatoes, corn bread and two eggs. After breakfast I walked two miles. At 11 A. M. the urine passed, was normal in color, specific gravity 1030. After standing there was no deposit of any kind; on a careful microscopic examination, I was unable to detect a single crystal of the oxalate of lime. I then ate four large oranges; at 1 P. M. I dined on a small quantity of roast beef, and whortle-berry and green currant pie. At 7 P. M. the urine passed, was of straw color, specific gravity 1036. After standing 30 minutes, a sediment was thrown down, consisting mainly of oxalate of lime in very large beautiful crystals. I think I never saw a specimen of urine in which it existed in greater abundance, or in which the crystals were larger. It also contained urate of ammonia, and an excess of urea. I placed some of it in a watch-glass, and added strong nitric acid; in a few moments it was almost a solid mass from the crystals of nitrate of urea. The urine passed the next morning at 7 o'clock had a specific gravity of 1030, and contained an excess of urea and uric acid and epithelial scales. At 11 P. M. the urine was normal. I then ate four more large oranges, and went to bed. The urine passed at 7 o'clock the next morning was loaded with the oxalates. These two experiments, one upon the urine of food, the other upon the urine of blood, seem to me to indicate, 1st, that oxalic acid may be produced from the ingesta; 2d, that oranges, and probably all fruits containing citric acid, may give rise to the oxalic diathesis.

The manner in which the transformation is effected is uncertain, nor is it a matter of much consequence. I venture, however, to present as a possible explanation the following formula:

$$
\text{6 at. of cit. acid} = \begin{matrix} \text{C.} & \text{H.} & \text{O.} \\ 24 & 10 & 80 \end{matrix} \Bigg\} = \left\{ \begin{matrix} \text{C.} & \text{H.} & \text{O.} \\ 12 & & 18 = 6 \text{ at oxalic acid.} \\ 12 & 10 & 10 = 2 \text{ at. lactic acid.} \\ & 2 & 2 = 2 \text{ at. of water.} \\ & 6 & \end{matrix} \right.
$$

We have remaining six atoms of hydrogen, which, united with 2 at. of nitrogen, would produce two at. of ammonia.

What influence have the organic acids in causing neuralgia through the derangement which they produce in the performance of the digestive functions. Do the neuralgic pains depend upon mechanical irritation, as I think may be possible, or do they depend upon perverted nutrition of the nervous structures, as I think more probable? These are interesting subjects of inquiry, but I have not the time to pursue them further.

From the Medical Times and Gazette.

Color-Blindness.

Dr. Wilson, of Edinburgh, in a paper in the *Athenæum*, refers to this subject as having an important bearing on the system of railway signalling by colors, more especially by red and green danger signals. This affection Dr. Wilson considers in three important practical relations: First, That the affection is much more prevalent than is generally imagined. Second, That red and green, the colors used for danger signals on our railways, are exactly those which are most frequently confounded with each other by the subjects of color-blindness. 3. That color-blindness implies not merely a confusion in distinguishing between two or more colors, but, at least in many cases, an imperfect appreciation or feeble hold of color altogether as a quality of bodies. Prevost says, that color-blindness occurs in one male among twenty. Seebeck (in Poggendorff, Annalen, xliii. 177) found five cases among forty youths in Berlin. Professor Kelland, of the University of Edinburgh, has this season found three examples among 150 students. In four of the cases which had come under Dr. Wilson's notice, none of them could be trusted to distinguish a red signal from a green one; and there was not only false vision of colors, but, in many instances, total color-blindness — so that the subjects of it doubted as to all colors, and would not swear, in a court of justice as to any color. These facts, in connection with the continually augmenting number of railway accidents occurring, must show the imperative necessity of strict examination being instituted as to the perfect vision of all railway servants.

From the London Lancet.

Observations on Chloroform and its administration. By W. Martin Coates, Esq., M.R.C.S. & L.S.A., *Surgeon to the Salisbury Infirmary.*

In the number of the Lancet published in May, 1851, will be found a paper written by me, under the above title. In that paper I cautioned the profession against suddenly saturating the patient's system with its vapour, and detailed an experiment to illustrate my opinion. I then stated my conviction, that the dose recommended (one fluid drachm at intervals) was unnecessarily and dangerously large, and that to be safely administered, it must be used in much smaller quantities. The fatal cases which have since been recorded are painful proofs that my fears were not groundless, nor my cautions unnecessary. By another experiment I showed in what order chloroform affected the three divisions of the nervous system when it was allowed to act progressively: 1st. The cerebral, producing loss of volition and anæsthesia; 2ndly. The true spinal, causing cessation of respiratory effort, and of general reflex action; and lastly, the ganglionic or organic, arresting the heart's action, and thus destroying life. I there announced that in the adult I had found that fifteen minims of chloroform inhaled every minute produced all the desired effect in a gradual and safe manner in from three to six doses. I have pursued this plan ever since with complete success, and I now feel in its administration no more anxiety than I do in that of any other stimulant or narcotic. In persons under fourteen years of age, ten minims are sufficient; under six, about five minims; in those under a year old, three to five minims. I have invariably found that intemperate persons are the most difficult to affect, and that the period of excitement usually occurring previous to anæsthesia is, in them, more prolonged, and the excitement more violent. I have used it in this way, both in private and hospital practice, and Mr. Wilkes, our house-surgeon, informs me that this plan has been generally adopted at the Salisbury Infirmary.

My manner of administering chloroform is as follows: The patient being ascertained to be free from affections of the brain, heart, and inflammatory affections of the lungs, &c., is freely purged the day before the operation, and his diet is limited on the morning appointed. Any article of clothing confining the throat or chest is let loose. The patient is desired to raise one hand, and to keep it raised as long as possible. Five minims is first given in Dr. Sibson's inhaler, to diminish the sensibility of the mucous membrane of the larnyx. After a minute has elapsed fifteen minims are added, and repeated every minute until the hand drops, and is not moved on the patient's being desired to raise it. I then commence the operation.

The person managing the chloroform watches the pulse and respiration. On the former becoming weak, or the latter stertorious, the inhalation is discontinued until they become normal. On any indication, on the other hand, of sensibility returning, ten minims are added.

Dr. Snow, in a paper published in the *London Journal of Medicine* for April, 1852, has proved by experiments on animals that if the air respired contain more than 8 per cent. of chloroform, the action of the heart ceases very suddenly, and sometimes before the breathing.

It would seem unnecessary to insist upon the necessity of using so potent an agent in the smallest possible quantity consistent with success. What intelligent practitioner would give an unnecessarily large dose of opium, calomel, or arsenic? The same rule applies to chloroform, and the more cogently, that when danger arises it comes so suddenly, that there is but little time for the application of treatment.

Chloroform inhaled in small quantities of five, ten, or fifteen minims, is a general stimulant, and the first two or three doses of fifteen minims usually render the pulse quicker and fuller. Whenever the pulse sinks in power, even slightly, the inhalation is too rapid, and the chloroform is accumulating too quickly, or has been continued too long. When this is the case it should be discontinued, for it is better to have an unsteady, or even a suffering, than a dying patient.

In natural labor I administer chloroform where the patient desires it, and circumstances do not forbid it. In operative midwifery I recommend it. Its effect is to diminish uterine action, and to relax the os uteri and external parts; so that what is lost in one direction is gained in another. Of course it destroys all voluntary effort. In natural labor I never commence its use until the latter severe pains begin. I cannot approve of the keeping a patient for many hours under its influence. I think it desirable in these cases (of natural labor,) to act upon the sensorium only, avoiding even more carefully the affecting the true spinal marrow, than in operations; this I do by giving first five minims, then, after the lapse of a minute, ten, and, if required, fifteen minims every succeeding minute, until the patient becomes unconscious; an occasional ten minims given when consciousness threatens to return, is sufficient to keep up the then existing freedom from suffering, without diminishing the uterine contractions to too great a degree. Patients who have been delivered under chloroform rarely suffer from after pain; so much is this the fact that I seldom have to give the usual opiate after such cases. The soreness of the labia and perinæum after labors is much diminished by the ease with which they yield, under the influence of chloroform, to the pressure of the head of the child. I am now in actual attendance on a lady, whom I delivered under chloroform at the birth of her last child, and who has requested me to pursue the same practice in her coming confinement, upon the ground that she had suffered so severely from soreness of the labia in all her confinements previous to her last, but had not done so then.

I believe that where this agent is used in the manner, and with the precautions I have recommended, no evil consequences will occur, but if it is administered in large doses, death will occur as in operations, and even where that catastrophe is avoided, labor may be indefinitely prolonged. In operative midwifery I administer the same quantities as in other operations, and I once kept a woman under the influence of chloroform during an hour and a quarter, without the slightest evil consequences.

In no case have I seen an unfavorable result, and in one case only have I been obliged to abstain, and as this case indicates a cause of danger not, I believe, noticed by others, and leads to an improvement in practice, I will relate it. I was about to use the forceps in a woman pregnant for the first time, aged upwards of forty years, and having a contracted pelvis. I placed fifteen minims of chloroform in the apparatus, but immediately on my bringing it to the mouth and nose, she had a sense of suffocation and croupy inspiration, with venous suffusion of the countenance, which symptoms forced me to desist. The chloroform had evidently excited spasm of the muscles closing the glottis, and I doubt not, had I persisted, my patient would have died asphyxiated. Since this case I have commenced, as stated, with five minims, and then proceeded to ten or fifteen. This plan has succeeded well, by gradually diminishing the excitability of the nerves of the mucous membrane of the larynx; it also prevents that painful sense of constriction about the throat and chest, which, I remember, was in my own case very unpleasant.

I think it right to state that, in experienced hands, a drachm of chloroform may be placed in the apparatus, and by carefully regulating the valves, a quantity not exceeding ten or fifteen minims, may be administered; but a proper apparatus is not within the reach of all. Therefore a plan was still a desideratum, by which a person only moderately skilled may be enabled to administer it safely and effectually. Such a one I feel that I have proposed. Ten minims every minute will frequently produce complete insensibility to pain, and in cases where absolute quiet is not requisite, or where there is any reason to fear syncope, such doses are the best, as they raise the pulse, and in that way would diminish the danger from loss of blood, or even from fatty degeneration of the heart. Indeed, I think that where ordinary syncope occurs from other causes, and where the patient cannot swallow ordinary stimulants, an inhalation of five or ten minims of chloroform might prove beneficial as a general stimulant.

Chloroform in repeated doses of fifteen minims is exceedingly useful in diminishing excessive uterine action, where, from its excess, or from rigidity of the external part, or from both, there is reason to fear rupture of the uterus or laceration of the perinæum. It is in its action, when given in the above quantities, the antithesis of the ergot, and is of course useful in directly opposite cases.

I have seen recommended by an eminent surgeon frequent stimulation of a patient in danger from chloroform. The following experiment seems full of meaning on this point. I placed two frogs under the influence of chloroform to the same degree. One I stimulated incessantly by irritating the skin; the other I left quiet. The former became more and more feeble, and would I think have died had I persevered; the other recovered in a few minutes.

As long as a patient has a good pulse and easy respiration he should be left quiet. A little cold water, after the conclusion of the operation, suddenly dashed on the face at intervals of a few minutes is all that is necessary or safe. If danger occurs, artificial respiration and galvanism seem to afford the best chance. In the absence of galvanism, the application of alternately very cold and very hot water at intervals, might excite deep inspirations. Too frequent stimulation would probably, as in the case of the frog, exhaust nervous energy.

There occurs sometimes after operations performed under the influence of chloroform, especially where stertor has been induced, vomiting, accompanied by great failure of pulse; for this the best treatment is a teaspoonful of pure brandy.

Notwithstanding the express opinion of Dr. Simpson, and other deservedly high authorities in their favor, I am satisfied that the handkerchief, piece of lint, and sponge, are inaccurate and dangerous chloroform inhalers. By them sometimes more, sometimes less is given than is intended or required. In truth, nobody can know what the quantity inhaled is; so much depends upon how the handkerchief is folded, what is the shape of the sponge, and the distance at which they are held from the mouth and nose.

An inhaler invented by Mr. Whitlock, of Salisbury, is far better than the handkerchief, sponge, or lint, and is very simple. It resembles a small mask enclosing the mouth and nose. It is composed of brass wire, the outer and convex part of which is covered with porous cloth, the concave surface is lined with lint, there being a small piece of sponge between the lint and wire. Whether Mr. Whitlock's instrument, the handkerchief, sponge, or lint is used, at least half the chloroform is blown by expiration into the room, to be inspired by the operator and his assistants.

In conclusion I earnestly call the attention of the profession to the plan I have recommended. I admit that it entails more care and trouble, but what conscientious surgeon would allow that to be a consideration? It occupies more time, but when life is at stake that cannot and will not be thought of as an objection. I am the more anxious, as I am convinced that, until some method is adopted by which a student may administer chloroform with safety, we shall hear occasionally of fatal cases.

From the N. W. Medical and Sugrical Journal.

Cold Water in Dysentery. *By* F. Blades, M.D.

If it be the accumulated experience of individuals which gives us our rules in the practice of medicine, every one ought to contribute his mite, if it be of any value. I am, therefore, prompted to send you a slice of my experience.

Last year I had many cases of dysentery to treat. Some of these "wore the livery" of the ordinary non-malignant variety, and were amenable to the usual remedial means; while others — the majority — were of the epidemic or malignant variety, and with surpassing stubbornness, "went their ways," heedless of cure, *i. e.*, by the most practised methods.

Now, we, who have not a reputation to live on after a defeat, cannot well afford — if I may use a sinister expression — to lose many patients consecutively, else we fall into disrepute, and strait-way lose our practice.

This motive, which was secondary to the heart-felt interest I had in the recovery of my patients, as also this latter motive, caused me to depart from the calomel and opium, etc., etc., *land marks* in treating the more malignant variety of dysentery. I have now in my mind a case, which, conjointly with Dr. Fowler, then my partner, I was called upon to treat. The malady "waxed exceeding sore" from its onset. The griping was positively excruciating; the straining extremely ardent and incessant; the stools exceedingly large, grayish and bloody, containing membranous-like shreds; the pulse was quite frequent, and not forcible. This is a rudely sketched outline of the condition of the case as was reported to me to have existed prior to my attendance. The doctor who was first called had treated the case with calomel and opium, q. s., castor oil and laudanum, as a laxative, once in twenty-four hours, with other adjuvantiæ now passed from memory, for three or four days, at which time I was called to see this case with him. The above-mentioned symptoms were said to be unabated. The pulse was now feeble and about 120; the tongue was covered with a thick brown fur, and dry, the edges were fiery and the whole tongue was dotted over with elevated papillæ — here and there protruding through ihe fur-coat. The stomach was so excessively irritable that it would scarcely rerain a tea-spoonful of water. I suggested an enema consisting of a *strong* solution of nitrate of silver, which was twice or thrice repeated during the ensuing twenty-four hours. Also camphor spts. and oil of turpentine, equal parts, to be applied, almost hot, to the abdomen. It was of no use. The disease increased in severity. We looked upon the mortal issue as being but a few hours in advance of us. Here was our extremity, and cold water was the straw caught at. What miraculous buoyancy there was in that dernier resort! We left off medicine entirely — little use was it when none would be retained in the stomach — and determined to try cold water. We wrapt the patient in a cold wet sheet, and thereupon — having previously passed a stool every ten or fifteen minutes — he lay one hour and a half without having desire to go to stool. At the end of this time the surface almost glowed with warmth, and there was the moisture of sweat about the face and neck. The patient was then wiped dry with towels and placed in a dry bed. This operation was thenceforward repeated every five or six hours for the next five days, after which time it was only used once or twice in twenty-four hours for two or three days longer. Instead of the warm fomentations, which had been constantly applied, cloths rung out of cold water were frequently repeated to the abdomen. As enemas we used cold water, simply—8 or 10 ounces immediately after every evacuation. In every case in the treatment of which we used cold water injections, it was found to be important that it should be administered immediately subsequent to every stool. They were borne without distress, and much longer. I ought, also, to mention that after the first day we used the cold Sitz-bath of the hydropathists. From the commencement of this treatment the irritability of the stomach was entirely appeased; the stools became less and less in frequency, and of a more natural appearance and consistence. As a diet, as well as an auxiliary in the treatment, we ordered the animal broths well salted.

Several other cases I have in my mind of a like character with the above. With the exception of one, however, none of them were so violently attacked. That case being of a more robust habit, the disease did not succumb so readily. I commenced treating with calomel, ipecac, and *one grain* of morphine every three hours — at the end of twenty-four hours giving a castor-oil laxative — warm fomentations to the abdomen; enemas of cold water and laudanum. This course was kept up with more or less modification until the expiration of a week. I was not flattered by the progress my patient had made for the better. I then resorted to the water treatment — carrying it out as in the first instance. Upon the first using of the wet sheet the bowels were quieted two hours — having been previously moved as often as from 15 to 30 minutes. The patient kept right on improving — steadily, yet I confess, slowly. It was gratifying to see the complete relief from the excruciating tormina and tenesmus which followed the " wet-sheet-packing."

In this case I used as often as once in four hours, the turpentine emulsion, strongly charged with laudanum. I also occasionally ordered laudanum in the injections.

In many cases, the cold, wet bandage and cold water injections were used as auxiliaries to other treatment, and with a highly gratifying effect.

I am so thoroughly convinced of the powerful efficacy of cold water in the treatment of dysentery that I do not hesitate to say I regard it as *one* of the chief remedies for combating that formidable disease.

Dr. Bennett, of this place a practitioner of many years standing, and a correct observer, after being repeatedly disappointed by depending upon the ordinary remedies alone, is, upon fair trial in many instances, enthusiastic in his confidence in cold water as a powerful auxiliary in treating dysentery.

It would be absurd to argue a general rule from such limited experience, yet its effects have been so highly gratifying in the hands of many practitioners, that it is hard to resist the conviction that cold water deserves a more honorable place among the therapia of dysentery than it has hitherto obtained.

EDITORIAL.

The Peninsular Quarterly and University Magazine.

We have received the first number of this humorous periodical. It is edited by J. S. Morton, Esq., and contains articles of much merit. It aims to give a channel of expression to the literary talent of the west. Those who rejoice to see the progress of our State, will be pleased at the advent of this magazine. The terms are one dollar a year. Letters should be addressed to Peninsular Quarterly, Ann Arbor.

We are indebted to Prof. Baird, of Washington, for valuable documents of the Smithsonian Institute.

Code of Medical Ethics. Concluded from page 96.

ART. IV.—Of the duties of Physicians in regard to Consultations.

Sec. 6. In conclusion, theoretical discussions should be avoided, as occasioning perplexity and loss of time. For there may be much diversity of opinion concerning speculative points, with perfect agreement in those modes of practice which are founded, not on hypothesis, but on experience and observation.

Sec. 7. All discussions in consultation should be secret and confidential. Neither by word or manner should any of the parties to a consultation assert or insinuate, that any part of the treatment pursued did not receive his assent. The responsibility must be equally divided between the medical attendants— they must equally share the credit of success as well as the blame of failure.

Sec. 8. Should an irreconcilable diversity of opinion occur when several physicians are called upon to consult together, the opinions of the majority should be considered as decisive; but if the numbers be equal on each side, then the decision should rest with the attending physician. It may, moreover, sometimes happen, that two physicians cannot agree in their views of the nature of a case, and the treatment to be pursued. This is a circumstance much to be deplored, and should always be avoided, if possible, by mutual concessions, as far as they can be justified by a conscientious regard for the dictates of judgment. But in the event of its occurrence, a third physician should, if practicable, be called to act as umpire, and if circumstances prevent the adoption of this course, it must be left to the patient to select the physician in whom he is most willing to confide. But as every physician relies upon the rectitude of his judgment, he should, when left in the minority, politely and consistently retire from any further deliberation in the consultation, or participation in the management of the case.

Sec. 9. As circumstances sometimes occur to render a *special consultation* desirable, when the continued attendance of two physicians might be objectionable to the patient, the member of the faculty whose assistance is required in such cases, should sedulously guard against all future unsolicited attendance. As such consultations require an extraordinary portion both of time and attention, at least a double honorarium may be reasonably expected.

Sec. 10. A physician who is called upon to consult, should observe the most honorable and scrupulous regard for the character and standing of the practitioner in attendance; the practice of the latter, if necessary, should be justified as far as it can be, consistently with a conscientious regard for truth, and no hint or insinuation should be thrown out, which could impair the confidence reposed in him, or affect his reputation. The consulting physician should also carefully refrain from any of those extraordinary attentions or assiduities, which are too often practiced by the dishonest for the base purpose of gaining applause, or ingratiating themselves into the favor of families and individuals.

ART. V.—*Duties of Physicians in Cases of Interference.*

Sec. 1. Medicine is a liberal profession, and those admitted into its ranks should found their expectations of practice upon the extent of their qualifications, not on intrigue or artifice.

Sec. 2. A physician, in his intercourse with a patient under the care of another practitioner, should observe the strictest caution and reserve. No meddling inquiries should be made ; no disingenious hints given relative to the nature and treatment of the disorder ; nor any course of conduct pursued that may directly or indirectly tend to diminish the trust reposed in the physician employed.

Sec. 3. The same circumspection and reserve should be observed, when from motives of business or friendship, a physician is prompted to visit an individual who is under the direction of another practitioner. Indeed, such visits should be avoided, except under peculiar circumstances, and when they are made, no particular inquiries should be instituted relative to the nature of the disease, or the remedies employed, but the topics of conversation should be as foreign to the case as circumstances will admit.

Sec. 4. A physician ought not to take charge of, or prescribe for a patient who has recently been under the care of another member of the faculty, except in cases of sudden emergency, or in consultation with the physician previously in attendance, or when the latter has relinquished the case or been regularly notified that his services are no longer desired. Under such circumstances no unjust and illiberal insinuations should be thrown out in relation to the conduct or practice previously pursued, which should be justified as far as candor and regard for truth and probity will permit ; for it often happens, that patients become dissatisfied when they do not experience immediate relief, and, as many diseases are naturally protracted, the want of success, in the first stage of treatment, affords no evidence of a lack of professional knowledge and skill.

Sec. 5. When a physician is called to an urgent case because the family attendant is not at hand, he ought, unless his assistance in consultation be desired, to resign the case of the patient to the latter immediately on his arrival.

Sec. 6. It often happens, in cases of sudden illness, or of recent accidents and injuries, owing to the alarm and anxiety of friends, that a number of physicians are simultaneously sent for. Under these circumstances courtesy should assign the patient to the first one who arrives, who should select from those present any additional assistance he may deem necessary. In all such cases, however, the practitioner who officiates should request the family physician, if there be one, to be called, and, unless his further attendance be requested, should resign the case to the latter on his arrival.

Sec. 7. When a physician is called to a patient of another practitioner, in consequence of the sickness or absence of the latter, he ought, on the return or recovery of the regular attendant, and with the consent of the patient, to surrender the case.

Sec. 8. A physician, when visiting a sick person in the country, may be desired to see a neighboring patient who is under the regular direction of another physician, in consequence of some sudden change or aggravation of symptoms. The conduct to be pursued on such an occasion is to give advice adapted to present circumstances : to interfere no farther than is absolutely necessary with the general plan of treatment, to assume no future direction, unless it be expressly desired ; and in this last case, to request an immediate consultation with the practitioner previously employed.

Sec. 9. A wealthy physician should not give advice *gratis* to the affluent; because his doing so is an injury to his professional brethren. The office of a physician can never be supported as an exclusively beneficent one, and it is defrauding, in some degree, the common funds for its support, when fees are dispensed with, which might justly be claimed.

Sec. 10. When a physician who has been engaged to attend a case of midwifery is absent, and another is sent for, if delivery is accomplished during the attendance of the latter, he is entitled to the fee, but should resign the patient to the practitioner first engaged.

ART. VI.—*Of Differences between Physicians.*

Sec. 1. Diversity of opinion and opposition of interest may, in the medical, as in other professions, sometimes occasion controversy and even contention. Whenever such cases unfortunately occur, and cannot be immediately terminated, they should be referred to the arbitration of a sufficient number of physicians, or a *court medical.*

Sec. 2. As peculiar reserve must be maintained by physicians towards the public, in regard to professional matters, and as there exist numerous points in medical ethics and etiquette through which the feelings of medical men may be painfully assailed in their intercourse with each other, and which cannot be understood or appreciated by general society, neither the subject matter of such differences nor the adjudication of the arbitrators should be made public, as publicity in a case of this nature may be personally injurious to the persons concerned, and can hardly fail to bring discredit on the faculty.

ART. VII —*Of Pecuniary Acknowledgments.*

Sec. 1. Some general rules should be adopted by the faculty, in every town or district, relative to pecuniary acknowledgments from their patients; and it should be deemed a point of honor to adhere to these rules with as much uniformity as varying circumstances will admit.

CHAPTER III.— OF THE DUTIES OF THE PROFESSION TO THE PUBLIC, AND OF THE OBLIGATIONS OF THE PUBLIC TO THE PROFESSION.

ART. I.—*Duties of the Profession to the Public.*

Sec. 1.—As good citizens, it is the duty of physicians to be ever vigilant for the welfare of the community, and to bear their part in sustaining its institutions and burdens; they should also be ever ready to give counsel to the public in matters especially appertaining to their professions, or on subjects of medical police, public hygiene, and legal medicine. It is their province to enlighten the public in regard to quarantine regulations—the location, arrangement, and dietaries of hospitals, asylums, schools, prisons, and similar institutions; in relation to the medical police of towns, as drainage, ventilation, &c.—and in regard to measures for the prevention of epidemic and contagious diseases; and when pestilence prevails, it is their duty to face the danger, and to continue their labors for the alleviation of the suffering, even at the jeopardy of their own lives.

Sec. 2. Medical men should also be always ready, when called on by the legally constituted authorities, to enlighten coroners' inquests and courts of justice, on subjects strictly medical—such as involve questions relating to sanity, legitimacy, murder by poisons or other violent means, and in regard to the various other subjects embraced in the science of medical jurisprudence. But in these cases, and especially where they are required to make a post-mortem examination, it is just, in consequence of the time, labor and skill required, and the responsibility and risk they incur, that the public should award them a proper honorarium.

Sec. 3. There is no profession, by the members of which eleemosynary services are more liberally dispensed, than the medical, but justice requires that some limits should be placed to the performance of such good offices. Poverty, professional brotherhood, and certain public duties referred to in sec. 1 of this chapter, should always be recognized as presenting valid claims for gratuitous services; but neither institutions endowed by the public or by rich individuals, societies for mutual benefit, for the insurance of lives or for analagous purposes, nor any profession or occupation, can be admitted to possess such privilege. Nor can it be justly expected of physicians to furnish certificates of inability to serve on juries, to perform militia duty, or to testify to the state of health of persons wishing to insure their lives, obtain pensions, or the like, without a pecuniary acknowledgment. But to individuals in indigent circumstances, such professional services should always be cheerfully and freely given.

Sec. 4. It is the duty of physicians, who are frequent witnesses of the enormities committed by quackery, and the injury to health and even destruction of life caused by the use of quack medicines, to enlighten the public on these subjects, to expose the injuries sustained by the unwary from the devices and pretensions of artful empirics and impostors. Physicians ought to use all the influence which they may possess, as professors in Colleges of Pharmacy, and by exercising their option in regard to the shops to which their prescriptions shall be sent, to discourage druggists and apothecaries from vending quack or secret medicines, or from being in any way engaged in their manufacture and sale.

ART. II.—*Obligations of the public to Physicians.*

Sec. 1. The benefits accruing to the public directly and indirectly from the active and unwearied beneficence of the profession, are so numerous and important, that physicians are justly entitled to the utmost consideration and respect from the community. The public ought likewise to entertain a just appreciation of medical qualifications; to make a proper discrimination between true science and the assumptions of ignorance and empiricism—to afford every encouragement and facility for the acquisition of medical education—and no longer to allow the statute books to exhibit the anomaly of exacting knowledge from physicians under liability to heavy penalties, and of making them obnoxious to punishment for resorting to the only means of obtaining it.

Proceedings of the American Association for the Advancement of Science.

This Association, as is known to our readers, was formed in 1840, under the title of the "Association of American Geologists and Naturalists." It held its meetings successively at different cities, once a year. In 1847 the title was changed to the "American Association for the Advancement of Science." Since then they have met at Philadelphia, Cambridge, Mass., Charlston, S. C., New Haven, Cincinnati and Albany. Last year they appointed a meeting at Cleveland, but from some reason or other it was postponed. The reason given was the prevalence of Cholera in some of the surrounding cities through which the members must pass on their way to Cleveland. That there was a little Cholera in some of these places is well known, but so little that the idea of being afraid to pass through them was simply ludicrous. To suppose that this was the only cause of the postponement would be to charge cowardice upon men whose whole lives would contradict the assertion. There were those who had faced the Vomito of Mexico and the Cholera of the States repeatedly — others who had braved the dangers of the Antarctic Exploring Expedition, and scarcely one who had not accustomed himself to more or less peril by land or by sea, in the pestilence of cities, or in the wildness of the forests. Men that had carried their packs to California by the land route, or sailed among icebergs on the shores of the Antarctic continent, could not be greatly terrified by a trip of a few hours to Cleveland. What the real cause of the postponement was we are not accurately informed, but we hope that next time they will get up a more substantial excuse. However, a year rolled around, and the Association this time came together, and a goodly meeting it was.

The session was opened on the 28th of July at 2 o'clock P. M., by the introduction of Prof. B. Pierce, of Cambridge, Mass., as President. Rev. G. B. Perry opened the session with prayer.

Prof. Agassiz, who was to have delivered the opening address, had contracted a malignant fever, while delving for new fishes among the marshes and rivers of the South, so that he nearly lost his life, and was not sufficiently recovered to attend. The President, Prof. Pierce, therefore delivered an opening address. Prof. Pierce is a distinguished mathematician. Personally, he is a little, dried up, dark complexioned man, who looks as though he had eliminated every particle of adipose tissue from his body. His straight black hair is parted with mathematical exactness over the saggital suture, and his face is furrowed with the lines of intense thought. Altogether he looks like the concentrated square root of a great man. Notwithstanding his dry look, however, his opening address displayed a full and luxuriant style of thought. Here it is.

OPENING ADDRESS.

Gentlemen of the American Association for the Advancement of Science:

WE are again met in the service of our high cause ; after the unusual interval of two years, we have again come together at our appointed rendezvous to make each other glad with the tidings of truth which we bring from the Heavens and the Earth ; and to re-animate our fainting zeal by the story of the successful search for the philosopher's stone, the true *elixir vitæ*, the fruit of the tree of knowledge, and the footprint of ¶Him of whom the earth is the footstool.

Gentlemen, from such an assembly, egotism shrinks abashed, and you will not reprove your President that he does not intrude his feelings of grateful pride at the honor which you have conferred upon him, and his profound sense of his incapacity to wear the robes of Redfield and Henry and Bache and Agassiz. His hopes of success in the discharge of his duties do not arise from the vigor of his own energy or the readiness of his own wisdom ; but from the manly hearts which surround him on all sides, hearty friends whose generous sympathy will easily forgive and correct the errors of an honest purpose.

Gentlemen, we are not convened for a light duty — our self-imposed task is not an amusing child's play ; and we have not accepted the liberally offered hospitalities. of this beautiful city for the enjoyment of a social festival. We have come to give and receive instruction and inspiration. We have come to the shores of this great Lake to admire and study the pebbles which our brethren may have picked up here and there with much labor, and to learn where or how they are to be found. We have brought our freights of knowledge to distribute them to the world that they may do good.

Gentlemen we have come to study our duty as scientific men, and especially as American scientific men. We are to learn the apparent, and not very pleasant paradox that America cannot keep pace with Europe in Science, except by going ahead of her. The New World must begin to build upon a level above that of the Old World, and it must build from its own materials. This is not asking too much. It is no more than was accomplished by the American Ship 'and the American Reaping Machine. The Yankee who picked the hardest lock of England and contrived a lock which all England could not pick, is but a type of American intellect. This was a work of mind, and we have a right to expect equal excellence in the higher and more abstract efforts of American genius. But, above all things, it is not to be forgotten that the Temple of Science, by whomever built, belongs to no country or clime. It is the World's Temple and all men are free of its communion. Let us not mar its beauty by writing our names upon its walls. The stone which we have inserted is not ours, it is not thine, it is not mine, but it is part of the Temple. The child picks up a shell, innocently admires its form and coloring and listens without a thought of self to the singing of the angels within it. It is the unconsciousness of the attitude which gives it its grace and beauty, and makes the child and the shell parts of the same divine thought, each forever belonging to the other, and both immortalized in the marble of the Artist.

Gentlemen, let us stand here reverently. This is holy ground. Let us not presume to make these walls resound with the bickerings of angry contention for superior distinction, and the foul complaints of mortified vanity. Let us not raise the money-changers' cry of mine and thine, lest the purifier come, and taking the royal jewel into his own possession, thrust us out into the ditch and turn our fame into infamy.

It has been observed by others, not of our number, that the meetings of the Association have been characterized by a generous appreciation of each others labors, and it has naturally contributed to the influence and power of our Society. May we continue this honorable harmony so fitting to our sublime studies, and be always open to the reception of new discoveries and new discoverers   But mutual admiration is not our only or our most necessary office. Mutual criticism is equally conducive to the best interests of the Association. We should exert ourselves to restrain vagueness and uncertainty of thought and expression, and to prevent the concealment of old truths under new forms. We must not permit erroneous statements to pass unchal-, lenged. It is our stern and solemn duty to criticise and expose all developments. whether they are intended, or the unintentional results of carelessness or ignorance This task may, and should be performed with delicacy and generosity, and the mode of performance will clearly manifest the spirit of the operator, and mainly determine the success of the operation. The knife, wielded with unsparing rudeness, is less effective than the touch of Ithuriel's spear. '

" For no falsehood can endure
Touch of celestial temper; but returned
Of force to its own likeness ; up it starts
Discovered and exposed."

Gentleman let us learn wisdom from the Poet,

There is another point to which I must allude before closing these opening remarks, which are already too much protracted. We have a constitution and laws, and it is our duty to observe them. If in any important respect we have deviated from our fundamental laws, we should either retrace our steps or amend our constitution — But let us not forget that unskilled lawyers may easily become pedants of law, and observe that this is an Association of gentlemen whose garments are intended for easy and graceful protection, and not a Bedlam, whose denizens are to be strictly confined within straight waistcoats.

And now, Gentlemen, without further delay, let us proceed to the business for which we have assembled.

The Association then proceeded with the business of the day. Ex-President Fillmore was elected a member, with a large number of others.

In looking around upon this assembly of over two hundred of the most eminent scientific men of the nation, we could not help noticing the casts of countenance which habits of life give. There sat President Fillmore, a great stately-looking man, with an unmistakable lawyer look upon his countenance. Lawyers have a look that belongs to them alone. Whoever has seen any national convocation of clergymen, cannot have failed to mark their aspect of calm and dignified solemnity. This scientific body had also its peculiar look, which it is difficult to describe. There was a sort of piercing concentration in their countenances, an air that made you feel as if they might look at you, and see instantly through every fibre of your body. There were very few *smooth* faces there — their features were knotted and twisted in every form, as though they had peered through microscopes, pried into the crevices of rocks, and figured and demonstrated until their very faces had come to express to mother Nature that her secrets were not safe. They were mostly young and middle aged men — many of them brawny with exposure, and sinewy with physical exertion. Among the men of note were Profs. Baird and Henry, of the Smithsonian Institute, Bache, of the Coast Survey, Lt. Wilkes, of the Exploring Expedition, Prof. Ridell, of New Orleans, St. John, E. Kirtland, of Cleveland, and many others. The Medical Profession was honorably represented, for indeed a very large proportion of the cultivators of natural science are always physicians. Mr. Redfield of New York, read an article on storms, and the value of the barometer in navigating our lakes. He maintains that the winds move not in straight lines, but in vast cycloids or whirls. In consequence of this form it is evident that the wind in opposite edges of a storm is moving in contrary directions, enclosing a calm space in the centre. Hence as the circle moves on, a vessel will have a breeze blowing briskly in one direction, then be overtaken by a calm, and soon afterwards be struck from the opposite direction by the other edge of the whirl.

The usefulness of the barometer consists in this. The centrifugal force of the circle causes the air to draw somewhat away from the centre, forming a slight tendency to a vacuum. In this part, therefore, a barometer sinks rapidly, showing that it is in the centre of a whirl, and that the passage of the circumference may soon be expected, and that with a violence and power directly in proportion to the amount of depression of the barometer. Too often the sailor, tempted by the favorable direction of the first part of the circle, ventures out, only to be hurled back on a lee shore by the onset of the second. Now a barometer, the gentleman maintained, kept on the vessel, and giving timely notice of what might be expected to follow, would enable the sailor to secure his safety while he was yet among the lighter breezes of the centre, and thus avoid the coming danger.

A convenient substitute for the barometer has lately come into use, which is called the Aneroid Barometer. It has advantages in compactness, and less liability to fatal injuries, with greater facility in reading its indications. On the other hand, it is liable to gradual changes in its standard readings; and hence requires an occasional reference to a good standard barometer for the purpose of new adjustment. With this needful precaution, I deem it for practical purposes equal to the common barometer, and well suited for lake navigation.

Prof. B. Pierce, of Cambridge, gave his views of the " *Stability of Saturn's Rings.*" At Cincinnati in 1851, Prof. Pierce took the position that Saturn's Ring was not solid, and that there " is no conceivable form of irregularity, and no conceivable combination of irregularities consistent with an actual ring, which would permit the ring to be permanently maintained by the primary if it were solid."

Other papers of great interest were also read, and then the Association adjourned until the following day.

On the second day the Convention divided itself into two sections, for the sake of expediting business. The following was the order of the day :'

SECTION A.

Mathematics and Physics.

On the Resistance of the Vertical Plates of Tubular Bridges. By Herman Haupt, Sup't of the Pennsylvania Central Railroad, Philadelphia.

On the Tides at Key West, Florida, from observations made in connection with the U. S. Coast Survey. By Prof. A. D. Bache, Sup't. Washington.

The Zodiacal Light. the periodical appearance of Meteors, and the point in space to which the motion of the Solar System is directed. By Daniel Vaughan, of Cincinnati.

On the South East Monsoon of Texas, the Northers of Texas and the Gulf of Mexico, and the Abnormal Movements of the North American continent generally. By Lorin Blodgett, of Washington.

Investigations in Analytical Morphology. No. 2 ; Stable and Unstable forms of Equilibrium. By Prof. B. Pierce, of Cambridge, Mass.

An investigation of the Storm Curve, deduced from the Relations existing between the direction of the Wind, and the rise and fall of the Barometer. By Prof. J. H. Coffin, of Easton. Pa.

Does the moon exert a sensible influence upon the clouds? By Prof. E. Loomis, of N. York.

On the Earthquake of April 29, 1852. By Lorin Blodgett, of Washington.

On the Rising of Water in Springs immediately before Rain. By Prof. John Brocklesby, of Trinity College, Hartford.

SECTION B.

Natural History and Geology, Mineralogy: Chemistry, Geography, and Ethnology.

A Geological Reconnoisance of the Arkansas River. By Dr. J. A. Warder, of Cincinnati.

On the Blood Corpuscle—holding Cells, and their relation to the Spleen. By Dr. W. I. Burnett, of Boston.

Origin of Quartz Pebbles in the Sandstone Conglomerate, and the formation of the Silicious Stratified Rocks. By Prof. J. Brainard, of Cleveland.

Indications of Weather, as shown by Animals and Plants. By W. H. B Thomas, of Cincinnati.

On the Geology of the Choctaw Bluff. By A. Winchell, Eutaw, Ala.

On six new species of Plants. By Prof. Alphonso Wood, of Cincinnati.

On a remarkable class of conjunct bases, containing Cobalt and the elements of Ammonia. By Dr. F. A. Genth and Dr. W. Gibbs.

On the Solidification of Coral Reefs of Florida, and the Source of Carbonate of Lime in the growth of Corals. By Prof. E. N. Horsford, of Cambridge.

On the fatal effect of Chloroform. By Prof. E. N. Horsford. of Cambridge, Mass.

Investigation of the power of the Greek Z, by means of Phonetic laws. By Prof. S. S. Haldeman, of Columbia. Pa,

On the Formation and mode of Development of the Renal Organs in Vertebrata. By Dr. W. I Burnett. of Boston.

Notes on the specimens of the bottom of the Ocean, brought up in recent explorations of the Gulf Stream, in connection with the Coast Survey, By L. F. Pourtales, Ass't. Presented by Prof. Bache, Sup't.

Most of the Medical men of course attended section B. In this section Dr. Burnett's article on the cells of the spleen, was very interesting, though we did not coincide in all his opinions. Prof. Brainard's article on pebbles was laughed at, being too ridiculous to be respectable ; and we were at first astonished to see such a paper seriously presented ; but from subsequent observations on the Ohio conglomerates, we find in them a certain uniformity which might make one who had not seen other localities think Prof.'s B.'s opinions plausible. His position was that nearly all stratified rocks were chemical precipitates from aquesus solutions, and that the quartz pebbles in conglomerate were chemical concretions, and not rolled fragments.

W. H. B. Thomas is a very young man, but acquitted himself creditably in laying down the facts he had observed respecting the predictions of weather founded on the instinctive actions of animals. Prof. Horsford's article on Chloroform touches upon a subject so important at the present time that we insert it entire :'

On the fatal effects of Chloroform. By Professor HORSFORD of Cambridge.

THE occasional deaths that have occurred in medical practice from the use of anæsthetic agents have within the last two years, attracted a large measure of attention. It was earnestly maintained by some in this country that Ether had been employed in all cases without injurious effects, and that the disastrous consequences were solely due to Chloroform ; while in England the two agents were held in the inverse order of esteem. Others in this country advocated the use of chloric ether, in the persuasion that it was safer ; while it was generally believed by those who had most to do with these agents, that the fatal results were due to diosyncracies of temperament on part of the patient, or in rare cases to want of attention and judgment on the part of the physician. There has been expressed the opinion * that the injurious effects of chloroform are due to a volatile body accompanying the chloroform and derived from the action of bleaching salt upon Fusel oil — a constituent of most inferior alcohols.— It was conceived that this body need be present only in a very small quantity to produce the fatal effects.

It was maintained by others † that chloroform was susceptible of undergoing spontaneous change and becoming thereby unsafe for respiration.

In the midst of this variety of explanations of the ill effects of anæsthetic agents, there appeared in the market from time to time, chloroform impossible to inhale from the presence of free chlorine and hydrochloric acid ; and another which, though not difficult to inhale, was found upon close examination to yield an offensive and unusual odor as of something putrid. The latter may be easily purified by repeated agitation with sulphuric acid, and was the subject of experiment by Gregory, to whom we are indebted for the method of its purification. The former variety has not hitherto, so far as I am aware been the subject of special experimental inquiry.

The following investigation was undertaken with a view to determine the nature of this variety of bad chloroform, under what circumstances it might be produced and how made pure — and further to determine how far the fatal effects of the administration were due to alleged impurities, and how far to other causes which have been suggested above.

The sample of bad chloroform which was made the subject of experiment, was received from Dr. Currie, an eminent Pharmaceutist of New York. It was contained in a ground stoppered bottle and was not quite full. The space above the liquid, and the liquid itself presented a yellowish green tinge. Floating upon the surface of the chloroform was a thin layer of deep yellow color of oleaginous consistency, which, when the vessel was agitated, separated into globules as oil would agitated with water. Upon opening the flask it yielded a strong odor of chlorine and hydrochloric acid.

A quantity of this bad chloroform placed in an inverted test-tube over mercury, yielded more and more gaseous products, at first of a decidedly greenish tinge, but becoming in a few days colorless displacing and forcing downward the chloroform, until now, after the lapse of nine months, several cubic inches have been evolved from a cubic inch of the liquid. As might have been expected, chlorine and hydrochloric acid could be entirely withdrawn by distillation from soda-lime. A quantity so purified nine months since, is now perfectly good.

Another quantity in contact with cotton fibre (candle wick), in a few days became perfectly pure and has so remained.

A better, and a thoroughly practical and simple‡ method, was discovered by the late Dr. Dwight, of Moscow, New York. Of this method I will speak more especially, further on.

It having been remarked in the letter accompanying the parcel from Dr. Currie, that the chloroform had been purified by Gregory's process, it occurred to me that the sulphuric acid might have contained a little nitric acid, and that this might have taken part in its tendency to decay. To ascertain if any form of sulphur might be present in the yellow oil floating on the surface, it was treated with fuming nitric acid and a soluble salt of baryta, but yielded no precipitate.

To ascertain if any nitrogen had, by possibility, taken on the form of ammonia, and were still present, other portions of the oily matter were, with some of the chloroform, carefully seperated and evaporated with platinum solution, to dryness. — They did not yield a trace of platina Salammoniac.

Unfortunately the quantity, too small at first for quantitative analysis, was only sufficient to enable me to observe that a portion of it crystalized under certain circumstances. As upon application to the gentlemen who had so kindly furnished the article experimented with, I found that no more was to be obtained, there remained only the alternative of attempting to reproduce the bad chloroform.

The atmosphere above the liquid, as above remarked, contained chlorine and hydrochloric acid, and the chloroform was colored pale yellow with a shade of green. These were the indications by which experiment was to be guided. Upon the hypothesis that this variety of bad chloroform was due to the presence of Fusel oil in the alcohol, chloroform was made with alcohol containing this oil in various proportions ; the water, alcohol and bleaching salt being taken in the proportion given by Dumas. In all cases the resulting chloroform was good.

The Fusel oil of the apothecaries, treated with water and bleaching salt in all res-

---

;* Dr. Charles T. Jackson. † Dr. A. A. Hayes.
‡ An eminent physician and surgeon who had, for more than a quarter of a century, pursued the successful practice of his profession in Moscow, N. Y., was lost at Norwalk, having within the previous week submitted an able paper on this subject to the American Medical Association. It is to be hoped that this paper, containing much valuable information and the results of careful experiment, will be given to the public.

pects as if it were alcohol, with a view to the production of chloroform, gave a product nearly like pure Fusel oil in smell, and having a specific gravity in these several preparations of —

0.8236
0.8225
0.8224

While that of pure Fusel oil is, 0.8124. It gave of chlorine, 1.35 per ct. when evaporated to dryness with soda lime, the chlorine in which had been previously determined. This was doubtless due to the chloroform derived from the trace of alcohol still present in the Fusel oil.

That such might have been expected as the result, will be evident when it is considered that Fusel oil is but slightly soluble in water, and would of course, from the outset, float on the surface of the mixture.

Experiments made with alcohol to which was added impure methyl alcohol (wood spirit) gave good chloroform.

Experiments with the product of distillation resulting from the mixture of pure Fusel oil, water and bleaching salt, upon man and inferior animals, were made under quite varied circumstances.

A practicing physician accustomed to the administration of chloroform, inhaled the vapor of this product for fourteen minutes without any marked anæsthetic effect, or any other effect than slight irritation of the bronchial tubes.

Two rats, one full grown, were successively subjected to the action of this agent, poured upon cotton to facilitate evaporation, the tuft of cotton and the animal being placed on the bottom of a covered becker glass. The air was renewed from time to time with the aid of a bellows. At the end of an hour no anæsthetic effect had been produced upon the full grown rat, and at the end of forty minutes none on the smaller animal. They were then exposed to the action of the vapor of chloroform. and in less than two minutes were insensible.

The experiment was repeated with kittens about a week old, with like results, except that they were longer in becoming insensible.

On a subsequent day two kittens were exposed to the vapor of the above body, each under a separate bell-glass, while two others, in all respects similarly situated, except that the latter breathed merely confined air, for one hour, without its being apparent that the vapor had produced any deleterious effect. When taken out, all appeared quite alike so far as activity was concerned, or disposition to seek legitimate nourishment.

At a period several weeks later, the experiments were repeated with the same kittens in the use of a fresh preparation of the above body, repeatedly distilled from chloride of calcium. There was in the course of an hour, an appreciable lethargic effect which was not so marked where confined air was alone inhaled, but in no instance attained such a degree that upon the removal of the bell-glasses, the animals did not at once resume unimpaired, the possession of all its powers.

These experiments led to the conviction that Fusel oil, when treated as in the manufacture of chloroform, substituting Fusel oil for alcohol, is not changed, and of course, that the Fusel oil present in alcohol in the ordinary manufacture of chloroform does not yield a poison, which taken with the chloroform has produced the fatal effects.

While the Fusel oil vapor and the impure chloroform which Gregory had recognized could be inhaled without difficulty, the article received from Dr. Currie, by its violent irritation, closed the glottis almost instantly.

Upon the presumption that the bad attribute was due to the mode of purification, a quantity of good chloroform was repeatedly distilled from concentrated sulphuric acid, and another from chloride of calcium. The products in both cases were perfectly good, and are so still, now nine months from the date of distillation.

Having tried alcohol of various degrees of purity and strength, and having subjected good chloroform repeatedly to different methods of purification, it remained to try different samples of bleaching salt with varying proportions of alcohol. Accordingly, several varieties in the market were procured, and a series of experiments undertaken by Mr. Gould, of the Laboratory of the Lawrence Scientific School.

The combinations of alcohol, bleaching salt, water, temperature, time and mode of distillation, made to meet the inquiry required above fifty successive preparations of chloroform, the detailed results of thirty-one of which will appear in the official proceedings of the Association.

From these and the foregoing series of experiments, it appears —

1st, that good chloroform does not spontaneously change in a period of nine months.

2nd. That the bad chloroform, containing free chlorine and hydrochloric acid, may be produced by using a bleaching salt of great strength with a quantity of alcohol disproportionately small.

3rd. That the bad chloroform may be produced by receiving the distillate into water, so as immediately to withdraw the alcohol from the chloroform.

4th. That the bad chloroform may be produced by passing chlorine directly into chloroform.

5th. That no formula for its manufacture can be relied upon as a guide, since bleaching salts vary in strength when derived from different factories, and vary with age. In the foregoing experiments the range is from 15 to 30 per cent.

6th. That quick lime added to the mixture does not promote the economy of manufacture.

7th. That the chlorine and hydrochloric acid of bad chloroform, as observed by Dr. Dwight, may be removed by agitation with a little alcohol.

8th. That the ill effects observed in the administration of chloroform are not due to the presence of chlorine as the irritation is such when it is attempted to inhale it, as to prevent inhalation altogether.

9th. That the ill effects are not due to any poisonous product arising from the action of bleaching salt on the small quantity of fusel oil, in the alcohol employed in the manufacture of chloroform.

10th. That the ill effects are due to peculiarities of constitution or temperament of some patients, and in a few rare cases to want of attention or judgment on the part of the person administering it.

Dr. Burnett's papers on the renal organs, alantois, etc., were interesting in matter, but inaccurate and very erroneous in the statement of facts.

The proceedings continued in the same style for five days, but a report of all the articles would be too voluminous. Prof. Ridell, of New Orleans, exhibited to the members his binocular microscope, which is so contrived that the rays of light, after passing through the object-glass, shall be divided into two beams by glass prisms, and reflected to the two eyes. This requires two eyeglasses. Objects thus seen present some striking views. They are clearer in consequence of the sensation from both eyes being more intense than from one, and also the object is seen, not as a flat shadow, but in relief, showing its depth as well as its breadth. Another advantage is that it prevents the *umating* which takes place where a person constantly uses one eye alone at the glass.

Prof. Ridell also read a paper on the "Histology of Red Blood." He showed drawings of the blood corpuscles of a Texan reptile, which being about the two hundredth part of an inch in diameter, are larger than those of any other animal. By the microscopic examination of these bodies, he discovers that they have each a nucleus enclosing several nucleoli, and that the space between the nucleus and the cell wall is filled with a quantity of very minute celules or vesicles, which, under a low power of the microscope, look like mere granules. Hence he infers that the granular matter in human blood corpuscles is celular in form, but too minute to be distinctly seen.

On Monday evening the citizens of Cleveland invited the members to meet them socially at the American Hotel. They repaired thither and found a company of the citizens with their ladies waiting to receive them, and a beautiful entertainment, both of social intercourse, and more material refreshments prepared for them.

On the fifth day the reading of papers was concluded. It had already been decided that the next annual meeting should be held at Washington. The Association then passed sundry votes of thanks, listened to some valedictory remarks, and adjourned.

Correction.

The following passage was accidently omitted in the last number, in the editorial concerning Chloroform. Its place is at the close of the article signed " G," page 91. As it contains the conclusion of the whole matter respecting the safety of Chloroform Inhalations, we insert it here.—ED.

We consider it (chloroform) about as safe to the patient as a journey by railroad or steamboat to the passengers. Our rule is never to use it in trivial cases, when the operation requires but a single stroke of the knife, or actually *recommend* it in any case. We make to our patients the above statement of its *comparative* safety, and if they elect, we administer it, taking due care that it is well mixed with atmospheric air, watching closely the pulse and respiration. With these cautions we bide our time, await our turn for an accident, and confess to a growing dread of the agent.　　　　　G.

THE

PENINSULAR
JOURNAL OF MEDICINE
AND THE COLLATERAL SCIENCES.

VOL. I.   OCTOBER, 1853.   NO. IV.

ORIGINAL COMMUNICATIONS.

Art. I.—*Notes of Travel.* By "X."

He that wants to know how a thing is, must go and see it. If you want to know how deep a stream is, there is no way so good as to go and measure it. So lately, upon a time, while jogging about in Michigan and the adjoining states, it occurred to me to take the dimensions by actual statistics, of that Jordan of Quackery which Behemoth Bullhead "trusteth that he can draw up in his *Corporal* mouth:" for this same Jordan has roared and foamed and sputtered, until many people suppose it to be exceeding deep and mighty, and if the Corporal and the Q. K. army purpose to precipitate themselves into any rash undertaking, we must hold on to their over-valiant coat tails, lest they be " devoured in battle." Moved by these humane considerations I took statistical notes of such places as I visited, or could obtain reliable information about. The brief result of my examination, is, that there is more foam than fact about the quack clans, and any body will do Corporal Bullhead a service, who will get enough of them together into one phalanx, to make it worth his while to charge them. The results of my inquiries may be found in the subjoined table. From various causes the numbers may contain some errors. Changes are frequent, and though but a few weeks have elapsed, removals have by this time, transferred some practitioners, and many quacks, to other locations; then there were men who had partly retired from practice, and it was not easy to say whether they were still to be classed as acting physicians or not, and there were quacks, who held themselves up to practice anything, and accommodated themselves to the whims of their patrons, so

· that it was a matter of difficulty, to know whether to call them Eclectics, Homœopaths, Botanists, or what. On account of these various sources of ambiguity, it was not possible to class them with perfect precision, but as a whole the table must be very nearly accurate. I have placed Homœopaths and Eclectics by themselves, because they boast the loudest of their numerical strength and supposed increase of power. All other quacks I put together under the head " Miscellaneous :"

TABLE.

Places.	Regulars.	Homœopathists.	Eclectics.	Miscellaneous.	Places.	Regulars.	Homœopathists.	Eclectics.	Miscellaneous.
Detroit,	40	8		6	Portland,	2			
Dearborn,	2				Sebewa,	1			1
Ypsilanti,	6	1		1	Lyons,	3	1		
Ann Arbor,	7	3			Ionia,	4			
Dexter,	3	2			Lowell,	1			
Jackson,	9	2		1	Grand Rapids,	7	1		
Albion,	8		1	1	Middleville,	1			
Marshall,	7	1	1	1	Hastings,	4			
Galesburg,	2			·	Schoolcraft,	2			1
Battle Creek,	8	1		3	Lawrence,	1			1
Kalamazoo,	10	2		3	Breedsville,	1			
Paw Paw,	3	2			Pontiac,	7	1		1
Niles,	6		1		Mt. Clemens,	5			1
Michigan City,	5			1	Utica,	2			2
Laporte, Ia.,	6	1	2		Washington,	2			1
S. Bend, Ia.,	7	1	4		Rochester,	3			
Mishawaka, In,	4		1		Romeo,	3			
White Pigeon,	2				Royal Oak,	3			
Coldwater,	9			3	Birmingham,	3			
Jonesville,	3	1			Constantine,	5			
Hillsdale,	7				Mottville,	2			
Adrian,	5	1	2	2	Centreville,	3			
Toledo, O.,	12	1		3	Union City,	4	1	1	
Monroe,	8					—	—	—	—
Eaton Rapids,	3	1	1		Total,	255	32	15	36
Lansing,	3			1					

Total of all Practitioners 338.

These places were taken at random, as specimens of the territory in which they lie, and probably give a pretty fair view of the relative strength of quackery in this region. I think the region as a whole, would not differ very widely from the percentages of the samples here given.

Of the entire number of practitioners, it will be seen by the table that about one in four is a Quack, about one in ten is a Homœopath, and one in twenty-two is an Eclectic.

The local distribution is also a curious point to be observed. Take the line of the Central Railroad from Detroit to Paw Paw, and it may be called the Homœopathic region, they being one-seventh of all the practitioners; while in the remainder they number only one in nineteen.— I commend these facts to the consideration of those who hear the loud boasts of this Homœopathic district, where little pill men talk and roar, as though this little patch of pillets were just on the verge of being a majority of the state. So far as I could discover, Homœopathy seeemed to be about stationary in actual numbers, and declining, if compared with the increase of population. I found a considerable number of large places where it had died out entirely.

On the Southern Railroad there is a similar patch of Eclectics. If you take from the table the places from Laporte, (Ind.) to Adrian, the Eclectics will be found to number about one-seventh of the practitioners, and the Homœopaths one-fifteenth.

The remaining quacks consisted of Botanics, Hydropaths, Root Doctors, etc., etc., all of which I have classed under the head "Miscellaneous." I found a small water-cure establishment at Coldwater, but no one seemed to know much about it. I was informed that it had eight or ten patients in it. A case of death by cold water took place there just before I arrived. A Thomsonian doctor, who had become partly converted to Hydropathy, was taken sick. He deemed that his valuable life required the potent virtues of two systems of quackery to save it, so he forthwith swallowed a goodly prescription of red pepper and whiskey, and then sent for the Water-Cure doctor to come and treat him. The Hydropath put him in a wet sheet, ordered him to drink very freely of cold water, and left him for the night. Not being very desirous to render to the bar of justice just then his soul's final account, he followed the directions vigorously. The nurse solemnly avers that she brought him two buckets of water in the night, and that he drank it all. How this is, I do not know, but one thing is certain, in the morning he "kicked the bucket," and went to settle his accounts with those of his patients, that had gone from his treatment to the other world before him. I saw in the same vicinity, a young man with a hopeless disease of the heart, brought on by cardiac rheumatism, transferred to that organ from other parts by cold water applications.

Those who watch the signs of the times in our profession, may, by help of the above table, mark one thing. The success of quack systems, is limited, localized, and interrupted by interference with each other; there is competition in the market, and *pathy* stocks must fall. There is a law of their rise and decline, which cannot be evaded. Once, patent medicines were all the rage, and enormous fortunes realized for a time by those who got them early enough into the market to get a universal circulation. This started up thousands of other nostrums-inventors from every corner of the land; each anxious to make a huge fortune by puffing his remedy into use. But this could not last. Secret remedies were no longer wonderful when every newspaper advertised fifty. In such a crowd, no one could be distinguished, so the whole fell into disrepute, and although abundance of nostrums are sold, their day of glory is over. The same principles now hold in regard to *pathies*. It is the day of *systems of remedies* now, the next natural step after the day of *single* remedies. But these are already too many to gain the highest glory,—they do not any of them go up with such eclat as did Brandreth's Pills,—and the machinery of propulsion for keeping them in motion is necessarily more ponderous and slow, but the principle is the same. If one *pathy* shines, a dozen more will spring up to share its money-making, and though they will live longer than patent medicines, their end is the same,—by multiplication they destroy each other. He that at this day invents a new quack system of practice, is a scoundrel it is true, but he is doing the world service. These are some of my hasty thoughts after surveying the field. I have dwelt entirely in my statistics on *numerical* strength, because that can be estimated in numbers, but the impression that remains upon my mind, of the intellectual and moral power of the profession of this region, as a body, cannot be thus expressed. There is in it a peculiar aspect of cool and calm strength, overlying an amount of science and attainment, and backed up by solid elements of power and influence, that make vapory nonsense of the clamors of our enemies. I can but be rejoiced at the present even, and exult for the coming future.

ART. II.—*The War with Quackery;—our Tactics.* By a HIGH PRIVATE of the Quack Killers.

I, EVEN I!—though of peaceful temper, and prone to run looking over my shoulder,—feel an inkling of an idea that—right about face and steady aim—would be more glorious than to have both friends and enemies worry themselves to death in searching for us.

But we have such fine sights on the rifles of our army, that we seldom get an aim at the flitting forms of our soulless foes, till they are out of reach on the popular side. These fine sights are of different construction, but false impressions of professional dignity are the material of nearly all. Corporal B. has noticed some of them. One is found in the code of ethics of the American Medical Association,—Sec. 3, of Art. 1, Chap. 2.—classing advertisements in public papers, with handbills, private cards and puffing of cures. We fancy this section would have been worded differently if the meeting at which it was passed, had been held west of the Catskill range. Settlers in new countries generally desire to employ a physician on whom they can rely, but often misjudge in the mode of selecting. They usually read attentively every word of the newspaper published nearest them, and expect to become acquainted with the location of the business men, through that medium. The lawyer, in the orthodoxy of his greatness, has his card in bold relief. The clergyman makes it the bearer of his appointments and address; and why should none but quack doctors record their names there? I know some do not understand the section referred to, as prohibitory to advertisements, but many, in the excess of their modesty do, and they are the ones we would order to present arms for inspection. The community find in the papers the names of Peter Perkem and Pompous Pillette, with the initials of *Miserable Deception* affixed; and Dr. Duckem has his location flatteringly described. The names and localities are retained, and if "Sally" sickens, "Simon" in haste flies,—not to inquire where competent aid can be found, but independently for those who hang out their flag. These facts are just as true in the older states, but are not as clearly developed.

Again, quacks of all sorts fire upon the people all manner of certificates of apparent or imaginary cures, which has an effect similar to sowing chaff among geese—*i e,* to make them greedy for the grain which seems to be promised.

Now Corporal B., what say you to turning some of their batteries, by publishing such facts as may tend to correct public opinion; to wit: Mrs F. would certify that she took sixteen bottles of *patent* Comp. Syrup of Sarsaparilla for salt rheum, without benefit of any sort. The relatives of Miss M. C., deceased, certify that she was evidently hastened to the tomb, by treatment in a popular water-cure establishment, and that she expressed her conviction of the fact before death. Mr. M. was slightly ill, and by order of a quack, was "packed" in a wet sheet— became appopletic and died the next day. *One* quack publishes *another* as a scoundrel and imposter—his patent a fraud, and his medicines dried humbugs. *Another* says *one* is a villain, self-dubbed M.D., and his nostrums a foul imitation; and these are probably the only truths in two whole books of puff and blast.

We ask why not use certificates thus "a la Hanneman,"—"for the healing of the nati"-ves.   EBENEZER.

ART. III.—*A Little Experience in Spiritual Writing, considered and analyzed physiologically.* By JOHN C. NORTON, M.D.

Seating myself one day by a table alone in my office, I determined to try an experiment. I had heard much and seen a little of the so-called

Spiritual Writing, and did not wish to cry out humbug, until I had fully investigated the matter, being well aware that though I might, by observing the operations of the mediums, and applying to them appro-priate tests, satisfy *myself* that the communications were not from the spirits of the dead, I could not form a definite opinion as to their real nature without testing the matter in my own person.

I had been told in one of the circles which I had had the curiosity to visit, that I was both a writing and a rapping medium. I therefore resolved to try my hand at conversing with the dead, if such a thing was possible, so taking my pen in hand, and placing it upon a sheet of paper before me, I called upon the spirits, if any were present, to move my hand. To my astonishment, my hand immediately began to move, but made no intelligible characters. I then said, if this is a spirit, write the letters A B &c. which was done until nearly the whole alphabet was written. My hand moved very slowly at first, but the movement was altogether involuntary. I did not stop here to inquire the cause of the movement, but my curiosity being fully aroused, I continued my invocations to the spirits. I asked the spirit to write its name, and at the word, in an old-fashioned hand, was written the name of B—— C——. I then asked, " is there any communication for me ?" when the following was written: " Come to Ireland, Wm. C—— is dead and has willed you all his prop-erty, amounting to £30,000." I did not stop to ask myself the question whether such a thing was possible or probable, but continued my con-versation with the supposed spirit. I was informed that on the next Monday evening I should receive a letter from the executor of the will, J. Crawford of Dublin, making me acquainted with all the circum-stances. In a short time I began to receive communications purporting to be from other spirits, suggesting that I might never receive the property after all, as the will would probably be destroyed. " Oh no !" says another spirit, " Crawford will never give up the will. It is safe in his hands." And so for my edification, the spirits would hold animated and lengthy discussions upon the subject, but soon came the announce-ment: " The will is destroyed and the property is taken." My spirit-friends, however, informed me that I might obtain possession of the legacy by commencing legal proceedings, and were kind enough to write for me the names of some fifteen or twenty different persons whom I must employ as witnesses in my great suit. Of these, the places of res-idence and occupations, were detailed with the greatest minuteness. I was not a little surprised to find among my list, the name of a college class-mate of yours, Mr Editor, (T. R. C) who I was informed was teaching in South Down, and who, you will, no doubt, be glad to learn from the spirits, is doing very well. Now came the important intelligence, that "Thomas Trumy," (the principal witness) " is dead; he has been thrown from a carriage and is now being carried home." I was shortly however convinced, that no more dependence can be placed upon the reports of the spiritual telegraphs, than upon our material ones in this lower world, for soon came the following despatch: " Thomas Trumy is not dead, he was only stunned and is now better." I should weary the patience of my readers if I were to mention one-tenth part of the communications that were written upon this one subject. The congratulations, the counsels, the plans for the future, the jokes, and the sober suggestions were without end.

In addition to these, I received a great number of communications, purporting to be prophecies of future events. I was told that the Millennium was shortly to dawn upon the world, and the glorious " Thousand Years" would commence in 1856; that before that time there would be wars, such as had never before been known. These wars would commence in Germany, and rapidly spread over Europe and Asia, and would result in the universal diffusion of civil and religious liberty. Kings and Emperors would be hurled from their thrones.— Louis Napoleon would be assassinated in his bed-chamber, and France be deluged again with blood. The Princes of the world were emphatically termed the Princes of the Power of Darkness, and that darkness was explained to be ignorance.

I was told that I must believe in the spirits and their philosophy. I requested that they would communicate to me that philosophy, and accordingly, I received six or seven communications, each covering from three to four pages of foolscap; each commencing with a series of aphorisms and closing with poetry; and I must be permitted to say that the idea, and the style of these productions, were of the most remarkable character. Many to whom I showed them, declared their decided conviction, that they could not be the composition of any human being. The style was not vivid merely, but fiery and tempestuous. I must confess that I was utterly bewildered, and knew not what to believe or say. I called upon different poets to write for me, upon subjects which I should designate, and in this way, in one afternoon I wrote more than ten pages of poetry, and that while I was engaged in conversation upon other subjects, unconnected with those upon which I was writing.

I also invoked the spirits to explain many obscure points in physiology, and explanations were immediately given. I supposed cases of disease, and prescriptions were forthwith given, with full directions for the management of the cases; upon my inquiry whether cancer was a curable disease, I was answered in the affirmative and was told that *sulphur* was the remedy.   I called for a formula for external cancer, and received the following, which was called

NORRIS' LARTIAN MIXTURE:

℞ Sulphur 2 oz.

Alcohol 1 oz.

Lard 4 oz ·

Tea and Spearmint, each ½ oz.

The spirits informed me that the two latter articles were useless in the formula, and should be left out.   The following formula was then given for the internal administration of the great cancer medicine:

Sulphur 3 oz.

Alcohol 16 oz.

Tea 3 oz.

Tinct. Thebaica 3 oz.

I called for the autographs of the Signers of the Declaration of Independence and of the deceased Presidents, as well as of many of my deceased friends, and in many instances the signatures thus obtained, were very good imitations of the true signatures.   So you see, Mr Editor, that I have had all the evidences, so far as writing is concerned, which were necessary to convince Charles Beecher of spiritual agency.   I may say, indeed, that I have had additional evidence, for he mentions nothing about this writing of autographs.   It may be asked, was I not convinced by them?   I answer I did not make up my mind in any way, until after I had taken time, calmly and carefully, to consider and compare all the circumstances.   I was engaged in writing these communications for about one week, during which time, it may well be supposed, that I was not in a condition for calm and sober reflection.   At the end of this time, I made up my mind to stop and post up, square my books and see where I stood.   I assure you, it was no easy matter for me to stop.   There was a kind of enchantment about it which it is impossible for me to describe, and I was bound by a spell more potent than that by which the son of Ulysses was kept upon Calypso's Isle.   But thanks to my watchful mentor, I did break away, and that entirely.   I now proceed to give you the result of my reflections and self-examinations.

I venture the assertion, Mr Editor, that no one has had any stronger evidence of spiritual intercourse than myself.   The writing was altogether *involuntary*, not only so, *but the mental operations which accompanied the writing, were equally involuntary.*   Almost any one unacquainted with the principles of Physiology and Psychology, would have unhesitatingly declared that neither the thoughts nor the writing were his own, and would have immediately attributed them to disembodied spirits; but my conclusions were far different.   It may be said that my mind was influenced by prejudice in forming my conclusions—that I had previously determined not to be convinced of the truth of spiritual communication; but I solemnly aver that this was not the case. On the contrary, I was disposed to treat the subject fairly, and was anxious to satisfy myself whether there was anything in it, or not. It seemed to me that if it were possible to hold converse with our departed friends, it would be the most pleasing thing in the world. But let us see how my conclusions were drawn, and what were the promises upon which they were founded.

In the first place, that the ideas originated in my own brain, was evidenced by the waste to which my whole nervous system was subjected, and the effect upon the process of nutrition and secretion throughout the body. Although engaged in writing only one week, during that time I lost ten pounds in weight; my whole nervous system was so affected that I could scarcely hold a pen. I was afflicted with palpitations and tremors, loss of appetite and constipation, disturbed sleep and frightful dreams. Involuntary muscular movements and inability to fix my attention, with giddiness and headache. Any one to have seen me would have said that I had passed through a long siege of sickness. In fact I am satisfied, by looking back upon my condition, that I was on the very borders of insanity. Every medical man knows that these are precisely the effects of long continued and severe mental exertion. Now if the motion of my hand was produced by the influence of spirits external to my body, I do not see how the effect upon my body and mind should have been so great. How should the mere exercise of moving my hand, when produced by the agency of another person, thus affect me? It may be said that I was frightened and that my nervous system was thus operated upon, but this was by no means the case. I could talk as familiarly with the supposed spirit as with an intimate acquaintance. I could joke as much as I pleased, and really enjoyed those conversations remarkably.

Secondly, I always knew what I was writing, and although the thoughts passed through my mind unbidden, I could always tell before I finished a sentence what it was to be, and often, when asked a question, I could answer it just as well without writing at all, as after writing the answer. Some may say that these were impressions made upon my mind by the spirits; I reply, it is an assumption to say that the spirits had any thing at all to do with these impressions, and I shall show further on, that they may be accounted for far more philosophically without refering them to any such source.

Thirdly, if I was requested to write a name which I did not know, I could not do it. I was told to call upon the spirit of Lewis Hanchett and request it to write its name. It was immediately written, "Lewis Hanchett." He had a middle name, says the person, tell him to write it. "Lewis George Hanchett." "Not correct." "Lewis William Hanchett." "Still wrong, the name commenced with B." "Lewis Benedict Hanchett." "Not right." "Lewis Burton Hanchett." "Wrong again, the name was Lewis Beebee Hanchett." It was then immediately written correctly. Numerous other experiments of the same kind were tried, and always with the same result; showing that it was absolutely necessary that I should have the idea in my mind before it could be written. Did not that spirit know its own name? If it did, why did it not write it without being told what it was? Here is another fact bearing upon the same point, which I have just been illustrating. In regard to the signatures which I wrote, whatever idea I had in my mind of those signatures, was faithfully written out. If I had formed a correct image within, that image was immediately transferred to paper, and in this instance the autograph was correct. On the contrary, if I had a wrong impression of the hand writing, the autograph would be wrong. If I never had seen the signature, the writing would be nearer like my own than any body's else. Hence it was that although some of the signatures were strikingly correct, a great majority bore not the least resemblance to the true one. Upon this principle we may account for the fact (if fact it be) that children and persons not knowing how to write, will make very good autographs, while calling upon the spirits. It is the idea which influences the muscles and thus imprints its image upon the paper.

Fourthly, to test the reliability of the prophecies, a record of the weather for a week to come, was called for and written. The sequel showed that either the spirits were most infamous *liars*, or else they were miserable almanack makers, for they did not come within forty rods of the mark. In fact my spirit friends never gave me one particle of information in regard to matters of which I was ignorant, upon which I could place the least dependence. I need not say, that the whole story about the legacy was a fabrication; the letter which I was to receive, somehow, never reached me, and the dead relative was only *spiritually* dead, for he is now alive and well. "Ah!" says the spiritualist, "I see you have been imposed upon by lying spirits." Very likely, but how, in the name of all that is sacred, am I to decide what the character of my communicating spirit is? I call upon the spirits of those whose character for veracity and candor on earth was unimpeachable, and relying upon their statements, I find myself most egregiously deceived. "By their fruits ye shall know them," says the spiritualist "True spirits speak of things Divine, false spirits talk of things of time." What you mean to say then is this, that those spirits who tells us of any thing we are capable of testing are *liars*, while those who tell us of something of which we shall never learn the truth or falsity till we pass to that bourne from which no traveler returns, are true spirits. But how do you know that even these are true! Does not Satan often transform himself into an angel of light! What useful information can we then obtain from the spirits. They lend us no assistance in ragard to the things of time and in regard to the weighty matter of eternity, they tear our *char* in pieces, take away our *anchor*, and leave us in the midst of a fearful storm to be driven about by the waves of conjecture among the rocks and shoals of error. But enough of this, let me not hear again the plea that there are lying spirits.

Fifthly, I have been told that if we called upon the spirit of a person still living we should get no answer. I can assert from positive experience that this statement is false. I have repeatedly called up the spirit of a person now living and held long conversation with it. The only reason then why mediums say they cannot converse with the spirits of the living is because they *think* they cannot, and therefore do not try. What does this show? To my mind it is conclusive evidence that we no more converse with the spirits of the dead than with those of the absent living, in other words, that we commune not with the dead at all!

Sixthly, I am satisfied that the ideas contained in my philosophy and poetry were my own, and one things that leads me to think so is the fact that I could recognize trains of thought that had formerly passed through my mind, moreover the style of the composition only differed from my own in being much more vivid and forcible. Besides my philosophy was unlike any other system of philosophy purporting to be from the spirits which I have seen. There were some ideas, it is true, in reference to mediums, spiritual intercourse, &c., which correspond very nearly with what we find in works upon spiritual philosophy, but those I had no doubt derived from others. One thing is worthy of particular notice. Take any two mediums unacquainted with the system of spiritual philosophy now in vogue, and let them, without any opportunity of comparing their views, call upon the spirits for a system of doctrines, and these systems will not only differ from the prevalent system but from each other, and that most materially; and this I have often remarked, a Universalist medium will obtain a Universalist philosophy, a Methodist medium, a Methodist philosophy, and so on. This is evidence that the doctrines obtained are not those of the spirits but those of the mediums.

A few words by way of explanation of the phenomena of spiritual writing. Being *careful to avoid* any *voluntary* acts, the will is placed in abeyance, and thus full play is given to emotional and other mental acts.

It must be remembered that emotions may have an internal as well as an external origin. Intellections give rise to emotions, and emotions in their turn, render the process of thought more rapid and clear. I have no doubt that much of the writing will come under the denomination of emotional action, and it may be a question whether the intellectual opera- tions which precede the writing do not in every instance influence the muscles through the medium of emotions. We have been heretofore accustomed to class these actions to which the mind gives rise under two heads, voluntary and emotional. Shall we introduce still another class, to cover those actions which are the direct result of intellection? I leave this question open for discussion. I beg leave, here, to refer my readers to the chapter on the Nervous System, in the fourth edition of Carpen- ter's Physiology, as they will find it reviewed in the July number of the British and Foreign Medical Chirological Review, where he takes the ground that there is such a thing as *involuntary cerebration,* as auto- matic thought. This idea is comparatively a new one, though I think not altogether so. I find in Upham's Mental Philosophy, under the head of "Dreaming," the following words: "A train of conceptions arise in the mind, and we are not conscious of any direction or control whatever over them. They exist whether we will or not." Here we have the same idea of involuntary cerebration, although expressed in a little different language from that which Carpenter used. Dr. Carpenter, however, goes still farther and takes the ground that cerebration may go on without either volition or consciousness. This would seem to be true with regard to the somnambulist, whose actions are doubtless the result of cerebration, although he is entirely unconscious of what he is doing. If he is unconscious, of course the actions must be involuntary, for there can be no volition without consciousness. The dreamer is con- scious of his intellectual operations, although he "possesses no control over them." The intellectual operations of the writing medium come under. the head of cerebration involuntary, but accompanied by consciousness. I say *involuntary,* but do not mean to be understood by this that the will is incapable of controlling those operations; I mean that the will stands aloof from them, as it were, and they go on without the direction of volition. The same remark will apply to the act of writing. It is in- voluntary only as the will is kept in abeyance, and the hand moves without its control. There was no time while I was engaged in writing, when I could not stop the motion of my pen and direct my thoughts into a different channel, if I chose to do so. I cannot help thinking that in my mental state, while receiving communications, there was something very analogous to dreaming, and that my involuntary muscular move- ments were much like those of the somnambulist. This assertion must of course be taken with some limitations.   What a beautiful dream was that of the Legacy!   Alas! it vanished just as all our dreams depart! The rapidity with which the long-forgotten thoughts of former years were recalled to my mind, the glowing colors in which these old thoughts, and the new ones which followed them were painted, go to show the activity of decomposition within my brain.

I said that I wrote much poetry; and this is just what might have been expected, when we consider that poetry is the language of strong emotions; and these were continually agitating my mind as the tempest stirs the ocean's waters.   I can now look back and see how in the storm of my mind, many principles of psychology were beautifully illustrated. Here, I may study at pleasure the operation of association and suggestion, memory and recollection, comparison and reasoning, doubting and dreaming, and all of those as going on without the control of the will.   Here, I may analyze the various emotions and view their connection with other mental actions.   When I look at all these things, Mr. Editor, and see what a boundless field of injury is thus opened up before me, I confess that I know not when to lay down my pen.   But remembering that I have already trespassed too much upon your good nature, I close without farther remarks.   JOHN C. NORTON.

ART. IV.—*Silk instead of Sponge for Laryngeal Peobangs.*   By J. H. B.

Having had occasion to use topical remedies within my own vocal organs, I was surprised at the apparent harshness of the finest sponge I could procure, and was induced to try a ball of silk floss or ravelings, well fastened by sewing through-and-through loosely.   It holds sufficient of any solution, and does not produce as much involuntary contraction as a sponge; hence it can be passed through the "rima glottidis" in most patients, in the first or second application to the throat, whereas a sponge often requires repeated trials, and is more painful than is necessary.

ART. V.—*Exposure of Secret Remedies.*

MR. EDITOR: The National Association, at their last meeting, had up the subject of the appointment of a national chemist, whose duty it should be to analyze patent medicines and secret remedies, and publish the result. This is certainly a good idea. Half the glory of secret remedies consists in that imaginative splendor with which people clothe an unknown and, as they suppose, unknowable thing. It is considered an unanswerable argument in favor of a thing, if nobody can find out what it is made of, and especially if the doctors have tried to penetrate the secret and failed. They will swallow such compounds with a ludicrously solemn reverence, when if they happened to know what commonplace materials it consisted of, they would turn up their noses in contempt. Such a chemist as is proposed would, by his labors, extinguish like magic the phantom glories that play around the pill-boxes of empiricism.

However, this measure, to be thoroughly carried out, would involve heavy expense, which there is no very obvious way of meeting. As a partial substitute for his labors, therefore, I beg leave to make the following suggestions, through your journal. Very many of the secret remedies are in fact no secrets at all, their compositions becoming known in various ways to individuals of the regular profession, but these physicians seeing that the best of them are not essentially different, nor a whit better than *extempore* prescriptions which they are making every day, laugh in their sleeves to see how the people are gulled, and think no more about it. Would it not be well in all such cases to publish the composition of the article, that it may be stripped of the false attractions derived from its secrecy. It would give a greater weight, too, to the opinion of physicians upon these remedies, were it understood that they were perfectly familiar with their composition, and that they spoke from knowledge, when they pronounced this, that or the other new wonder a very common-place preparation. The glory departs from patent pill boxes, in most men's eyes, when you enumerate to them, article by article, the things that are in it.

I do not know as you will consider this suggestion as worth your notice; but if you do, here is a formula to begin with, which I am informed is that of Ayer's Cherry Pectoral:

℞.—Morph. Acetas,	gr. iv.
Tinct. Sanguinariae,	ʒ ij.
Wine of Antimony,	ʒ iij.
Wine of Ipecac,	ʒ iij.
Syrup of Wild Cherry Bark,	℥ iij.

ART. VI.—*The Birds of Michigan. By* CHARLES FOX, Lecturer on Agriculture in the State University and senior editor of the " Farmer's Companion and Horticultural Gazette."

It is believed that no complete list of the birds found in Michigan has ever yet been published. Dr. A. Sager, of the University, Ann Arbor, printed a synopsis of our birds, as then discovered, in the Second annual Report of the State Geologist,1839 ; but since that period large accessions to the number have been made. Dr. Hoy, of Racine, Wis., has lately published in the "Proceedings of the Academy of Natural Sciences of Philadelphia," a list of the Wisconsin birds, in which we find between twenty and thirty more species than have yet been met with in Michigan, though many of them will probably still be found within the boundaries of this State. The geographical distribution of this class of animals, however, appears, so far as is at present known, to be essentially different on the eastern and western sides of Lake Michigan; on the latter, southern birds proceed further to the north, and northern birds further southwards than on the former.

As Zoology, in all its departments, is daily becoming a more popular study it is trusted that this list—the result of many years' labor—will be of interest and value.

A large proportion of the birds named below have been procured on Grosse Isle, Wayne Co., an island about ten miles in length, the southern end of which forms the mouth of the Detroit River, and which appears to be a more than usually favorable position for the capture of our migratory birds. The species marked thus (*) are given on the authority of Dr. Sager; and (†) on that of Audubon, in his " Synopsis of the Birds of North America." In a few cases the localities are especially designated in a note. The numbers at the end of each genus are intended to designate the number of other species which will propably yet be found in Michigan. Stuffed specimens of most of those procured by Dr. Sager may be seen in the museum of the State University.

It is unfortunate for the interests of natural science in Michigan, that those who pursue the study are so far separated. In such cases associa. tion is an almost necessary element of success. At the late meeting at Cleveland, a wish was expressed by the naturalists of several of our Western States, for the formation of a society, so that those of similar tastes might occasionally meet, correspond, and perhaps publish their transactions. No steps towards such an organization have yet been taken, but it is hoped that before long, something of the kind may be originated, as it is, we scarcely know who in the west is a student of nature.

More, perhaps, in our own State, has been accomplished, in Botany, than in any other department; next to this, ornathology has attracted attention; some slight progress has been made towards collecting our reptiles; seventeen species of snakes are known to be indigenous to Michigan, and Dr. Sager has a fine collection of our lizards and tortoises. During the last two years between 50 and 60 species of our fishes have been collected, and are now in the possession of Prof. BAIRD, of the Smithsonian Institution, Washington, D. C., but our Shells and Quadrupeds are little known, and our Insects, we believe, not at all. In the vast department of animalculæ, and infusorial forms, nothing has been attempted. Here, then, are wide fields sufficient to occupy the time and tax the industry of the present generation, as well as afford that greatest of pleasures to the naturalist, the discovery of new or rare species, while our Eastern friends are making such rapid progress in such studies, it surely becomes us to show at least some signs of vitality.

We cannot conclude without reminding our readers of Prof. AGASSIZ's visit to Lake Superior; which resulted in the publication of a thick octavo volume; nor without mentioning that Dr. Kirtland and Prof. BAIRD spent a week in our State this summer, and succeeded in procuring many new and interesting species of fishes and reptiles.

Black Vulture	Cathartes atratus 1
Hen Hawk	Buteo Borealis
Common Buzzard	" vulgaris (?)
Red breasted Hawk	" lineatus
* Roughed legged Buzzard	" lagopus 1
Bald Eagle (*)	Haliaetus leucocephalus
Osprey	Pandion Haliaetus
* Dutch Hawk	Falco peregrinus
Pigeon Hawk	" columbarius
Sparrow Hawk	" sparverius
Merlin (?) (*Swainson*)	" æsolon (?)
* Coopers Hawk	astur Cooperi
Sharp shinned Hawk	" fuscus 1
Harrier	Circus cyaneus
* Hawk Owl	Surnia funerea
* Snowy Owl	" nyctea
* Little owl	Ulula acadica 2
Barred owl	Syrnium nebulosum
* Long eared owl	Otus vulgaris
* Short eared owl	" brachyotus
Virginian owl	Bubo Virginianus 1
Whip-poor-will	Caprimulgus vociferus
Night Hawk	Chordeiles Virginianus
Chimney Swallow	Chœtura pelasgia
Purple Martin	Hirundo purpurea
White bellied Swallow	" bicolor
Cliff Swallow	" fulva
Barn Swallow	" rustica
Bank Swallow	" riparia 1

(*) The late Rev. Mr. Wright had a live Golden Eagle, Aquila Chrysaltos, taken near Toledo, Ohio, in 1851.

King Bird	Muscicapa Tyrannus
Great crested Flycatcher	" crinita
* Cooper's Flycatcher	" Cooperi
Say's Flycatcher (a)	" Saya
Yellow-bellied Flycatcher	" flaviventris
Short legged Flycatcher	" Phœbe
* Green crested Flycatcher	" acadica
Pewee Flycatcher	" fusca
Wood Pewee	" virens
* Traill's Flycatcher	" Traillii
Redstart	" Ruticilla 2
* Blue-grey Gnat-catcher	Culicivora cœrulea
* Hooded Warbler	Myiodioctes mitratus
* Spotted Warbler	" Canadensis
* Wilson's Warbler	" Wilsonii
YellowRump Warbler	Sylvicola coronata
* Bay-breasted Warbler	" castanea
* Chestnut-sided Warbler	" icterocephala
* Pine-creeping Warbler	" pinus
* Black-throated Warbler	" virens
Cœrulean Warbler	" cœrulea
* Blackburnian Warbler	" Blackburniæ
Yellow Poll Warbler	" æstiva
* Yellow-backed Warbler	" Americana
* Prairie Warbler	" discolor 8
* Maryland Yellow Throat	Trichas Marilandica
Gold wing Swamp Warbler (c)	Helinaia chrysoptera
* Nashville Swamp Warbler	" rubricapilla 7
Black & White Creeping Warbler	Mniotilta varia
Tree Creeper	Certhia familiaris
Carolina Wren	Troglodytes ludovicianus
Wood Wren	" Americanus
House Wren	" ædon
* Winter Wren	" hyemalis
Marsh Wren	" palustris 2
Black-cap Tit	Parus atricapillus
Carolina Tit	" Carolinecsis 2
Gold crested Kinglet (d)	Regulus Satrapa 1
Blue Bird	Sialia Wilsoni
* Mocking Bird	Orpheus polyglottus
Cat Bird	" Carolinensis
Brown Thrush	" rufus
Robin	Turdus migratorius
Wood Thrush	" mustelinus
Hermit Thrush	" solitarius
Dwarf Thrush	" nanus
Gold crowned wagtail	Seiurus aurocapillus
Aquatic wagtail (e)	" Novœboracensis.
Pipit	Anthus ludovicianus
* Horned Lark	Alauda alpestris
Snow Bunting	Plectrophanes nivalis 2
* Black throated Bunting	Emberiza Americana
* Bay-winged Bunting	" graminea
* Savannah Bunting	" Savanna
Field Sparrow	" pusilla
Chipping Sparrow	" socialis
Tree Sparrow	" Canadensis 3
Snow Bird	Niphœa hyemalis
Oregon Snow Bird	" Oregona
Indigo Bird	Spiza cyanea
* Swamp Sparrow	Ammodramus palustris
Mealy Redpoll	Linaria borealis
Lesser Redpoll	" minor
Pine Linnet	" pinus

(a) Killed near Owasso, Shiawassee Co., July, 1853.
(c) Breeding on Cedar Creek, Lansing 1853.
(d) One specimen can be seen at Howell, Livingston Co., July, 1853.
(e) Common in Shiawassee Co., where it breeds. Rare on the Detroit River.

Goldfinch	Carduelis tristis
Song Finch	Fringilla melodia
White-throated Finch	" Pennsylvanica
Whtie-crowned Finch	" leucophrys 1
Towhe Bunting	Pipilo erythrophthalmus
Purple Finch	Erythrospiza purpurea
Rose-breasted Grosbeak	Coccoborus ludovicianus
Black-headed Grosbeak (*f*)	" melanocephalus 1
Evening Grosbeak (*g*)	Coccothraustes vespertina ·
Scarlet Red Bird	Pyranga rubra
Bob-o-link	Dolichonyx orizivora
Cow Bird	Molothrus pecoris
Red-winged Blackbird	Agelaius phœniceus
Baltimore ·Hangnest	Icterus Baltimore
Orchard Hangnest	" spurius
Crow Blackbird	Quiscalus versicolor
Rusty Grakle	" ferrugineus
Meadow Lark	Sturnella Ludoviciana
Raven	Corvus Corax
Crow	" Americanus
Magpie (*h*)	Pica melanoleuca
Blue Jay	Garrulus cristatus
Canada Jay (*i*)	" Canadensis
Great Shrike	Lanius borealis
Yellow-throated Greenlet	Vireo flavifrons
* White-eyed Greenlet	" noveberaucensis
Red-eyed Greenlet	" olivaceus
Bartram's Greenlet	" Bartramii 2
Yellow-breasted Chat	Icteria viridis
Bohemian Chatterer	Bombycilla garrula
Cherry Bird	" Corolinensis
White-breasted Nuthatch	Sitta Carolinensis
Red-bellied Nuthatch	" Canadensis
Common Hummingbird	Trochilus Colubris
Kingfisher	Alcedo alsyon
Logcock	Picus pileatus
Canada woodpecker	" Canadensis
Hairy woodpecker	" villosus
Downy woodpecker	" pubescens
Yellow-bellied woodpecker	" varius
Red-bellied woodpecker	" Carolinus
Red-headed woodpecker	" erythrocephalus
Flicker	" auratus 5
* Yellow-billed Cuckoo	Coccyzus Americanus
* Black-billed Cuckoo	" erythrophthalmus
Pigeon	Ectopistes migratoria
Dove	" Carolinensis
Turkey	Meleagris Gallopavo
Partridge (Quail)	Ortyx Virginiana
Pheasant (Partridge)	Tetrao umbellus
* Canada Grouse	" Canadensis
* Prairie Hen	" Cupido 2
Gallinule	Gallinula Chloropus
Coot	Fulica Americana
Yellow-breasted Rail	Orty-gometra noveboracensis 1
Virginian Rail	Rallus Virginianus 1
Sand Hill Crane	Grus Americana
Black-bellied Plover	Charadrius Helveticus
Golden Plover	" marmoratus
Killdeer	" vociferus
Ring Plover	" semipalmatus 1
* Turnstone	Strepsilas Interpres

(*f*) A young male killed near Owasso, July, 1853, now in possession of the Smithsonian Institution, Washington.
(*g*) Not yet detected south of Lake Superior, but common in South Wisconsin.
(*h*) Lake Superior and Wisconsin, rare.
(*i*) Lake Superior.

* Bartram's Sandpiper	Tringa Bartramia
✦ Knot	" Islandica
* Pectoral Sandpiper	" pectoralis
Schinz's Sandpiper	Schnii
✦ Little Sandpiper	·· pusilla
Long legged Sandpiper	'· Himantopus 5
Spotted Sandpiper	Totanus macularius
Solitary Sandpiper	" solitarius
Yellow Shanks	" flavipes
Tell-tale	" vociferus 1
* Marbled Godwit	Limosa Fedoa
English Snipe	Scolopax Wilsonii
Red-breasted Snipe (*j*)	" noveboracensis
Woodcock (breeds on Grosse Isle)	Microptera Americana
Bittern (Stump driver)	Ardea lentiginosa
Least Bittern	" exilis
Great Heron	" Herodias
✦ Great White Egret	" Egretta 5
Canada Goose	Anser Canadensis
* Snow Goose	" hyperboreus 1
Swan	Cygnus Bucinator 1
Mallard	Anas Boschas
* Dusky Duck	" obscura
Gadwall	" strepera
Widgeon	" Americana
Pintail	" acuta
Wood Duck	·· Sponsa
Green-winged Teal	" Carolinensis
Blue-winged Teal	" discors
* Shoveller	" clypeata
Canvass Back (*Carooge*)	Fuligula Valisneriana
Red-head Duck	" Ferina
Scaup Duck	" marila .
✦ Ring necked Duck	" rufitorques
Butter Ball	albesla
Long-tailed Duck	" glacialis 1
Goosander	Mergus merganser
✦ Red-breasted Merganser	" serrator
✦ Hooded Merganser	" cucullatus
Pelecan (?) (*k*)	Pelecanus Americanus
Common Tern	Sterna Hirundo
† Arctic Tern	" arctica
† Roseate Tern	" Dougallii
Black Tern	" nigra
Least Tern	" minuta 1
✦ Bonaparte's Gull	Larus Bonapartii
Black-headed Gull	" articilla
* Ring-billed Gull	" zonorhynchus
† Herring Gull	" argentatus
* Glaucous Gull	" glaucus
† Black backed Gull	" marinus 2
Loon	Colymbus glacialis
† Black-throated Diver	" arcticus
* Crested Grebe	Podiceps cristatus
* Red necked Grebe	" rubicollis
Horned Grebe	" cornutus
* Dobchick	Carolinensis

(Two hundred and twelve species)

(*j*) Port Huron, August, 1853.

Besides the Pine Finch, (*Corythus Enucleator ;*) the Crossbills (*Loxia curvirostca and leucoptera ;*) Cardinal Grossbeak (*Pitytus Cardinalis ;*) 2 species of Ptarmigan (*Lagopus ;*) Red Phalarope (*Phalaropus fulicarius;*) Wilson's Lobefoot (*Lobipes wilsonii;*) Avocet (*R. Americana;*) 2 species of Curlewo (*Numenius*) and Glossy Ibis (*J. Falcinelus*) will probably be met with in some part of the State, and we may expect occcasional visits from Oregon and Californian birds. The north shore of Lake Superior will undoubtedly prove rich in Arctic genera

(*k*) This is *said* to reach Lake Superior, but we do not know of any specimen being killed there. We are credibly informed that it was shot within 2 or 3 years near Port Sarnia in Canada, opposite Port Huron on the St. Clair River. It is occasionally seen in Wisconsin.

SELECTIONS.

From the American Jour. of Med. Sciences.

Anæsthetic Properties of the Lycoperdon Proteus—Common Puff-Ball.

The number of the *Medical Times and Gazette*, for June 11, just received, contains an abstract of a paper read before the Med. Society of London, on the anæsthetic properties of the Lycoperdon proteus. The author's attention had been directed to the fact, that the smoke of the common puff-ball was used in the country for stupefying bees, and the idea struck him, that it would be worth while to ascertain if the same agent would produce narcotism in higher classes of animals. Several weeks since, he commenced a series of experiments with the fumes of the fungus, and had continued them to the present time. He found it possible to produce the most perfect anæsthesia with the fumes. His experiments had been made on dogs, cats, and rabbits, and had been witnessed by Dr. Wills, Crisp, Cormac, Snow, and several others. He had administered the narcotic fumes in the impure state, and in a clarified state obtained by passing them through a solution of caustic potass. When an animal was exposed to a large quantity of the narcotic vapour, the narcotism came on very speedily, and the insensibility was most decided, but recovery soon took place. Dr. Willis and Mr. Richardson had removed a large tumor from the abdomen of a dog that had been placed under the influence of the narcotic. No sign of pain was shown during the operation, and the animal did well afterwards. The fumes were obtained by burning the fungus. When a moderate quantity was inhaled slowly, the narcotism came on and passed off slowly, the animal exhibiting all the symptoms of intoxication, with convulsions, and sometimes vomiting. Several animals had been intentionally destroyed by the narcotic. It destroyed life slowly; a dog would often inhale the fumes for twenty minutes or half an hour, after being completely narcotized, previous to expiring. The heart's beat, in all cases, survived the respirations. The lungs, after death, were pale; there was no sign of congestion in any organ; the blood retained its red color, but did not coagulate quickly; cadaveric rigidity set in in two or three hours. During recovery from a protracted narcotism, an animal would sometimes be quite conscious, but insensible to pain. Mr. Richardson had himself inhaled the clarified fumes of the fungus; they produced in him symptoms of intoxication and drowsiness, but he did not breathe them long enough to become completely narcotized. Mr. Richardson was able to afford but little information as to the nature of the narcotic agent contained in the fumes. Many of the fungi possessed narcotic properties, and had been supposed to possess an alkaloid resembling morphia; but the subject had never been thoroughly investigated. He should only say, concerning the narcotic principle contained in the puff-ball—1st. That it was of a most volatile nature; 2dly. That it was not absorbed by alcohol, water, or strong alkaline solution; 3dly. That if the fungus was burned in oxygen gas, the narcotic principle still remained in the fumes, and produced its effect, if free oxygen was breathed with it. The fungus had been given internally to two animals without effect. In Italy, it was fried and eaten as food.— In conclusion, Mr. Richardson said, that he had been anxious only to show that a volatile narcotic principle, capable of causing anæthesia by inhalation, did exist in one of the fungi; it remained to be seen whether other fungi possessed a similar principle, and whether from a fungus an anæsthetic could be obtained that might be used in practice, with as little trouble to the operator and with less danger to the patient than ether or chloroform.

Dr. Snow corroborated Mr. Richardson's observations, having witnessed several of his experiments. There could be no doubt that the fungus did possess a very volatile narcotic principle, capable of causing insensibility to pain. As yet, however, the narcotic was not so practicable as chloroform. The subject deserved and required farther research.

From the Southern Journal of Medical and Physical Sciences.

On the use of Ext. Belladonna in the Treatment of Obstinate Vomitings in Pregnant Women. By R. L. SCRUGGS, M.D., of Louisiana.

It is not a little surprising that an article capable of promptly arresting so grave a disease as the obstinate, and even dangerous vomiting, which often supervene in the course of pregnancy should have been so entirely neglected or overlooked by the profession generally; particularly when it is remembered that M. Bretonneau, more than eight years ago, announced the important fact to the profession in Europe, and pointed out the circumstances under which it ought to be used, and the manner of applying it, &c. In the many recent discussions and papers read upon the subject of the propriety of inducing premature labor for this disease, I am surprised to see no allusion made to this remedy whatever. Even in that excellent and unique work, published in 1851, by Chas. D. Meigs, upon "women and her diseases," no mention is made of it, notwithstanding he says that the affection is so untractable as to justify the induction of premature labor. M. Trousseau, in a clinical lecture, delivered at the

Hospital Neckar, in January, 1848, thus alludes to M. Bretonneau's theory and practice in these cases.*

"Five years ago," remarked the professor, "a lady, pregnant for the first time, who, for six weeks, had vomited both liquids and solids, called in M. Bretonneau. He found the patient in a most alarming state—the affection progressed rapidly, and threatened to become inevitably fatal.— This woman, when questioned, complained of sharp uterine pains. In a primipara, the fibres of the uteras are not broken in, if you will allow the expression, and not habituated to the process, and allow themselves to be distended with difficulty; and it is this which causes the pain. M. Bretonneau thought that the uterine pains were the cause of the other symptoms, and that if he succeeded in mastering them, he would overcome the sympathetic vomitings of the patient. Acting upon this idea, he covered the hypogastrum repeatedly with a mixture of belladonna; the vomitings ceased the same day, and recovery ensued. Sometime afterwards, he had occasion to observe another case, where the pains of the uterus did not exist; but he thought that even if the brain did not perceive the pains of the uterus, the ganglia might take note of them, and reaction occur. To modify these accidents, he believed it to be sufficient to prescribe the belladonna mixture, and was again gratified with complete success. The result of these and similar cases justifies him, he thinks, in laying down the following principle:

"Whenever, in a woman, pregnant for the first time, or many times, vomitings supervene during the course of gestation, frictions should be made upon the hypogastrium with a mixture of belladonna, and the vomitings will cease.

The Professor then asks, "In what manner does the belladonna act? I confess it is impossible to determine. Can it be supposed that the fœtus, in being developed, painfully distends the fibres of the uterus; that the vomitings are sympathetic, like those which supervene in cystitis, for example? This is possible. Whether it be this or something else, it is upon this hypothesis that M. Bretonneau has employed his remedy. He has promulgated his theory, and has endeavored to confirm it by facts. The fœtus distends the uterus, the nervous ganglia takes cognizance of it, and sympathetic vomitings are the consequence. This is the theory, which you may adopt or not, but which must be admitted to conform, with marvellous exactness to the therapeutical results."

I had but just seen these opinions of M. Bretonneau announced, when I had an opportunity of making a practical application of them. My first patient, however, presented other symptoms than those described by him, for the relief of which he prescribed the belladonna mixture with such confidence and success. The result in this instance was equally fortunate.

Called in consultation, July 14th, 1848, to Mrs. L. W. D., aet. 24.— This lady had been married about two years, and had miscarried once during the time, at about the fourth month of utero-gestation. She had been attended for several days before I saw her, by an experienced and

---

*Yandell's Letters from Paris.

scientific physician, who, failing in his efforts to relieve her of a most distressing cough, solicited my assistance.

Pregnancy, at the time of my visit, had not been suspected; but upon a more thorough examination of the case, assisted by the answers elicited from her by questions in reference to this condition, we satisfied ourselves of the existence of pregnancy. I immediately suggested to my colleague the theory of M. Bretonneau, and asked, if this theory be correct, might not the sympathetic irritation produced by the distended and fretted uterine fibres react as well upon the bronchial mucous membrane—thus producing cough—as upon the stomach? He caught at the idea at once, and we directed equal parts of ext. belladonna and lard to be rubbed together, and frictions made with the mixture, every four hours until our return. The next morning we were much gratified to find that the cough had entirely disappeared, and the patient feeling, of course, greatly relieved. She got up in a short time, and continued to enjoy moderately good health until she removed to Memphis when we lost sight of her, but understood shs was taken ill some months afterwards, and after suffering for several days, was delivered of a dead fœtus, at about the seventh month of utero-gestation. Having repeatedly seen the vomiting return after having been arrested by the application of belladonna over the hypogastrium, and again arrested by the same means, as promptly as at first, I am inclined to think now, that had the belladonna been used again in her case she might have gone to her full term, and possibly borne a living child.

Since the occurrence of this case, I have had repeated opportunities of testing the virtue of this article in similar cases, and in no instance has it failed to relieve the patient. It may be proper to remark, however, that any complications that may be found to co-exist with this condition, such as gastritis, gastro-enteritis, constipation, &c., ought to be treated with their appropriate remedies; and when the vomiting has continued for a considerable time, I have usually applied cups, fomentations, &c., under the impression that the excessive vomiting itself had excited inflammation of the gastric mucous membrane. But this has probably been an unnecessary proceeding, since it would appear from the observations of some of the most distinguished physicians of Europe, that no such condition of the mucous membrane of the stomach has been found to exist in subjects examined after death from this disease. My own observations tend also to establish this fact. At least, I have repeatedly found that the most active means that could be used for the subduction of the supposed gastric inflammation, proved altogether unavailing until the belladonna was applied over the hypogastrium, when the vomiting has invariably ceased. Very recently I delivered a young married lady of a healthy female child, who, about the middle of December last, was taken with excessive vomiting, attended with such violent straining, that when I arrived, I found that the matters ejected from the stomach were streaked with blood. The stomach being also tender to the touch, I proposed at once, the application of the cups. But no persuasion could induce her to allow scarifications, nor even dry cupping. Failing in this, I ordered a purgative enema, a stimulating foot bath, a mustard cataplasm over the stomach, and used a variety of anti-emetic mixtures, but all to no purpose. I then applied a belladonna plaister over the hypogastrium, and very soon she was relieved of her nausea and vomiting, and had no return of it for eight or ten days, when the plaister was again resorted to, which relieved her as promptly as at first, and she had no return of it afterwards.

· I have now under my charge a young married lady, pregnant about six months, who suffered for a considerable time before she applied to me for relief. The belladonna here, as usual, was prompt and effectual in stopping the vomiting. She made use of it once or twice afterwards upon feeling slight nausea, but she is now, and has been for several weeks, perfectly healthy and free from any trouble of that sort. ·

M. Dubois, while upon the subject of the "induction of abortion in the vomiting of pregnant women," during a recent discussion in the Academie de Medicine, "stated the results of his experience in relation to obstinate vomiting in pregnancy. In proof that this is oftener a more dangerous occurrence than is usually supposed, he stated that in the course of thirteen years, he had met with twenty cases in which it had proved fatal. That obstinate vomiting is but the exaggeration of the natural sympathetic vomiting of pregnancy, and not due to any special lesion, is proved by the facts that at the autopsies nothing is found, and that when the process of gestation becomes arrested, whether spontaneously or artificially, the vomiting is ordinarily put an end to, although the woman may not be delivered until several days after, of a dead child, and may yet die of the effects of what she has undergone." (Amer. Journal of the Medical Sciences, Jan., 1853.)

The observations of Dubois, Bretonneau, Ems, Duclos, Trousseau, and others, seem to go to establish the fact, that, no matter how violent or continued the vomitings are in these cases, there is no real inflammation of the stomach produced by them, and consequently any anti-phlogistic measures resorted to in view of this condition of the stomach, would appear to be, to say the least of it, unnecessary. Notwithstanding my own observations tend to establish the same fact, yet I cannot recommend an entire neglect of such adjuvant measures as would naturally suggest themselves to the intelligent physician. The bowels, of course, ought to be attended to, and the cups, fomentations, poultices, &c., may, I think, be justifiably resorted to upon a mere suspicion of gastric inflammation, for the patient is but slightly inconvenienced by them, and they will certainly relieve any inflammation that may exist. But I must protest against the blister. It will do no good at the time, and prove a source of great annoyance to the patient afterwards.

I have also used the belladonna ointment in cases of painful menstruation, with apparent benefit, but my experience with it, in the treatment of these latter cases, is too limited to justify me in recommending it with any great confidence. ·

I have used it recently in a very violent case of dismenorrhœa, and it appeared to assist in relieving the pain; but so many other measures were resorted to, at the time, for the relief of this young lady, that it is impossible to determine what part, if any, the belladonna acted in giving the relief. I think, however, it is worthy a still further trial in these cases.

In conclusion, I would suggest that it may be applied much more conveniently, and with equal efficiency, to the hypogastrium, by spreading the extract, undiluted, upon soft leather, in the manner of using the exp. cantharides, than by the plan originally suggested, of rubbing it on with the hand. This plan has the advantage, first, of being more cleanly, and secondly, may be re-applied by the patient herself, at any time when pain or nausea is felt.

From Philosophical Transactions, 1852.

Discovery that the Veins of the Bat's Wing (which are furnished with valves) are endowed with Rythmical Contractibility, and that the onward flow of blood is accelerated by such contraction. By T. WHARTON JONES.

In entering on the investigation of the state of the blood and the blood-vessels in inflammation excited in the web of the bat's wing, I applied myself, in the first place, to the study of the distribution, structure, and endowments of the arteries, capillaries and veins of the part, and of the phenomena of the circulation in them.

I had not observed the circulation under the microscope long, before I was struck with something peculiar in the flow of blood in the veins; I therefore directed my attention to them, and discovered that they contracted and dilated rythmically. Following the veins for some extent in their course, I further discovered them to be provided with valves, some of which completely opposed regurgitation of blood, others only partially.

The cause of the peculiarity in the flow of blood in the veins was thus no longer doubtful; but some continued observation was required before I was able to make out exactly its mode of operation.

The act of contraction of the vein is manifested by progressive constriction of its caliber and increasing thickness of its wall; the relaxation of the vessel, by a return to the former width of caliber and thickness of wall.

The rythmical contractions and dilatations of the veins are, in the natural state, continually going on; but sometimes with greater, sometimes with less rapidity, and sometimes to a greater, sometimes to a less extent. The average number of contractions in a minute, I have found to be ten. I have on some occasions counted only seven or eight, and on other occasions as many as twelve or thirteen. Most usually, the numbers were nine and eleven. The supervening dilatations take place rather more quickly than the contraction. The amount of constriction of one of the larger veins,—one about 1-300th or 1-400th of an inch in width when dilated,—at each contraction of its walls, may be put down at a fourth or fifth of its whole width when in a state of dilatation; I have sometimes estimated it at nearly a third, sometimes at not more than a sixth.

The contractions *centrad* and *distad* of a valve appeared to be simultaneous, as did also the dilitations.

The smaller veins, those of the first and second order, proceeding from the radicals, contract, but not in a very marked manner, and are destitute of valves.

During contraction, the flow of blood in the vein is accelerated. On the cessation of the contraction, the flow is checked, and a tendency to regurgitation of the blood takes place, which brings the valves into play. Where the valves are perfect, the backward movement of the blood is at once stopped by their closure; but where the valves are not complete, the blood regurgitates more or less freely.* But this check to the onward flow of the blood is usually only for a moment or two. Already, even while the vein is in the act of again becoming dilated, the onward flow of blood recommences and goes on, though comparatively slowly, until dilatation is completed and contraction supervenes; whereupon accelera- tion of the flow takes place as before.

It is to be observed, that in determining the flow of blood in the veins (the phenomena of which I have now described,) the action of the heart is concerned as well as the contractions of the veins themselves. It ap- pears to be the heart's action which maintains the onward flow of blood during the dilatation of the vein, whilst it is the contraction of the vein, coming in aid of the heart's action, which causes the acceleration. Some- times the *vis a tergo* is sufficient to keep up a pretty steady flow in the veins, this being only accelerated at each contraction of these vessels.

The check to the flow of blood in the veins takes place at the comple- tion of the contraction or commencement of the dilatation. The num- ber of checks observable in a minute, therefore, corresponds with the number of contractions. In one case, while an assistant marked the time by a seconds' watch, I observed that a complete valve checked the tend- ency to regurgitation nine times in a minute; and on counting the num- ber of contractions of the same vessel, I found them also nine in a minute. In another case, eleven checks and eleven contractions were counted; and so on repeatedly. Though I quote these little experiments, I would re- mark that, after some practice in the observation, the eye is quite able to take in at a glance the succession and relations of the two phenomena.

The valves of the veins are composed sometimes of but a single flap, sometimes of two. In the situation of a valve, and *centrad* of the in- sertion of its flaps, the veins present the usual dilatations or sinuses cor- responding to the sinuses of Valsalva at the origin of the pulmonary artery and aorta. These sinuses are best seen when the valve happens to present its flaps edgeways to the observer.

Valves are found close to the entrance of a large branch, but distad of it. They are also found at intermediate parts of the veins. Tracing the veins from radicles to trunks, the first valves I have noticed were at the junction of the second order of veins to form the third.

In watching the circulation, it is interesting to observe the backward eddy of blood-corpuscles into the sinuses of the valves, when the blood issues from the narrow valvular opening into the wide part of the vein beyond.

In structure, the valves are seen to be a reduplication of the clear in- nermost coat of the vein, with sometimes a pretty evident layer of fibrous tissue intervening.

---

* Sometimes, as for example, into a venous branch with an incomplete valve, a retrograde flow of blood takes place from a large vein, at the moment this latter is contracting and propelling its blood onwards.—May 7, 1852.

Each vein is closely accompanied by an artery, a nerve only intervening. The average diameter of a vein is to that of its accompanying artery as about 3 to 2.

The contractility of the arteries is altogether different in its nature from that of the veins. It is *conic contractility, not rythmical.* ·· On the application of pressure over an artery, this vessel may be seen to become constricted, sometimes even to temporary obliteration of its caliber, and that uniformly throughout some extent of its course, both above and below the point where the pressure was applied; or, the constriction is greater or less at intervals, so that the vessel presents a varicose appearance. This tonic contraction of the arteries of the bat's wing does not take place quite so quickly as the same phenomenon ·in the frog's web, and, ordinarily, continues a longer time.

The pulsation of a vein so affects its accompanying artery as to push the latter, as a whole, to and fro. That the movement of the artery referred to is really owing to this cause, and not to any pulsation or rythmical contraction and dilatation of its own walls, is evident from this, that the movements are synchronous with the contractions and dilatations of the vein, and that *both sides of the artery move in the same direction,* not approximating and receding from each other, so as to constrict or dilate the caliber, as in the case of the vein.

I have not been able to observe unequivocal evidences of tonic contractility of veins in addition to their rythmical contractility. When pressure is, at the same time, applied over the vein as well as the artery, the vein is not found to become tonically constricted in the same manner as the artery, upward and downward. At the place where the vein was pressed on, a mechanical indentation of its wall may perhaps be seen.— And, in addition to this, there may often be observed an appearance of great and abrupt constriction. This appearance, however, is not owing to contraction of the walls of the vein, but to a deposit of a viscid-looking grayish granular lymph within the vessel at the place, obstructing its channel and narrowing the stream of blood. On watching, I have seen portions of this deposit detached and carried away by the stream of blood, with corresponding enlargement of the channel, and again an additional deposit with renewed narrowing of the stream. When the pressure has been considerable, I have seen the vein become for a time wholly obstructed by the deposit. A similar deposit of lymph takes place in the artery. In one case, I observed that the artery, at the place pressed on, was actually not so much constricted as above and below, though, on account of the narrowness of the stream of blood from the presence of the lymphy deposit, it appears as much so at first sight.

Having subjected the web to the galvanic influence from a single pair of plates, I found all the smaller arteries of the part in a state of considerable tonic constriction, but the larger arteries constricted in a less degree. The effect of galvanism on the veins appeared to be to render their rythmical contractions somewhat more brisk, they having been previously rather languid. On cutting a vein across, I did not observe tonic constriction of it, any more than in the frog,

After the application of a drop of vinum opii to the web, the veins were found dilated as well as the arteries, and their rythmical contractions appeared to be suspended.

. It has been stated, by an authority not liable to err, that, on mechanical irritation, both artery and vein of the bat's web gradually contract and
close, and, by and by, dilate wider than before. And, again, that in
bats, contraction of veins is quite as well marked as that of arteries.

These statements, it will be observed, imply tonic contractility of the
veins.

Notwithstanding my attention has been repeatedly directed to the point,
I have not, as previously stated, been able to observe unequivocal evidences of tonic contractility of veins, in addition to their rythmical contractility. For this reason, I cannot help venturing on the supposition
that Mr. Paget must have made his statements either from a hasty and
imperfect observation of the proper rythmical contractions of the veins;
or, seeing that in rythmical contraction of the veins, the constriction is never
to closure, like that of the arteries, under some such misapprehension as
to the nature of the vessel observed as he certainly must have labored
under when he supposed that arteries and veins of the second and third
order open directly into each other without any intermedium of capillaries.

The arteries and their subdivisions anastomose freely with each other,
forming a network all through the web, the meshes of which go on to
diminish towards the free margin. Each artery, and each subdivision of
an artery, is closely accompanied by a vein; and these veins, like the
arteries they accompany, anastomose with each other. But it is to be remarked, that nowhere do the arteries and veins directly communicate.—
The only communication is the usual one through the medium of capillaries. The capillaries, the walls of which are destitute of contractility
receive the blood from small arterial twigs, which arise from the arternal
network, and return it to the venous radicles which open into corresponding veins. These arterial twigs, capillaries, and venous radicles, form
networks within the meshes of the great vascular network, and a looped
network at a margin of the web.

The observations recorded in the preceding pages were made principally with one-eighth of an inch object-glass, and the two lowest eye-
pieces, affording magnifying powers of 370 and 550 diameter.

The web of the wing was stretched out on the object-plate, wetted on
both sides with water, and covered with a thin plate of glass at the spot
to be examined.

Appendix to the foregoing Paper.

In consequence of the dark pigment in the cells of the epidermis of
the web of the bat's wing, the structure of the vessels cannot be well
made out except by dissection.

A small piece of the web containing vessels being detached and disposed in a drop of water, under the simple microscope, the two layers of
skin may be readily torn from each other with needles, and the artery
and vein, with their accompanying nerve, which lies between the two,
separated in one bundle.

In pieces cut out of a web which had been dried, the bundle of vessels and nerve was, after tearing away the skin, left surrounded by a
sheath of cellular and elastic fibres disposed longitudinally; but in pieces

cut out from the living web and directly examined, this sheath was always detached along with the skin,' and the vessels, with their accompanying nerve, at once laid bare.

Both artery and vein are seen to have a middle coat of circularly disposed muscular fibres; but the appearance of the fibres is different in the two vessels.

The fibres of the vein are about 1-3600dths of an inch broad, pale, grayish, semi-transparent, and granular-looking. In general aspect they very much resemble the muscular fibres of the lymphatic hearts of the frog.— In none of the muscular fibres of the vein, however, did I detect an unequivocal appearance of transverse marking.

The fibres of the middle coat of the artery are not so pale-looking as those of the middle coat of the vein, are clearer, and exhibit a 'more strongly marked contour.

Second Appendix.

From a microscopical examination of the blood vessels and circulation in the ears of the long-eared bat, I have ascertained that, different from what I discovered to be the case in the wings, the veins of the ears are unfurnished with valves, and are not endowed with rythmical contractility, and that the onward flow of blood in them is consequently uniform. I ought, perhaps, to qualify the statement that the veins of the ears are not endowed with rythmical contractility, by saying, that I think I noticed a very slight tendency to it here and there in a vein, but so slight as not to have the smallest effect on the flow of blood.

This observation regarding the ear of the bat illustrates how that the heart's action is sufficient of itself for the circulation of the blood in the body generally; but that being sufficient for that only, the supplementary force of rythmical contractility of veins, supported by the presence of valves, is called forth to promote the flow of blood in the wings, which on account of their extent, are, as regards their circulation, in a considerable degree, though not entirely, beyond the sphere of the heart's influence.

I may take this opportunity to mention, that I have also found the veins of the mesentery of the mouse destitute of rythmical contractility.

From the New York Journal of Medicine.

A Treatise on Epidemic Erysipelatous Fever, etc.
(Continued from page 81.)

The course and terminations of these two forms are considerably different. In the more superficial variety there are rarely seen those large bullæ, containing a thin yellowish serum, which are so common when the deeper seated tissues are involved; nor do we ever find in this form those gangrenous eschars in the early stages of the disease, which always imply a great degree of malignancy in the character of the malady. The desquamation is also less abundant, and we do not see that distention of the capillaries remaining, which if upon the face, gives to the person an unusually florid appearance and turgescence of the features after convalescence and even perfect health are established. The degree of redness also varies much according to the depth to which the inflammation extends, and to the part of the body upon which it is located. In the superficial erysipelas it is either pale or rose-colored, presenting a very uniform tint over the whole part affected; and in this form I have never seen it assume that livid hue which is so common when the whole structure of the dermis is inflamed. When situated upon the face, the redness is generally more intense than upon other parts of the body; and in the progress of the disease from the face and scalp to the neck and breast, the shade becomes lighter, more rose-colored. It is an assertion of most authors upon the subject of Erysipelas, that the redness disappears upon pressure, and soon returns when the pressure is removed. According to my own experience this is not true of those cases in which the coloration is intense; pressure may modify but by no means effaces for a moment the eryspelatous hue except in the superficial rose-colored variety.

There is one other form of cutaneous erysipelas, several instances of which I witnessed during the epidemic which prevailed in this town, and what is a little remarkable, its seat in every case was limited to a circumscribed portion of the skin bordering upon the eyes, giving to the patients a most singular expression of the physiognomy. The dermis and subjacent tissues are tumefied, the skin exhibiting a smooth shining appearance, with a very light shade of red, and although it does not pit upon pressure, yet is evidently in an œdematous state, arising from an early serous effusion from the cellular tissues. Incisions or punctures made in the part, exude a large quantity of sanguinolent serum, which will continue to flow for some time by the aid of an occasional application of tepid water.

All these varieties do not differ materially, so far as external visible signs are concerned, from the vareties of sporadic erysipelas described by various authors in general treatises on disease.

In a considerable proportion of cases of this malady, we have a different train of local lesions seated in the integuments of the body, more especially the deeper layers and masses of areolar tissue in various regions, one of the most common being that of the axilla. Diffuse inflammation and suppuration of the axillary and sub-pectoral cellular tissues formed the principal local lesion in one-twelfth of the cases which have occurred under my observation. After the premonitory pyrexial symptoms, together with the anginose affection already referred to, the patient experiences a distinct rigor of longer or shorter duration. This is followed by an exacerbation of the febrile movement, together with sharp darting pains in the part about to be the seat of the diffuse inflammation. At first there is no perceptible tumefaction, and this may not occur for several days, so as to be distinguished by the eye; but the part is exceedingly tender to pressure, and muscular motion is much impeded and painful. As the disease progresses, the tumefaction becomes visible, and after a long period, varying from two to six weeks, an abscess may point and discharge upon opening a thin pus mingled with serum, together with large pieces of dead cellular membrane. These abscesses are many times very extensive, reaching deep under the pectoral muscles forward, and the latissimus dorsi backward, and destroying a large portion of the areolar tissue of these regions. These cases are universally of protracted duration, the supperation continuing weeks and months, and many times producing, from injury done to the muscular fasciæ, permanent obstruction to the free motion of the arm.

This inflammation and suppuration of the deeper seated areolar textures, is common to all parts of the body and occurs in several at the same time. I have seen it, commencing in the axilla, spread over the entire trunk, the tumefaction producing an enormous increase in the circumference of the body at certain points. The disease of these tissues extends often to the inter-muscular areolar membranes terminating rapidly in gangrene of the member, or if suppuration is established, dissecting out the muscles by destroying their investing membranes. I have seen the termination in gangrene take place in eighteen hours from the commencement of the attack.

In reference to the effects of these lesions, as they occurred under their own observation, Drs. Hall and Dexter remark, that "the disorganization which was the result, detached all connection between the skin and muscles, and in not a few fatal cases, the muscles and bones; and there was formed a large quantity of a semi-putrid, thin fluid, in which the disorganized cellular membrane, seemed to float, and when openings were made into the skin for the purpose of letting out this fluid, long strips of the cellular membrane protruded, resembling pieces of wet rotton linen which could be drawn out by the forceps. In like manner, portion of disorganized glands and other substances were brought away. So corroding and acrid was the fluid discharged, *that the hardest steel was directly penetrated by it as by nitric acid*, and instruments used in opening an abscess, or in detaching the membrane, were found after being laid by a few hours, to be entirely eaten through, and unfit for further use. This distructive process in the cellular tissue was unlike the gathering of an abscess; it was without any defined boundary, the skin over it assuming a deep red color, and in some cases was checkered with petechiæ, and when punctured with a lancet, bubbles of fetid gas escaped from the opening.

The lesions already enumerated, are the least formidable of those which attend this disease at various stages of its progress. The internal mucous and serous membranes, as well as the tissues of the lungs, have been the frequent seat of inflammations of a peculiar character, and where these occur, the mortality is very great.

The first which I shall attempt to describe is the specific form of pneumonia, which is a common lesion in all epidemics of this character. Dr. Sutton makes mention of it, and observes: "These two diseases have been so intimately connected in my practice, and wherever I can hear of the epidemic prevailing, that it has been a question with me, whether the last was not a pulmonic erysipelas. The premonitory symtoms in each disease were alike; the character of the fever in each was the same; it was often the case that one form of the disease changed into the other, and we frequently had, in different members of the same family, the two forms of the disease at the same time." This statement corresponds in every particular with my own experience.

The anginia is generally an antecedent of this as of all other organic lesions which occur in this disease. "After the chill, which was usually very protracted," says Dr. Sutton, "there were generally severe neuralgic pains in some part of the system; somtimes darting down the arm and side, without any tenderness of the spine that I could discover. From the pain alone, I should frequently have had difficulty in deciding whether the disease was a pleuralgia or pleuritis; however, in most cases besides the neuralgia which was very acute and lancinating, there was a constant deep-seated pain in the side, of an obtuse character. This neuralgia in many cases was very severe, and attacked various parts as one of the toes, darting from thence into the leg; the fingers, arms, heels, knee, elbow, shoulder, and the side of the neck. It generally subsided in the course of twenty-four or forty-eight hours, sometimes continuing in the arm or the foot until the limb became swollen and an erysipelas made its appearance in the part. There was generally great prostration of strength; in most cases a few ounces of blood drawn from a large orifice, produced complete syncope, followed by a profuse perspiration. The blood in nearly every instance which I saw was buffy. The cough was sometimes spasmodic at first, though not generally so; it was nearly always connected with the expectoration of a thick, ropy sputum, frequently tinged with blood. The crepitating rale at first was generally very distinct, assuming more of a mucous character after a few days; percussion after the third day, nearly always yielded a dull sound, and in several cases at the very commencement of the disease. There was generally dyspnœa, and an inability to expand the chest by a full inspiration, without aggravating the pain."

The above account of the characteristic features of this form of pneumonia, is the most perfect which I can find, and accords well with my own experience. In the cases which I have observed, the crepitating rale was mingled at the very onset with the mucous, and was soon wholly lost in the abundance of the latter. The respiration was extremely hurried, almost panting, and the pulse corresponded in frequency. It is my opinion that these cases do not proceed to perfect hepatization, as in ordinary pneumonia, and do not at all follow the order of lesions peculiar to non-specific inflammation of the pulmonic tissue. This pneumonia appears often to be a mere extention of the pharyngeal inflammation, involving in its progress the whole texture of the lungs, as well the bronchial mucous membrane as the parenchymatous tissue, and proving fatal in a large majority of cases.

The next lesion in order of frequency I believe to be that of the serous membranes, lining the various cavities of the body. Any one of these or several at the same time, may become implicated. The pleura, the peritoneum, the cerebral meninges, are each and all the frequent seat of this peculiar inflammation.

The cases of pleuritis are attended by general symptoms very similar to those above described as occurring in the pneumonia: voilent neuralgic pains in different parts of the body, especially of the joints, together with an intense pain in the side affected. The respiration is also hurried and painful, and the pulse frequent and bounding. I verified my diagnosis of one case of this character, a double pleuritis by a *post mortem* examination. The right lung was adherent to the thoracic wall by means of loose pseudo-membranous adhesions, apparently the product of the costal pleura, which presented a diffused redness, while the visceral pleura, after the removal of the pseudo-membranous productions, appeared nearly normal. Upon the left side there were no adhesions, but an effusion of a sanguineous serum to the amount of eight ounces, and the visceral serous membrane was of a dark red throughout its whole extent. The lungs on both sides were crepitant, and were evidently very little altered from the normal condition.

This is the only case to which I am able to refer, where a *post mortem* was instituted; neither am I able, from all the sources of information within my reach, to point out any other signs or symptoms which may distinguish this from the ordinary form of pleuritis.

The cerebral meninges are occasionally the seat of this inflammation. I met with two cases of this character in our own epidemic, in both of which these membranes were attacked subsequently to the appearance of the anginia and of the cutaneous erysipelas. The cases were both protracted in their duration, and the patients died with all the symptoms of effusion upon the brain. In each the external efflorescence disappeared several days before death, but not before the meningeal disease was well established.

The peritoneum is a frequent point of attack, both in the non-puerperal and puerperal states, and this is of all others the most formidable lesion to which patients are liable in this malady. I am not aware that these two forms present any striking symptomatic differences, with the exception that the latter is rarely accompanied by the anginose affection, so universal in all other forms of the disease.

In the non-puerperal state, the patients after undergoing the premonitory symptoms, and frequently after other inflammatory lesions, are seized suddenly with extreme pain in some part of the abdomen, accompanied by vomiting and diarrhœa. The pulse increases in frequency, being rarely less than 130 or 140 per minute; the abdomen becomes tumefied and very tender to pressure. As the case progresses, the hands and feet grow cold, the features are shrunken, the body is bathed in a cold clammy perspiration, and death closes the scene in from 24 to 72 hours after the attack.

An autopsy exhibits the peritoneum dark and injected, its cavity containing a thick dark serum evolving a most loathsome odor, in which are occasionally found floating patches of recent formed membrane. Slight adhesions to the viscera sometimes occur, but they are loose and easily broken up. The viscera themselves are often softened, of a dark color and highly congested with blood.

In the post-puerperal state the attack is ushered in by a severe chill, which almost invariably takes place within 48 hours after delivery. So certain is this, that in the epidemic in this town, I was in the habit of saying to females who escaped beyond this period that they were perfectly safe, and in no instance was my prediction invalidated. This chill may be of longer or shorter duration, and often a succession of rigors is observed during the first 24 hours. These are soon followed by a vio-lent reaction, a frequent small and wiry pulse, acute pains in the abdo-men and region of the uterus and its appendages, a sighing respiration, and great prostration of the muscular powers. In rare instances of this disease there is no pain whatever, no tympanism of the abdomen, and the lochial discharge and the secretion of milk continue almost to the hour of death. The progress of this form of puerperal peritonitis is very rapid, its duration rarely extending beyond one week, where the case is fatal, and a majority dying within five days from the attack. Occasionally death takes place within 24 hours, the patient never rallying from the over-whelming onset. In these latter cases the chill is protracted, the pulse de-pressed and extremely frequent, 140 to 160 per minute, the body bathed in a profuse warm or cold perspiration, usually the former, the pupil of the eye contracted, the features shrunken, and the intellect clear to almost the last moment. In cases more protracted, when the abdomen becomes enormously distended, when the respiration is hurried and sighing, deliri-um generally supervenes toward the close of the scene. In the rare instances of recovery, the favorable change is nearly always due to the appearance of the disease in some other part, generally upon the surface of the body.

The internal mucous membranes are also sometimes the evident seat of structural lesion. I have already mentioned that of the mouth and throat. The mucous surface of the bladder, urethra and kidneys is said to suffer, producing suppression of urine and spontaneous hemor-rhage from the urethra. I have no doubt, also, that the mucous mem-brane of the alimentary canal is often involved at the same time with the peritoneum, all the symptoms indicating this. The gastric irritability, nausea, vomiting and diarrhœa, all point to the gastroenteric mucous coat. In the case which I examined after death, although there had been no sypmtoms upon the part of the first passages, the follicular patches were preternaturally developed for two or three feet above the ileo-cæcal valve, and as is usual in all developments of this kind, the nearer the ter-mination of the ileum the greater the change. At a distance of thirty inches from the valve, the patches were slightly raised above the sur-rounding mucous membrane, and of a bright rose color. As I approached the valve they were more prominent, and studded with dark points, but none were in a state of ulceration. The spleen was of its natural size and consistence. The mesenteric glands were healthy.

Progress and duration of the disease.—It is impossible to define any regular order of succession as regards the local affections which arise in this protean malady. They take place sometimes singly, but more often in groups. The character of the accompanying fever, which is very gener-ally of a typoid type, is but little modified by any intercurrent complica-tions, but the latter are universally modified by the former. The anginose affection is the only local lesion which very uniformly marks the commence-ment of the disease, and is many times the only one which is manifested. In cases of this character the duration of the disease is usually short, rarely exceeding ten days; on the other hand, where the cutaneous efflorescence occurs, the case may be protracted to several weeks. After the continu-ance of the pyrexial symptoms and the anginia, for a period varying from one to fifteen days, the efflorescence makes its appearance upon some point of the skin, more often upon the face, and rapidly extends from thence in various directions, occasionally passing in succession over the whole surface of the body. While the cutaneous disease is progressing, the patient complains very little of the disease of the throat, but I am satisfied by actual inspection of the parts, that it is not in consequence of the resolution of the anginia, but upon the principle *duobus doloribus*, &c. The pulse is at this time very frequent, the skin dry and hot, rarely jaundiced, the urine scanty and high colored, often depositing a dark brown sediment. The neuralgic symptoms to which reference has been heretofore made, usually precede and accompany the efflorescence, and so general are they in many cases that it would seem as if the whole system were penetrated by an irritating poison operating upon the sentient extremities of the nerves. Some patients complain of a severe *neuralgic shock*, as if they were subjected to the operation of a powerful electrical machine.

When the case progresses to a favorable termination, the efflorescence begins in a few days to grow paler, an amendment is perceptible on the part of the circulation and excretions, an abundant desquamation takes place from the diseased surfaces, and numerous small abscesses are formed. As convalescence is established, the hair often falls out, and if the face has been the seat of the erysipelas, it retains for a considerable period a florid hue, which is much increased by exposure to extremes of heat and cold. If, on the other hand, the case proceeds towards an unfavorable termination the efflorescence assumes a leaden hue, small gangrenous eschars form and soon slough out, leaving ill-looking ulcers with abrupt edges, their bases formed of dead cellular membrane. The pulse is small and frequent, the tongue dark brown, the urine scanty, diarrhœa, low muttering delirum, and death generally in about ten days from the first appearance of the external erysipelas.

The progress of those cases in which inflammations of the deeper-seated areolar textures occur, is usually more tardy, and the duration more protracted, unless speedily terminated by gangrene. Deep-seated pains in the part about to be attacked, are the forerunners of these inflammations. They are alleged by some to be of a neuralgic character; but I think, under the circumstances, they may be more reasonably considered the result of the incipient inflammatory process. Tumefaction is soon perceptible, and after a long period, during which the constitutional symptoms continue with a fixed character, suppuration is established, not, however in the form of a circumscribed abscess, but diffuse, and involving a large extent of the cellular tissue, a description of which has heretofore been given under the head of symptoms. Convalescence is exceedingly slow, and months pass by before perfect health is restored. The termination in gangrene may vary from twenty-four hours to ten days from the commencement of the attack. I do not know that any particular train of symptoms can forewarn us of this event. It supervenes suddenly, and when no visible signs forebode such a catastrophe.

The duration of those cases in which the vicera become involved, excepting, perhaps, lesions of the cerebral meninges, is very brief, rarely exceeding five days, the termination being in death. In the only two cases which I witnessed of the extention of the disease to the membranes of the brain, death took place in one instance in seven, and in the other in four days after the manifestation of cerebral symptoms.

Prognosis.—This depends upon the form which the disease assumes, the type of fever, the age and constitution of the patient, and above all upon the extent and variety of the local lesions. In the cases accompanied by the angina alone, death is very rare. In the epidemic in this town not a single fatal case occurred. The next most favorable condition is that in which the inflammatory lesions occur upon the surface and in the deeper areolar tissues. Although these sometimes terminate fatally, it is either the result of the occurrence of gangrene, or of exhaustion, produced by long continued suppuration and extensive textural disorganizations. The instances of death, however, are rare compared with the number of cases of this character. By far the most fatal are those in which the internal organs, the serous and mucous membranes are attacked. The mortality in puerperal peritonitis is fearful. In the county of Caledonia, Vt., says Drs. Hall and Dexter, thirty cases occurred, *only one of which recovered.* In Bath, twenty mothers died of puerperal peritonitis. In Michigan City, out of ten cases only one escaped. In this town out of fifteen cases only one escaped, From all the information which I can gather, I believe the mortality in this form of the disease may be fairly estimated at 90 per cent.

Physical character of individuals attacked.—It has been the remark of more than one who has witnessed this disease, that it seems especially to single out the old, the infirm, those afflicted with other maladies, and those of anæmic appearance and lax fibre. My own experience is decidedly of this character. Out of the fourteen who died under my care, from an aggregate of eighty cases, five of them were persons over sixty-five years of age, and three others were laboring under chronic organic affections. Children are less liable than adults to this disease; and, if we consider the cases of puerperal peritonitis, females suffer much more frequently than males. Infants appear to be almost entirely exempt, except those born of mothers who become the subjects of the peritoneal inflammation. Dr. Sutton states, that " children under two years of age almost universally escape the disease."

It was the observation of my uncle, Dr. E. P. Bennett, as well as of myself, that those females who suffer from the puerperal disease, were very uniformly of an anæmic appearance, of delicate constitution and lax fibre, and I believe that in no single instance in this town, was a female of florid countenance, firm fibre, and robust health, the subject of this fearful malady.

Is the disease contagious?—This question, which is one of so great importance, although difficult to settle definitively, has yet many facts connected with it, which lead almost inevitably to an affirmative solution. Dr. Peebles, in his account of the disease in Petersburg, Va., narrates the following facts, which are worth more than a volume of special pleading. The first case occurred in a healthy young man, named Stevens. A brother of this individual had made a visit to a town sixty miles distant from Petersburg, where the disease was at that time prevailing, and returned home sick, with his face red and swollen, and Stevens had been in constant communication with him.' On the second week of Stevens' illness, a man named Petway and several of a family named Jones, all living in the same neighborhood, were attacked with the disease. The neighbors generally, from a fear of contagion, had refused to visit Stevens, but these persons had all seen him, most of them several times a day. A young woman sister to Petway, came six miles from her residence in the country, to act as his nurse. After continuing with him two weeks, she was herself taken down. She went to her home in the country and died in a few days of erysipelas. Two others of the family died in quick succession, and there were six cases of erysipelas in this neighborhood, all occuring in persons who had visited the Petways.

Returning to the family of Jones, in Petersburg, who had visited young Petway, all had the disease, and Mrs. Jones died. The body of the deceased was conveyed fourteen miles in the country for interment, at the residence of her brother. Her nephew, the only member of her brother's family who had visited her during her illness, accompanied the corpse, and on the seventh day from the time he had seen his aunt, this young man broke out with erysipelas. Fourteen cases in all occurred in this family and neighborhood, in every case the period of incubation being about seven days. The next case which occurred in Petersburg was among a better class, and in the person of a Mr. V———, a merchant of that place. The attack was a severe and troublesome one, and two nurses who attended him had the disease. In addition to these, two other persons, those who were most frequently in the sick room were attacked, besides Dr. Peebles himself. He suffered severely with symptoms of a poisoned wound created by dressing the patient's face when there was a slight abrasion upon one of his fingers. While in the room with this patient Dr. P. received a hasty summons to a female in labor. The lady was in the hands of a female accoucheur, and the Dr. merely bled the patient and withdrew, soon after which she had a safe and easy delivery. On the morning of the second day after this occurrence, the lady was seized with a severe rigor, and perished on the fourth day of her attack with puerperal peritonitis. This melancholy case had for its sequel facts of still further interest. The mother-in-law of the deceased and a young lady, a resident of the house, fell ill on the day of her burial. Upon these two had fallen the burden of constantly nursing the unfortunate lady, and both of these cases proved to be erysipelas. Nor did it stop with them, for two other young ladies, attendants in their sick room, and also inmates of the same house, long before their convalescence became affected with the same disease.

The next case of erysipelas occurred in a very different quarter of the town, but in accordance with its previous character, its appearance there could be fairly traced to Mrs. P.'s residence. It occurred in the person of a lady who had visited her during her illness, and who had taken her child in charge after her death. As usual, her husband, the other members of her family, and those persons besides who were most frequently in the sick room, had erysipelas. Her mother and sister, living apart and in different quarters of the town, carried the disease to their respective homes, where it ran through both their families.

" Setting aside entirely the question of their dependence upon each other," says Dr. Peebles, " the reader must be struck with the manner in which the cases we have detailed up to this time progressed, the one succeeding the other in regular gradation. Fully six weeks had elapsed after the breaking out of Mr. V.'s case, during which erysipelas had only advanced thus far on its course. This, therefore, it must be understood, was the manner it progressed. It is true, many simultaneous cases afterwards occurred, but never till the disease had made various lodgments in different quarters." And I may add, that in the whole range of medical literature, I know of no narration which stamps upon disease the seal of contagion more forcibly and indelibly than this.

The evidence was very strongly in favor of the contagious nature of the disease during its prevalence in this vicinity. The first case was in the person of a gentleman, who had an attack of the characteristic angina. An old lady visiting at his house, returned home, and died in a few days of erysipelas. Four other cases occurred in the same family, three of the anginose character, and the other a fatal pleuritis, to which I have before referred. A young lady, a near neighbor of this family, who was frequently in the sick room of the old lady, was soon seized with the premonitory symptoms, and broke out with cutaneous erysipelas of the face and scalp, terminating eventually in inflammation of the cerebral meninges and effusion upon the brain.

An old gentleman, in another part of the town, who had had no connection with the other cases, died of erysipelas of the arm and face, and three of his children contracted the disease, all residing in the same house.

Two ladies from a healthy district, came some distance to watch with an acquaintance suffering from erysipelas of the face; they returned home after remaining but about twelve hours, and upon the third day after, were both seized with the usual symptoms of the epidemic. It would be useless to enumerate all the circumstances of this character; the evidence in favor of contagion was certainly startling, and popular opinion became fixed in that direction. One other striking instance, which occurred a few miles west of Danbury, in which quarter our epidemic receded, is, perhaps, worthy of record. A gentleman who labored under an extensive erysipelas of one thigh, was attended by a physician who resided some seven or eight miles distant, in a locality where the disease had not prevailed. This gentleman died, and the physician above mentioned was soon seized with the characteristic anginose inflammation, which progressively extended to the lungs, producing the peculiar form of pneumonia heretofore described, and rapidly terminating in death.— Two other members of this physician's family were seized with the disease, which here again displayed itself in the form of cutaneous erysipelas.

It is the opinion of all those who have had intimate relations with this disease, that the poison is conveyed to puerperal females by the hand and clothes of the practitioner. Many facts are related which certainly tend to give strength to this opinion. During the epidemic in this town, however, some circumstances connected with the course pursued by myself and my uncle, Dr. E. P. Bennet, have a peculiarly opposite bearing. Conceiving that all precautions which I could take, engaged as I was, day and night, in constant attendance upon those sick with the epidemic disease in all its forms, would be wholly unavailing, I went freely and unhesitatingly from the bedside of a patient laboring under cutaneous erysipelas to that of the lying-in woman. During the whole period of the prevalence of the disease, I lost but three females in this state, the number of accouchments falling to my hands being upwards of 40. On the other hand, my uncle took the utmost precaution, not only to wash his person thoroughly, but also to change his apparel, before visiting a lying-in woman. The disease followed him like a spectre from house to house, and in a short time he had lost ten females in the puerperal condition. Being called again to a lady in labor, he stripped himself from head to foot, washed himself thoroughly with soap and water, changed his entire apparel to that which he had never worn, and attended his patient. In twenty-four hours after delivery she was seized with the disease, and in a few days died. In despair of accomplishing any thing by such precautionary measures, he abandoned them entirely, went from the bedside of this same patient while dying of erysipelatous peritonitis, and delivered two other females in rapid succession. Both of these did well, and from that period not another case occurred in his practice.

It is worthy of remark in connection with this narration, that this gentleman himself had an attack of erysipelas of the face during the prevalence of the epidemic, and that it was previous to, and immediately succeeding this attack, that nearly all of his cases of peritonitis took place. It will be remembered also that the case mentioned by Dr. Peebles occurred while he was indisposed from a similar cause. Is it possible that individuals may imbibe and evolve from their persons, the poison, the morbific cause of an infectious malady, even before they feel its effects upon themselves or when it is incapable of exerting upon them its specific action? This is a question which I believe deserves an attentive consideration, and its hypothetical affirmation is in my opinion as rational as the supposition that the poison merely adheres to the cuticle or to the garments of the person exposed to it.

Pathology.—No disease presents a greater variety of local lesions, and at the same time a more uniform train of general symptoms than that which I have attempted to describe in the foregoing pages. In one case we have a simple angina, preceded and accompanied by more or less constitutional disturbance; in another the angina is complicated with erysipelas of the face; in a third the previous local difficulties may be still further complicated with diffuse cellular inflammation of a limb, with a meningitis, with a pleuritis, &c. So various are these lesions, that some writers have asserted that every tissue of the body is liable to be attacked. The multiform grouping of the different local inflammations in particular cases, proves most conclusively the identity of their nature, as well as the unity of their cause. In all epidemics of erysipelatous fever, numerous cases are presented in which various groups of topical inflammations are manifest. So frequent is a succession and combination of structural lesions in the same case, that it is unsafe to make a favorable prognosis, except in the mildest forms of the disease.

I have some years since intimated the view which I entertain, explanatory of this great diversity of local lesion—to wit, *that the areolar tissue is the primary seat of every true erysipelatous inflammation,* whether occurring in the more simple or complex structures; that an erysipelatous inflammation of the dermoid system is identical in its anatomical elements with the same disease in the subcutaneous cellular membrane; that whenever the cerebral meninges, the pleura, the peritoneum, or the viscera are involved it is still the areolar component. In order to illustrate this view it may be well to advert briefly to the varieties and general diffusion of this tissue.

The areolar membrane is the most widely diffused of any of the tissues of the body, forming not only the envelope of all the organs, but serving also as the cement of their various parts, and filling up their interstices. This tissue, so widely diffused, is at the same time a continuous tissue, and its continuity is scarcely interrupted, being subject only to the circumstances of greater or less density according to the location which it occupies, or the office which it subserves. The subcutaneous areolar tissue is of loose texture, capable of great distention in various pathological conditions, while that which forms the envelope of the muscular bundles, is condensed and possessed of a much greater degree of firmness. The membranes termed serous are acknowledged to be but a mere modification, a condensed form of areolar tissue. The fascias, the peritoneum, the pleura, the cerebral and rachidian meninges, are a series of envelopes composed of the same anatomical elements. In a healthy state they all secrete a fluid similar in physical properties and chemical composition.

The hypothesis that this tissue is the primary anatomical seat of the local inflammations developed in the course of the disease termed epidemic erysipelas, or erysipelatous fever, readily accounts for the great topical diversity of these inflammations. Conceive that it is the areolar tissue for which the poison producing erysipelas has an elective affinity, and you are led at once to conceive also every location for its morbid products. The sub-mucous tissues of the throat may form the point of departure for erysipelatous angina, and this idea receives confirmation from the appearance of the fauces in certain cases in which the parts appear tumefied, pale and semi-transparent, the evident result of a serous effusion from the areolar tissue, and precisely similar to external œdematous erysipelas. The face is peculiarly liable to erysipelatous inflammation, and here the abundance of the cellular membrane is remarkable. In short, every portion of the body in which this tissue exists, is liable to be attacked by the disease. The skin and mucous membranes, into the composition of which the areolar structure enters largely, the serous membranes, the fascias, &c. &c., are alike subject to its invasion. Diffusion is a peculiar characteristic of erysipelatous inflammation, and the continuity of the cellular membrane is eminently adapted to this character.

It is contrary to analogy to suppose that erysipelas attacks indiscriminately all the elementary tissues of the body. Specific inflammations manifest strong affinities for particular structures, and erysipelas certainly discovers a marked preference for those parts of the body in which the areolar tissue abounds. The face is pre-eminently the most frequent seat of the disease, and from hence it many times spreads over the entire dermoid system, exhibiting the most striking marks of propagation by continuity of tissue, the inflammation declining in parts contiguous to the point of departure long before the most distant have become involved. Is any other tissue so well adapted as the areolar, to this progressive lesion? The dissection of a case of phlegmonous erysipelas recorded by Gendrin in his *Histoire Anatomique des Inflammations,* admirably illustrates in some points the extension and adherence of this inflammation to the minutest distribution of the areolar element. He says, " Some arterioles and nervous filets traversed the purulent deposit. The laminous tissue which surrounded the former (arterioles) was dense, red, friable, it was resolved in a soft pulp in contact with the pus, and then gradually approximated the natural state, which it preserved immediately about the vascular canal. The nervous filets appeared to us healthy; notwithstanding, they were reddish, and we thought that *the cellular tissue which enters into their composition, was inflamed; at least it appeared so under the lens; but the nervous tissue properly so called, appeared to us in a state of integrity.*"

The connection between erysipelas and a very fatal form of puerperal peritonitis, is positively established by the concurrent testimony of numerous writers not only in this country but in Europe. The hypothesis which I have advanced appears to afford a ready explanation of this latter phenomenon, the most important connected with the whole subject. The peritoneum being almost entirely a membrane of condensed areolar tissue, and having a less compact substratum of the same anatomical element, is placed by the process of parturition in a state eminently capable of taking on diseased action, and is the first to suffer in the lying-in woman who becomes infected with the poison of erysipelas. The epidemic in this town gave a most conclusive proof of the identity of this form of puerperal fever and erysipelas. Out of thirteen infants born of mothers who succumbed to puerperal peritonitis no less than five died, at periods varying from three to eight days after birth, with well marked cutaneous erysipelas, and one after a longer period, of extensive inflammation and disorganization of the subcutaneous cellular tissue, *while not a single infant born of a healthy mother contracted the disease.* Is it possible to evade the conclusion that the poison which infected the mother, was identical with that which destroyed the child?

I cannot but refer here to some remarks upon this subject, by Dr. Meigs, in his letters on *Females and their diseases.* In the forty-first letter he mentions the startling fact, that in the practice of Dr. Rutter fifteen children died of erysipelas out of ninety-five born of mothers who suffered from puerperal fever, and yet without an effort to explain this striking coincidence, he proceeds in a subsequent part of the letter, to assert that "there is not and cannot be any identity between erysipelas, a dermal disease, and the deadly inflammation of the peritoneum observed in lying-in women." If, however, we adopt the hypothesis that erysipelas of the skin consists in a specific inflammation of its areolar woof, instead of that which maintains that " it is always an *angeio-leucite,*" it would not be " absolute nonsense" to say that a lying-in

woman " has an erysipelas of the serous lining of her belly." The coincidence of erysipelas of the dermis and post-puerperal information of the
peritoneum is incontestable, and the pathological views which I have
advanced constitute them a direct relation of cause and effect.

The uniformty in the general symptoms of erysipelatous fever, has
been a subject of remark for all who have witnessed it, and it is an incontrovertible fact, that the febrile phenomena in this affection are not modified to any extent by the varieties of local lesion which may occur
during its progress. It matters not whether it be an external erysipelas,
or subcutaneous cellular imflammation, a pharyngitis, an arachnitis, a
peritonitis (except the puerperal,) they all occur *under the direction* of
the peculiar genius of the disease, and the characters of the febrile movement are unchanged by them. While the most appreciable differences between one case and another of similar intensity, are the local lesions
developed, and while these may be widely divergent, the general phenomena receive from them no special stamp, but impress upon them
certain characteristics not to be mistaken.

In the case of puerperal peritonitis, there is a special modification of
the symptoms, and a determination of locality, dependent upon the
peculiar condition of the organism during the reproductive process; so
that while the disease still adheres to its favorite tissue, it is directed to
the peritoneum by a secondary influence, which also changes in a measure the general aspect of the symptoms.

I believe that every impartial observer, who views the facts set forth
in the foregoing pages, through a medium unobscured by prejudice, will
be struck with the plausibility of the hypothesis offered in explanation
of these facts, and I leave it for close anatomical and microscopic investigations hereafter to corroborate or invalidate this view.

Treatment.—The treatment of this disease has been almost as varied
as the number of practitioners who have treated it. According to the
account of Dr. Jewett in reference to the disease as it prevailed in Caledonia Co., Vt., the most successful mode of treatment in those cases
which commenced or were soon followed by chills, was to place the
patient in bed, give warm mild drinks, such as sage, balm, hemlock,
spearmint, &c., as fancy or necessity dictated; apply heat externally, give
the patient acetate of ammonia, from ʒij. to ʒiij. every three hours
until free perspiration ensued. He uniformly applied counter-irritants,
but seldom so as to produce vesication. To aid the perspiration and
procure quiet, he early and repeatedly gave Dover's powder, applying
at the same time sinapisms to various parts, when pain, numbness or
cold supervened. " In some few cases," says Dr. Jewett, " emetics were
used early in the disease, and occasionally a cathartic at first, but the
more general and successful practice was not to give an emetic or cathartic until the expiration of from twelve to twenty-four hours, and then
move the bowels gently with oleum ricinni. Bleeding has been seldom
practiced by myself or either of the physicians in this county who have
had much experience in the disease; and though there has been some
discrepancy of opinion among medical men in this section, I speak
advisedly when I say that the phyicians who have done altogether the
greatest share of business, have seldom practiced bleeding, or scarcely

ever commenced treatment by an emetic or cathartic." This view of the treatment was entertained by other practitioners in the same section; Drs. Hall and Dexter, however, maintain that where the anginose affection is accompanied early by severe constitutional symptoms, "*bleeding*, prompt and efficient bleeding is the only remedy to be depended upon, and in their hands the only one which succeeded." They add, "that a delay of a few hours in such a condition of affairs is fatal. *Full bleeding*, reducing the action of the heart and arteries, followed by either an emetic or cathartic, has rarely failed in our hands of arresting the disease when applied in season. And in not a few cases where there has been but little affection of this membrane, but much efflorescence upon the skin, has one bleeding arrested the disease and the patient become convalescent in a few days." The authority of Dr. Sutton, of Indiana, corresponds in a measure with that above quoted. "If there has been any remedy in the course of treatment," says this physician, "that has caused the disease to be less fatal in this neighborhood, than it has in other parts of the country over which it pased, it has been the prompt exhibition of an emetic after venesection, making a decided impression upon the disease at its very onset, without prostrating the system." He adds, however, in another part of his paper, that "*a large blood-letting from a small orifice*, seldom failed to produce injurious effects, neither did patients bear a second venesection well, particularly in the pneumonia.

Dr. Shipman's estimate of the efficacy of blood-letting, is not materially different from that of Dr. Sutton. He contends that the venesection should be *early*, as soon as reaction is fully established. "If this golden opportunity is lost, and the tendency to collapse is apparent," says Dr. Shipman, "or if the fluids have become greatly deteriorated, and gangrene is on the point of taking place, then bleeding should never be thought of. Those cases tolerate venesection best, where there is violent pain in the occipital region, a full bounding pulse, and early cerebral disturbance, or where the pleura or peritoneum is implicated." He thinks, however, the use of blood-letting should be restricted, and says, that "in those cases where deep seated abscesses form, I do not think that venesection *practised at any period* is of service, but will generally be detrimental i wasting the vital energies, without mitigating or controlling the subsequent suppuration. When the tonsils or the mucous membrane of the throat alone is affected, or there is simply the eruption on the surface, bleeding I deem not indicated, and may do harm, and in puerperal peritonitis, although it has been practiced to the greatest extent by every practitioner who has had occasion to treat it, yet the success attending it does not speak very highly in its favor."

Dr. Peebles, speaking in reference to treatment, remarks that bleeding was only called for in a small minority of cases, and that its requirement in any case, for two obvious reasons, was always unfortunate. In the first place it implied the dangerous and malignant character of the attack; in the next, while it removed immediate danger, its ultimate result might be disadvantageous, since the system, weakened by its employment, had still to bear the course of the disease and eliminate the morbid poison.

It must be evident to every one who has had experience in the treatment of epidemic diseases, that no rule of practice can be established applicable to all cases. The practitioner must be governed by the age, constitution and habits of his patient, together with the circumstances attending the attack. My own experience has nothing to add in favor of blood-letting, for even in the cases of puerperal peritonitis, where it would seem above all to be indicated, success has not followed its employment nor even arrested the progress of the disease. I have uniformly conducted my treatment upon general principles, and according to the circumstances of the case. In those of an anginose character, unaccompanied by any other local inflammations, my success was perfect and unattended with the loss of a single patient. The course of medication consisted in the first place of an emetico-cathartic, formed by combining the ordinary antimonial solution, with a strong decoction of eupatorium perfoliatum, the latter to be drank freely during the intervals of taking the emetic solution. This method of giving these medicines, scarcely failed in a single instance, of producing an emetico-cathartic effect, and to afford at least temporary relief to the patient. Vesications upon the neck with emp. cantharidis, was the remedy next in order, and many times acted like a charm in relieving the excessive soreness of the throat. Frequently I applied also a strong solution of nitrate of silver directly to the inflamed mucous surfaces. This constituted the principal part of the treatment in a majority of the anginose cases; but in some in which there was a continuance of the fever after the abatement of the local difficulty, I administered freely an infusion of bark with evident advantage. In the more malignant cases accompanied with the erysipelatous eruption and diffuse cellular inflammation, I also mainly depended upon bark, with an infusion of serpentaria and mild laxatives during the first stages, and afterwards upon the more powerful stimulants, such as ammonia, wine, brandy, &c. In short, although frequently perturbative at the onset, my treatment was in the main decidedly tonic and stimulating; and it was only in the cases of serous inflammation that I departed from this plan. In these I used calomel and opium largely, but without success, excepting one case of puerperal peritonitis. In this I have no doubt that the free use of the mercurial combined with opium and digitalis saved my patient. With reference to external applications to the erysipelatous efflorescence, I at first made use of a favorite remedy, namely, nitrate of silver in strong solution; but perceiving no benefit whatever, I abandoned all external remedies with the exception of cooling lotions to allay the heat and smarting of the inflamed parts, in a case of glandular engorgement of the neck, which I succeeded in resolving, I administered bark internally, applied the vesicatory to the tumor, and afterwards rubbed with ointment of iodide of potassium.

EDITORIAL AND MISCELLANEOUS.

To Subscribers.

This is our fourth number. The good sense and energy of the physicians of this State and the adjoining region which led them to call into existence such an organ for their use, has also seconded its efforts to extend its circulation so that for a new Journal its subscription list is doing well, but at the same time we beg leave to remind those of our friends who are in arrears that it is important that they forward their remittances with the least possible delay, as nothing is more necessary to the prosperity of a Journal than that it be kept free from financial embarrassments. We have no doubt this hint will meet with a kind and substantial response.

Physicians' Visiting List for 1854.

This useful little blank book has been laid on our table, published by Lindsay & Blakiston, Philadelphia. To those who have not used it a description may not be amiss:

It is so arranged under printed heads that a physician may visit twenty-five to fifty patients a day constantly and at the end of the year have a perfect record so far as is necessary for accounts in his pocket memorandum book, of the entire number, with the addresses of the patients, record of obstetric cases, general memoranda, &c. There is also an Almanac and a list of poisons and antidotes for sudden reference in emergencies. Lindsay & Blakiston send it by mail free of postage to any one ordering it. Prices fifty cents to one dollar, according to binding and size.

The annual announcement of the Medical Department of the Pennsylvania College is before us, and shows that institution to be in a prosperous condition with a gratifying increase of numbers.

Motorpathy.

Some ass has sent us a work with the above title, advocating a new system of cure by motion. It appears that there is an establishment in Rochester, N. Y. for Motorpathic treatment of females. The author advocates exercise *of all kinds* for them but the chief remedy is what he calls "statuminating vitolizing motion." This operation he declines to explain in print but says it must be performed by the practitioner *in person*. The word "statuminating" is evidently from the Latin *statuminatio*, which signifies propping up with a stake. Now we haven't the slightest idea what the operation upon the female can be, which the quack does not like to explain, which he must perform in person, and which is compared to propping up with a stake, but it is our belief that the City Marshal of Detroit some years ago pulled down a very similar establishment, at the order of the Common Council. We advise the police of Rochester to keep an eye upon that Institution.

Dr. Drake's Discourses.

This is a little work by the late distinguished Dr. Drake of Cincinnati, who used facetiously to boast that he had been appointed too, and turned out of more professor's chairs than any other man in North America.

With ome peculiarities that stood in the way of his own success, he was beyond dispute, one of the greatest men in the west. The discourses were delivered before the Cincinnati Medical Library Association, and contain an account of the first origin and subsequent history of medical practice in Ohio. Dr. Drake was the first medical student that ever studied in Cincinnati. He came there in the year 1800, so that he had a personal knowledge of almost the entire medical history of the State. Among the early medical men of the earlier times in the army he enumerates President Harrison, who studied in Virginia, and attended lectures at the University of Pennsylvania. His military tastes however induced him to take the field, but his knowledge was frequently and efficiently brought into service for the benefit of those who could not otherwise have had medical advice. This little work is a valuable contribution to the professional history of the west.

Transactions of the Tennessee State Medical Society.

A copy of the transactions of this society is before us. The meeting was held at Nashville and was small in numbers, but we presume of good grit. The power of licensing all practitoners for the State of Tennessee is in their hands, and they have been in existence since 1830.

Transactions of the Medical Society of the State of N. Y.

This is a bulky document of about three hundred and fifty pages. It contains much valuable matter, and, among other things, an article on the registration of births, deaths and marriages, a subject now attracting considerable attention. The whole is got up in handsome style and several of the articles in it exhibit great care and research.

Epidemic Diseases of Ohio, Indiana and Michigan.

[We call attention to the following circular, and we trust that all who are in possession of any valuable information on the subject alluded too, will respond to the call.—Ed.]

At the late meeting of the American Medical Association the undersigned was re-appointed chairman of a committee to report upon the Epidemic Disease of Ohio, Indiana and Michigan at the next meeting of the Association to be held in St. Louis, in May next. In fulfilling the object enjoined upon the chairman, he has appointed N Johnson M. D., of Cambridge City, Ind; Z. Pitcher, M. D., of Detroit, Michigan ; D. Tilden, M. D.. of Sandusky, Ohio ; and J. Adams Allen, M. D., of Michigan, as members of the committee. It is desirable that as complete a report as possible be made, and the co-operation of the profession in these States is therefore most earnestly requested. Information is especially desired on the following subjects:

Epidemic Cholera.	Typhus and Tyhoid Fevers
Cholera Infantum.	Hooping Cough.
Diarrhœa.	Influenza.
Dysentery.	Measles.
Erysipelas	Scarlet Fever.
Intermittent and Remittent Fevers.	Small Pox, &c.

Any other form of disease appearing as an epidemic will be understood as being included along with the above.

The points of greatest interest to which attention is particularly invited are, Causes giving rise to and favoring the propagation of diseases or checking its progress ; Prophylactics ; influence of Age, Sex and Nativity ; Prominent Symptoms ; Extent of Prevalence ; Proportional Mortality ; Post mortem appearances ; Treatment ; Duration of individual cases of disease ; and any other points that may in any way bear upon the subject, such as Soil ; Geological formations (illustrated by a map when practicable,) Natural productions ; Condition as to improvements ; Water ; Meteorological Observations, &c.

It is preferred that reports be made to January 1st, 1854, including the previous year. If any remarkable visitation of disease should have occurred previously to that time an account of them will be acceptable, carefully designating the date of occurrence.

General Medical History, also of the *changes* which have occurred in particular districts in disease since the settlement of the country will be gladly received.

It is desirable that all reports made to the committee, may be forwarded so that they may be in the hands of the chairman by the 15th of January 1854.

The chairman takes this method of thanking those physicians who sent him contributions for previous years, and hopes that they may repeat them for the present year.

It is hoped that this appeal to the profession will be responded to, and that every member will feel himself called upon to contribute something to the general fund of knowledge on these subjects.

Contributions may be sent to   GEO. MENDENHALL, M. D., *Chm'n.*
    Cincinnati, Ohio.
    Z. PITCHER, M. D., Detroit, Mich.
    N. JOHNSON, M. D., Cambridge City,
    [Wayne Co. Ia.
    D. TILDEN, M. D., Sandusky, Ohio.
    J. ADAMS ALLEN, M. D., Ann Arbor,
    Michigan.

P. S. The committee would respectfully solicit the aid of the County and other Medical Societies; which can be efficiently rendered by members making brief reports to the secretaries, who can condense them, and furnish the result to the committee. Especial attention is also requested to the furnishing of geological maps of countries and districts when practicable.

Removal of a Nail from the Lungs by Tracheotomy. By PAUL F. EVE, M.D., Prof. of Surgery in Nashville University.

On the 20th of June, the Rev. Mr. Lane, residing near Talladega, Alabama, came to Augusta, seeking professional advice for his little son; who, two weeks previously, had placed a four-penny nail in the hole of a cotton spool with the design of making a whistle, but unfortunately in taking a deep inspiration, it passed with the air into the windpipe. There was evidence that this foreign body was still in or near one of the bronchi. The child is five years old, of excellent constitution and good health.

The usual distressing symptoms followed the introduction of this extraneous substance into the air passages, and efforts were immediately taken for its expulsion. Emetics were given; the patient was held up by the heels, and stricken repeatedly between the shoulders and on the sternum; but these means failed.

Drs. Ford, McKie, J. A. Eve, Henry and Robert Campbell were the consulting physicians called into the case here. There was a large bronchial rhronchus, distinct at a distance, in both lungs, but chiefly in the left. There were also degrees of sibilant rhonchus, alternating with the moist. This examination could not, however, be critically made, owing to the extreme repugnance of the patient and his consequent restlessness. The foreign body was not large enough to occlude one bronchus; and besides, the irritation created by it might readily have extended into both, in the space of two weeks, that interval having now elapsed since the accident occurred—so that the exact location of the nail could not thus be determined. There was a cough like some expectoration every morning, and occasional dyspnœa, especially after exercise. The disturbance to his general system was but slight; his appetite was good and he went about as a child without restraint.

After watching the case for a few days, we came gradually but unanimously to the conclusion, to recommend the operation of tracheotomy for the removal of the nail. It is proper to state that the possibility of acting upon it through the agency of magnetism was duly considered and experiments performed with this object, but leading to no available practical results. The forceps used in the case was magnetised, but exercised no perceptible influence in the extraction of the foreign body.

On the 27th, kindly and efficiently aided by the professional gentlemen above named, and by Prof. Means, who administered chloroform, Drs. Broadhurst, Dearing and Simmons, the operation was performed as follows:—The patient having the neck made prominent by a pillow under it, the intgeuments were raised in a fold over the *trachea* and divided from within outwards to about 2 1-2 inches in length. The dissection was then cautiously continued upon the median line with the handle of the knife forceps and director; passing the platisma myoides (not recognized however,) cellular tissue and adipose matter; between the sterno-hyoid and sterno-thyroid muscles; and opening the trachael fascia described by Porter of Dublin, the windpipe was exposed at about its 5th cartilaginous ring. At this point of the operation the two middle thyroid veins, running directly from the thyroid body or gland as it is commonly called, into the venæ innomentæ were greatly exposed, and at every struggle of the patient or difficult respiration would become largely distended. By means of blunt hooks all the soft parts were carefully held aside, and no important vessel was injurrd. The whole bleeding was probably less than an ounce, and proceeded from the first or superficial incision. It was quite a bloodless operation, considering the region involved, and may be attributed to acting rigidly upon the principles to keep directly upon the median line; to have the cutting edge of the knife always turned upwards; and to be chary even with its point in laying here the trachea. Thus fully exposed, a hook secured the windpipe, while some three or four of its rings were rapidly slit open with a small knife, turning its back as much as possible towards the vertibræ. Trousseau's tracheal forceps were now introduced, and between its expanded blades other curved forceps were passed down into the right bronchus. These latter instruments were made in this city by Mr. J. D. Smith; are of different lengths, varying from 3 to 7 inches in their narrow legs, and have considerable curvature near the handles or rings. Each introduction of them was attended with slight spasm, but which the subsequent manipulation (gentle of course,) in the bronchial tubes did not increase.— Closed and used as a probe, these forceps were carried into the right bronchus, but their handles coming in contact with Trousseau's instrument holding up the wound, I could not determine if the nail had been touched. Calling for a probe, Dr. H. Campbell passed it down and readily detected it on the left side, where it was at once seized and extacted with the forceps.— From my position to the right of the patient, and the hand sustaining his head being placed under the right side of his chin, the right bronchus was easiest penetrated. To find the object searched for, I had to request the assistant holding the patient's head to withdraw his hand, while I passed my right hand carrying the forceps to the right of the neck. I am thus particular to prove that the nail must have been in the *left* bronchus and not in the right, as is almost invariably the case with extraneous substances passing down the windpipe, especially if they be, like this one, ponderous. The body removed could not have been more than two inches below the top of the sternum; was at an angle with the perpendicular line; and situated more anteriorly than I expected to find it. Its head was downwards, and is very rough. It measures nearly an inch and a half in length and is slightly oxydized.

The patient was about half an hour on the table, some portion of which time was consumed waiting for all bleeding to cease before the trachea was opened, and also by his vomiting freely; the stomach having been filled by misplaced kindness to prepare him for the operation, and contrary to all expeciation. For success in the case, I am greatly indebted to *chloroform*, which was admirably regulated to an extent sufficient for all purposes, yet never once producing stertorous breathing—to Dr. Ford for insisting that the extracting forceps should be curved greater than I intended—to Dr. Henry Campbell for so readily touching the nail with a probe—and to Trousseau's trachael for keeping the parts dilated when cut open. Climate and season too, no doubt had their influence over the happy result. The operation was performed in an open piazza with the thermometer at 84°.

TO BE CONTINUED.

THE

PENINSULAR
JOURNAL OF MEDICINE
AND THE COLLATERAL SCIENCES.

| VOL. I. | NOVEMBER, 1853. | NO. V. |

ORIGINAL COMMUNICATIONS.

ART. I.—*Are Typhus and Typhoid Fevers Identical?* Being a
Report read by Z. PITCHER, M. D., before the Detroit Medical
Society, and published by its request.

I do not design this evening, merely by the collation of authorities, to
attempt the settlement of the question whether Typhus and Typhoid
fevers are identical, or the equally difficult task of showing, by the same
process, that they are generically or specifically distinct, independent in
origin, propagated by different laws, amenable in certain stages to opposite methods of treatment, but intend rather to give the result of my
own observations on the subject under discuss, made at the bed-side of
the sick, in the hovels of the needy and afflicted, and to draw, if need be,
from other observers, such sketches of the aspects of these forms of disease, as will ensure fidelity in the description of phenomena which may
be peculiar to one or the other, or common to both.

My first opportunity for practically studying the subject of Typhus
Fever, occurred at Fort Brady in this State. This fort is a simple rec-
tangular stockade, built on the bank of the river, close to the foot of the
falls or Sault de Ste. Marie. The quarters are of wood, arranged in the
form of a square, and rest directly upon the ground, having been constructed expressly with a view to exclude the cold of a northern winter.
The troops were abundantly supplied with wholesome provisions, had
fresh beef twice a week, and the only fatigue service performed by them,

except by a small party detached for lumber, was in procuring their own fuel, which was obtained at no great distance from the fort. Large bodies of snow fell this season (1826 and 1827) as early as November, and continued till late in the spring. The winter was a cold one, the thermometer many times sinking below zero, and on one occasion, the mercury congealed in the bulb. These degrees of cold made it necessary to take the sentinels off their posts, and prevented that attention to personal cleanliness by bathing, which the soldier is required, at less inclement periods of the year to give. Notwithstanding we enjoyed so many circumstances favorable to health, Typhus Fever broke out in the autumn of 1826, and continued through the winter of 1827. Our first cases occurred in the family of an officer, which occupied quarters on the east side of the square. This family, very late in the season, after losing one of its number, left the post. One of its members, a child, sickened on the road—it suffered for a long time, but ultimately recovered. This was the only instance in which the disease was communicated by occupants of the fort from the sick to the well. The range of quarters on the south side of the fort, exclusively appropriated to officers and constructed similarly to those in which the disease commenced, produced no case of fever during the winter. The grounds on which the infected quarters were erected were naturally a little lower than the other sides of the square, and had been filled up in 1822, when the work was built. In other respects, there was no appreciable difference in the quarters infected, and those that were not, unless it be in the fact that the uninfected quarters fronted the river, and the others rested upon it perpendicularly.

At that time the commerce of the Sault consisted in the shipment of a few packs of furs, a few barrels of white fish, and a few tons, in mococks, of maple sugar, and the receipt of the annual supplies for the troops, and the pork and flour necessary to feed some two or three hundred citizens and Indians. I make this allusion to the commerce of the place with a view to exclude from the mind the idea that the disease could have been introduced through the channels of trade, for there was at that time no arrivals, except from the ports of Buffalo and Detroit, and those places on Lake Erie whence the commissary and Quarter-master's stores were received. I ought, however, to remark here, that late in the fall, a large family arrived from the colony of Lord Selkirk, on the Red River of the north, in which the fever broke out about the time the first cases originated inside the fort. Between this family and that of the officer's first affected, there had been no communication, as could be ascertained.

As the season advanced the disease extended to the soldiers' barracks, and prevailed most among the men of (B) company, which occupied rooms at the north end of the same range of quarters in which it first appeared.

There was no instance, among those who remained at the post, where the fever was communicated by those under treatment, either to the nurses or other occupants of the same apartments. All the cases in the family from Selkirk's colony, as well as the three in the family of Captain C——, became sick about the same time, as if they had originated in a commom cause, the influence of which was limited to the residences of those who fell sick. Those originating in the soldiers' quarters were sent immediately to the Hospital for treatment, from whence there were no cases of its extension by contagion. This immunity from the ordinary effects of the contagion of typhus, we ascribed to the measures adopted to remove the fomites by ventilation, ablution, and the use of disinfectants. The company barracks having been constructed with a view to exclude the rigors of a northern winter, and being occupied by so many persons, particularly at night, could not be so thoroughly purified. The physiognomy of this disease was so strikingly distinct from the Remittent Fever I had seen on the Saginaw River in 1823, appearing in the midst of hyperborean snows, as it did, that it made a strong impression upon my mind, but not more ineffaceable than the evident fact, that the materies morbi which produced this extraordinary picture, consisted in emanations from bodies still in apparent health.

We had no evidence, if we except the case before mentioned, in the strict sense of the word, of the contagiousness of this disease. Sufficient proofs having been furnished in its history, in other countries and climates, of its ability to propagate itself, and which should also be inferred from the manner of its origination at the present time, we leave the question of contagion untouched, believing it settled. The cases were individually tedious. One continued sixty days; and this was the only one in which there was any special local affection of severity or any particular sign of dothinenteritic inflammation, which was confined to the pharynx. There were no opportunities afforded us for making post mortem examinations. Only two of our cases terminated fatally. One an aged female from the Pembina settlement, whose death was occasioned apparently by the sloughing of a blistered surface, an epispastic having been applied to arouse her from a state of coma, and the other, a child, which I now think was literally starved to death. The gentleman (now deceased) who was associated with me in the treatment of this case, had been a pupil of the venerated Dr. Nathan Smith, and his plan of low diet, and cold water, was carried to such an extent, that death ensued from starvation. Two others, in the same family, on the verge of dissolution, were then put upon the use of wine and animal food, with such an immediate change in their symptoms, and followed by so rapid a convalescence, that we felt conscious of having made a fatal mistake. There was nothing in the symptoms of those cases which terminated fatally, or of those which recovered that led me to suspect the existence of organic lesion in any portion of the alimentary canal. This, of course, is mere opinion.

I have given this general account of the Typhus of Fort Brady in advance of the description which I propose to copy from my memoranda, for the purpose of bringing into closer proximity the parthognomy, if the term may be applied to morbid expression, of this disease, of the ship fever of 1848 and 1851, and the typhoid fever of the present time. The treatment of the cases in the family of Captain C—— was dictated by my colleague up to the time of the death of the member above alluded to, consequently, I have no notes of the symptoms which they exhibited in the first stages of their illness. At this time the removal of my colleague fromt he post left me in charge of the Hospital, and rendered it necessary for me to assume the charge of the sick. From this time I took personally the oversight of all the cases of disease which occurred at the Sault that winter, and can consequently, from my own observation, speak of the manner of their approach, of their period of incubation, their physiognomy, when fully developed, the duration and termination of the individual cases, but not so explicitly of the anatomical character of this disease as I could wish. From this time, all the cases which came from the company quarters, if we date their sickness from the period of their admission into the Hospital,had had a protracted period of incubation,marked by a feeling of muscular languor and mental torpidity, aversion to food and pain in the head or vertego. In most cases, as this period passed away, slight rigors would precede the more perfectly formed stages of the fever, which were never marked by such decided chills as characterize the advent of diseases ushered in by the agency of some accidental or suddenly disturbing cause. After this, the heat of the body increased and the pain of the head became more severe. The organs of secretion being embarrassed either primarily through the condition of the blood or from a paralyzed state of the nerves of organic life, the urine would become scanty and turbid, the alvine dejections dark and fœtid, and the expectoration dark and offensive. When the disease was fully developed the skin would become more dry and hot, giving to the hand a sensation of pungency—the pulse frequent and feeble, being more than a hundred per minute,—the respiration embarrassed owing to the rapid movements of the heart and the imperfect manner in which the mucous membrane performed its function as an excreting surface. The mucous surface of the lungs coinciding in action with the parched and heated skin, caused the tongue and teeth to be covered with sordes, and the fauces dry and disordered. The pain in the head so usually a premonitory indication of the approach of the disease, was soon followed by pains in the back and limbs, indicative of a general disturbance of the nervous function; and the mental hebetude which characterized an earlier stage, was soon followed by intellectual confusion, delirium and coma.   Deafness supervened in some cases, in others a morbid sensibility of the retina and of the skin, and subsultus tendium was a common symptom; but what most particularly attracted the eye of the physician was the general aspect or physiognomy of the patient—the Hippocratic expression and the rufous hue of the cheek, followed in a majority of cases by a maculated state of the general surface, which obeyed no special law, as to the time of its appearance.   This is a general view of the St. Mary's typhus.   A daguerreotype of an individual case might serve to fix the phenomena more permanently in the mind.

The famine of Ireland and the crowded state of the emigrant ships arriving in New York and Quebec in the summer of 1848, brought us a modified, yet undoubted form of Typhus Fever.

The coincidence of want and the impure air of a crowded ship-hold shortened sensibly the period of incubation and increased the tendency to diarrhœa.   The perturbations of the system, occasioned by atmospheric exposure and errors in diet on landing in America, developed a form of Bronchitis and an intestinal irritation analagous to Dysentery, some of which collapsed like cholera.   Such cases, owing to the sympathies of the skin with the mucous surface, were attended with a more decided eruption and terminated fatally after a briefer existence.   As should be expected from the nature of the exciting causes, we had more emphatic intestinal meteoration, more violent delirium, more frequent epistaxis and more evidences of arachnoid irritation and effusion than in 1827.   Nurses contracting the disease this season had decided chills, more perfectly developed and active febrile symptoms, and a wilder state of delirium, so much so as to require venesection to mitigate the violence of the cerebral excitement.

Although not written for that purpose especially, the foregoing remarks show the importance in our attempts to settle the pathological character of diseases analogous or identical, of looking more to the etiology and less exclusively to the phenomena presented at the dead house.

During the winter of 1847 and 1848 the inhabitants of Michigan were visited by an epidemic known as the Brain or Spotted Fever, which proved to be an erysipelatous affection of the cerebro-spinal meninges, from which the population of Detroit suffered more than their rural neighbors.

In 1849, the cholera was epidemic in Detroit, and in a milder degree in 1850.

The summer of 1851 brought us other cases of typhus modified by erysipelas.   The general aspect of the disease did not differ from the fever of 1848. Some of the cases took on the appearance of brain fever and terminated suddenly. In others convalescence was protracted by erysipelatous inflammation of the parotid glands and of the parts subjected to pressure, as around bed sores and on the elbows.

In 1852, the cases of cholera may be said to have been sporadic, but of unusual violence. Some of these, where reaction took place, were followed by typhoid fever. Cases of cholera and typhoid fever would sometimes occur in the same house, particularly in the German part of the city, and in the latter part of the autumn, as the cholera disappeared Typhoid Fevers became more common, and have continued to occur up to the present time.

This leads us to the other part of our subject, the consideration of Typhoid Fever.

Before proceeding, however, I will take occasion to remark, that from the time I left Fort Brady in 1828, I had seen nothing more of Typhus Fever till the summer of 1848, when I met with it at this place; and that although between those dates, I had seen much of fever in all its grades of intensity, in various climates, at Fort Gratiot in 1829, at Fort Gibson on the Arkansas River and the lower tributaries of the Mississippi in 1830, 1831, 1832, and 1833, at the emboucheures of York and James Rivers, in Virginia, in 1834 and 1835, and at this place again in 1837, I had never seen its analogue, the Typhoid Fever, till the adynamic epidemic, known as the Brain Fever of 1847 and 1848 had passed over our country, leaving its trail in the air, and lending its livery to every form of disease which has followed in its wake down to the present time. Having seen so much of the diseases peculiar to large sections of the country, and having noticed how many of them are common to all, varying only in degree, without meeting either with Typhus Fever or the disease I now recognize as Typhoid Fever, I not only embraced the opinion of Dr. Dewers as to the northern origin of Typhus Fever, but had been led gradually to believe, that the only cases of Typhoid Fever to be found were such cases of synochus as had been neglected in the early stage, and become adynamic in consequence of the retention in the circulation of the effete materials of the tissues, which should have been liberated by the chemistry of the organism.

Typhoid Fever, in its intense form and when fully developed, you will find graphically described by Louis. For the sake of brevity I refer you to that elegant work, "Louis on Typhus," for a more perfect sketch of the physiognomy of Typhoid Fever than I could possibly give you. I shall, therefore, give you only such brief notes on this head as will enable you to comprehend the views I entertain on the question for the evening, "Are Typhus and Typoid Fever identical?"

The father of medicine seemed to comprehend the existence of a pervading atmospheric agency, which at the time, gives character to the diseases of a season and may continue to be felt for several succeeding years. This Sydenham spoke of, under the name of intemperament of the air; and such an influence, occult though it be, has been recognized under different names down to the present day. So obvious was the effect of such an agency in the time of Dr. Rush, that from the omnipresence of its effects, he no doubt evolved the idea of the unigenous origin of disease, and hence his conception of the unity of its character. Such diatheses move in cycles, of which we had the beginning of one in 1847, the influence of which we yet see in the peculiar tone and type of our diseases of to-day. Hence, in the order of time, there appears an evident periodicity in the return of some of our graver epidemics, as we have seen in the case of the spotted fever of New England and New York, in 1811 to 1814, and again in this region in 1847 and 1848, on both of which occasions it has been followed by Typhoid Fever, of which it is in fact the most malignant form.

The Epidemic Erysipelas and the Epidemic Cholera having faded away and left their place to be occupied by Typhoid Fever, by Dengue, or Break Bone Fever, whichever name you may choose to call it by, it would be profitable, if we had the time and requisite ability, to proceed to show how the types of disease in the first place blend, and then gradually become converted, one into the other. Nosologists in their attempts to fix the character of genera, to limit the boundary of species, and thereby give symmetry to their plans of arrangement, have looked to the plan of creation for their types, expecting to find the same permanency of order, the same fidelity to the law of procreation in the morbid as in the natural world, and have made insufficient allowance for the co-operation of two or more disturbing causes, acting at the same time, upon the human organism. We all know from daily observation, that in districts highly charged with malaria the fever of Catarrh, of Small Pox, of Measles and of Scarlatina is sensibly remittent; and that even the Hectic of Phthisis is modified by its presence, but not enough so in these particular cases to establish the doctrine of hybridity. Still, the analogies in the two cases should lead us to suspect, what we think observation confirms, that nosological hybrids result from the co-equal operation of causes which if left to act singly would produce far different results. Of this kind of mixed progeny we believe Typhoid Fever to be one, its paternity on one side being traceable to malaria, hence its tendency to intermit in its first stages, and on the other to an epidemic meteoration which has changed the tone of disease, not only in this place, but throughout the country, in a striking manner, for the last ten years. I would gladly enlarge upon this topic, but feel restrained by the shortness of your sessions, and pass from this part of my subject to a description of Typhoid Fever as at present to be seen in Detroit.

Firstly, of its period of incubation. This is notably shorter than the forming stage of Ship or Typhus Fever. After a period, varying from one day to one week, in which the patient has a feeling of languor, with pains in the head and loins and a sense of fullness in the hypochondriac regions or else a slight diarrhœa, he will be seized with a very decided chill or else a succession of rigors; nausea and vomiting occur, the diarrhœa becomes more painful, and perhaps passing into a form of dysentery, either with or without tenesmus, during which time the body grows hot, with an increase of pain in the head and bones, and thirst and restlessness. This is his condition the first day after the occurrence of chills. Then there is an exacerbation, with recurrence perhaps of rigors, with increase of heat, extending to the extremities, which may have remained till this time cold, calor mordax, dry and dark tongue. The time taken to confirm the grade of reaction which ensues, varies in each individual case, after that, the tendency to intermit is not so perceptible, except in the milder cases. After the heat has become general, then we have burning of the hands and feet, a rose colored rash appears about the neck and chest, regulated in quantity by the degree of bronchial irritation. The patient coughs, has apistaxis, and sometimes bloody sputa. The tongue becomes more dry and dark, the teeth incrusted with sordes, the pulse smaller and more frequent, delirium passes into coma, with deafness and subsultus tendinum, the discharges take place involuntarily, the urine being scanty and ammoniacal and the stools ochreous and liquid. This is the general concourse of symptoms, not precisely their order of occurrence.

If the skin of the patient is examined after the chills, there will be seen a congested state of the capillaries, indicated by a livid color of the extremities, which deepens to a purple about the neck. Pressure upon the back of the hand leaves a white spot into which the blood slowly returns, and on the chest a similar displacement of the blood from the skin will be succeeded by a stripe of crimson, which increases with the intensity of the febrile excitement, and in many cases looks more like scarletina than the maculae of Typhus Fever. From the symptoms as well as from the recognized existence of cutaneo-intestinal sympathies, we believe that a similarly congested state takes place in the mucous membrane of the lungs and alimentary canal, owing no doubt to a paralysis of the nerves of organic life. The diarrhœa and vomiting are probably attributable to the sensibility remaining in the colon and duodenum which are in part supplied with nerves coming from the dominion of the encephalon. The dothinenteritis which takes place in a later stage of this disease and gives origin to its severer symptoms, as well as to the morbid changes in the alimentary canal, considered by many as the anatomical seat of Typhoid Fever, is the natural result of the phenomena we have just been considering, unless appropriate measures are adopted at an early period, to restore the action of the skin and the functions of the alimentary mucous surface. How this is done we will speak of hereafter.

Having spoken of the periodic tendency in the early stage of Typhoid Fever, I ask leave to introduce here a case or two illustrative of that tendency, as well as by a reference to treatment, to show that its course can be abridged by remedies not adapted to Ship or Typhus Fever.

W——d, a sailor, was sent to St. Mary's Hospital the fourth day of his attack, having chilled twice, without a solution of the paroxysm of fever by perspiration, after either. On the day of admission he had a pungently hot skin, with a crimson rash about the neck and chest, his pulse was small and frequent, without force, his tongue was covered with a dry, short, but not very brown coat, he complained of head-ache, pain in the limbs and back, and tenderness over the right hypochondriac space. His bowels were confined and urine scanty.

4th day—prescription, Sulphate Quinine jj gr., Hydrarg. cum creta j gr., every four hours, warm drinks, hot applications to the extremeties, and a blister over the region of the liver.

5th day—Heat of the body more equal, but not diminished. The feet have become warm, but he is deaf and comatose. Prescription continued.

6th day—Medicine has effected the bowels. Evacuations made in bed. Pulse rather fuller. Other symptoms much the same. Continue prescription.

7th day—Medicine still operating. Is conscious—will protrude the tongue if the act is performed before him, to indicate what we wish him to do. Skin is soft and pulse less frequent. As the stools are yet dark and not too liquid, give him Rhei and Magnesia.

8th day—Cathartic has operated well. Patient hears and answers questions, briefly. Tongue and skin moist. Rash disappearing. Urine more copious. Prescribe spirits mendererus.

9th day—Ward is convalescent.

Lest the question might be raised whether the foregoing case was not one of pernicious miasmatic fever, I add another, attended with haemorrhagic symptoms:

Cherodot, a laborer, as we learned after he became conscious, was admitted on the eighth day of his illness. He did not recollect having been much unwell before he was seized with a violent chill, which was followed by a daily exacerbation of fever up to the time he lost his hearing and recollection, three days before he came to the hospital. When I first saw him, he had epistaxis, bloody expectoration, discharges of blood from the bowels and occasional vomiting. His pulse was small and frequent. His head and body hot, but legs and feet and hands were cold. He was delirious and inclined to rise from his bed. He had a dry and brown tongue and the crimson eruption upon his chest.

9th day.—Directions for the attendent—Sponge the limbs with tincture of capsicum—make cold applications to the head and hot ones to the feet, and lay a large epispastic over the stomach and liver. Give jj gr. Quinine, j gr. Gum camphor and j gr. Hydrarg. cum creta, every three hours and let him drink hot mint tea.

This plan of treatment was continued till the eleventh day of fever, when the skin relaxed, the vomiting and loss of blood from the mucous surface of the nose, lungs and intestines had ceased, and the rash began to disappear. Under the use of Mendererus' Spirit and Wine whey, he convalesced rapidly, and in another ten days returned to his labor.

The following case gives a veiw of one of the modifying circumstances in this grade of fever, if it be not in fact the cause of its adynamic character.

H—— M—— had a chill only two days before admission, at which time there was a stronger scarlet hue than usual in these cases, of the face, neck and chest, with intense heat of the skin, dry cough, vomiting and slight diarrhœa, with scanty and high colored urine. His pulse small and very frequent, with slight epistaxis—tongue red and dry and great tenderness over the stomach and liver—violent pain in the limbs and head, with slight delirium and subsultus tendinum.

3d day.—As the cutaneous congestion seemed already to be passing away, I ordered an epispastis to be applied over the stomach and liver and that he should take jjj gr. Carbonate of ammonia, j gr. Hydrarg. cum creta and j gr. Gum camphor every three hours with tepid drinks.

4th day—Vomiting is relieved, but he passed a restless night.

5th day.—Evacuations have improved, delirium succeeded by coma. Continue prescription and apply a blister to the nape of the neck.

6th day—Symptoms every way relieved by the appearance of an erysipelatous eruption, extending from the blister on the neck to the one on the abdomen. From this time he was convalescent.

The case of Conrad Scanlon gives another phase of this epidemic.

When brought to the hospital his surface was very livid and cold, except about the head and thorax, where the color deepened to crimson. He had no diarrhœa, but vomited freely; had hiccough, and the kind of coma of a man heavily drunk. His pulse was scarcely to be felt at the wrist. Tongue coated, but not yet dry. No apparent secretion of urine. Showed signs of pain when pressure was made over the stomach and right hypochondriac region. Measures were taken to restore warmth to the surface, but reaction was never perfectly restored. He took, until partial reaction was brought about, such remedies as hot sling, camphor and ammonia. Then an epispastic was applied over the liver, which enabled him to take and retain small doses of Quinine and Hydrarg. cum creta, alternated with liquid acetate of ammonia. The evacuations procured by these means were passed in bed. The man improved for a week very slowly. The pulse became more natural as well as the temperature of the skin, but the coma never sensibly diminished, until he was aroused from it (not completely) by neuralgia along the left sciatic nerve, which was soon followed by erysipelas of the leg. Purpura to a considerable extent, appeared on the other leg, and shortly before death erysipelas was developed in the parotid glands. Before death the tongue, teeth and fauces had the appearance of a patient in the last stage of Typhus Gravior.

I will add but a brief sketch of one case more, in which there were genuine petechiæ, both on the cutaneous and intestinal surface.

Miss. A. B——, a resident inmate of the hospital, complained of pain in the head on Saturday, which was hot, whilst her hands and feet were icy cold. She was costive and took a blue pill. Her fever increased slowly, but remitted for the first week, the exacerbation being preceded by slight rigors. In spite of treatment the fever became more persistent—vomiting and diarrhœa ensued—dryness of the tongue—delirium—subsultus tendinum, petechiæ, at length coma, then convulsions and death, on the twenty-first day. On making the post mortem examination we found no ulceration, but an irritated state of the duodenum and lower portion of the ilium, with distinct points of extravasation under the mucous coat of that intestine and under the cuticle.

I could multiply illustrations of the modifications which this disease is made to undergo almost indefinitely, but as my aim is rather to make myself understood than to change the views of others, I will detain the society by the citation of cases no longer this evening.

Until I had witnessed the change which took place in the type of our autumnal diseases, between the year 1837, when the billious remittent fever prevailed as an epidemic with ardent synochal sypmtoms on Jefferson avenue, and 1847, when the Spotted Fever made our city desolate, I had lived in the belief that Typhus and Typhoid fever were identical.— On revising my opinions in the light of facts, which I have endeavored to make intelligible to the members of the Society this evening, and comparing them with the experience, and regulating them by the reasoning of others, I have been led to reverse the judgment I had heretofore deliberately formed on this subject.

If the validity of the statements I have made this evening is not called in question, I think we are compelled to adopt one of two opinions—either that Typhus Fever, when the symptoms of a patient imbued with its fomites are so far changed by coming into an atmosphere of malaria as to be with difficulty recognized, until it has arrived at maturity; or else, that there is, at irregularly recurring periods, such an epidemic influence superadded to the effects of malaria, that diminishes to such a degree the reactions of the vital powers, when they are disturbed by some exciting cause as to give the disease thus developed an adynamic character. Of the two, we find the least difficulty in adopting the latter. For we have seen in the first part of this report, a brief description of unquestionable Typhus Fever, occurring north of the 46° of north latitude, where no case of Intermittent Fever has ever been known to originate; among a people not enervated by hunger and in the midst of winter, when the local determinations which would give complexity to it, usually take place in the respiratory organs, and that either from the absence of these modifying causes or from the inherent nature of the disease, there was no reason to suspect the existence of ulceration in the plates of the ilium or the glands of Peyer in the duodenum, or the deposit of "typhus matter" in either of the cavities. For we have also seen how famine, the heat of summer, with errors in diet, promoted the tendency to mucous irritation in the abdominal cavity in 1848, whereby the apparent identity of Typhus and Typhoid Fever were greatly increased; and still further, how three years later a new feature was added by the interfusion of erysipelas; but in no instance has the primitive type of the disease been so far modified as to cause it to assume a remittent form in any period of its duration. If Typhoid Fever is remittent in either of its stages, of which we think we have abundant proof, and amenable to remedies which are antiperiodic in their modus operandi, there must exist, in a nosological sense, the two forms of fever we have been speaking of, no matter what their analogies in the latter periods of their progress, when remittent fever, pneumonia, erysipelas, and even the small pox, if we leave out of view its peculiar eruption, so blend or assimilate as to be scarcely distinguishable; or what others consider of great importance, how nearly related by their post mortem results. With becoming deference for the opinions of others, which I think not incompatible with the exercise of individual judgment, I would inculcate the idea that we ought to learn to distinguish diseases by their exhibition of vital phenomena, and not postpone our decision in mere matters of specific distinction, until the scalpel has made its revelations through the dead-room examination.   Having thus hurriedly given the results of my individual experience on a subject which engages and divides medical opinion, an experience which varies so much from that of gentlemen of acknowledged eminence in the profession, that I should do violence to my own sense of duty, and injustice to those learned men who have labored so much for our instruction, if I passed the subject by, without making some reference to what they have said, either for the purpose of reconciling discrepanices or of defending opinions adverse to theirs.

If our differences of opinion were speculative merely and carried no practical consequences in their train, then our indulgence in medical polemics would be a harmless passtime, which might serve to sharpen our wits and try our armor; but when dietetic restrictions, which should be imposed upon cases of dothinenteritic inflammation are enjoined, (as happened in the case of my juvenile patient who sank from inanition,) upon the subjects of Typhus Fever, like that of Fort Brady, where the functions of the skin and mucous tissue seemed to be suspended rather than exalted, under a misapprehension of the nature of the case, clearly resulting from the teachings of an authority (confessedly superior) who had seen but one of the forms of this disease, it becomes the duty of every man, however humble, to examine carefully the foundation of his own opinions.

My first opinions of the nature and my first thoughts on the revolution of the great epidemics, were suggested by a perusal of Rush's edition of Sydenham, and my earliest ideas of Typhus Fever were drawn from his edition of Pringle, on Diseases of the Army.   My impressions of the nature and origin of typhus, thus derived, were confirmed and strengthened by my experience in 1827, and my reflections on the revolution of epidemics, if not followed by convictions of the regularity of their return, have led to the belief that they follow each other in a certain order, because of the degree of consanguinity, the closeness of the relationship which obtains between them.   Since 1848, I have seen a kind of cholera unknown to me before, collapsing with fewer stools, the last of which were small and bloody.   Since then I have met with cases of dysentery not to be distinguished in the later stages from the cholera above referred to, and a form of puerperal fever of unwonted malignancy, attended with dysenteric symptoms.   I have seen the reactions, which rarely took place after these cases, followed by Typhoid Fever.   I have seen in these cases erysipelatous inflammation of the parotid and mammary glands, such as complicated the Typhus of 1851. And I have seen these more malignant forms of disease gradually shading into Typhoid Fevers, of which now and then one with graver cerebral symptoms would collapse into a condition intermediate to the cholera, and the Brain Fever of 1848.— Within this period we have had cases of disease which some would call scarlet fever and others erysipelas, and in some sections of the State, numerous other cases' which seemed to occupy a position midway between Variola and Erysipelas.

These same excentricities manifested themselves in the time of Sydenham, as if a pervading element either of meteoric or telluric origin had stepped in to give a tint or tone to the diseases of the era, or else by laying a general foundation and allowing the exciting causes to construct a superstructure at their will. In his chapter on the epidemic constitution of part of year 1669, and of the years 1670, 1671, and 1672, at London, he remarks:

"In the begining of August, 1669, the cholera morbus, the dry gripes, and likewise a dysentery that rarely appeared during the ten preceding years, began to rage. But though the cholera morbus proved more epidemic than I had ever known it before, yet nevertheless it terminated this year in August; but the dry gripes continued to the end of autumn. But upon the coming in of winter, this disorder likewise vanished, whereas the dysentery became more epidemic.

"Between these gripes and the above-mentioned dysentery, which raged very universally, a new kind of fever arose, and attended both diseases, and not only attacked such as had been afflicted with either of the former, but even those who had hitherto escaped them, unless that sometimes, though very seldom, it was accompanied with slight gripings, sometimes with stools, and at others without. Upon the approach of winter, the dysentery vanished for a time, but the dysenteric fever raged more violently.

"In the beginning of the following year, the measles succeeded.

"This kind of measles introduced a kind of small pox, which I was not hitherto acquainted with, so that to distinguish it from the other kinds I choose to entitle it—the anomolous or irregular small pox of the dysenteric constitution.

"It must further be observed that as each epidemic disease is attended with its periods of increase, height, and decline, in every subject, so likewise, every general constitution of years that has a tendency to produce some particular epidemic, has its periods according to the time it presides; for it grows every day more violent till it comes to its height, and then abates in nearly the same degree, till it becomes extinct and yields to another."

This blending of the forms of disease, through the instrumentality of an atmospheric influence, independent of its sensible qualities, so clearly seen by the "English Hippocrates," was noticed also by Armstrong, and became, with Dr. Rush, a leading and controlling idea. Dr. Armstrong in his chapter on the modifications of "Common Continued Fever," makes these remarks: "If it be the fact, as I am inclined to believe, that genuine typhus always originates from contagion, how can the present epidemic be accounted for, which has raged in so many parts of the United Kingdom for at least the last three years? My own observations would lead me to infer that what has been so generally called *the* Epidemic is not one specific fever, but three fevers, especially different in their exciting causes; and these fevers are, namely, typhus, proceeding from a specific contagion, the common continued fever, proceeding mostly from atmospheric influences, and a peculiar fever which arises from the huddling together of many human beings, in confined and filthy situations."—Page 162, Leland's edition, 1829.

Cullen's love of system, which happened to lead him in a direction opposite to that taken by Sauvages, who magnified symptoms into species, evidently blinded him to the most obvious distinctions. Otherwise it would be difficult to account for the emanation of the following remark from so distinguished a source: "The most common form of continued fevers, in this climate, seems to be a combination of these two genera; (the inflammatory and nervous,) and I have therefore given such a genus a place in our Nosology, under the title of Synochus. At the same time, I think that the limits between the Synochus and Typhus will be with difficulty assigned; and I am disposed to believe that the synochus arises from the same causes as the Typhus, and is therefore only a variety of it."—lxix. Reid's edition.

Dr. Mackintosh, whose position must have afforded him abundant opportunities for observing the phenomena of Typhus and Typhoid Fevers, seems to have been led by his contempt for definitions to the rejection of nearly all the distinctions made by authors on the subject of fever, particularly the numerical attenuations of Dr. I. Mason Good. His silence on the subject of Typhoid Fever, I should more naturally have imputed to the absence of an epidemic manifestation in Scotland during his period of professional activity, had not his cotemporary, Dr. Perry of Glasgow, have written very fully on that subject. The observations made by Dr. Mackintosh on the relations of the maculæ in adynamic fevers, to the condition of the mucous tissue of the lungs, coincide so nearly with remarks made by myself that I insert them: "In all the fevers which are called putrid, and which are accompanied by dark-colored spots on the surface of the body termed petechiæ, it will be found, I am almost inclined to say, invariably, that bronchitis prevails to a great extent.— The circumscribed and somewhat livid redness which is seen so often in the fevers called Typhoid, is principally owing to the embarrassed state of the lungs."

In the English edition of Marshall Hall's Practice of Medicine, a similar degree of confusion is found to exist.   The obscurities in that work
in regard to the duality of Typhus and Typhoid Fever, have been effectually cleared away by his American annotators, Drs. Bigelow and Holmes,
of Boston.

A reperusal of Southwood Smith, since being engaged in the preparation of this report, has caused me to doubt his familiarity with the
Typhus of Pringle, for many of his cases given in illustration of the different degrees of Typhus fever are certainly well described instances of Typhoid disease, originating from malaria and epidemic causation : more
sudden in its attack, more violent in its course, and more abrupt in its
termination.   In this opinion I know I dissent from excellent authority,
[Dr. Bartlett.]   Speaking of typhus mitior, with acute cerebral affections,
he says, "during its progress, erysipelas, first appearing on the face, then extending over the scalp, and often down the shoulders and back, is very
apt to occur."   Among the 'accidental events' which occur in the progress of fever, he adds, " in severe and protracted cases, and often coming
to destroy the hope that was beginning to spring up in favor of the patient, erysipelas is no unusual visitant.   It is the outward and visible sign
of an inward and always most formidable disease."

This I venture to assert is never an attendant upon true Typhus, unless
the patient after being imbued with the fomites of this disease, is exposed
to an atmosphere pregnant with the poison of Erysipelas.   Such cases then
so much more nearly resemble those of Typhoid Fever, that the diagnosis
becomes exceedingly difficult.   This, the poison of Erpsiyelas, is the element which converts the paludal fevers of this country into cases of Typhoid Fever.   This is the principle which occasions the adynamic form
of inflammations, from whence effusions take place into various portions of the cellular tissue, and gives the sizy (not buffy) coat to the blood
in pneumonia Typhoides, sometimes the contagious character to Typhoid
Fever, and to Typhus Fever the appearance of an epidemic.

In order to show that the views I have taken of this subject, the distinctness of Typhus and Typhoid Fevers and the cause of that distinctness,
and which veiws I have labored in this report to enforce, are not heretical
though announced less explicitly by any one else, I have gleaned the
following remarks from the writings of others, extracted from such sources
as I happened to have at command, chiefly from the Transactions of the
American Medical Association, and have placed them in their present relation to each other for that purpose as well as to show how a common
cause of disease, such for example as malaria, when influenced by atmospheric variations, by epidemic metorations, by violations of Hygienic
laws, or by the temperament of the individual affected, may produce

varied, and to the uninitiated observer, apparently contradictory results. The histories of epidemics, as far back as the time of Hippocrates, have furnished instances of a reigning power in some one form of disease, which, like the Rod of Aaron, swallowed up or incorporated into itself all its cotemporaries, inspiring dread and impressing its name upon the era in which it appeared.

" During the prevalence of spotted fever in New England, the *typhus* (typhoid) fever was also more frequently met with than usual, appearing in many instances with its ordinary symptoms; in others the symptoms resembled those of the former disease."—Copland, vol. 1, page 1179.

" In some parts of the country, when complicated with bronchial affection, it (Spotted Fever) went under the name of *Typhoid Pneumonia.*" Copland vol., page 1180.

" Since the disappearance of the *Spotted Fever* in 1812, Typhus has prevailed sporadically, to a greater or less extent, over the whole of New England; assuming, however, a variety of grades and forms, but answering to a common type." Copland, vol. i, page 1191.

" It (Typhoid Fever) sometimes occurs at the same time that an epidemic or autumnal remittent or Typhus exists." Gerhard.

" In a good paper upon the diseases of Dallas County, Alabama, we find a disease of low type, called Typhoid Fever, in which the very marked remissions and the early convalescence or death induce us to have a doubt of the correctness of the diagnosis." Trans. Amer. Med. Association vol. iii, p. 133.

" When I see the two forms of disease, Typhoid Fever and Dysentery, intermingled in the same epidemic, in the same family, at the same time; and when I observe the exposure of persons in health to the disease in one form, followed by its appearance in the other form, I cannot resist the conviction that they are essentially the same disease."—Joseph Reynolds, M.D., Transactions of the American, Med. Association, vol. p 143.

Dr. Fenner, in the 4th volume of the Transactions of the American Medical Association, after expressing the opinion that *Yellow Fever* is not a disease, *sui generis*, but *only one of the varieties of endemic malarious fever*, asks this pertinent question, " Has any new and distinct disease made its appearance in these places? " alluding to the cities of Charleston, Augusta, New Orleans, Mobile, Natches and Vicksburgh. " Or have we only witnessed *a slight modification of our customary endemic fevers, which, though extensively prevalent, have been unusually mild?* In my opinion, the latter is the true position." This in reference to the diseases of 1848.

" In 1849, the general character of the endemic fevers was much the same and went mostly by the same name—nearly all the cases that recovered were called *dengue ;* and nearly all that proved *fatal,* were called *Yellow Fever.*"

To give an idea of the protean form of this disease called Dengue,

Breakbone Fever, and Neuralgic Fever, in America, and, by Drs. Cocke and Copland, Scarletina Rheumatica, it will be sufficient to introduce the names given to the eruption which was one of the characteristic symptoms, according to Professor Dickson, although by no means a diagnostic sign. This accomplished teacher and writer arranges his description of the eruption under the following heads: *Scarlatinous, Rubeolous, Erysipelatous, Variolous or Varicellous, Lichenoid, Papulous, Phelgmonoid, Miliary, Urticarious and Purpurous.*

The same elegant author, in his essay " On the Blending and Conversion of Types in Fever," remarks, " but this *blending* is not confined to these connate types of fever. " Holland describes a mild form of Typhus, with intermittent symptoms, both tertian and quotidian in type, and often very regular in period, the tendency to which seemed more common when the disease was abating." He also quotes Lempriere, who admits the existence of a distinct disease in the West Indies, usually showing itself in crowded ships, partaking of the character of both yellow fever and typhus, and, like the latter, contagious.

" We are now prepared to appreciate correctly the phenomena of apparent *conversion* of types. Of numerous attacks which commence in the same way, the course, history, and ultimate termination may be strikingly diverse. Invading with the ordinary symptoms of climatorial, autumnal bilious fever, one shall retain its periodical malarious character, ending as it begun with the symptoms of a simple remittent. Another losing these features in a protracted course, shall grow more and more continuous, and ultimately put on all the appearances of maculated typhus; or present the meteorism and abdominal disorder of typhoid, with intestinal ulceration, shown *post mortem;* and a third shall sink promptly into profound collapse, dying with orange-yellow skin and eyes, and black vomit." (Dickson.)

I can myself bear testimony to the truthfulness of the learned Professor's sketch, and unite with him in the exhibition of fact, but must separate from him in the matter of opinion. What he would consider as cases of conversion, I should regard as instances of the blending of symptoms, occasioned by the meeting of distinct morbific agents, by which not only the type of the fever, but the grade of action may be regulated.

The committee on epidemics, for New Jersey, in 1852, (Dr. Parrish,) remarks, "From four of the counties in this region, reports have been received which state that the diseases of the last year have been of a typhoid type, and that dysentery, was, in some localities, especially fatal."

In the same report Dr. I. Henry Clark, of Newark, N. J., speaks of what he calls " The Winter Miasmatic Fever," which he likens to the dengue of South Carolina; sometimes having dysenteric symptoms, at others those of influenza, but adynamic in character, and prone to take on a typhoid condition.

Following through the reports of the committees on epidemics for 1852, from Pennsylvania to Louisiana, including Delaware, Maryland, South Carolina, Georgia, Alabama, Kentucky, Tennessee, Ohio, Indiana, Michigan, Mississippi, Arkansas and Texas, we find constant mention of the subject of Typhoid Fever, either as prevalent in certain localities, or as appearing in others in connection with Erysipelas, with Pneumonia, Dysentery, Cholera, Parotitis, with Dengue, and even with Yellow Fever.

This consociation, so generally noticed, of diseases nosologically distinct, in such an extent of territory, either proves that an interfusion of species, of genera, and even of orders, according to some arrangements, do take place under the concurring influence of general and local causes, educing new forms of morbosity; or else, that the professional mind of the whole country is involved in worse than Babelonian confusion. The latter proposition is too absurd to be entertained.

It is known that the geology of a country influences and gives character to its vegetation, that the food of plants will change the tints of their inflorescence and affect the quality of their fruits; and we have equal reason for believing, that in diseases, where the same fidelity to caste is not to be looked for that we find in the vegetable creation, we should look to the climate of the country in which it may occur, to the mode of living of its inhabitants, the epidemic influences which may be prevailing therein at the time, for such modifying influences as would render the most faithful description of a particular form of disease to be found in one portion of a country, extended like ours, in many respects unsuited to another.

Although it may appear presumptious in an unpracticed writer like myself to call in question the accuracy of opinions expressed by gentlemen so distinguished in the profession, as Mackintosh, J. M. Smith, Marshall Hall, Gerhard, and Southwood Smith, on a subject so important, as that which engages our attention this evening; still when the authority of bright names may lead through the guidance of speculative ideas to errors in practice, we deem it to be a duty to call the attention of junior members of the profession to the discrepancies in opinion to be found among physicians, with a view to reconcile them to each other, or explain away their injurious effects.

Our reasons why Cullen and Mackintosh adopted certain generic names have already been hinted at. The other gentlemen we think have written without having had the same opportunities for comparing these forms of disease with each other, as have fallen to our humble lot; and this I apprehend to be true of the learned author of the Report on Practical Medicine, [Prof. J. M. Smith,] made to the National Medical Association in 1848. He has undoubtedly had ample opportunities for the study of Typhus Fever in the harbor of New York, but I doubt very much whether the Typhoid Fever of rural districts has ever prevailed as an epidemic to any considerable extent in that city, during the years to which his personal recollections extend. In his remarks on the nature of Typhus, he omits one important means of arriving at a correct judgment, and that is a consideration of its etiology; an omission which might have been excused in a less popular writer and a less practical teacher if engaged in the same labor of striving to establish the identity of Typhus and Typhoid Fevers.* Leaving behind him the enquiry into the causes of both these forms of disease, he proceeeds to combat the anatomical doctrine of M. Louis, so ably defended by Dr. Gerhard, and succeeds pretty effectually in overturning the foundations on which that school of pathologists has built its distinctions.

Forced then by the testimony of others into the same position, we were led by our own experience and reflections to re-affirm our belief, and repeat the declaration, that there is an adynamic form of fever, arising from an animal poison, and an adynamic form of fever arising from malaria, and modified by an epidemic meteoration, or originating from an epidemic cause and modified by malaria, which being distinct in origin, must be so far distinct in nature as to require in their earlier stages different modes of treatment, no matter how closely they may approximate each other, when they have each had time to pass from Synocha to Typhus, under the influences of the effete materials retained in the tissues, the secretions or the circulation.

Detroit, Oct. 4, 1853.

---

* In a more recent paper, the report of the Committee on Public Hygiene, addressed to the American Medical Association, Dr. Smith has dwelt upon the origin and causes of Typhus Fever, in such a manner as fully to atone for his former silence. In this report he remarks, " as the theme of his contribution to the present report, the chairman of the Committee has selected the sources of Typhus Fever, and the means suited to their extinction. His design is to show that the disease originates from human excretions."

After carefully estimating the amount of matters excreted from the skin, the pulmonary surface, and the other outlets of the human body, in health, for a given time, which from their nature have not the diffusible force inherent in gases, and are consequently slow of dispersion; he proceeds to show how soon an apartment of specified capacity, occupied by a given number of persons, would become unfit for the wholesome support of animal life, its inmates sources of disease to themselves and radiating points for the poison of Typhus Fever. This principle he applies to communities—Remarks upon Hospitals— and shows how the sick may communicate disease to those in health; and adds, " it is then the excrementious matters thrown off from the skin and lungs of diseased persons that the poison of Typhus is mostly traceable." A process of reasoning by which it would be difficult to account for the origin of the cases of Typhoid Fever, which extended in 1852, from the Arostook to the Rio-Grande.

ART. II. — *Pervious Foramen Ovale, with Emphysema, at sixty-six years of age.*

September 6th, 1853. Post-mortem examination of Mr. IRA BRONSON, six hours after death, æ. 66. Undertaker's measure—length six feet, breadth one and a-half feet. Body not emaciated. Skin and epithelium generally of a dark modena hue. Rigor mortis complete. — Chest presenting the usual extreme rotundity of asthmatics and abnormally sonorous. Precordial dullness below usual situation, *i. e.* from lower edge of fourth rib downwards. Abdomen tumid but not tympanitic. Some general anasarcous effusion. The blood was fluid and flowed profusely at each stroke of the scalpel. All the cartilages were free from ossification, except the seventh of the right side. Lungs seemed held down by the walls of the thorax — pressing forward on removing the sternum. No adhesions of the pleura pulmonalis were found. Color of lungs generally livid, but exhibiting considerable carbonaceous deposit in the tissues. (His occupation was a tinsmith, and he had worked several years without a pipe to his furnace.)

The costal surface of the left lung presented several cicatrices from half an inch to one and a-half inches in diameter. The emphysema was both lobular and inter-lobular. The air vesicles both dilated, hypertrophied and broken down. Considerable serum was found in all the cavities, but was not separately measured, blood from the several veins having early flowed into the first cavity opened.

The whole amount of blood and serum removed during the examination, was about ten quarts. The blood coagulated feebly on exposure to air. The pericardium appeared healthy, except some abnormal adhesions infero-posteriorly. It contained about 4 3 fl. of serum. The external surface of the heart appeared healthy, having about the usual amount of adipose tissue. Some fibrinous shreds existed in both ventricles, and in the right auricle. The right heart was slightly enlarged in capacity. The tricuspid valves seemed atrophied and the chordæ tendiniæ attached, attenuated. Regurgitation must have been constant upon the contraction of the right ventricle. The fossa ovalis presented a deep sulcus on its right auricular surface, occupying the inner half of its elipsis; and at the bottom of this sulcus a round opening about the size of a crow-quill. The left heart was natural, except the reception of the above opening by the auricle.

Abdomen—Slight peritoneal adhesions retained the serum, effused in distinct portions. The spleen was pear-shaped, flattened, and curved laterally; its texture dark and friable; its length three inches, breadth two and a-half inches, thickness one and a-quarter inches; the liver small, *i. e.*, about seven inches in breadth, five and a-half in length, and three inches thick; rather hard, friable, and dark chocolate color.

Kidneys— No evidences of disease appeared to us. Bladder contracted and easily torn; inner surface dull white color, not appearing coated with mucous, but what we think would be called *pulpy*. Intestines exhibited no essentially unhealthy feature on peritoneal aspect, although an inguinal hernia existed on either side. The intestinal canal was not opened.

Previous history subsequently gathered.

Of the early life nothing is known, except that at nine years of age he suffered severe pneumonia, from which he was slow in recovering. Before adult age, hernia upon one side was produced by an apparently slight cause. At about 45 years, acquaintances observed sighing, and expressions of uneasiness in left side, and about this time he used to complain of great fatigue on ascending stairs. These symptoms may have existed long before. Flatulence was always productive of severe distress, and hence he was habitually careful in diet. Hearing became obtuse at about fifty-five years. Powerful stimulants uniformly afforded signal relief from dyspnœa and angina. Resisting with conscientious firmness an habitual use of alcoholic beverages, he sometimes spoke with apparent surprise and regret of the charming effects of good brandy. Under the care of Dr. S. S. Cutler, who had been his physician for several years, and who was present at the examination, ferri. carb. præc. had been the most reliable remedy. The general appearance of the deceased led people to suppose him much farther advanced in years.—There seemed to have been premature senility, in which all but the osseous system participated. The symptoms had gradually augmented in severity for several weeks. He walked out of doors three days before death, which, as described to us, must have been by asthenia. It is a remarkable fact, that, from the first of his dyspnœa, until the last few weeks of his life, he always breathed easily in the recumbent position, and finally it was only changed as symptoms of serous effusion appeared.   J. H. BEECH.

Coldwater, Sept. 16, 1853.

ART. III.— *To the Editor of the Peninsular Journal of Medicine.*

SIR:—In looking over the medical profession at the present time, and comparing her experience and discoveries of three thousand years and over, to say nothing of the sanction it has received from men of giant minds and profound erudition, one might well be struck with astonishment to see the little confidence that community has in her theory and practice. When we look at the practice of her disciples, conducted as it is with the most profound secrecy — her theory and medicines buried beneath its compound medical language — then we need not wonder that the community have so little confidence, and that we have *quackery* and *isms* of every shape and hue, from aeripathy down to spiritpathy. This state of things will continue so long as the great mass are ignorant of the elementary principles of medicine. The question is, how to obviate the present difficulty. Let every man when called upon to prescribe for a patient, give the friends a full description of the disease, and explain the effects the medicines should produce in order to effect a cure. This course, in connection with a weekly paper, devoted to medicine and general science, well sustained and properly placed before the community, will create confidence and intelligence — and quackery and empiricism will vanish before the meridian sun of Allopathy. W. M. H.

SELECTIONS.

From the Boston Medical and Surgical Journal.

Aphonia of Twenty Months' Standing, relieved by Iodine Inhalation.
By EDWARD B. STEVENS, M.D., Lebanon, O.

IN a communication to the American Medical Association, in its volume of Transactions for 1850, Prof. Pancoast has given the record of two cases of loss of voice — the one of six, the other of seven months' standing — both cured by inhalation of a dilut. chlorine vapor.

In connection with these cases, Dr. Pancoast remarks: — "The form of aphonia here alluded to, is that which practitioners must have met with, following an ordinary cold, without leaving any perceptible organic lesion in the pulmonary apparatus. The voice is reduced to a faint, hoarse whisper, distinguishable only at the distance of a few feet, and at continued attempt to talk, though it gives no pain, becomes quickly attended with a feeling of fatigue, as though there was some obstruction to the passage of air through the larynx. In breathing merely, there is little or no difficulty, in these cases, as the individuals are capable of undergoing considerable exertion without any unusual signs of fatigue. The difficulty has appeared to me to be in the paralyzed condition of the muscles of the larynx, whose business it is to dilate the rima glottidis, during the act of articulation."

The conclusion of Dr. Pancoast is, that such agent as will excite a healthy and proper degree of stimulation in the affected structure ought rationally to restore the power of articulation. He consequently used the dilut. chlorine vapor, with entire success in the two cases referred to — at the same time suggesting that iodine, or other similar agents, would doubtless produce a similar effect.

The following case of this kind lately occurred in my practice, chiefly remarkable from the long duration of absence of voice, being twenty months, in other respects similar to those related by Dr. Pancoast.

April 6, 1853. — Miss ———— applied for medical advice and treatment, in a case of loss of voice, of twenty months' standing, supervening upon a slight attack of influenza. Has been subject to brief attacks of hoarseness, lasting for a few days at a time, for several years. General health delicate. Since the present attack, has been subject to a great variety of treatment, including the application of nit. silv. in strong solution, within the larynx, by means of the sponge probang. Nothing, however, produced any effect upon the voice. I find, upon careful examination, no especial evidence of disease in the fauces; there is an entire inability to produce sound of any description with the proper vocal organs; all attempts at speaking are made with the lips — *whispering.* But not being able to divest myself of the idea that a follicular inflammation of the throat and bronchial tubes was the cause of the mischief in some way, I commenced the treatment by directing the inhalation of nit. silv. prepared with the lycopodium, as an impalpable powder, and inhaled by means of the apparatus introduced by Dr. Ira Warren. This treatment was faithfully persevered in for one month, with no better results than the previously-tried remedies.

May 7. — Acting upon the idea suggested by Prof. Pancoast, of paralysis of the muscles of the larynx, I now determined to try the iodine vapor. I accordingly selected an apparatus, consisting of a metalic vase or urn, with a close-fitting cover, flexible tube, and mouth-piece attached, (used some years since for breathing medicated vapors in the treatment of consumption.) I directed my patient, after filling the vessel half full of hot water, to drop in twenty drops *tinct. iodine*, and inhale the vapor produced by the heated water. Inhalation to be repeated once to thrice daily, according to the irritation or effects, otherwise produced. The first inhalation produced great nausea for a short time, and copious bloody expectoration, but accompanied by an almost immediate, though partial, restoration of voice. The dose of iodine was directed to be reduced to fifteen drops; and thereafter no unpleasant effects were produced. The voice continued to improve steadily under this treatment, until, at the end of a week, it had acquired the natural fullness and distinctness of tone.

June 15. — More than a month has elapsed since the restoration of voice; it continues distinct and natural. — *Western Lancet.*

From the New York Journal of Medicine.

Remarks on Milk-sickness and Trembles. By I. N. CONVERSE, M. D. (Submitted to the Faculty of Starling Medical College, Columbus, Ohio, as an Inaugural Thesis for the Degree of M. D.)

THIS disease may truly be called one of a malignant character. It prevails in many places in the western part of the United States, and generally during the summer and autumnal months, commencing about the first of July, and terminating as soon as vegetation is destroyed by frost. It commences earlier, and is more general and more malignant, in dry, hot seasons than in others.

The cause of milk-sickness, in its primitive form, is not easily settled, In fact, it is as yet almost entirely unknown. In the horse or cow, may be found a perfect sample in the earliest form of its development. In other animals and man is another form (secondary) of the same disease, which seldom varies from the first, but is produced from the milk or flesh of animals, and has never been known to change or lose its character, though transmitted through other animals; its first development is, however, confined to the lower animals that feed npon vege-

tation. It has been supposed by some that malaria alone is capable
of producing it; others believe that vegetables may; among which the
Rhus is supposed to be the chief cause; others ascribe the disease to
minerals, others still to water, &c. I believe, so far as I have yet learned,
that no cause has been suggested but what serious objections may be
urged against it, and for the very reason that many peculiarities connected with its development are not yet understood.

The particular localities where the disease generally or always prevails is along the borders of streams passing through level countries,
timbered chiefly with white elm and soft maple, interspersed with numerous small prairies; along their borders it is said to be always found,
but it entirely disappears as soon as the timber is removed and the
land cultivated. That the cause exists in such places is proved by the
fact that when cattle and horses are brought from high and healthy
pastures and confined in narrow limits in those localities, they soon
fall victims to the disease. Hay cut in or near such places and fed
the following winter has produced it, and this is the only way that
it has ever been known to exist after vegetation was destroyed by
freezing.

Cattle brought from healthy pastures and allowed to pasture in these
dangerous places, are more liable to fall victims to the disease than
cattle which have been raised there; young and fat cattle are more
subject to it than others, and cattle more than horses. During lactation the disease is never found, so far as my observation or knowledge
extends. Farmers living in districts where the cause of trembles exists,
have taken much care to study the cause, and it has been found that a
few precautions will obviate very much the danger of the disease.
Where animals are not permitted to feed upon the grass while the dew
is upon it, there is but little if any danger, and more especially if you
give them good, healthy water, plenty of salt, and afford a well ventilated
place for sleeping.

The length of time between taking the poison (for such it is) and
the development of the disease, varies according to the quantity taken
by the animal. Some animals have been exposed for a length of time,
then taken into healthy pastures, and some weeks after the disease was
developed. This is done often by warming the bood of the animal by
worrying, running or exciting it. Hence the custom among cattle
merchants and especially butchers, to worry and run cattle before purchasing, where there is the least suspicion, which is regarded as a sure
test. At other times animals are attacked soon after receiving the
poison, for I have known many cattle die in a few days after having
escaped for only a few hours from a healthy pasture into an infected
district. I think it is generally developed earlier when taken from the
milk or flesh of poisoned animals. One instance occurred in the central part of Ohio, where poisoned meat was used for dinner, from which
five persons died; among whom was a physician from the state of New
York, who called to dinner, ate freely of the beef, was attacked with
vomiting at the table, and died in twelve hours with many symptoms
of narcotic poison; the others did not die so soon, although within a
few days.

The question whether the system has the power to eliminate the poison has been frequently asked. There is no doubt in my mind but the system has this power when small quantities are taken, or not enough to bring the system immediately under its influence. In this case, as in other cases of poison, the proper requisites or conditions are necessary, such as energetic vital forces, or reaction, rest, &c. It has been ascertained that one animal poisoned is capable of poisoning many more. Each pound of his flesh is capable of poisoning many other animals, and these as many more, &c. I have no doubt, the same poison may be propagated thus in succession to any number of animals.

Malaria is also named as a cause of trembles. This is not certainly known to be a cause, although many forms of bilious disease exist where sick stomach or milk-sickness prevails. If it arises from malaria, why is it often latent until winter in hay, butter, &c., and not always prevalent when there is the greatest amount of decomposition going on? If vegetation is the cause, among which the *Rhus Toxicodendron* stands first, why is it that fields and woods abound with it in many places and the disease is not known? Or why, in confining cattle in small lots where the *Rhus* has never been seen, do they soon fall a victim to the disease? It is also said that minerals or mineral waters produce the poison. Some springs that have been charged with producing it, causing much excitement, have afterwards been found to be good, healthy springs, and have been used safely for many years. As soon as the country was improved, the cause of trembles, milk-sickness, sick stomach &c., disappeared. Good water, a healthy, ventilated place for sleeping, &c., are no doubt necessary for the health of both man and beast.

It has been supposed by some observers that mineral agents, effluvia, or some poison, may mingle with the dew that collects upon the vegetation, which is permitted to escape when the dew evaporates, but which may be taken into the system by feeding upon the plants while the dew is upon them.

When the disease is found in the lower order of animals and produced from the primary or unknown cause, the symptoms are, first, general lassitude, a great relaxation of the nervous and muscular power; in a few days, and sometimes in a few hours, the patient is unable to stand, followed by tremors (hence the name trembles) which continue till death; or, if the patient recovers, he is subject to the same trembling for many years, when over done or excited; the eyes are sunken, there is a profuse flow of saliva, circulation at first small, is soon followed by reaction; the bowels first constipated, but, upon reaction are unloaded freely, a profuse discharge continues, inflammation of stomach and bowels increase rapidly; the patient drinks much, and becomes insensible to surrounding objects; loss of nervous energy, relaxation of sphincters, gangrene and death often follow.

The treatment is principally confined to dry corn and salt in the early state of trembles, which is said to give relief, and which the animal willl take freely, having an abnormal appetite so great as to eat almost any thing given. The lower order of animals that take the poison from milk or flesh, &c., die from similar symptoms, rather more aggravated, and which terminate sooner, and cannot as often, if ever, be cured. It is produced oftener perhaps in places where the trembles are found, by feeding cats and dogs with milk at night, for the purpose of testing its condition, which will show itself before morning if poison . be in it. This is done in many before using the milk otherwise, and is said to be a true test.

In man the true milk-sickness or sick stomach is, I believe, invariably produced by the milk, flesh, butter, &c., of the animals that have already recieved the poison into their systems. It is contended by some that the disease is produced by contagion; this is probably not the case, although many forms of bilious diseases are found where and whenever the milk-sickness prevails.

The *first symptoms* that are calculated to excite suspicion are a loss of nervous energy, general lassitude with nausea. Sometimes a number of days pass in this way, followed by a loss of appetite, great constipation of the bowels, disposition to sleep, dull headache, pulse small, tense and frequent. The symptoms may exist for a greater or less length of time, when the patient is suddenly seized with vomiting, continued and severe, the discharge is a thin mucus, sometimes tinged with bile; the patient is disposed to excite vomiting which generally gives momentary relief, the tongue at first is covered with a white thin coat which soon passes off, leaving it red, dry and swollen, the secretions are very scanty, &c. As soon as the patient is attacked with severe vomiting, a reaction takes place in the circulation, the pulse is full and frequent, the eyes are sunken, and the vessels are distended with blood, great thirst, aversion to every thing but the coldest drinks, inflammation goes on to ulceration; gangrene and death follow. About the fifth, seventh, or ninth day, they frequently become insensible to all surrounding objects, with a total suspension of nervous influence.

The symptoms are very characteristic, such as severe vomiting, constipated state of the bowels, with a loss of nervous energy; the vomiting is accounted for from the irritation and subsequent inflammation of the mucous membrane of the stomach, from the action of the poison.

Constipation of the bowels does not seem to depend so much upon the presence of hardened fœces (as they are seldom found in the early stage of the disease, though Dr. McIlheny claims hardened fœces to be the only cause of the constipation) as upon a suspension of nervous influence, which necessarily lessens the peristaltic motion, and paralyzes the muscles connected with defaction; and they are so perfectly paralyzed that the patient has no more control over them than if he were dead. Their power is invariably restored as soon as a free operation upon the bowels takes place, which may be regarded as the effect perhaps rather than the cause. The paralysis is doubtless the effect of the narcotic influence of the poison. I should state that a peculiar odor is given off during vomiting, which is always readily recognized by all who have once noticed it, the same smell can be detected in the lower animals, when under the influence of the poison, and frequently in the perspiration for a long time afterwards.

When children are attacked with milk-sickness, which is generally from milk, the train of premonitory symptoms cannot be so readily detected as in adults; vomiting is first discovered, followed by many symptoms of narcotic poison, and death is the result generally. I believe I have never known a case of this kind to recover.

The *treatment* of milk-sickness has been a question of much importance among the physicians living in the districts where the disease is found. I believe that all acknowledge that, as soon as the bowels are opened, the greatest difficulty is overcome, particularly if inflammation has gone too far. The different modes by which this is to be accomplished have been numerous.

In the first settlement of the western country, the common practice was to commence with calomel as soon as vomiting began, and continue its use, in from twenty to sixty grain doses, every two or four hours, until an operation was produced, or until one fourth or one *half a pound* was taken; if the bowels were not moved by this time the case was considered a hard one, and *severer means* must be used, and then one half pound of quicksilver was given, which soon found its way through the patient and seldom failed *to kill.* I have known a few cases of this kind recover, treated upon general principles afterwards. Others recommended the use of Epsom salts, dissolved in mucilage, given in small quantities, at regular intervals, which, it was said, acted as a febrifuge, and also called from the neighboring tissues into the stomach the poison to be evacuated by vomiting, always an urgent symptom, and thus unloaded the system of its contents; at the same time it urged its way along the canal, and eventually effected catharsis, the main object sought to be attained. Many families have treated themselves successfully in this way in its milder forms, believing that though they called a physician they should die; these means were aided, of course, by fomentations, counter-irritants, etc. Many other methods of treatment have served their turn as hobbies, such as frequent blood-letting, warm bathing, spirits, turpentine, table salt, etc.; these have mostly fallen into disuse.

The more recent course of treatment, amongst learned and judicious practitioners, seems to be based upon a more intelligent appreciation of symptoms, and corresponds more nearly with common-sense principles.

, I do not know as I can better define my views of the treatment of milk-sickness, than to relate the treatment given by Dr. J. A. Skinner, of South Charleston, Clark Co., Ohio, in a letter to me upon the subject some time since. " It consists," he says, " in the first place, in moderating the arterial circulation by venesection, when the pulse is found frequent and full, then take sulphate magnesia one ounce, aqua ammonia half an ounce, *boiling water* four ounces; of this mixture give a teaspoonful once in fifteen or twenty minutes, until it operates as a cathartic. This composition will usually arrest the vomiting in from twenty minutes to half an hour perfectly; and I administer no other medicine until catharsis is procured, after which alterative doses of sub. mur., hydrarg., may be advantagiously used, to excite the hepatic secretion, which is usually all that is required, except the precautions usual to convalescence." He further adds, in the same communication,

" that there is a number of circumstances in the history and propagation of this disease of peculiar interest. And, first, as to the Rhus Toxicodendron's being the origin of the disease, why does not the disease exist in western New York, where the Rhus grows in abundance, and where no such disease was ever known in man or brute. Second, in the southern parts of Huron and Lorain counties, Ohio, the cause is supposed to reside in water or poisonous exhalations. But if such is the cause, why are not brutes as well as man, subject to the disease? But no such disease was ever known there among the cattle as trembles, though the disease prevailed extensively among the early settlers and hundreds died with it before the country became settled; since that time, I believe, the disease has entirely disappeared. The true cause of this disease may never be satisfactorily ascertained, and the above treatment originated with me on the supposition that the system was laboring under the influence of poison, and that a diffusive alkali would neutralize it, which subsequent treatment has fully proved. I have, for some years previous to this, been in the habit of using the aqua ammonia with sulph. mag., as above, in cases of poison by the ivy; and frequently, when cases occurred in persons without knowing by what agent, I have used this preparation with the happiest effects; and in those cases I depend upon this compound alone."

I have no doubt but what the disease may be treated successfully upon general principles, applicable to the treatment of most diseases.

The want of post-mortem investigations in this disease, still leaves the pathology much in the dark.

In making the few suggestions that are presented here, I have attempted to sustain nothing but what I have either tested myself or have derived from those in whose veracity I could put full confidence. And if I shall hereby benefit one individual in any one respect, I shall be fully rewarded for my labor.

From the Ohio Medical and Surgical Journal.

Case of Extensive Osteo-Sarcoma. Read before the Stark County Medical Society, by L. M. WHITING, M.D., of Canton, Ohio.

The following case is especially interesting by reason of the character and amount of morbid anatomy, presented on examination of the cadaver. But the train of distressing symptoms which attended the decline of the patient, and the mode adopted for the relief of some of the most pressing difficulties, it is thought may also be regarded as worthy of record. Its history, however, is necessarily meagre, for the reason, that like a thousand other individuals in trouble with obscure maladies, he "run the gauntlet" through files of doctors—some of whom may not inaptly be denominated savages, and his sufferings during this ordeal were not a whit behind those of the victims subjected to this aboriginal mode of torture amongst our North American Indians.

The first diseased manifestations were those common to malarious districts. The patient was a man 29 years of age, of nervous temperament and by trade a tailor. After being harrassed with intermittent fever, more or less, during a residence of some years on the Ohio canal, in the village of Fulton, in this county, he fell into a condition in which attacks of what are called by " the world's people" *bilious* trouble, were frequent, and for the relief of which he took " Anti-bilious pills," and various nostrums—but finally resorted on these occasions to the use of Calomel; the effect of which was temporary freedom, and ability to continue his occupation. In the fall of 1851 he was engaged in an active political campaign, and being a candidate for office, rode much in the heat of the sun during some weeks, and of course was in an excited state most of the time. He now began to have frequent attacks of diarrhœa, for the relief of which opiates and astringents were taken repeatedly. Being elected to the office of Clerk in the district court for this county, he removed to this town in February, 1852. He was now enfeebled and pale, and suffered with pain in the rectum, where he discovered some kind of obstruction. After some time spent in tampering with various forms of quackery, for " Piles," he visited Cleveland, and consulted Prof. Delamater, the elder; but (as he said) obtained no satisfactory information in regard to the character of his disease, or relief from his sufferings. Some further time was consumed in fruitless quacking; then he went to Wheeling, where he remained some weeks under tne care of Dr. Hullihen, who adds to his brilliant reputation as a dental-surgeon, fame in other departments of operative surgery. But he returned from his wandering still the prey of unmitigated disease. The autumn came, and with its falling leaves our poor invalid found himself steadily inclining earthward. His attempts at locomotion were attended with but indifferent success on account of a painful stiffness experienced in the left hip in the locality of which he noticed thickening of the soft-solids. A new prospect of entire relief now appeared in the shape of a burly "*Fellow*," who assured him that by a purely " Botanic" plan he would very soon be eased of all his troubles.— A couple of months proved the pretender to be so near right that it was deemed unnecessary to retain his services longer in order to insure the fulfilment of his prediction.

On the 12th day of January, present year, I was requested to visit the sufferer. Found him barely able to traverse his room with the help of a cane, and complaining of very severe pain in the left leg—in the lower part of the back, and in the bowels from whence it had become a matter of great difficulty to procure any evacuation whatever. In general aspect he was white, haggard and emaciated, yet his appetite was good and his respiration free. On manipulating the lower abdomen and pelvis, the attention was arrested by the presence of a large and very solid growth aising from and filling entirely the left Iliac fossa, and projecting boldly from thence in a round tower shape into the corresponding hypochondrium. Passing the hand over on the dorsum of the left ilium it was found covered thickly with the same non-elastic tissue. In the right Illiac fossa was another tumor of the same character as that on the left side, but occupying only the pelvis. On the upper, and frontal aspect of the trunk were discovered several of the same degenerations. Four or five, varying from the size of a filbert to that of a pigeon's egg, were scattered over the anterior and superior surface of the thorax and neck. On the left temple was situated one of these indurations of the size of a hickory nut, and a much smaller one on the occipital protuberance. A careful examination of the liver detected a feeling of extraordinary hardness in the free border of the large lobe. A digital exploration per anum announced the existence of an induration and thickening in the parietes of the rectum about $1\frac{3}{4}$ inches from the anus. This seemed to be a complete investiture of the organ, and produced nearly or quite entire occlusion when in a quiescent state. By firm pressure which produced much pain, an opening could be forced through the natural channel about $\frac{3}{8}$th of an inch in diameter. This change in the structure of the rectal wall seemed strikingly like the enlargements more exposed and was believed to be the same in character. By some it was pronounced *scirrhus*—but it was *too hard* for scirrhus. The intellect was clear—the tongue clean and digestion seemed to be performed with integrity. My prognosis was *death*—and warning was given the patient to look for it under circumstances the most aggravating. The irritation by pressure of the morbid growths upon the large nerves supplying the lower extremity of the left side was already such as to induce not merely pain, but intense agony; and the constant recurrence of violent spasmodic contraction of the muscular coats of the intestinal canal, by reason of inflation from pent up gasses, produced intolerable *colics*. Any attempt to relieve these sufferings by either the forms of opium which are in common use—or which he had tried, was followed by the most prostrating nausea, vomiting, and almost irretrievable constipation. To guard against entire occlusion of the obstructed portion of the alimentary tube, by which he and his advisers were kept in constant terror. His mouth, œsophagus, stomach, small and large intestines were made the constant thoroughfare of all manner of pills, potions, boluses and cathartic compounds; and yet the awful climax seemed constantly approaching. As the hopes of the victim were now fast fading away in all remedial means, and entirely extinguished, so far as boasting charlatanism was concerned, he requested me to take the entire charge of him and make such appliances as I deemed judicious, and most conducive to his comfortable exit from what was to him emphatically a "a vale of tears."

For present relief chloroform was prescribed—in liniment over all the painful limb, and inhalation of the pure article to "Point comfort." For permanent and reliable means of relief, I had—

1st. To substitute for McMunn's elixir of opium, prepared after the formula given in Braithwaite's Ret.

2d. To counteract the constipating effects of this drug, he was directed to take ℥ij each day of *ox gall*, and confine himself to such articles of liquid diet as contribute to a soluble state of the bowels.

3d. To be ready in all emergencies for relieving the bowels from undue accumulations, I constructed catheters and bougies, of appropriate size, of *gutta percha*, which were passed through the constricted portion of the canal, the former being made the duct for alvine evacuations. By the adoption of this plan he was soon brought into a state of comparative comfort. The opiate was taken without regard to quantity, but was graduated by the degree of pain, and the Fel. Bovin. acted like a charm as a solvent of the contents of the alimentary canal. Indeed, it was not long after he commenced the free use of the latter article, before he found himself able to disregard dietetic regulations to a great extent, and eat and drink that which was most agreeable; and yet by the use of a pump for injecting warm water, followed soon after by a gutta percha conductor, procure daily and copious liquid discharges.

But daily and hourly did the process of morbid change go on in the localities heretofore specified. Steadily the tumefaction increased, especially in the pelvis, the abdomen, and on the temple. At length there came a stage when the remaining soft-solid tissue belonging to the patient, began to disappear with astonishing rapidity, and the fluid secretions of the internal organs to run off without "let or hindrance." Although to all beholders he appeared almost a living skeleton before, he was now seen manifestly to *grow poor* from hour to hour. In a few days a shadow was all that was left of our friend, and he succumbed to the great destroyer, with his mental eyes wide open, but a striking instance of human attenuation. His death occurred on the last day of April, late in the afternoon, and a post obit. examination was made at 10 o'clock the following morning, in presence of Drs. Hurxthal and Whiting of Massillon, Dr. Slusser, of Fulton, and Dr. McAbee and myself, of this town. The following notes were made of the autopsy:.

External appearance, that of a skeleton, with integument drawn tightly over each individual bone.

Tumor in left temporal region first dissected out. It was found firmly adherent, apparently growing upon the bones of the skull, which it covered. The periosteum was entirely gone underneath the mass, yet the structure of the bones was not materially changed. There was, however, slight softening of the external table of the os frontis. On an incision being made through the integument the growth appeared enclosed in a non-adherent envelope, which appeared to be the temporal fascia. In its longest axis (antero-posterior) the tumor measured two and a half inches, vertically two inches, and had an average thickness of one inch. Structure, *osseous* and *spiculated*; the spiculæ standing at nearly right angles with the plane of the bones from whence they sprung. The abdominal and pelvic cavities being exposed, the most prominent feature which presented itself, was a large body with a smooth and shining surface, filling the left half of the upper portion of the cavity of the pelvis and rising boldly into a great promontory in the hypochondrium of that side. This was exceedingly indurated, and on attempting its removal was found to be connected with the entire inner surface of the left illium in precisely the same manner as the tumor on the head was with the bones of the skull. Its structure was osseous, and spiculated like the former. Its color yellowish white. This pathological specimen measured before removal six and a half inches in its vertical axis, and three and a half antero-posteriorly. In the right illiac fossa was another growth of precisely similar pathological character, and attached to the bone of that side in the same way as the two already described. This measured three inches in its vertical axis, and one and a half in average thickness. Scattered along over the frontal aspect of the last two lumbar and sacral vertebræ were indurated growths bearing the same general character as the larger ones, and varying in size from that of a pea to a hickory nut. They were osseous. The presence of so large a quantity of foreign material in the cavity of the pelvis, of course reduced its capacity to retain in a natural position its appropriate contents, and much suffering was the result.— The bladder was covered on its exterior surface with reddish colored indurations, varying from the size of a small shot to that of a pea, very hard, but not yet bony.

The rectum, although firmly secured by adhesions, was carefully taken out of its place, and found to be thickened throughout its entire extent.— At the distance of one inch and three-fourths from the anus it was found invested in its entire circuit with a very hard deposit three-eights of an inch in thickness, and extending from the point already designated, one inch and a half upward in the long axis of the tube. This we believe to be *osteo-sarcoma*, for although the osseous structure was not so manifest as in the larger tumors, yet on cutting through the diseased mass the cracking sound as of fracture in minute spiculæ of bone was distinctly heard, moreover crepitus was also perceived on pressure between the fingers, and the roughness of incipient ossification could be felt.

The liver was studded over most of its convex surface, and much on its opposite side, with degenerations. These were lenticular in form, and varied in size, from that of a split pea to a large sized seed of the strychnos nux vomica, which last body in many respects they strikingly resembled. All these degenerations had raised margins and depressed centres, forming little basins. The impression created by a view of them was, that a purulent fluid had existed underneath the envelope of the liver; that this had been nearly absorbed, and the covering raised by the presence of this fluid, had fallen back into the pit which the absorption had created. But all were alike solid, and all parts of each individual degeneration were alike solid, and all approximated bony structure so clearly as to be pronounced the same in pathological character with those portions of the decidedly osseous tumors which had not yet become converted into that tissue. The free border of the large lobe of this organ was entirely changed. Color, pearly; texture, apparently cartilaginous; but upon handling and cutting we discovered the same impassability and crepitus, (the latter very slight) which characterized all the other morbid specimens not *decidedly* osseous. The gall bladder was much thickened, and the walls *solid.* This morbid character of the structure of the liver extended upward upon and through it to the height of three inches, and in some points nearly four.

The diaphragm was covered upon its inferior surface with the same reddish colored elvations as those found distributed over the urinary bladder. In the pancreas was found an unequivocal osseous formation in size equal to a small garden bean, and similar in form. Adhesions abounded throughout the entire abdomen and pelvis, which of course rendered the dissection tedious, and a perfect exposure of the pathological anatomy difficult.

I would, however, take occasion in this place to express my sense of obligation of my young friend, Dr. H. M. McAbee, who kindly took upon himself most of the labor, and who so performed it, that we have

been enabled to preserve a number of very valuable pathological specimens, which I have the pleasure to present for your inspection. The induration and enlargement on the dorsum of the left illium was not removed; but a dissection was made over the crest of that bone, which
exposed a fan-shaped expansion of the diseased tissue connecting the
mass within the cavity with that upon the external surface of its parietes.
This external tumor was large, and had all the characteristics of that
described as springing from the opposite side of the same bone, and no
doubt was *osseous.* The same was undoubtedly true of those located
on the superior and anterior portion of the thorax and neck, as also that
upon the occiput.

To sum up this already protracted and somewhat verbose report, permit
me to remark, that I regard the case as a very remarkable one. I know
of none on record in which such a vast amount of osteo-sarcoma is described as existing at all in a single individual; then the extreme rapidity with which the large masses of this material increased, is matter
of surprise to me. Other items of interest will suggest themselves to
your minds.

I close this paper with the enquiry, whether with a full knowledge
of this proclivity to morbid osseous development in the human body,
it might not be made to cease, if in its early stages this perverse disposition was subjected to such remedial means as would be the result of a
thorough knowledge of the *chemistry of man.*

From the Medical Examiner.

On the Influence of the Mineral Kingdom on Disease. — By J. P.
Hiester, M.D.

Reading, Pa., June 8th, 1853.

To the Editors: — In the January No. for 1852, you did me the
honor to publish a short communication on the above subject, which
had been read before the Berks County Medical Society. I there endeavored to show, by established facts and a course of reasoning, the
influence exerted by inorganic matter, as presented in the natural state,
upon organized beings.

A sufficient number of facts were adduced to prove the influence of
soil upon vegetables, and the probable effect of soil and water, or *minerals in solution,* upon the lower order of animals and fishes. From
analogical reasoning it was conjectured, that the higher orders of animals were also subjected to a greater influence by mineral agents than
we are, in the present state of our knowledge, prepared to admit.

It was farther concluded, from the activity of many of the mineral
agents that are known to enter into the composition of the animal organism, either necessarily or adventitiously, that their influence might,
and probably did, produce decidedly pathological conditions, or at least
such changes as would strongly predispose to disease; and that even deficiences of many mineral substances in certain soils, might produce such

conditions or predispositions. Iodine, which late observation has shown to be far more extensively distributed than was formerly supposed, was particularly referred to as one of these active agents.

In verification of the above conjectures, I would beg leave to call the attention of your readers to the following well-authenticated and interesting facts contained in a communication made to the French Academy of Sciences. extracted from the May No., 1853, of the Journal de Medicine et de Chirurgie Pratique.

" M. Chatin communicated to the Academy the following extremely curious facts :—

" Fully and Saillon are two contiguous villages, situated in the midst of the vineyards that border the right bank of the Rhone. Fully, where the whole population is goiterous, is remarkable for its great number of Cretins; Saillon, on the contrary, was renowned in the Vallais for the fine health of its inhabitants, who were scarcely ever attacked by goitre, and more rarely still by cretinism. The contrast was the more marked as the conditions of altitude, aeration, exposure, &c., are as nearly alike as is possible in the two villages.

" But within a few years Saillon has lost the happy exemption which it enjoyed ;—goitre and cretinism have increased to a degree that scarcely leaves Fully any room for envy. The observations made by M. Moulin, President of Saillon, prove that the progress of goitre and cretinism date from the time when, in defiance of the counsel of M. Barmont, brother of the Swiss Ambassador at Paris, the commune took the water, destined for the use of the village, formerly received from a lower point of the torrent, ('the Salente,) from a point where it is precipitated in a cascade from the glacier of the mountain. Between these two points, a strong thermal spring (temperature about 28 C.) falls into the torrent, constituting nearly a sixtieth part of its waters.

" From my analysis it results —

" 1. That water taken from above the point where the hot spring enters the torrent, and which is that at present used in Saillon, is destitute of *Iodine*, like that of Fully, and of the greater part of the districts of the Vallais.

" 2. That the water taken from the point whence Saillon was formerly supplied is more iodized than the water used in Paris.

" 3. That the water of the thermal spring above referred to, is a true mineral water, containing at least sixty times more iodine than the water of Paris, and that of most of the countries where goitre is unknown.

" These facts go to prove —

" 1. The existence and nature of a *local* cause of goitre and cretinism.

" 2. The possibility of introducing iodized water as a prophylactic in these maladies, both as a regimen for man, and for animals producing meat, milk, &c."

From the Medico Chirurgical Review.

Regeneration of Nerves.

" Dr. Augustus Waller has been engaged in a very interesting series of investigations on the regeneration of nerves. ' While previous observers were contented with examining the nerve tubes at the point of section, or in the cicatrix, this author has pursued the investigation to the peripheral ends ; and has arrived at the interesting and unexpected result, *that the old fibres of a divided nerve never recover their original functions, and that reproduction of a nerve takes place not only in the cicatrix itself, but throughout the terminal ramifications.* The vagus of a dog having been divided, was examined after twelve days, when it was found that the inferior segment was completely disorganized, the fibres being all converted into black or irregular and opake parcels, and the membranous tubes destroyed. At the end of a month the condition was different: almost all the disorganized substance had been removed: new fibres were found in place of the old, possessing all the characters of young fibres, and being very difficult of recognition, owing to their grey color, intimate adherance, and want of double contour; but on the addition of organic acids — concentrated acetic especially — they were readily recognized as embryonic fibres. The disorganized nerve presents nothing similar, there being only an amorphous tissue, which dissolves readily in acetic acid, without any residue.

The author thinks that the neurilemma plays an important part in the regeneration of nerve fibres; it remains intact during the changes thus described. The results of section applied to the sympathetic fibres show that regeneration takes place in them in a similar manner. The following remarkable results were observed with regard to nerves in connection with ganglia: the roots of a spinal nerve were laid bare, and cut above the ganglion, in such a way as to leave a portion of them in connection with it: the animal was again examined after twelve days, when it was found that the sensitive part of the root attached to the superior part of the ganglion was altogether disorganized, in the same manner as when a nerve is cut in its peripheral portion. The nerve, followed into the ganglion, exhibited its branches disorganized, subdividing in the body, and mixing with fibres altogether normal, and appearing to terminate in a collection of ganglionic structures equally altered. All the fibres which passed out of the ganglion preserved their normal condition, the state of the fibres being found the same, after a month or more, as at first. The regeneration of the superior fibres between the ganglion and the spinal marrow takes place in the ordinary manner. The motor fibres were completely altered and disorganized to their extremities.

Report on the Surgery of Cortland County.

We cut the following practical extract from the " Transactions of the Medical Association of Southern Central New York," held at Ithaca, June, 1853.—ED.

The question arises, is there no therapeutical agent which can supplant the knife in the treatment of enlarged tonsils? I answer, in brief, that after repeated trials of nitrate of silver, iodine and other medical treatment, and after marking the experience of other surgeons for the relief of this affection by medicines, and comparing the results with the effects of the knife, I can say most emphatically, that for safety, promptness and efficiency, the knife is superior to all other means employed.

Another question frequently put to the surgeon by patients, and sometimes by physicians too, is, "Do the tonsils grow again, after amputation ?" Prof. Hamilton, in an able article on enlarged tonsils, in the third volume of the Buffalo Medical Journal, says [page 195] that according to his experience, when the whole or two-thirds of the gland is cut away, no more trouble is experienced from it, but that when one-half or one-third is removed, the ballance does not generally disappear, and, not unfrequently it again enlarges. This is not in accordance with the experience of many surgeons, nor with my own. Dr. Hyde has seen it but once. My opinion is, that in nearly all the cases of supposed regrowth, it is an appearance and not a reality. Dr. J. Mason Warren, of Boston, in an able article on "Enlargement of the Tonsils, attended with certain deformities of the Chest," published in 1839, [Am. Jour. Med. Sci., Aug., 1839, p. 525,] mentions one case in a list of nineteen, where, at the end of a short period after amputation, an appearance was presented as if they had been re-generated. This, he remarks arose from the original shape of the tonsil, in which the base was very broad, and extended some distance down the throat. The appearance of reproduction arose from the upper and lower portions rising or curling up, as it were, after the apex was removed.

This leads me to speak of lobed tonsils. I have had two cases in which the tonsils were each divided for about two-thirds of their lateral depth into two lobes. In the first of these cases, both lobes stood out prominently from the arches of the palate, so that I removed them by operating twice on each tonsil—each lobe being about the ordinary size of a hypertrophied tonsil, the remaining portion atrophied ; and an entire relief of the symptoms, for which removal was demanded, was the result. In the other case, I was not aware of the existence of the posterior lobes, until some days after the amputation of the anterior ones. At the end of that time, the patient, a young lady, presented herself again, saying that her tonsils had grown again, and to my astonishment, I found, on looking into her throat, two plump looking tonsils as ever need be, standing out about three-quarters of an inch from the edges of the palate. It was twilight, and I did not like to yield my opinion, previously expressed, in reference to the reproduction of amputated tonsils, until I could have more light upon the subject. The next day, by a strong light, I examined the throat, and found at the base of the "new" tonsil the cicatrix left by the amputation of the anterior lobe. The difficulty was at one explained. The anterior lobes had pushed the posterior ones backwards and downwards along the side of the pharynx, so that their existence was not suspected before operation, and at the time of it they were obscured by the coagulæ, which immediately formed about the divided surface of the first lobes. When the pressure of the anterior lobes was removed, the posterior ones resumed the usual position, and we had a marked instance of what is supposed to be a regrowth of the tonsil.

I am willing, however, to subscribe, in part to Dr. Hamilton's views on this subject, for I believe that if only a *small* portion of the gland is removed, the same condition of the organ remains—the morbid vascularity is kept up, and the tonsil *continues* to enlarge.

The conditions which contra-indicate amputation, where for other reasons it is desirable, are inflammation of the substance of the tonsil, and the hemorrhagic diathesis.

As to results of the operation, I must say that they have, in my experience, been almost uniformly gratifying. I cannot recall to mind one instance where I think injury was done to the throat by the operation, and but two instances in which no benefit was derived. I have witnessed profuse bleeding in but one instance. This was in the person of a young man with whose constitutional peculiarities I supposed myself acquainted, and so did not make the inquiry, which I rarely omit, whether he was apt to bleed much for slight wounds. In this case, I found the patient to be of a decidedly hemorrhagic tendency, and in ten or fifteen minutes after the operation, I found him in a state of partial syncope, and it was not until a minute afterwards that I was aware of the extent of the hemorrhage, for immediately after the operation he reclined upon a settee, and in that position, instead of disgorging the effused blood, he swollowed it, and when faintness came on, he vomited a large quantity of coagulæ. I immediately applied the neck-cloth, filled with pounded ice, and the bleeding was promptly arrested. This, by the way, is the most efficient remedy for this accident which we possess.

My strong conviction is, that this operation ought to be resorted to much oftener than it is by a majority of practitioners. There is no doubt that some operators have made this a surgical hobby, and see an indication for cutting in every throat, but the mass of practitioners, so far as my observation and acquaintance extends, are willing to let the matter go, if they can be excused from operating, or, perhaps, in many instances, they do not appreciate the indications for the removal of enlarged tonsils.

There are several other subjects which might be alluded to in this report, but I have already occupied too much of your time.

It may be well, however, before closing the report, to enumerate the inferences which justly follow from the cases and remarks here presented:

1st. That lumbar abscess is not necessarily a scrofulous disease; that, to be fatal, it need not involve the bones; that in a majority of instances the disease commences in the investment of the psoas magnus muscle; and that, in a large majority of cases, the disease is so far advanced before the surgeon sees them, that the treatment is directed rather to palliation than cure.

2d. That in treating fractures of the fore arm, the graduated compress should be so applied as not to press upon the pronator quadratus muscle.

3d. That diagnosis of fractures of the lower end of the radius is sometimes difficult, and that the direction of the fragment, as well as the recurrence of the deformity after reduction in fracture, are the diagnostics.

4th. That in many cases of hemorrhage, from wounds where pressure is the means resorted to for its suppression, bandaging the limb so as to control entirely the muscular action, is an important and indispensable item of treatment.

5th. That we may be encouraged to persevere in the treatment of very unpromising cases of morbous coxarius.

6th. That simple hydrops articuli can be converted into an irreparable injury, by bad management and unwarrantable interference.

7th. That, in some cases of traumatic hemorrhage, the best surgical procedure is to put the part into as quite a position as possible, and expose the wound entirely to the action of the air.

8th. That the mode of extension, by adhesive straps, is invaluable in compound and other fractures of the lower extremities.

9th. That, among the indications for the excision of enlarged tonsils, are the tendency to frequent attacks of tonsillitis and pharyngitis; the fear of croup in certain cases; the difficult and exhausting respiration during sleep in young children.

. 10th. That amputation of the tonsil is vastly preferable to the attempt to reduce the hypetrophy by medicinal treatment.

11th. That re-growth of the tonsil rarely if ever occurs, and that this occurrence is apparent rather than real, and is often caused by a lobed form of the tonsil.

12th. That the main contra-indications for the amputation, other things being equal, are, an inflamed condition of the tonsil, and the hemorragic diathesis.

13th. That in hemorrhage after excision, pounded ice, worn in a neck-cloth, applied to the throat, is the remedy.

14th. That the results of amputation are gratifying.

15th. That this operation is not resorted to with sufficient frequency.

Removal of a Nail from the Lungs by Tracheotomy.　By PAUL F. EVE, M.D., Professor of Surgery in Nashville University.

(Concluded from page 192.)

The after treatment of the case was of the simplest character. Two sutures applied to the skin had to be removed on account of threatened emphysema, and all dressing to the wound omitted, owing to the alarm of the patient recovering from chloroform. Two hours after the operation, he was taken in a carriage to his boarding-house, distant from mine two and a half squares.— During the after part of the day, bloody mucus was still discharged with air through the tracheal factitious opening whenever he fretted or cried; but when composed he breathed altogether *per vias naturales.* At 8 o'clock P. M., he was sleeping quietly and had less mucous rattle.

June 28th, 6 o'clock.—Has had a good night. Has very little fever. The wound was partially closed at 11, and effectually at 7 P. M., with isinglass plaster. The lungs are much freer and the respiration improved. The diet, up to this period, has been ice-lemmonade, and milk and sugar, the latter his favorite and accustomed nourishment.

29th, 7 A. M.—Is doing well; but at 11 has considerable fever. Prescribed calcined with the sulphate of magnesia. This being vomited, salt water enemata were directed. 8 P. M., the fever has abated, but the prescriptions have not been carried out, and there has been no action yet in the bowels.— The wound remains closed and his cough has ceased.

30th.—The patient is down stairs and it is difficult to keep him in doors. His bowels have been moved twice. The wound was dressed, found healed internally leaving the skin ununited.

July 1st.—Has left by railroad for the country.

2d.—Came in to have the wound dressed—it is nearly healed, but the cicatrix is a little irregular. 4th.—Left for home.

Recapitulation of case.—Patient aged five years. Gets a four-penny or shingle-nail into the left bronchus, from which it is removed through an opening in the trachea by forceps three weeks after its sojourn in the air passages. Within four days after the operation he goes into the country and fully recovers, for he has been heard from several times after the above date.— *—Nashville Journal of Medicine.*

EDITORIAL AND MISCELLANEOUS.

Our October and November numbers are delayed by accidents beyond our control, but which will not be likely to occur again. Those of our patrons who feared that the Journal had come to a fatal termination, and that they should "never see it more," may rest assured that there is not the least danger of any such catastrophe. We intend that it shall live until we are too old and gray to occupy its chair efficiently, and then we expect to hand it over to the next generation, as vigorous as it ever was. The delay that has occurred, was from no cause that threatened our prosperity, but from a combination of circumstances of an entirely different nature.

We are often inquired of for copies of number one. We have ordered number one to be reprinted, the first edition having been exhausted. The delay of number four and five caused a delay in the reprint, but it will be out before long, and will be sent on to those who have it not.

The Second Semi-Annual Meeting of the South-Western Medical Association of Michigan, will be held at Kalamazoo, on the second Tuesday of December, 1853, at the Court House.

We insert the following Circular with great pleasure. The work of Medical organization goes bravely on:

[CIRCULAR.]

Without pretending to determine what the future may demand in the administration of the trust confided to us as a profession, I may be permitted to enumerate certain of the duties imposed, and the privileges implied, in our organization.

It is our duty to use all proper measures to enhance our numbers; to devise ways and means for the furtherance of our objects — the advancement of Medical Science and the elevation of the Profession: and to this end, to appoint standing committees upon the several branches of Science connected with medicine, to control private pupilage, so far as private instruction may become the duty of our members; to sustain our Peninsular Journal of Med.

icine, to devise ways and means for the publication of Medical Literature adapted to the general reader.

In meeting together from time to time we will not only become socialized, as a profession, but fraternized as brethren of a great scientific family, where each will contribute to the interest of all, and all return to each the joint results of their labors.

This truly would be ample remuneration for all the time, money and effort spent in obtaining so desirable a result.

We live in an age emphatically progressive, an age in which mind in contact with mind are producing results in variety and execution, outstripping the imagination. " An age in which men think as gods, and hold converse through the instrumentality of the electrical spirit of the Universe ; an age in which men run to and fro as on chariots of fire, and in which knowledge is increased."

We live in a State emphatically great — Michigan, as yet but an infant of days — the first page of whose history is written in the present century — has exhibited a spectacle in the rapidity of her progress which challenges the world for a parallel. Living in such an age, under the benign influence of the freest government in the world, untrammeled by the despotism of Kings and Colleges, enjoying freedom of speech and thought. The sciences and arts, religion and politics, making mighty and rapid progress, increasing their strength by union of effort and concert of action. Shall we be content to stand still as idle beneficiaries of the past and present?

This cannot be so. Are we not all indebted to the past for much of the blessings we now enjoy? And should we not, as individuals, bestir ourselves, adding strength to our activity by the power of association?

We draw much of what we now enjoy of the blessings of the sciences from other countries and other parts of our own country, and shall we not show a willingness to act as co-laborers, if not progressives and revolutionists' in the domains of science?

William M. Wood says that " the enlarged sphere of duty pertaining to the profession of medicine, can only be promptly met by professional organization.

The people have their most solemn interest concerned in sustaining the organization, and how much reason to suspect those who affect to be independent of it. Medical men who voluntarily refrain from the work, are either behind the age, ignorant of their duties and of what the profession is doing, or else are seeking to hide sinister designs and selfish purposes under the affectation of individual independence, just as all do who profess to be independent of the general laws of society.

It is an easy mode of getting rid of wholesome obligations and restraints, by assuming to be entirely independent of it, and the people who cheer on such lawless spirits, must not complain if they find themselves the victims of lawlessness."

Let no ordinary business prevent you from attending, and come prepared to report some case from your practice. Yours, truly,
B. P. WELLS,
Dated Niles, October 29th, 1853. Corresponding Secretary.

We call the attention of all our friends in the Southwest, to the above Circular. Let there be a grand Mass-Meeting of the Profession in that part of the State. Union in peace is power, in war it is victory, and the goodly work of organization which is now going forward in every part of the State, is the forerunner of honor and renown to the profession, and of destruction to its enemies. From the signs of vigor in the local organizations, we predict a large and enthusiastic meeting of the State Society next spring. Once again, therefore, arouse, ye strong men of the Southwest !

———

The following Circular was sent us by Dr. Taylor of Mt. Clemens, who is on important Committees, both in the National Association and the State Society. Dr. Taylor is an active and efficient investigator of the Medical Sciences and a staunch defender of the Profession. We hope that Physicians in every part of this and adjoining States, will, without fail, communicate to him all the facts which may be in their possession respecting the subjects mentioned in the Circular. It should be remembered that it is not *remarkable* facts alone that are useful to the Committee, but *all* facts. We hope, therefore, that all who have the cause of Science at heart, will lose no time in communicating to Dr. Taylor, diseases that prevail in their particular vicinity, particularly all the facts respecting Dysentery. It is only by prompt response from individual physicians that such a Committee can come in possession of the information which they require.

[C I R C U L A R.]

(For the Peninsular Journal.)

At a meeting of the State Medical Society I was appointed to report on the geographical distribution of diseases in this region.

I was also appointed Chairman of a Committee to report on the disease Dysentery, by the American Medical Association, at its last meeting.

The peculiar character of Dysentery as presented in the last few years, has been a subject of much interest to the Medical practitioner, and it is hoped that inquiry may bring to light some useful discovery regarding the nature or cure of this troublesome complaint.

The undersigned, therefore, takes this course to call out the investigations of Physicians upon this matter, and assures them that they will confer a high obligation by corresponding with him upon either of the above named subjects.

Please address H. Taylor, M.D., Mt. Clemens, Mich.

H. TAYLOR.

———

Transactions of the Medical Association of Southern Central N. Y.

This body held its seventh annual meeting at Ithaca, in June. The papers read were of an unusually interesting character, consisting, principally, of reports on the Surgery of the several counties in the district and also the epidemics. A body that can produce such a report of proceedings, must occupy a high and honorable standing both in the profession, and before the community. We hope to give our readers some extracts at a future time.

Proceedings of the American Pharmaceutical Association.

The American Pharmaceutical Association held its last annual meeting in Boston on the 24th, 25th and 26th of August. Many of the reports are able, and the tone and spirit of the meeting was worthy of all commendation.

Suspension of Lectures at Geneva.

The lectures at Geneva Medical College, as most of our readers are doubt-less aware, are suspended, probably never to be resumed. It is to be regret-ted that an institution which has run so honorable and useful a career, should have become extinct; but its geographical position rendered it impossible to meet the competition of rival schools. After continuing the lectures a week or two, the number of students was only about twenty, and it was judged best, both by the faculty and students, to disperse; which was accordingly done.

The Yellow Fever at New Orleans.

We have as yet no full and scientific summing up of the course of this scourge. The N. Orleans Medical Register, speaking of its causes, attributes its severity to the filthiness of the foreign population, and the want of clean-ness in the streets and vacant grounds. The Register says:—

" We have a fruitful element of disease in our midst in the growth and in-crease of our foreign population. They bring with them not only bodies sus-ceptible by their foreign birth to our endemial disorders, but habits and cus-toms as unlike and unsuited to our climate and usages. They come from wretched crowded hovels, where want and filth produce pestilence to our cities and towns, where they cluster in numbers as thick, and live amid filth as gross as that they have escaped from. They come to find employment and ready remuneration for their labor, and they live like persons just escaped from the pains of famine. They eat and drink to excess. They violate by day and night every maxim of prudence—every safeguard of health. Surely the fault can not be theirs — poverty and oppression at home may have caused much of this huge evil. They know no better. All the traditions of home and family record no variety to their woes. It was want, and privation, and filth before their day. It is the heritage they derive from their parents and friends; it is the sole accompaniment, the invariable attendant upon them in their pilgrimage to our shores. We must look to their domestic relations, therefore; we must subject their social irregularities to control and discipline if we wish to do them good service, and to exempt ourselves from the destroy-ing ravages of a cruel pestilence. They must be taught to value not only the blessings of political freedom which they gain by coming to our shores, but to learn how to value the higher blessings and comforts of a good, well ordered, and salubrious home. One means to insure this will be to discourage by stringent laws the habit of subleases to tenants, which leads to over-crowding and to all the consequent ills."

" This has become too common an abuse of property. A landlord rents his house and lot to one person, who subleases it to a dozen or more families, the more the better for the original lessee -- no matter what abuses result therefrom, and how other interests are made to suffer. Generally, too, it is old decaying property, whose rafters are undermined by time, and grown green with mould, that falls into the occupancy of this class. As long as it continues decent, or comfortable, or safe, they are excluded by high rents and a better class, from its use. But let it wear by time and neglect till it totters, let it grow dank and unwholesome, let it become but little better than the sheds which house our cattle, and then it becomes the fit habitation for that portion of our population who are content with all these discomforts, and who seek shelter there as naturally as bats do crannies and dark holes. But enough have we said on this topic. It makes the heart sick to witness the great suffering among this unhappy class. The neglect of society, the indifference of our laws, the aversion of our people to them, conspire with their disorganized condition and mischievous habits, to keep perpetual the elements requisite to give malignancy to disease and facility to its spread. We have space to allude to but one more nuisance, and that a huge and monstrous one. This is the manner in which our city authorities sanction the filling up of the land reclaimed by changes of our river bed. A viler compost, one more abounding in disgusting, offensive nuisances, can not be found anywhere.-- Standing in the evening after sunset on any portion of our levee, one might realize something of the disgust of Coleridge at Cologne--

> " He might count two-and-seventy stenches,
> All well defined and genuine stinks."

so thick and reeking are the odors escaping from these foul spots. They are the burial places of all dead animals—from a mouse to a horse, the common receptacle of all the offals from every cook shop and kitchen, of the refuse vegetables, bones and garbage of our market houses, and the sweepings of our streets. If the art of man could contrive anything worse than this, we should like to see it. Yet we breathe this foul air—worse than the abattoirs of Paris, and wonder that we sicken and die. Rouse up ' we must set our household in order if the future is to be spanned with brighter hopes, and stronger assurances. We will have to look more closely into our domestic habits, more narrowly into our social vices, more determinedly on the negligence of our laws, if we are to be anything besides the immense lazar-house the late pestilence has made us."

So far as we can learn about the peculiarities of this visitation of yellow fever, it is well marked and clear, but does not bear the same treatment that the previous one did. Then the administration of large doses of quinine succeeded best, while in the present epidemic, that mode of treatment fails entirely. We shall post up our readers on this epidemic thoroughly, when its results are better analysed. The deaths from yellow fever alone, in one month, were four thousand seven hundred and ninety-eight.

NOTICES OF WORKS.

MANUAL OF OBSTETRICS. By T. F. COCK, M.D., Physician to the New York Lying in Asylum, Physician to the Bellevue Hospital, etc.

This is a small work, intended as a hand-book for students and young practitioner. It is a brief compendium of the *facts* of obstetrics, and will be an excellent companion in the lecture room.

It comprises the anatomy of the pelvis — natural and abnormal; the anatomy of the organs of generation; menstruation — natural and diseased; pregnancy, with its accidents and complications; labor — natural and abnormal; and the diseases, remedies, and operations incident to parturient females.

Those who wish a work of this nature to refresh their memories, will find it a valuable assistant. It is published by S. S. & Wm. Wood, 261 Pearl-street, N. Y. Also to be obtained from A. B. Wood, Ann Arbor, Mich.

PRESCRIBER'S PHARMACOPŒIA. Third American, from the fourth London edition; revised by T. F. COCK, M.D.

This little book contains the entire pharmacopœia in a form to be easily carried in the pocket. It contains the name, dose, and uses of each medicine, together with tables of weights and measures, poisons and their antidotes, special formulæ, and directions for the diet of the sick. A very useful pocket companion. Published by S. S. & Wm. Wood, 261, Pearl-street, New York. It can be obtained also of A. B. Wood, Ann Arbor, Mich.

MEDICAL FORMULARY.

This valuable work has reached its tenth edition. It consists of an admirable collection of prescriptions, collected from various authorities, together with dietetic preparations and poisons, with their antidotes, to which is added an appendix on the endermic use of medicine and the use of ether and chloroform.

We recommend this work to all physicains as eminently a practical one. It is published by Blanchard and Lea, Philadelphia.

EXCHANGES.

The American Journal of Insanity, published by the New York State Lunatic Asylum, Utica. A valuable periodical, from which we will present our readers some interesting extracts at a future time.

The American Journal of Dental Science, edited by C. A. Harris M.D., D.D.S., Alfred A. Blandy, M.D., D.D.S., and A. S. Pigott, M.D. Address Drs. Harris, Blandy, & Piggot, Baltimore, Md.

Annals of Science, conducted by Hamilton L. Smith, A.M., Cleveland, Ohio.

The Boston Medical and Surgical Journal, · Edited by J. V. C. Smith, M.D.

The British and Foreign Medico-Chirurgical Review, or Quarterly Journal of Practical Medicine and Surgery, republished by S. S.& W. Wood, 261 Pearl-street, N. Y.

The Buffalo Medical Journal and Monthly Review of Medical and Surgical Science, edited by Austin Flint, M.D., and S. B. Hunt, M.D.

The Charleston Medical Journal and Review, edited and published by J. D. Cain, M.D., Lecturer on the Principles and Practice of Medicine in the Charleston Preparatory Medical School, and F. Peyer Porcher, M.D., Lecturer on Materia Medica and Therapeutics in the Charleston Preparatory Medical School;—Bi-monthly. Charleston, S. C.

Iowa Medical Journal, conducted by the Faculty of the Medical Department of Iowa University, Keokuk, Iowa.

Kentucky Medical Recorder, edited by H. M. Bullitt, M.D., and R. J. Breckinbridge, M.D., Louisville, Ky.

Materia Medica, or Pharmacology and Therapeutics, by Wm. Tully, M.D., Springfield Mass.

The London Lancet, edited by Thomas Wakley, Surgeon; republished by Stringer & Townsend, N. Y.

The Medical Examiner and Record of Medical Science, edited by Prof. Francis Gurney Smith, M.D., and Prof. John B. Biddle, M.D., Philadelphia.

Memphis Medical Recorder, published bi-monthly by the Memphis Medical College; edited by Prof. A. P. Merrill, M.D., and Prof. C. T. Quintard, M.D., Memphis, Tenn.

The New Jersey Medical Reporter and Transactions of the New Jersey Medical Society; edited by Joseph Parish, M.D., Burlington, N. J.

The New Hampshire Journal of Medicine, edited by Edward Parker, A.M., M.D., Concord, N. H.

The Philadelphia Medical and Surgical Journal, edited by James Bryan, A.M., M.D., Philadelphia.

The Northwestern Medical & Surgical Journal, edited by Prof. W. B. Herrick, and H. A. Johnson, A.M., M.D., Chicago, Ill. A first rate periodical, and conducted by two of the ablest men in the West.

Ranking's Half-Yearly Abstracts. Philadelphia, Pa.

Nashville Journal of Medicine and Surgery, edited by Professor W. K. Bowling, M.D., assisted by Professor Paul F. Eve, M.D., Nashville, Tennessee. Got up in handsome style and very ably sustained.

Southern Medical and Surgical Journal, edited by Professor L. A. Dugas, M.D., Augusta, Ga.

The New York Journal of Medicine and the Collateral Sciences, edited by Samuel Purple, M.D., and Steven Smith, M,D. Sustained in a superior style.

The Virginia Medical and Surgical Journal, edited by Geo. A. Otis, M.D. and Howell L. Thomas, M.D., Richmond, Va.

The Western Journal of Medicine and Surgery, edited by Professor Lunsford, P. Yandell, M.D. and T. S. Bell, M.D., Louisville, Kentucky.

The Western Lancet, edited by L. M. Lawson, M.D., and T. Wood, M.D., Cincinnati, Ohio.

NONPROFESSIONAL EXCHANGES.

The Western Literary Cabinet, edited by Mrs. Electa M. Sheldon, Detroit, Michigan.

Independent Press, Waukesha, Wisconsin, edited by S. A. Bean and E. H. Baxter.

Michigan State Journal, edited by G. W. Peck, Lansing, Mich.

The Washtenaw Whig, edited by S. B. M'Crachen, Ann Arbor, M.

The Michigan Argus, edited by Cole and Gardiner, Ann Arbor, M.

The Independent Register, edited by M. C. Read, Hudson, O.

The Ancient Landmark, Mt. Clemens, Mich.

THE

PENINSULAR

JOURNAL OF MEDICINE

AND THE COLLATERAL SCIENCES.

| VOL. I. | DECEMBER, 1853. | NO. VI. |

ORIGINAL COMMUNICATIONS.

ART. I.—*Occlusion of Vagina, Operation for relief of.* By JOSEPH BRIGGS, M. D., of Schoolcraft, Kal. Co., Michigan.

I was called, May 23d, 1852, to visit Mrs. W———, farmer's wife, aged 51 years, the mother of five children, the youngest aged nine years.

Found the patient sitting up, able to walk about the house, countenance pale, indicating poverty of the blood, complained of pains resembling labor pains, rather more continuous, sensation of weight in lower part of abdomen, and pressure upon the bladder, making a necessity for frequent micturition, which was attended with considerable pain. Patient said there was some obstruction to the discharges from the womb.

Upon examination, vagina, per vaginam, found about midway, firm adhesions of the walls of vagina, producing entire closure of that passage; the parts up to this obstruction appeared healthy, entirely free from ulcers or excoriations, or indications that there had been ulcers in this portion of the vagina. Upon passing the finger into the bowel, a large and inelastic (very firm) tumor could be felt, apparently filling the cavity of the pelvis, the sensation to the finger, as to bulk, resembling the touch of the head of a fœtus, at full term, in the pelvic cavity. The uterus could be felt above the os pubis, firm, and, in shape well defined, appearing about as large as it would at the seventh month of gestation, the organ, however, not having that easy rounded feel, but more elongated and pointed than in pregnancy.

Previous history, as obtained from patient and husband. She had been in the enjoyment of very good health since the birth of her youngest child until the preceding autumn, had been healthy with her catamenial periods until the preceding November, when she was taken with what she supposed, severe uterine hæmorrhage, as the patient states positively that the fluid never coagulated, it was probably not hæmorrhagic, but a case of excessive menstruation, the discharges continued at times very profuse, at others much less, but never an entire cessation, until in the early part of February, it suddenly ceased. She thinks there never was any pus passed with the fluid, nothing resembling it, except once or twice, there was something like white mucus mixed up with it just previous to the cessation, (it is, however, not probable that she would analyze the discharges very closely) she has no recollection of having suffered from pain or sores in the vagina during this period.

Her general health, previous to February, had suffered very much, to such an extent that her life had been almost despaired of by her friends and medical attendant. After the cessation of the menstrual flux, her health had gradually improved, up to within a short period of the time I saw her; she was still, as I before remarked, to a certain degree anæmic; she had suffered some pain about the pelvis, at her menstrual period in March, still more in April, and again, the symptoms were more aggravated when I was called in May.

From the previous history, and present condition of the patient, it was evident that the case was one of accumulated menstrual fluid in uterus, and that portion of vagina above the point of obstruction, and the means for relief, (an operation to re-open vagina) appeared to be immediately called for.

May 27th—Operated upon patient, assisted by Doctors William and Chas. Mottram. Chloroform administered by Dr. C. Mottram. The bowels having been previously emptied by castor oil, the patient was placed upon a table, as in operation for Lithotomy, a catheter was passed into the bladder, for a two fold object, viz: to empty that viscus and learn if in its natural position, or displaced by the previous disease; an assistant with an abdominal tractor being placed upon each side of patient to hold apart the sides of vagina and support the knees, the operation was then commenced with a small knife, by carefully dissecting in direction of the vaginal passage; by occasionally introducing a finger into the bowel, the relation of parts could be very accurately kept in mind. I had intended to operate after the manner of Dr. Warren, (see report

American Journal of Medicine, &c., July, 1851) and after cutting far enough to feel the tumor through the part, to finish the operation by pushing a trocar forward into the tumor, but being able to follow the tract of vagina very accurately, I continued with the knife until it entered the tumor; this was followed by a gush of very dark and tenacious fluid. The opening was then enlarged by an anal knife, directed by the finger, to about three-fourths of an inch in diameter, the adhesions occupied nearly one and a-half inches of the vaginal canal. The amount of fluid discharged was about three quarts. The parts were then washed, and a sponge tent, covered with oiled silk, was introduced into the opening, with a string attached, to prevent its slipping into the cavity beyond the stricture, which was yet large.

May 28.—Patient slept well, and had slight uterine pains during the night; the tent had been removed, followed by about one quart of fluid; as before, had urinated without pain. Pulse 100.

May 29th.—Removed the tent, which was followed by the discharge of a small quantity of like fluid as before; uterus still perceptible above the os pubis, slight contractions, a little tenderness in vicinity of uterus; slightly restless. Pulse 100.

May 30.—Patient much worse; had severe rigors in latter part of night, followed by fever; dry and hot skin, pulse 120, whole surface of abdomen painful, tender to the touch, complains of most pain in left ilio-abdominal region, countenance indicating suffering and anxiety. Removed tent again; no unusual tenderness about wound; some little discharge still.

It will not be necessary to enter into a description of symptoms from day to day, but instead, give a general outline of the course of the inflammatory attack. Nor will it be necessary to give the treatment, further than to say that the patient was treated upon general principles, as the general health of patient seemed to contra-indicate the abstraction of blood. Reliance was placed principally upon calomel and opium, counter-irritants and mild aperients.

From the time of this attack the fever ran on without intermission, almost an entire suppression of the appetite, hot and dry skin, dry tongue, pulse about 130. The inflammatory action in the bowels gradually became circumscribed to certain limits, forming a well-defined tumor at a point near where the colon passes into the pelvis, the pain centering at this point, producing, when touched, or when the bowels moved, most intense suffering. This inflammatory action ending in the formation of an abscess, and very favorably opening into the bowels and passing off through the rectum upon the eleventh day from operation.

From this time the unfavorable symptoms subsided, the appetite returned, the abscess continued to discharge for about a week, the tumor becoming less in size, and less tender and painful. She rapidly improved in health from this time, and at the end of six weeks she was able to attend to her household duties.

A few remarks may be made in relation to the opening made into vagina. I found it necessary during the severity of the inflammatory fever to remove the tent entirely and trust to the occasional introduction of the finger, to keep the parts from again closing. The consequence of having to leave the opening without the tent, the parts closed so as to leave only a space sufficient to introduce a common sized catheter. But this answers all purposes as to her own health, never having given her any trouble but once, when it became plugged up a short time with some tenacious meterial, which gave way from the accumulation, without other interference, up to the present time, September 17th, 1853.

Remarks.—This case presents some points of interest that do not usually belong to cases of the kind. In the first place, in what manner were these adhesions brought about, between surfaces so obnoxious to such accidents, without any of the antecedents that would lead one to suspect that danger? I am satisfied that it was not from long or deep ulcerations, nor from harsh or unusual treatment from the medical attendant. If an opinion might be hazarded, was it not probably brought about by the irritating quality of the fluids passing over their surfaces, producing simply exconations or abrasions of the mucous coat, happening at just that time when the original disease had spent its force and the discharge was subsiding, by which the abraded surfaces were brought into contact and united by (if it would be proper to say,) the first intention? This view is confirmed somewhat by there being no very deep cicatrices, nor large fibrous bands seen in operation.

In the second place, from what cause was the abscess formed? Was it from the general inflammation of peritoneum which finally centered and spent its force upon a single point, or was it produced by previous disease in the ovary, which had also played a conspicuous part in the menorrhogia? Or was it from the forcing of the contained fluid from the uterus back through the ovarian tube into the ovary, enlarging the same, or bursting some of its delicate parts, forming a nucleus around which the inflammatory process was subsequently set up?

As I was unable to satisfy myself in relation to this, I shall leave the reader to form his own opinion from the symptoms previously detailed.

ART. II.—*Diagnosis and Treatment of Thecal Abscess, etc.*

Having during the last eighteen or twenty months been cutting my way through a furunculoid epidemic, in which local diagnosis has sometimes been a desideratum, I read with eagerness an article on Thecal Abscess in the September number of the Peninsular Journal of Medicine, &c., copied from the London Lancet, and beg leave to add a few more hints on the subject.

There is no doubt of the usefulness of free incisions in all active inflammations existing below the palmar, and plantar fasciæ, and it is still more important when the theca, tendon, or bone is involved.

Early incisions or scarifications, before pus is formed, relieves the painful tension, empties the surcharged vascular apparatus, and often prevents suppuration—a perfect cure resulting in seventy hours, without a tender cicatrix. But who is not liable to drive the unrelenting steel to the very bone, when all the disease is in the tissues of the corium? or, what is worse, only scarify when the mischief lurks far below? To guard against such accidents we are informed that "straightening the finger gives pain in the thecal abscess," and we aver most confidently that it does the same when the cutis is made tense by superficial inflammation, and the amount of complaint made depends on your patient's power of endurance.— Again, the writer states that "fluctuation in thecal abscess may be felt laterally."

But the period at which such fluctuation may be felt is many hours later than the incision might be advantageously made, as we will cite one case to show. Fluctuation is also felt "from one side to the other in some superficial abscesses." Our means of diagnosis are as follows:— Bend the wrist and hand as far back as can be done *without pain.* Then press upon the muscle in the fore-arm to which the suspected tendon belongs, and if its theca is inflamed, you will seldom be left in doubt, while superficial abscess will not feel it. 2d. We bring the finger, whose phalanx, or whose metacarpal is suspected, as near straight as can be done *without severe pain*, and then push or strike gently against the end. If the bone is inflamed the hurt will inform most patients that the citadel is stormed. 3d. If the part has been poulticed, scrape off the softened cuticle, and if not shave it thin with a keen instrument. Take a wide, well-polished scalpel or razor, and hold the edge perpendicular to— and touching lightly—the surface. Let the sun, or a strong artificial light shine upon the farther side, and you can see well down into the translucent tissues. If the disease is superficial, a zone of congested vessels around the point of attack will often tell to what depth you need to cut. This being ascertained, we take a narrow, well-pointed knife, usually the club-foot knife, and introduce it p·rpendicularly, *quantum opus est*, cut towards the distal extremity freely.

It is true we usually manipulate laterally, vertically, and longitudinally as much as our patients can reasonably bear; but the above are the most reliable diagnostics.

After the incision has been made in the part first inflamed, we some-- times arrest the progress upwards by applying a pleget of lint, saturated with a strong tincture of iodine over the newly invaded portion.

An emolient and anodyne poultice is always necessary after opening, as before. The dregs and filter of tr. opii. make a good application. The case promised, was E. B., an adult, possessing considerable powers of endurance, felt some pain in the second phalanx of ring finger, about 9 A. M. April 9th, 1851, the hands were kept in warm suds during most of the forenoon. While setting dinner table, she became faint from pain and was compelled to give up business. I was called at 3 P. M., and im- mediately laid open the theca nearly the whole length of the phalanx. Gramous blood and a drop of yellowish mucous, but no pus, escaped. Warmth and moisture were applied. Patient slept well the first night, and the incision healed almost by first intention.

June 3d, 1853, the same lady called me about midnight, and stated that five or six days before, she "felt another felon coming" on the second phalanx of one thumb. She had previously shown it to a physician, who advised her to "*wait.*" I laid it open as before described, finding exit to considerable pus. We applied an anodyne poultice. Two days after she returned with the back of the thumb tender, and inflammation extending nearly to carpus.

℞ Sal. Rochelle ℥i. immediately. Emp. vesc. to dorsal surface of metacarpipolicis. This was kept on twelve hours with no effect on the cutis or the disease.

A pleget of lint as large as a penny, wet with a saturated tincture of iodine, was applied in place of the emp. vesc. After one hour the pain abated, and soon the surface was found to be blistered. From this time convalescence was uninterrupted, but slow; a cicatrix, which was for sometime tender, being formed—making about three weeks' duration to a disease, whose accession was less severe than that which was cured in about as many days.

J. H. B.

ART. III.—*To the Editor of the Peninsular Journal of Medicine.*

DEAR SIR·—Permit a boy,—a mere novice, as it were, in the science of medicine,—to intrude upon the quietude of your 'sanctum' by presenting the following rare, and, to *me*, very interesting case, which occurred to my personal notice:

Mrs R ——, aged seventy-two, and descended from a line of long-lived ancestors, with an otherwise naturally strong constitution, was, from early youth, subject to a severe cough, and at times some pain in the region of the left lung. This state of things continued with occasional intermissions of cough and pain, and as her health was otherwise good she performed much labor. Married at the age of twenty-one and became the mother of four healthy children. At the age of forty a small tumor made its appearance on the left shoulder, in the region of the supra scapular muscle. This continued to enlarge, becoming at times exceedingly painful, and as it did so, the cough and irritation of the lung gradually lessened until they were hardly perceptible. The tumor was shown to Professor Thomas Spencer, late of Geneva, N. Y., who pronounced it to be an incipient carcinomatous enlargement, and as its removal was advised, the operation was cheerfully submitted to, and it was extirpated by the above-named Professor.

After the wound healed, the cough returned with its former intensity, and continued to trouble her until about six months previous to her decease, which occurred in November, 1852. During the interval which elapsed from the extirpation of the tumor and the relapse or last attack, which terminated her life, she enjoyed excellent health, save the cough and the troublesome irritation felt in the left lung.

She expectorated freely a kind of glazy, frothy matter, which she described as tasting very salt, but having no other peculiarity. About one year previous to her death, she noticed a slight soreness of one of the glands of the left breast, just below the nipple, which continued to increase; the gland at the same time began to enlarge and assume a leaden color, and when of the size of a butternut lancinating pains were felt shooting from the tumor to the lung, and *vice versa*. These pains increased in intensity, the countenance became haggard and sallow, while the tumor rapidly enlarged, assumed the shape of a damask rose, and at length appeared of nearly the same color. At this stage of the disease, an occasional diarrhœa, frequent tenesmus, and oft-repeated attempts to vomit, were among the most prominent occurrences.

About six months previous to her death, the cough gradually began to lessen, and continued to do so for three months, when it ceased entirely. At this time the tumor, which was now as large as a tea-saucer, *burst*, discharging a very fetid sanious matter, offensive to the patient and disgusting to her attendants. The swelling now *decreased* as rapidly as it *increased* before, until there was but a small portion left. The fetor was partially controlled by a solution of nitras argentii, or pulverized tannin and sulph. quinine, applied to the part affected, and the *intense* pain by morphine administered internally, or applied to the surface of the ulcer.

Active hemorrhage would often succeed the rupture of a vessel, as its coats were corroded and eaten away by the disease, but the bleeding was always easily suppressed.

Anæsthetics were frequently administered with happy results, until death closed the sufferings of the patient, whose last hours were peaceful and happy.

The following post mortem appearances were observed, *viz:*

The principal seat of the disease appeared to be the superior lobe of the left lung, although the inferior lobe was much diseased, as well as the superior and middle ones of the right.

Fibrous white bands, or feeders, were seen running in every direction, from the superior lobe of the left lung to the tumor, right lung, pleura, mediastinum. The heart and other internal organs appeared to be uninjured. From the above, which is a fair exposition of the case, it appears very evident to my own mind, that, contrary to the established opinion of the mass of physicians and surgeons of the past and present day, other structures than those of a glandular nature, are, and may be, the seat of cancerous degeneration. For my own part, I have long been of the opinion that there was such a disease as *cancer of the lungs*, a fact to which I wish to call the attention of the medical faculty, of this state *especially*, and in proof of the position which I have taken, I would refer to the above case of Mrs. R——. That her's was a case of *pulmonary cancer* cannot reasonably be doubted. That it originated in the substance of the *lung itself* is *self-evident*: first, from the fact of the lung being diseased long before any outward manifestations of cancer had made their appearance; and secondly, that as soon as the tumor had attained any considerable size, in the first instance, or had *burst*, in the second, that the cough and expectoration partially ceased in one, and entirely in the other.

If you deem the above worthy a place in your Journal, you are at liberty to publish it, with such corrections as you may deem it to require, or if not worthy of appearing in print, you will please throw it under your table.

If the cause of humanity will be benefitted by the truthful exposition of the case which I have given, the aim of the writer will have been attained.

With asking your pardon for intruding myself into your notice, I remain your most obedient servant, M. F. PALMER.

COLUMBIA, Jackson Co., Mich., Sept. 5th, 1863.

ART. IV.—*Report of a case of Carinoma of the Stomach.* Read before the Detroit Medical Society, by E. P. CHRISTIAN, M.D.

I have here, for the inspection of the Society, the stomach, a portion of the right lobe of the liver, part of the left lung, and a section of the diaphragm with pericardium attached, showing very extensive carcinomatous disease. It had not only invaded these parts, but had involved all the contiguous parts to some extent — among others, the aorta and duodenum were notably diseased.

These were taken from a patient of St. Mary's Hospital, at a postmortem made by Dr. Pitcher, myself assisting, on the 8th of this month, (October.) The history of the patient is as follows: About three months previous to his death he entered the hospital for a supposed injury of the ribs. No injury could be discovered on examination, but bandages were applied, as in fractures of these bones, and treatment adopted accordingly. There was no other indication of disordered condition at that time, but want of appetite. His health had been previously good, and he presented no indications whatever of organic disease.

About one month after his entrance, he began to be troubled with pains, of no very acute character, after eating, and vomiting of his food, which came up in a macerated condition. This continued in an aggravated manner until his death. It was accompanied by a very torpid condition of the bowels, their motions occurring not oftener than once in nine or ten days. This constipation was owing to the lack of their natural stimulus of food, and perhaps in a slight degree to a depravation of, or lessened secretion of bile, owing to the implication of the liver in the disease; for the bowels, when examined, were found like a mere cord, having adapted themselves to their contents by their tonic contractility. He became very much emaciated, presenting also that peculiar pale straw color complexion spoken of as peculiar to the cancerous cachexia. These then were all the diagnostic symptoms exhibited at any time of carcinoma of the stomach, and these all within two months of its fatal termination. 1st. Pain in the epigastrium after eating; 2nd, vomiting of food soon after its ingestion; 3rd, constipation of the bowels; 4th, the peculiar pale straw color complexion; 5th, great emaciation. There was at no time the piercing, lancinating pain spoken of as one, though of the least constant diagnostic symptoms of carinoma. There was no vomiting of blood or bloody matters, no diarrhœa at any stage, nor anasarca.

The peculiarity of this case is in the fact that it should have progressed so far; involving the stomach and all contiguous viscera to such an extent, before manifesting itself by diagnostic symptoms, and even in this advanced stage, manifesting symptoms so little indicative of the amount of disease and destruction; or else it is singular in the rapidity of its progress after the latent seeds of the disease were once set in action by the injury received just previous to entering the hospital.

Now, which of these was in reality the case? Whatever evidence is afforded by the history of the case itself, would certainly lead us to the latter conclusion; for, on his first examination there was not, nor could it be ascertained that there had been at any time previous, any indications of organic disease; neither his sensations, appearance, nor functions, presented anything abnormal.

To be sure, this is only negative evidence, but it is such evidence as should prevent us deciding on the previous existence of the disease without positive proofs. On the other hand, the well known difficulty of diagnosing this disease; the fact that carcinoma of the stomach has been known in repeated cases to have existed for a long period without special symptoms to draw attention to the part, justifies the opinion that this was of that character.

Tweedie says, "There is no one symptom pathognomonic of the disease, and our judgment must depend upon their concurrence." Gerhard says, "The diagnosis of cancer of the stomach is always doubtful, unless there should be positive proof of the presence of a tumor." And Watson remarks of this disease, " Carcinoma of the stomach has sometimes no symptoms at all, or none which the most sagacious practitioner would refer to the stomach." This is convincingly shown by one of his cases, that of the young woman with a pulsating tumor of the abdomen, which was taken for an aneurism, until having subsided very much by free purgation; it was then supposed by some that it was formed by an accumulation of feces in the transverse colon. The woman died, and it was then discovered to be cancer of the stomach. There was no sickness nor any one symptom to draw attention to the stomach. But there are numerous other cases recorded, showing how insidiously the disease may sometimes progress; and with such evidence, I think we may rightly consider this case as one of that character, up to the time of its becoming so extensive as to offer a mechanical impediment to the passage of food from the stomach downward. The other symptoms, constipation and emaciation, and finally death following as a consequence of the occlusion of the pylorus.

ART. V.—*Aphonia of Four Years' Standing, cured by Electro-Magnetism,* By F. K. BAILEY, M.D., Almont.

Mrs. S——, aged 79, in the spring of 1849, had a severe attack of Bronchitis, which was relieved by appropriate treatment.

On regaining her general strength, however, her voice was at times very hoarse, and at the close of the day it was difficult to speak loud at all. In the course of six months from the first attack, there was a complete Aphonia, which continued until last April.

At that time she was induced to make trial of Electro-Magnetism. In a few days after this means was tried, her voice became more distinct, but very rough at first. In the course of a week or two speech was natural, and has continued until the present time.

The favorable result in this case may lead to the use of Electro-Magnetism in other affections produced by want of proper innervation. I will add, the apparatus used was one manufactured by Charles Crosman, Detroit.

October, 1853.

ART. VI.—*Researches upon a new Function of the Liver, considered as a Sugar-producing organ in Man and in Animals.* By M. CLAUDE BERNARD. Translated from the French, by Prof. A. SAGER.

INTRODUCTORY.

I will establish in this work that animals as well as vegetables possess the faculty of producing sugar. I will show, moreover, that this animal function, which until now has been unknown, has its localization in the liver.

The unexpected results to which I have arrived, relative to this singular production of sugar in the liver, will appear, I trust, to be supported by incontrovertible proof. But before entering upon a description of the special facts of this question, I deem it useful to indicate by what ideas I was guided in these physiological researches. This exposition, which will show the successive steps of the investigation, will prove, moreover, that the discovery which was the object of this memoire, is entirely due to experimental physiology—that is to say, the only possible means of arriving at the result was, by direct experiments upon living animals.

Indeed, how would it be possible to ascertain by anatomy alone that the liver produced a saccharine matter, which is constantly introduced into the blood to supply a want of nutrition? No induction drawn from the form or structure of the organ would furnish us with a hint, nor would the most minute microscopic investigation of the cells and vessels of the organ ever lead us to a knowledge of this function.

The rapid progress of organic chemistry, and the fruitful physiological impulse given to that science by modern chemists, and especially by Dumas in France, Liebig in Germany, &c., have thrown great light upon many questions touching animal nutrition. But even the splendid torch of chemistry would have illuminated only the surface of the phenomena of life if the aid of experimental physiology had not been secured to enable it to penetrate into the interior of our organs, and into the midst of those interior functions, many of which still remain enveloped in much mystery. Aided by this powerful resource, I have succeeded in demonstrating the existence, in ourselves, as well as in all other animal bodies, of a process of sugar-formation, the phenomena of which were so profoundly concealed as never to have been suspected, and which revealed itself by no external manifestation.

Comparative observations upon the nutritive functions of animals and vegetables, on the contrary, led to the conclusion that the organism of the former was incapable of generating saccharine matter. Indeed, the sugar and starch which is formed in considerable quantity in the vegetable kingdom, are incessantly destroyed by animals in the process of self-nutrition. There are, therefore, two apparently correlative phenomena constantly taking place under our observation—viz: 1st. An abundant production of saccharoid matter by vegetables. 2d. A rapid and incessant destruction of the same products for the subsistence of animals.

Chemical science also confirmed this idea, for hitherto fermentable sugar (glucose) has been only formed through the transformation of another vegetable product, viz. fecula. The belief, therefore, that the saccharine principles we meet with in animals were derived exclusively from saccharine and farinaceous aliments of vegetable origin seemed to be but a just and logical conclusion.

Yet there were phenomena presented by that singular disease known as diabets mellitus, which were quite inexplicable. That remarkable affection is characterized, as is well known, by such an abundant production of sugar in the organism, that the blood is surcharged with it, that all the tissues are penetrated by it, and the urine especially, sometimes contains an enormous quantity of it. But in cases of this kind, and more especially when the disease exists in an intense degree, the quantity of sugar in the diabetic excretion always exceeds that which could be produced from the saccharine and farinaceous substances contained in the aliment, and the presence of sugar in the blood and in the urine is never completely arrested, even when articles containing sugar or fecula are entirely discontinued for food.

It was from careful consideration of the phenomena presented by the subjects of that disease, and which, moreover, are known to all physicians, that I was led to the conclusion that there might exist in the animal organism, conditions unknown to chemists and physiologists, capable of giving use to the formation of sugar from other substances besides those of a farinaceous character. These facts, from the year 1843, induced me to make it a subject of physiological investigation.

But the impossibility of making direct experiments upon the *production* of sugar in the animal organism, will be readily understood. In its normal condition I could detect no trace of the existence of that function; it presented itself only as a pathological and temporary condition in the subjects of diabetes, while in those animals upon which it was possible to make experiments, it entirely concealed itself from observation.

On the other hand, the *destruction* of the sugar of food was a physiological fact at once evident, and easily determined by direct experiment. In order to ascertain the mechanism of this phenomenon, and to discover its cause, it is only necessary to introduce a certain amount of saccharine matter into the circulation of a healthy animal, and to trace it, mingled with the blood, until by transformation into other products, it is destroyed and entirely disappears. By thus determining the tissue or organ in which the sugar disappeared, we should be able to give a precise location to the organ, or assimulatory agent, by which, in living animals, the transformation was effected. Then, the organ being known, I intend to prosecute the comparative study of its function in both carnivorous and herbivorous animals, and then, if possible, to suppress it; for the purpose of ascertaining whether an artificial diabetes mellitus could be produced, and to exhibit whatever evidence might present itself of the formation of sugar in the animal organism, &c.

Such was, according to my recollection, the plan of somewhat indirect and circuitous experiment that I had conceived for surmounting the difficulties of the problem that I had proposed to myself to solve, to determine whether in the animal economy sugar was ever produced without the intervention of saccharine or farinaceous food. But when we deal with phenomena as complex as those that take place in living bodies, there are always a great number of elements, that, in our experimental combinations, escape our observation simply from being unknown to us.

An experimentalist, whose opinions were either undecided or preconceived, on meeting these elements unexpectedly, might, without doubt, be disconcerted or misled by them. For the docile and unprejudiced observer, they are, on the other hand, new elements of knowledge, which by giving origin to new ideas, often induces him to make a thorough revision of his former modes of investigation. This was verified in my own experience in this particular case. I soon found it necessary to abandon my former position, for the enquiry respecting the existence of a sugar-producing organ, which I had regarded as the most difficult of physiological attainment, was on the contrary revealed the first, and as it were, spontaneously, at the commencement of my investigations, as the history of the following experiment will show:

I fed a healthy adult dog with food containing a large proportion of sugar. Every day he got two dishes of milk soup, to which bread and sugar was added. It was evident that the animal, thus supported, absorbed by its abdominal veins sugar derived from three sources. 1st, sugar contained in the milk. 2d, sugar derived from the digestion of bread. 3d, cane sugar, which was added to the soup.

The object of this experiment was to follow, as it were, step by step, the saccharine material derived from the food through the entire circulatory system, tracing it from its primary absorption, at first through the liver, then in the lungs, and finally in all the tissues of the body.

The question to determine then, is, whether the sugar will be destroyed in passing through the liver, which is the first organ by which it can be acted upon after its absorption by the branches of the portal vein? To answer this question, after seven days' feeding in the manner above stated, the dog was sacrificed by division of the medulla ollangata during digestion. In order to discover whether sugar existed in the blood of the hepatic vein, I immediately, and as quickly as possible, opened the thorax and abdomen of the animal. I easily obtained the most decisive proof of the existence of a great quantity of sugar (glucose) in the blood of the hepatic veins near its entrance into the vena cava ascendens.

There was nothing in this result that need to appear surprising at first sight. The presence of sugar in the organism of the dog admits of easy explanation in view of the nature of its food, and the presence of the saccharine principle in the blood that flows from the liver seems clearly to indicate that this organ is not the agent by which its destruction is effected.

It was necessary to verify the correctness of the result thus obtained by other and decisive experiments. In order to demonstrate conclusively that the sugar found in the blood of that dog was derived from his ingesta which had escaped destruction in its transit through the liver, it was necessary to prove that sugar does not exist in the blood of the hepatic vein of a dog fed exclusively upon meat or other food destitute of saccharoid matter. This comparative method of experimenting is the best means of avoiding the sources of error in the study of the complex phenomena of living beings, and in this instance it has led to the discovery of new facts, which it is my purpose at present to communicate.

As a test experiment, another healthy and adult dog was fed exclusively for seven days upon meat, (sheep's head,) of which he ate *ad libitum;* he was then killed as in the former instance by a section of the medulla oblongata during digestion. To apply the test, I immediately collected the blood of the hepatic vein, and what was my surprise at finding here, in the hepatic blood of a dog which had been fed upon meat, and deprived of all saccharine matter for seven days, as undoubted evidence of the existence of sugar in considerable quantity as in the dog which, during a corresponding period, had been supplied with food containing an abundance of that principle.

A result so unexpected and so important, could not be received without hesitation. To remove my doubts I subjected two more dogs to the same differential regimen. The result of this second comparative experiment was precisely the same as in the former, to-wit: sugar was clearly detected in the blood of both the dogs, notwithstanding the great difference of their food. To complete the demonstration of this astonishing fact, I ascertained by autopsic inspection that in all respects the conditions of the experiments were unexceptionable. I found a considerable quantity of sugar in the contents of the stomach and intestines of the dog that had been fed with farinaceous and saccharine matters, while not a trace of sugar could be found in the contents of the digestive apparatus of the dog submitted to an exclusively azotized food, and yet, I repeat, the blood of the hepatic vein of both animals was most distinctly saccharine.

It will now be readily understood why I at once abandoned my first plan of investigation, to follow the indication presented by this new fact which completely embodied the gist of the question. In fact the detection of sugar in animals which feed only upon flesh, furnished an indication of a sugar-producing function in the organism in a physiological condition, and that, it will be recollected, was the final object of my researches. From that moment the destruction of sugar became a ques-, tion of quite secondary importance, the chief question being to determine the source and origin of the sugar found in the blood of the hepatic vein of an animal nourished exclusively upon flesh or azotized food.

I was naturally led to seek for the source of the saccharine element in the abdominal viscera, since the hepatic vein through which it brought to the abdominal vena cava is, as it were, a supplement to the portal system of veins.

The only remaining question was to determine which of the viscera of the abdomen was capable of producing that element.

That it was not in the intestinal canal I had previously ascertained by an examination of the residual contents of that viscus, and further deri- ved confirmatory evidence by testing the blood of the mesenteric veins, which was found equally destitute of saccharine matter.

Neither was it the spleen, for the blood of the splenic vein contained no sugar; it was neither the pancreas nor the mesenteric ganglia, for in the blood that flowed through these organs no trace of sugar could be detected.

Finally, after making many trials, and meeting many deceptive ap- pearances, which repeated experiments alone enabled me to correct, I sat- isfied myself of the correctness of this conclusion: that, in flesh-fed dogs, the blood of the portal system of veins contains no sugar prior to its entrance into the liver; the same blood while flowing into the vena cava through the hepatic vein, exhibits a notable quantity of that ele- ment, (glucose.)

I was, therefore, driven to the conclusion, that, in traversing the tissues of the liver, the blood acquired its saccharine quality, and also to admit that the sugar-producing power is a special function of that organ.

Furthermore, a chemical examination of the hepatic tissue, led directly to the same conclusion.

On boiling a portion of the liver of a dog, — which had been fed solely on flesh for fourteen days, — in a little water, I obtained a decoction, in which it was easy to demonstrate the presence of sugar.

No other tissue or organ of the body, treated in the same manner, yielded the same result.

From these experiments, sufficiently numerous and varied, the demon- stration may be regarded as complete, — *that sugar may exist in the animal organism, independently of farinaceous food, and that the for- mation of sugar is a special function of the liver.*

Since I published my first results in 1848, I have considerably ex- tended my observations and researches on this new function of the liver, which consists of a true generation or secretion of sugar from the blood that flows through the hepatic tissues. I have proved that this function, which no one before me had recognised, or even suspected, is universal in the animal kingdom. I have, moreover, shown, that if we must regard the formation of this element as essentially a chemical result of the metamorphosis of certain elements of the blood of the liver, to produce glucose, we must, nevertheless, admit, that like other secretions derived from the blood, it is a chemical phenomenon peculiar to living animals. That, in fact, without the nervous influence, it cannot be accomplished, and in this respect, there is, perhaps, no other function as much under the direct influence of nervous action, as the secretion of sugar by the liver. I have elsewhere shown, that by acting on certain parts of the nervous system, we may, at pleasure, suppress the formation of sugar by the liver, or so increase it as to render the animal artificially diabetic.

I had the honor of demonstrating these facts before a committee of the Academy of Sciences, which awarded to my work, " On the Origin of Sugar in the Animal Economy," its prize for experimental physiology, in 1850.

Many foreign savans have also witnessed the results of my experiments, which have since been repeated and confirmed by many experimentalists, especially by Van Denbrock, Froerichs, Lehman, Baumert, Gibbs, A. Mitchell, &c.

After having proved that animals possess the power of sugar-formation, independant of the nature of their food, the question of its office and destination in the animal economy very naturally presents itself. Neither that which is formed by the liver, nor that which is derived from the food directly, is in the normal state of the organism destined to accumulate in the system or to be excreted from it. On the contrary, it should be either assimilated constantly, or be transformed into other products.

All these subjects have engaged my attention for several years past, and the collective results of the numerous physiological investigations that I have made may now be embodied in a single essay.

Each of the individual facts which were published separately in the order of their discovery will here be connected in their natural relation, and each experiment, when described in detail, will draw its own correction, and furnish a reply to some premature criticisms, even from the narration of the circumstances in which they will be established.

As I at present view the subject, the process of sugar-formation, as it occurs in man and animals, should be regarded in three different aspects, which require as many different modes of demonstration, viz.; 1st. The experimental demonstration and physiological history of the production of sugar in man and animals, considered by itself and as a special and normal function of the liver.

2nd. The demonstration of the mechanism by which the destruction and disappearance of the sugar is effected, and the uses to which it is applied in the animal organism.

3rd. The demonstration of the direct influence of the nerve-force on the production of sugar in the economy. This question is undoubtedly one of the most interesting that the physiology of the nutritive functions presents, as it furnishes an instructive example of the modifying influence of vitality over phenomena that are entirely chemical in their intimate nature.

Now so widely different are the ideas and considerations that naturally group themselves around these propositions, and they are moreover so comprehensive in themselves that they require to be treated of in distinct essays.

In the present one I propose to limit myself to the consideration of the first question, viz.: The function through which in the animal economy there is a production of saccharine matter constantly occurring in the liver.

All my demonstrations will be purely physiological, nevertheless, for the benefit of those who may desire to repeat the experiments for themselves, I will add a few remarks upon the nature of the sugar formed by the liver, as well as the means of investigation, and the quantity I employed.

TO BE CONTINUED.

SELECTIONS.

From the New Orleans Medical and Surgical Journal.

Yellow Fever Epidemic of 1853 *in New Orleans.*

About the 26th of May last, the first case of yellow fever entered the Charity Hospital, and after death black vomit was found in the stomach. The first fever cases originated among the shipping along the Levee, in the Fourth District, from which point it extended rapidly through the adjacent portion of the town. A large population of unacclimated persons, living in wooden huts, with floors and timbers soaked in water, and half decayed, were seized with the disease in the most malignant form. For some time previously rain had fallen almost daily, and this, added to a hot, burning sun, seemed to give strength to the poison, and lent intensity to the disease. The streets in this vicinity, for the most part, were unpaved, or planked, and the culverts gutters, etc., were filled with water, saturated with filth, and decaying vegetable and animal matter,— The crowded state of these huts and low wooden tenements, with their floors steeped in mud and water, is admirably calculated to generate and propagate the germ of a disease which had already been sown in their midst.

The habits of these people (being chiefly Irish and German laborers,) notoriously negligent and filthy, and utterly indifferent to all those precautionary measures which a limited knowledge of the laws of hygiene should suggest, served only to add fuel to the conflagration which was destined to extend its ravages to every portion of our devoted city.— Hence, for some time, the yellow fever confined its work of death within particular localities; but, by and by, gaining strength by what it fed upon, it began to travel to other and more distant points—to extend its arms, so to speak, in every direction, until it grasped the Four Districts within its deadly embrace. For some time the hope was entertained that those who paid proper regard to personal comfort and cleanliness, who dwelt in high, airy, and well-ventilated apartments, might escape the disease; but this proved a delusion. It soon became apparent that, as heretofore, the epidemic fever was no respecter of persons; the master was stricken down with the servant the mistress with the maid, the proud and wealthy were brought to a level with the humble and needy. All who had not passed through some one of our epidemic seasons were exposed to attacks from the disease. As has been already mentioned, the fever made its appearance in the latter part of May, at least a month and a half earlier than usual, and from the first case up to the present, it steadily increased almost daily, until the mortality per diem exceeded that produced by any epidemic know in the annals of our sanitary history. In recording the fearful ravages of the present epidemic, we must not forget that we have remained exempt from any such visitation since 1847; and during this time an immense population of unacclimated persons, both from Europe and the north-western part of our own country, have been accumulating in our city. The number of unacclimated persons in the city, at the breaking out of the epidemic, has been estimated at 30,000 souls; but many of these, it is fair to suppose, have left the city to escape the disease.

The type of the epidemic differs but little from that to which we have been subject in former years, and the belief that persons had died of the disease in six and eight hours from the moment of seizure can readily be explained by a better knowledge of the antecedent history of the case; for, on inquiry, it would generally be found that such individuals have had slight fever, and other symptoms of the epidemic, for two or three days previous to taking their bed and calling in medical aid. This surmise gains additional strength from the fact, that the attack, in many instances, has been so insidious and destitute of alarming symptoms, that it is with difficulty such persons could be persuaded to submit to the usual restrictive treatment.

It is not strange, therefore, that such cases, which had been neglected for two or three days in the early and curable stage of attack, should terminate in fatal black vomit in a few hours after the physician is summoned to the bedside of his patient. So much for the apparent malignity of the present epidemic. In making the foregoing explanation, we aim not to deny the existence of an occasional case of extreme severity; so severe, indeed, as to terminate in death in a few hours, in spite of the best efforts of the most skilful physician, and the most careful nursing.

In some instances, the system seems so thoroughly saturated with the poison of the disease, from the very moment of the seizure, that no system of medicine, as yet suggested, seems able to cope with and stay the fatal tendency of the fever. Every medical man, who has had much experience in the disease, must remember occasional instance of this kind.

The disease, this season, though essentially the same in many of its most prominent features, exacts, perhaps, on the part of physician and nurse, more care, diligence and precaution, to terminate favorably, than usual in our epidemics. The slightest imprudence, either in diet, exposure, or excitement of any kind is almost certain to superinduce a relapse, from which state it is usually very difficult to extricate the patient. Hence, the great mortality among those who are not only ignorant of the peculiarities of the disease, but who are also unable, and in some instances unwilling, to pay for the requisite medical aid and attendance.

We refer to our table below, furnished by Dr. Simonds, the active Secretary of the Board of Health, for a full account af the deaths, and other particulars which have occurred since the epidemic broke out.

By this it will be seen that yellow fever has done terrible e_xecut_ion among our unacclimated population, has produced a mortality unparalleled in the history of our ill-fated city. Even while penning these lines the fever is sweeping off over *two hundred per diem*, and from present appearances, it is likely to continue its fearful ravages for perhaps weeks to come.

Our quondam associate, Dr. Fenner, will, in due time, give us a full and detailed history of this épidemic, as he did that of 1847, when the disease shall have run its course, and done its work of death.

Below we give the mortality produced by the epidemic, in the city of New Orleans, from the 28th of May, up to the 26th of August, inclusive, for 1853.

The Epidemic.—Total number of deaths by yellow fever and other diseases, from May 28 till date:

Week ending	Total.	Yellow Fever.	Other Dis.	Not stated.
May 28	140-- 140	1-- 1	139-- 199	..
June 4	157	1	156	..
June 11	154	4	150	
June 18	147	7	140	
June 25	167-- 625	9-- 21	158-- 604	..
July 2	177	25	152	
July 9	188	59	129	..
July 16	344	204	140	..
July 23	617	435	182	..
July 31	884—2210	704--1427	133-- 741	42
Aug. 1	142	106	25	11
" 2	135	115	14	6
" 3	146	124	17	9
" 4	166	135	15	10
" 5	150	128	9	13
" 6	238	194	30	14
" 7	209--1186	165-- 957	40-- 150	4--69
" 8	219	187	23	9
" 9	201	166	21	14
" 10	230	193	33	4
" 11	233	192	13	18
" 12	207	180	25	2
" 13	214	179	22	13
" 14	232--1526	191--1288	26— 163	16--75
" 15	217	187	24	6
" 16	193	163	19	11
" 17	219	191	21	7
" 18	219	188	22	9
" 19	234	203	15	16
" 20	224	184	29	11
" 21	269--1575	230--1346	24-- 153	15--75
" 22	283	239	29	1[.
" 23	258	220	24	14
" 24	222	188	23	11
" 25	218	186	19	13
" 26	193--1074	151-- 884	29-- 124	13--66
Total	8336	5934	2075	327

N, B. The returns from St. Patrick's Cemetery, since the 31st July, not having been duly made, cannot be relied on, except for two weeks, when the books were resorted to by the Secretary, to enable him to make a weekly report.

Quinia in Yellow Fever.

The editor of the " New Orleans Medical and Surgical Journal," states (No. for Sept. 1853,) that his " experience during the present epidemic, with the sulphate of quinia, has convinced him that large doses of this salt cannot be relied on in the early stages of the attack.

" In the commencement of the epidemic, the advocates of large doses of quinia soon found that this article, when given in sedative doses, failed to accomplish a cure, although the febrile symptoms gradually gave way to its use.

" As the epidemic progressed, and its type and characteristic symptoms became better known, few, as far as we can learn, ventured to give large and repeated doses of this salt, except in perticular instances. In our previous epidemic of yellow fever, the quinia practice succeeded best; but it is generally conceded, as far as we could ascertain, that this season it failed in a majority of cases to sustain its previous high reputation as a powerful curative agent. Hereafter, we shall have more to say on this subject."

From the London Lancet, May 14, 1853.

On the questionable utility of Tracheotomy in the treatment of any kind of Epilepsy. By Dr. RADCLIFFE, Assistant-Physician to the Westminster Hospital.

IN order to arrive at a proper decision upon this question, I have deemed it desirable to collect the cases in which Dr. Marshall Hall's views have been tested practically, and submit them to the judgment of the profession: and this more particularly as the reviewal of this evidence has led me to adopt the title which heads this paper. With this object, therefore, I beg to present these cases and a few comments arising out of them.

Mr. Cane's Case.—The patient was a boatman, aged twenty-four, who had been epileptic for seven or eight years. The fits were severe and frequent. The operation was performed during a fit, in consequence of a state of asphyxial-coma that had lasted nineteen hours. The relief was immediate, and no fits have followed the operation. The habits of the patient were very irregular and intemperate, and he was discharged from his employment on this account about ten months ago. The tube is still worn, and curiously enough, it is worn with a cork in the opening.

Mr. Anderson's Case.— The patient in this case was a stout, thickset, muscular female, æt. thirty-six, the daughter of an epileptic father, and herself epileptic for twenty-four years. Her complexion was ruined by the former use of nitrate of silver. The operation was performed

in March, 1851, and the tube was worn until her death, which happened in a fit about four months ago. After the operation the fits continued as before — possibly a little less frequently and severely, but decidedly of the same character. Her health and spirits also are said to
have undergone some slight improvement, and she lost a numbness in
the right arm which had previously distressed her, but those who knew
her best doubt the existence of any appreciable change of this kind until
about two or three months before her death — sixteen months after the
operation. The following notes of the final seizure are from Mr. Anderson:— "Eight A. M.: Had been up and dressed; heard to fall heavily.
A woman removed the inner tube from the trachea as she was in a fit
apparently more severe than usual. She 'snorted loudly;' nails of a
deeper color. She was placed on the bed as the woman thought she
would recover as usual." The woman here referred to says the patient
was black in the face and violently convulsed, and that death must have
taken place within ten minutes. The body was examined twenty-four
hours after death, and the following are the particulars supplied by Mr.
Anderson: "Body extremely muscular; cadaverous rigidity still present;
not much fat. Head: Vessels of scalp much congested; skull thick,
and dura mater so universally adherent that the skull-cap could not be
removed until the dura mater was divided. The sinuses were filled with
dark blood, and on the removal of the brain an unusual quantity of
dark blood flowed from the spinal canal. On either side of the longi-
tudinal sinus, and on the inner side of the frontal bone, two or three
growths of bone were found, and to these the dura mater was so firmly
adherent that on attempting to separate it, it was torn through, and portions remained attached. The largest of the exostoses was about an
inch and a-half in circumference, and projected about half an inch from
the surface of the bone. No alteration was observed in the corresponding portion of the cerebrum. The brain was softer than natural, and
the puncta were more than usually distinct. There was little fluid in
the ventricles, but the choroid plexuses were congested. Lungs: These
organs were collapsed, occupying but little more than a third of the thoracic cavity, and somewhat congested at their posterior margin; structure healthy. Heart: Larger than usual (perhaps a fourth;) cavities,
especially the left, distended with blood. It was surrounded with fat,
and its structure flabby;* valves healthy. Liver, kidneys, and spleen:
Highly congested. Uterus natural, but cysts containing viscid fluid in
the ovaries. Small intestines (especially lower part of the ilium) congested, and the mesenteric glands enlarged. Internal jugular, above the
level of the omohyoid, almost empty."

Mr. Mackarsie's Case.— R. W——, aged forty, and epileptic for
twenty years. Latterly the fits have become much more frequent and
severe, the subsequent torpor much prolonged, and the mind much impaired. His complexion had a congested, mahogany-like tint. Two
years previously he had had two attacks of paralysis, but his present

---

* Dr. Jenner examined a portion of this heart microscopically, and found some slight degree
of fatty degeneration.

health, apart from the fits, is pretty good. Tracheotomy was performed on the 24th of August, 1852, by means of the tracheotome. On the day following the operation inflammatory action began in the lungs, and continued until the 6th of September. Thus,—August 25th; "A large quantity of mucus has passed from the tube." 26th: "The patient has been hot and feverish and passed a restless night; tongue furred; pulse 100; a large quantity of mucus passing through the tube." 27th: "Pulse 100, full and hard." 28th: "Tongue still furred." 31st: "Violent hemoptysis." Sept. 1st: "Violent return of hemoptysis; left lung congested, dull on percussion, and respiratory murmur feeble." 2d: "Expectorates bloody mucus; dulness on percussion not so marked; respiratory murmur more audible." 3d: "Still bloody expectoration." 4th: "Pulse 90 and soft." 6th: "Pulse 75, soft; respiration free; dulness on percussion gone." Again, on the 20th of September, and for some days afterwards, there was feverishness, attended with bilious vomiting, and required salines, calomel, and prussic acid. The fits, however, kept away until the second week in October, when four or five slight ones happened. After this true fits made their appearance, and continued to recur with their usual frequency, though in a mitigated form, until about two months ago, when the tube was withdrawn by the patient's wife, (who throughout has been greatly opposed to, and dissatisfied with the operation,) since which time the fits are as bad as ever, and the mental condition worse than ever. Mr. Mackarsie is of opinion that during the time the tube was in the trachea the mind was more active, the complexion less congested, and the fits less severe, though there was no alteration in the subsequent sopor.

Mr. J. A. Lockhart Clark's Case.— In this case the patient was a female, twenty-three years of age, who had been epileptic for twelve years. The fits were very violent and very frequent. Laryngotomy, not tracheotomy, was performed about three months ago, and the tube worn until recently, when it was removed, in consequence of there being no perceptible alteration either in the frequency or in the severity of the fits.

Mr. Henry Thompson's Case.— The main facts of this case are substantially these: the patient was an epileptic of twenty years' standing, whose intellect had suffered considerably. Tracheotomy was performed nearly three months ago. Before the operation the fits were frequent and violent, and the subsequent sopor prolonged; since the operation the fits have altered little in frequency and violence, but the subsequent sopor is greatly abridged. The general health also is improved, and the mind clearer than it was.

Dr. Tyler Smith's Case.— Sarah B——, the wife of a game-keeper at Debden in Essex, and the mother of four children. She has been epileptic since puberty, and chiefly about the menstrual period. The numbers of the fits during the month were sometimes as many as twenty, but generally not more than five or six. The fits themselves were usually preceded by the scream and attended with much lividity of the head and neck; the convulsions were very violent and the subsequent sopor protracted. The mental state was one of great inanity. There had been several paroxysms of insanity, and twice the patient had been in a lunatic asylum. During the month that she remained in the hospital before the operation, there were nine fits; during the month after the operation there were five fits. The operation itself was performed on the 13th of Feb. by Mr. Lane. On the 15th, 16th, and 17th, she was restless, wakeful, and unruly, with heat of skin, raised pulse, and furred tongue. She threw a glass at the nurse, and persisted in attempting to withdraw the tube from the neck, and her state required constant watching. Three weeks after this time she was greatly depressed, her pulse feeble and wretched, her countenance anxious, and much viscid, fetid phlegm passed from the tube; and this state continued for the greater part of a week. Since this time she has rallied, and now her mental condition is much better than it was during the month before the operation; her fits also are less severe, the period of sopor is lessened, and the cry is lost; but still the convulsion is violent, the venous turgescence of the head and neck considerable, though less than it was, and once at least the tongue has been bitten.

Dr. Andrea Verga's Case.— This case cannot strictly be classed with the former cases, for the operation was performed unintentionally, and by the patient himself; but in all other respects it fulfils the required predicaments. It was originally reported in one of the Lombard journals, and copied thence into an early number of Schmidt's *Jahrbuch* for 1852. The main particulars are the following: A. B——, aged twenty-five, was admitted into the great hospital at Milan, with his throat cut and his genitals severely mutilated, in consequence of a determined attempt at suicide. Six months afterwards the wounds had healed, with the exception of a free fistulous opening in the trachea; but the fits and despondency had undergone no change. The breath passed freely in and out of the artificial opening, and the fits recurred with equal frequency and force whether that opening were closed or not. In this state he was removed to a madhouse, and there he remained for three years, when he died of tabes, the fistula continuing open and the fits unabated up to the end. After death the brain and skin were found congested and the bowels somewhat ulcerated.

Comments.— Such are the clinical data upon which as yet the remedial value of tracheotomy in epilepsy has to be tested, and the question is, whether or not they realize Dr. Hall's expectations, and justify the comments which have been passed upon them.

What of Mr. Cane's case? Here undoubtedly the results seem most marked, but do they not prove too much? There are no fits whatever after the operation, and this is not to be expected even on Dr. Hall's own premises. Moreover, fits do happen in all the other cases, and in some of them very severe fits, and this fact gives a probability of at least seven to one that the fits in this case did not keep away in consequence of the operation. It is to be remembered, also, that the wearing of the cork in the tracheal tube did in fact place the patient in the same predicament as that in which he was before the windpipe was opened. Why the fits kept away it is not necessary to inquire, for nothing is more certain than that epilepsy may suddenly disappear, and keep away for a long time, without any apparent cause.

What of Mr. Anderson's case? Here the main questions are as to the character of the fits, the state of general health, and the cause of death. Were the fits improved in character? Possibly, but not probably. Dr. M. Hall, in his lectures at the College of Physicians, allowed that a fit had followed very shortly after the operation, in which the tongue had been bitten. A Mrs. Dwellie, living in the adjoining garret to the patient's, and who frequently went to the patient's assistance when she heard the noise and struggle of the fit, states explicitly that the convulsions were as frequent and violent, and the subsequent sopor as prolonged, after the operation as before it. A Mrs. Smith, also, an aunt of the patient, who had known her from childhood, and who saw her several times a week during the whole of her life, makes the same statement. Miss Lewis, on the contrary, who lives on the first floor of the house in the garret of which the patient lived, thinks the fits after the operation were not so severe or frequent as before it; but why she thinks so is not very evident. She saw her in but few fits, and in none (there is reason to believe) from the commencement. Indeed, it is to be understood that this witness was infirm and half crippled, and often quite an invalid; that she had to be fetched from the top of the house, and then to mount up two flights of stairs before she could get to the place where the patient was; so that the fit must have been far from its commencement before she could see it. The last fit, also, which was evidently of great violence, is spoken of only as "apparently more severe than usual," showing that the ordinary fits were severe, and the patient was "expected to recover as usual," showing that death occurred unexpectedly in what was regarded as an ordinary fit. Concerning the state of the general health there was two opinions. Miss Lewis says this was better; Mrs. Dwellie and Mrs. Smith say there was no perceptible improvement until within two or three months from her death, fifteen or sixteen months after the operation. The cause of death is very obscure. It could not be, however, from the strangulation of laryngismus, for the inner tube was removed at the beginning of the last fit, as it was in all the fits in which the patient was watched. Indeed there was never any neglect or mismanagement about the tube (which reflects the highest credit on Mr. Anderson's mechanical ingenuity,) and the patient herself had so schooled herself to it that she could remove and cleanse it, and did so remove and cleanse it many times a day. The fatty state of the heart, as Dr. Hall supposes, might have had something to do with death, for death happened shortly after the commencement of the seizure; but, on the other hand, it is not to be forgotten that there was stertorous breathing, blackness and turgescence of the head and neck, with distended sinuses, distinct cerebral puncta, and other signs showing that death might have been caused by coma.

What of Mr. Mackarsie's case? Here it is not difficult to imagine that the pulmonary inflammation and the subsequent febrile action may have had something to do with the absence of the fits during the first two months after the operation, for inflammation and fever are not only uncongenial to, but incompatible with epilepsy. This inflammation, also, even after its cessation, may have had something to do with the amelioration of the fits, by acting derivatively in regard to that mischief in the brain, the existence of which is to be argued from the two former attacks of paralysis. The fact, however, is not to be doubted, that the fits were "mitigated" and the mental state ameliorated after the operation. This is undeniable. Still the fits were true fits, and not mere warnings, and there is little if any reason for supposing that they gave up the characters of epilepsia gravior for those of epilepsia mitior; nor is it clear that the mind was not invigorated by hope or some other psychical stimulus, and that the fits were not subdued by the mind thus invigorated, the tracheal tube all the while acting merely as a charm by which to propitiate hope and her allies; nor is it clear that any diminished sopor after the fit, may not have been the consequence rather than the cause of the mental invigoration. Time must elapse before these doubts can be resolved, and in the mean time it must not be forgotten that the wife of the patient was dissatisfied with the operation.

What of Mr. Clark's case? Nothing favorable to the operation.

What of Mr. Henry Thompson's case? In this case the fits recur as frequently as before, but the subsequent sopor and intermediate stupor are greatly diminished. Still it is by no means certain or even probable that the fits after the operation were of the character of epilepsia mitior, or that the diminished sopor and stupor were not the consequences of faith in the operation rather than of the operation itself.

What of Dr. Tyler Smith's case? In this case it is more than improbable that the fits underwent that modification which they ought to have done, or that any improvement in the symptoms is really due to the operation. All the fits after the operation were certainly not of the type of epilepsia mitior, for the convulsions were severe, and once at least the tongue was bitten. It is doubtful also whether the fits were really less frequent. During the first month of hospital life there were, it is true, nine fits, but this was a time when the patient was exposed to the agitating publicity of a hospital ward, with the fear of an operation before her eyes. The usual number of fits during the month would also seem to be from five to six, though occasionally ranging so high as twenty, and these numbers correspond with the numbers after the operation. It is clear also that as yet little can be said about mental improvement after the operation, seeing that a paroxysm of insanity and a week of extreme mental inanity, form a part of this period. This being the case, it is not necessary to speculate whether such improvement is psychically or somatically the result of the operation.

What of Dr. Andrea Verga's case? Possibly very little, but certainly nothing in favor of the operation.

On looking over these cases, therefore, one conclusion is inevitable — namely, that severe fits have followed the operation — fits in which the tongue has been bitten, and one fit in which death has happened. Almost uniformly the convulsion has been as bad as ever. In Mr. Anderson's, Mr. Clark's, Mr. Mackarsie's, and possibly Dr. Andrea Verga's case, the sopor after the fit, and the torpor between the fits, were unaffected; in Mr. Henry Thompson's and possibly in Dr. Tyler Smith's cases, they were relieved, though *how* they were relieved remains a matter of doubt. As judged, therefore, by the results of the cases in which it has been practically tested, the utility of tracheotomy in epilepsy would seem to be extremely doubtful; so doubtful, indeed, as to render it a matter of paramount and imperative necessity to pause and ponder well upon the evidence before again resorting to it, and this all the more because it is by no means certain that the remedy is not more dangerous than the disease, and because the inevitable result of the operation is to convert the patient into a dumb, whistling wretch, whose every breath is an annoyance to himself and others. In order to do this it will be necessary to examine epileptics, whose windpipes are sound as well as those whose windpipes are not sound. It will be necessary to determine how much of the epileptic asphyxia depends upon spasmodic "setting" of the whole chest, and how far this "setting" will negative the results of an opening in the windpipe. It will be necessary to go to the root of the matter, and determine whether, apart from organic disease, the larynx does close spasmodically in epilepsy, and whether such closure can exist at the time of life when epilepsy happens. In the mean time the absence of any stridulous inspiration in epilepsy, such as is heard in laryngismus stridulus, in hooping-cough, and in certain organic diseases of the larynx, would seem to be a serious, if not fatal objection to the existence of laryngismus in epilepsy. The age of epileptics — namely, youth and manhood — is also an objection to the same effect; for, judging from the history of laryngismus stridulus and hooping-cough, pure spasmodic closure of the larynx is confined to the period antecedent to that at which epilepsy commences; indeed, as a rule, laryngismus stridulus is an affection of teething, and hooping-cough loses its characteristic hoop before puberty. This deduction is also borne out by the results which follow the division of the laryngeal nerves in dogs and cats; for in these experiments the young animal is immediately suffocated by the closure of the glottidean chink, whereas the old animal goes on breathing without any evident diminution in the current of air.

RESPONSE

BY OLIVER WENDELL HOLMES, M.D.,

To the following Toast, proposed at the Entertainment given to the American Medical Association, by the Physicians of the city of New York, at the Metropolitan Hall, on the 5th of May, 1853 : —

TOAST.— "The Union of Science and Literature — A happy marriage, the fruits of which are nowhere seen to better advantage than in our American HOLMES."

I hold a letter in my hand —
    A flattering letter — more's the pity —
By some contriving junto planned,
        And signed, *per order of Committee*;

A Medical Poem.

It touches every tenderest spot —
   My patriotic predilections —
My well-known — something — don't know what —
   My poor old songs — my kind affections : —

They make a feast on Thursday next,
   And hope to make the feasters merry —
They own they're something more perplext
   For poets than for port and sherry —
They want the men of — (word torn out) ;
   Our friends will come with anxious faces,
(To see our blankets off, no doubt,
   And trot us out and show our paces).

They hint that papers by the score
   Are rather musty kind of rations :
They don't exactly mean a bore,
   But only trying to the patience ;
That such as — you know who I mean —
   Distinguished for their — what d'y call 'em ? —
Should bring the dews of Hippocrene
   To sprinkle on the faces solemn.

— The same old story ; that's the chaff
   To catch the birds that sing the ditties ;
Upon my soul, it makes me laugh
   To read these letters from Committees !
They're all *so* loving and *so* fair —
   All for *your* sake such kind compunction —
'Twould save your carriage half it's wear
   To grease the wheels with such an unction !

Why, who am I, to lift me here
   And beg such learned folks to listen —
Ask a smile or coax a tear
   Beneath these stoic lids to glisten ?
— As well might some arterial thread
   To ask the whole frame to feel it gushing,
While throbbing fierce from heel to head
   The vast aortic tide was rushing.

As well some hair-like nerve might strain
   To set its special streamlet going,
While through the myriad-channeled brain
   The burning flood of thought was flowing —

Or trembling fibre strive to keep
　The springing haunches gathered shorter,
While the scourged racer, leap on leap,
　Was stretching through the last hot quarter!

Ah me! you take the bud that came
　Self-sown in your poor garden's borders,
And hand it to the stately dame
　That florists breed for, all she orders;
She thanks you — it was kindly meant —
　(A pale affair not worth the keeping)
Good morning; — and your bud is sent
　To join the tea-leaves used for sweeping.

Not always so, kind hearts and true —
　For such I know are round me beating —
Is not the bud I offer you —
　Fresh gathered for the hour of meeting —
Pale though its outer leaves may be,
　Rose-red in all the inner petals,
Where the warm life we cannot see —
　The life of love that gave it, settles?

We meet from regions far away
　Like rills from distant mountains streaming;
The sun is on Francisco's bay,
　O'er Chesapeake the lighthouse gleaming:
While summer skirts the still bayou
　With every leaf that makes it brighter,
Monadnock sees the sky grow blue,
　And clasps his crystal bracelet tighter.

Yet Nature bears the self-same heart
　Beneath her russet-mantled bosom,
And where, with burning lips apart,
　She breathes, and white magnolias blossom:
Ay! many a check is kindled here
　With morning's fire as richly laden
As ever Sultan of Cachemere
　Kissed from a sun-enameled maiden!

I give you *Home!* its crossing lines
　United in one golden suture,
And showing every day that shines
　The present growing to the future —

A flag that bears a *hundred* stars
In one bright ring, with love for centre,
Fenced round with white and crimson bars,
No prowling treason dares to enter!

Oh brothers, home may be a word
To make affection's living treasure —
The wave an angel might have stirred --
A stagnant pool of selfish pleasure ;
HOME ! It is where the day-star springs
And where the evening sun reposes,
Where'er the eagle spreads his wings
From Northern pines to Southern roses!

---*Virginia Medical and Surgical Jour.*

From the British and Foreign Medical Chirurgical Review.

Treatment of Cancer.

M. DEVAY, (*Gaz. Med.* 1852, No. 52,) of the Hotel Dieu, Lyon, has long been engaged in investigating the therapeutical properties of conium in cancer, being of opinion that Storck's experiments should be resumed with the aid of the improved chemical knowledge of the present period. He finds the best preparations to be an extract and balsam, containing one per cent. of conicine, made from the seeds of the plant, gathered when at maturity, of full weight, and of an ash-gray color.— As the result of his researches, he states : 1st, that an ointment, applied externally, in chronic enlargements of scrofulous glands, possesses a resolvent power greater than that of any other substance. 2nd, in engorgements of the uterus, or inflammatory hypertrophy of the organ — so frequently complicating its prolapsus or deviation — this medicine, employed internally and externally, is of great service. 3d, in cancerous affections it exerts remarkable calming effects, and in some cases even cures seem to have resulted from its employment, especially in the atrophied form of scirrhus. Its use is less satisfactory in soft and rapidly increasing tumors; but the progress of some of these has seemed to be retarded. In other cases, it has diminished the size of secondary tumors, rendering the primary ones more amendable to surgical operation. As a means of assuaging the suffering, whether used topically or taken internally, it is invariably preferred by the patients to opium, and all other narcotics.

M. Manec, surgeon to the Saltpetriere, has just obtained a recompense of 2,000 francs from the Academie des Sciences, (Gaz. Med. 1853, No. 10) for the perseverance he has shown in investigating the action of Frere Comes' Arsenical Paste in more than one-hundred and fifty cases

of cancer, in some of which, he obtained unhoped-for results. His experience leads him to these conclusions: 1st, that the arsenical paste
penetrates the cancerous tissue by a sort of special action which is limited
to it.   This action is not simply escharotic, for beneath the superficial,
blackish layer, which the caustic has immediately disorganized, the subjacent morbid tissue seems struck with death though it may retain its
proper texture, and almost its ordinary appearance.   Later, the cancerous mass is separated by the eliminatory inflammation which is set up
around its limits.   The same paste, which extends its action more than
six centimetres deep in a cancer of close texture, when applied to superficial gnawing ulcers, usually only destroys the morbid texture, however
superficial this may be, and respects the sound parts.   2nd, the absorption of arsenic is proportionate to the extent of surface to which it is
applied; and as long as this does not exceed a two-franc piece in size,
there is no danger from this source.   A large surface should only be
attacked by successive applications.   3d, arsenic which is absorbed is
chiefly eliminated by the kidneys, during a space of time of not less
than five, and not more than eight days, as amply demonstrated by Pe-
louze.   Thus, if we allow nine or ten days to intervene between successive applications, all danger from absorption may be avoided.

M. Gozzi, (*Bull. delle Sc. Med.* xx. p. 231) strongly recommends the
following caustic for the destruction of cancerous growths: Corrosive
subl. one scruple; caustic potass ome drachm; arsenic and cerussa aa,
gr. vj.; to be made into a paste with starch and white of egg.   While
using this or other caustics, emollient poultices, ointments, &c., should be
avoided, as diminishing their effects, unless the irritation produced by
their application has been excessive.   M. Gozzi objects to the usual plan
of destroying the tumor, layer by layer, from the apex to the base, the
latter becoming very indurated after these repeated applications, and
offering great obstacles to the approximation of surrounding granulations
and their cicatrization.   He prefers applying the caustic laterally, in the
direction where the tumor seems most inclined to separate

Extracts from PROFESSOR ALLEN'S *Introductory Address.*

We want, and like Diogenes we would search for them with a lantern,
Men — men not only rich in professional lore, but so prepared by nature,
study, discipline and cultivation, that out of the barbaric profusion of
medical literature and rubbish, they may, as by occult masonic skill,
construct a new Temple, where Science shall sit enshrined, and the
priests of Art go up with confidence to quaff inspiration.

We want the zealous student, not the studious zealot.

We want — but space and time forbid enumeration of our needs,
which shame the line,—

> " Man wants but little here below."

Yet, there is reason for wonder, that, amid the confusion of search and the blindness of the seekers, so much has been wrested from ignorance.

The laws of nature and of art, spring, like the waters of the Nile, from obscure fountains in regions peopled by fancy with strange forms and fantastic fleeting, changeful shadows, yet the accumulating waters irrigate the waste desert, and by art assisted flow out upon the otherwise arid plains, causing the wilderness to blossom like the rose, and the parched sands to bring forth foodful plants. Thus although the origin of our profession is lost in the dim clouds of mythic record, and ruins have marked its advance, and the false and the deceitful still entangle and weaken it, nevertheless there is within all a truth which must prevail, and a genetic force that will beget ever new and beneficent results. In this belief let us await with confidence and assurance its future destiny, meeting, with merited scorn, all attempts to smuggle even Truth into general acceptance by attiring it in the garish robes of Falsehood.

Let old Saturn devour his puny children; whilst young Jupiter supplies an Olympus of potential agencies.

The discordant mutterings of the voices coming up from the depths of an obscure antiquity, impress some even more than the voice coming down from the throne of the Omniscient; whilst others mistake the lengthened shadows of the Orient for the noontide revelation. Nevertheless the Old and the New are not as the conflicting principles of the Manichæan system, but rather the Isis and Osisis of Egyptian myth, prolific of the beautiful, the useful and the true.

Finally, and forever, let this be borne uppermost, that the eye and ear, yea, all the senses fail when mind is at fault; then that mind itself, whatever its power, may not arrive at truth in Medicine, unless elevated by appropriate instruction, enlarged by liberal acquirements, strengthened by suitable discipline, it can seize and maintain the true and right STAND POINT OF VIEW.

Dr. Cormack on the Galactagogue and Emmenagogue Effects of Warm and Stimulating Applications to the Mammæ.[*]

Dr. J. O. M'William published in the *Lancet* of September 7, 1850, some very interesting details, regarding the use, among the natives of the Cape de Verd Islands, of fomentations with the leaves of the Ricinus Communis and Jatropha Curcus, for the purpose of accelerating and bringing on, or increasing the flow of milk when the secretion was tardy or deficient after childbirth; and in the *London Journal of Medicine* for October, 1850, Dr. Tyler Smith described some trials made by him with the leaves of the ricinus communis, for the purpose of showing that similar galactagogue effects might be produced in London as in Boa Vista, by adopting measures similar to those employed by the natives of that island. The method adopted by Dr. Tyler Smith was essentially that detailed by Dr. M'William.

From a number of observations which Dr. Cormack has made at various times, and in cases of very different character, he is fully satisfied

[*] Galactagogue and Emmenagogue Effects of Warm and Stimulating Applications to the Mammæ, by Dr. Cormack Association Medical Journal, March 25, 1853.

that the cases of Drs. M'William and Tyler Smith do not in any way support the notion of a special galactagogue power belonging to the leaves of any particular plants. It will.be found, he thinks, that simple warmth, still more hot fomentations, and in a yet higher degree stimulating embrocations and cataplasms, have an extraordinary power in exciting the mammary glands to the secretion of milk, even in circumstances apparently the most adverse to the performance of their function. The leaves of the ricinus communis and of the jatropha curcus, when applied to the mammæ, produce decided stimulation, as we might expect, when we remember that they belong to the natural family Euporbiaceæ, of which acridity is the leading character. This acridity exists in a very high degree even in the seeds of the ricinus communis;' and Pereira quotes, along with similar cases, the case of a girl, eighteen years of age, who died of gastroenteritis, from eating about twenty of these seeds.

The author's object is to establish, by the brief narration of a few facts, the following propositions:—

1st. That warmth and stimulants applied to the mammæ often act powerfully as *galactagogues.*

2d. That warmth and stimulants applied to the mammæ often act powerfully as *emmenagogues.*

3d. That the leaves of the bofareira (or ricinus communis) and jotrapha curcas act as galactagogues and emmenagogues; but not by virtue of any peculiar or specific power.

I. *Warmth and Stimulants applied to the Mammæ often act powerfully as Galactagogues.*— CASE 1. *Milk restored to the Mammæ by Hot Fomentations.*— Last month, a lady, when nursing her infant about seven months old, was attacked with acute bronchitis of moderate severity, which was successfully treated by low diet and tartar emetic in small doses. At the end of four days, the bronchitis was cured; but the milk, which had previously been failing, almost entirely left the breasts. On the fifth day, from exposure to cold, she experienced a relapse of the bronchial affection. As she had been considerably weakened by the previous attack, and as the symptoms of the relapse were not sufficiently severe to justify recourse a second time to antimony, I ordered her to take a draught containing ammonia and chloroform, as an anodyne, expectorant, and diaphoretic, every eight hours; and to carry out similar intentions, I also directed a succession of pillow-cases, filled with heated moist bran, to be applied to the chest. When I saw her on the following day, after this treatment had been employed, she told me that she had profusely perspired for some hours; she was (after copious expectoration) free from cough and pain in the chest; and, what was equally a source of pleasure and surprise to her, *her breasts had become distended with milk.* This lady was able to resume nursing, and to continue it, with the assistance of a suitable diet.

CASE 2. *Effects of a Sinapism applied to one of the Mammæ of a Lady, five months advanced in Pregnancy; Effects of Warmth in the same Case.*— A lady was under my care for bronchitis, at the same time as the patient whose case I have just sketched. She was directed one night to apply a sinapism over the sternum, which she did, but having fallen asleep, it slipped to the side, and remained undisturbed for about an hour upon one of the breasts. For some days this mamma was very much larger in size than the other, and its areola was also much darker. From the delicacy of this lady and the unusual severity of the weather, I directed her to wear a double flannel jacket and a wadded wrapper round the chest. She tells me that *the breasts are larger, and the areolæ much deeper in color than they ever were in any of her ten previous pregnancies, even at the full time;* and these conditions were established while her general health was exceedingly depressed by illness.

CASE 3. *Stimulating Embrocation increasing the Supply of Milk.*— A lady, though in excellent health, had a very scanty supply of milk for her infant, when it was a few weeks old. She consulted me as to the use of means to remedy this evil; and I advised her to rub the mammæ gently every six or eight hours with an embrocation containing a small quantity of tincture of cantharides and oil of thyme, and to sheath the mammæ very warmly in wadding. *In a few days the milk was abundant.*

CASE 4. *Hot Poultices keeping up the Secretion of· Milk when this was not desired.*— A lady suffered, after her confinement, from a succession of abscesses and abortive abscesses in the breast. The surgeon who attended her treated her by antiphlogistic medicines, under which discipline she passed some wretched months, from mental and bodily depression, aggravated by hysterical attacks. The local affection did not seem to make any satisfactory progress; and the great obstacle to a cure was stated to be the impossibility of getting rid of the milk, in spite of saline purges being freely administered. The mammæ during the whole of the period to which I refer, had been ceaselessly treated, night and day, with hot poultices and medicated fomentations. These applications were abandoned, and a generous diet prescribed. *In a few days there was not a drop of milk in the breasts;* and the abscesses, actual and threatening, had ceased to give any pain, and had, in fact, almost disappeared.

These cases, which have occurred within the last few months, are considered sufficient to establish the first proposition, viz: that *warmth and stimulants applied to the mammæ often act powerfully as galactagogues.* Dr. Cormack also adds, that along with the use of such means, the regular application of an infant to the breast will greatly assist in reproducing lactation, as, according to the testimony of various authors, this stimulus has of itself proved sufficient to restore the secretion of milk, and has actually caused it to flow, not only from virgins and other women who had never been pregnant, but even from males.* Excitement and sanguineous turgescence of the gland is induced; and these conditions afford to the organ both a power and a stimulus to perform its previously dormant function.

II. *Warmth and Stimulants applied to the Mammæ often act powerfully as Emmenagogues.*— Warm clothing of the abdomen and limbs, hot hip-baths, and medicines which stimulate the bladder and rectum,

---

* Cases in which men have suckled children are on record. The essential character of the gland is the same in both sexes.

(such as ergot, canthardes, and aloes,) have undoubted emmenagogue powers in properly-selected cases of retarded or suppressed catamenia; and, indeed, they constitute, in various combinations, the principal measures by which the physician usually endeavors to excite the ovarian nisus upon which menstruation depends. The observant physician knows well, that while his treatment is directed to the uterus through the ovaries, the effects produced upon the mammæ are generally very striking, and the first indications which he expects to find of the uterus being roused from its torpor are turgescence and tingling of the mammæ — phenomena which also usually precede normal menstruation. It is equally true, though not so familiarly understood, that measures which act directly and primarily upon the breasts, such as warm clothing to the bust and the application of stimulants, not only cause them to swell and throb, but likewise stimulate the ovaries, and cause the menses to flow. The practice adopted by some practitioners, of applying leeches to the mammæ in amenorrhœa, owes its efficacy to fomentations used, and the irritation of the bites.

In 1834, Dr. Charles Patterson published, in the *Dublin Journal of Medicine*, a paper in which he described the emmenagogue power of irritation of the mammæ by sinapisms. This paper, continues Dr. Cormack, fell into his hands at the time of its appearance, when he was an Edinburgh dispensary pupil, practising, he believes, with more zeal than knowledge, and using, often with more confidence than discrimination, that plan of treatment which he had seen most recently or most enthusiastically recommended. In these circumstances, he successfully employed Dr. C. Patterson's method in amenorrhœa. The beneficial results which he then obtained, produced a very strong impression upon his mind as to the efficacy of irritation of the mammæ in producing menstruation; and the experience of nineteen maturer years has confirmed this impression.

As Dr. Patterson's facts do not seem to be referred to by subsequent writers, and as the practice which he recommends is so little noticed by autors, I subjoin an extract from his paper. Dr. Patterson writes as follows:

Mary Reardon, aged 24, of moderately corpulent habit, was admitted into the Rathkeale Hospital on the 10th of August, 1832. She labored under slight synochial fever, which in a few days yielded to venesection and purgatives. On the 19th of August, symptoms which were considered of an hysterical character presented themselves, with pain in the upper and outer part of the right side of the chest. For the latter affection, a small sinapism was prescribed; but from inattention of the nurse, it was made so large, that it covered a considerable portion of the mamma. The sinapism remained on for half an hour. At the visit on the following morning, the 20th August, Reardon complained that the right breast was exceedingly painful—the pain being very different in its character from that which she had before experienced. On examination, the whole side of the chest was found considerably swollen; there was slight diffused redness of the skin; and though the mamma itself was enlarged to four or five times its natural bulk, yet there was no circumscribed hardness, nor any tendency to superative inflammation. On the 21st August, the right mamma and adjoining parts of the chest were found much more enlarged than they had been at the preceding visit. The left mamma and side of the thorax were unaffected; and it was announced by the nurse that the catamenia had that morning appeared, and were then in considerable quantity. This discharge, which, as the patient stated, had been for two years and a half wholly suppressed, continued to flow for two days; and then began to decline, and with it the tumefaction of the mamma gradually disappeared. (Pp. 193—194.)

Dr. Patterson's attention having thus accidentally been directed to mammary irritation as an excitant of the tarpid uterus, he resolved to try its efficacy when a suitable opportunity presented itself. His next case is thus described:

Catherine Power, aged 19, applied to me on the 14th September, 1832. She complained of headache, languor, loss of appetite, and inability to attend to her usual business, that of a servant. She stated that about the middle of April, the menstrual discharge being then present, she incautiously exposed herself to cold in washing clothes at a river. The catamenia then suddenly ceased, and had not since returned; and from that period she had been constantly subject to ill-health. She had consulted different medical gentlemen, and taken a great variety of medicine, with little advantage. I directed that the clavicular half of the right mamma should be covered with a sinapism. It was allowed to remain on for thirty minutes; and on visiting her in six or seven hours after its removal, I found the whole right breast considerably swollen, hot and painful. The next morning, the enlargement of the mamma was very much increased, the tumefaction having extended to the clavicle and axilla of the irritated side. There was no hard circumscribed or prominent tumor, but a painful, diffuse, elastic distension of the mammary gland and surrounding cellular substance. On the evening of the day next succeeding the application of the sinapism, this poor girl with much joy reported that the catamenia had appeared. The flux having continued for two or three days in moderate quantity, she then found herself greatly relieved of the headache and other most distressing symptoms; and in a week her health was so far restored, that she ceased to require any farther attendance. (Pp. 194—195.)

Dr. Cormack is disposed to regard irritation of the mammæ as a convenient and rapid agency for the induction of menstruation, but one which must neither be rashly nor indiscriminately employed. In numerous cases it may be used alone, but, generally speaking, it may be advantageously combined with other means.

In cases of acute suppression of the menses, he is in the habit of prescribing, along with sinapisms to the mammæ, warm clothing of the bust and limbs, and the hot hip-bath every twelve hours.

In anæmic amenorrhœa, it need hardly be stated that irritation of the mammæ is only calculated to do good in conjunction with, or after a course of a metallic medicine, such as some of the preparations of iron, manganese, or arsenic. In such cases, where we can trace a monthly ovarian nisus, though there be no catamenial flow, these periods should be seized as the appropriate times for using the sinapisms, and then also we may sometimes, by venturing a few doses of forcing medicine, such as cantharides and ergot, bring the case at once to a favorable issue.

The emmenagogue effects ascribed to the application of the leaves of the ricinis communis, by Drs. M'William and Tyler Smith, can easily be understood, when we remember their irritative character, and the consequences which we have found to be induced by irritation of the mammæ caused by other stimulants.

" When the breast " says Dr. M'William, " are small and shrivelled, the plant is said to act more upon the uterine system, bringing on the menses if their period be distant, or causing their immoderate flow if their advent be near."

In the subjoined case, related by Dr. Tyler Smith, the effect produced may have been owing partly to the application to the breasts, and partly to the application to the genitals.

" I have used," says Dr. Tyler Smith, " the remedy in a case of scanty menstruation of a remarkable kind. Owing to exposure to marsh malaria some years ago, the patient had scarcely a sign of colored discharge at the usual catamenial periods. She used the infusion of the leaves of the red bofareira at the date of her period, applying the infusion and leaves to her breasts, and the vapor to the genitals, with the effect of producing, in two days, a considerable flow of the catamenia."

III. *The Leaves of the Bofareira do not produce their Galactagogue and Emmenagogue Effects in Virtue of any Specific Property.* The facts which have been already cited, point out pretty plainly that the effect of the leaves of the bofareira does not depend upon any specific property possessed by them, but simply on the determination produced by warmth and the irritative juices which they contain. That a good deal depends upon the mere warmth of the poultices, is sufficiently obvious. Dr. Cormack has seen frequent examples in his own practice. He does not, however, enter into the particulars of these cases; but concludes by mentioning two circumstances which thoroughly corroborate this view.

In the *Boletin de Medicina, Cirujia, y Farmacia* of 14th November, 1852, a short abstract was given of Dr. M'William's paper. In the same journal of the 19th December following, a correspondent writes to say, that in consequence of the notice which had appeared of Dr. M'William's paper, he had used fomentations of fig-leaves *(hojas de higuera)* to promote the secretion of milk in three cases in which it had wholly or nearly ceased. In all the cases, the benefit was decided. The Spanish practitioner wrote to confirm the practice recommended by Dr. M'William, but he has in reality, by using the wrong leaves, shown very clearly the galactagogue effects of poultices and fomentations, even when destitute of stimulating properties. He likewise states, upon the authority of a Spanish lady, (with whom he conversed on this subject a few days ago) that in Cadiz, women are in the habit of bringing back the milk to their breasts after it has left them in consequence of weaning the child, or of any other cause, by means of drinking an infusion of the wild lupin *(Altramuz)* and applying to the mammæ fomentations made with the same plant. This plant has no stimulant or irritative quality, and the efficacy of the poultices made with it must, as in the case of the fig-leaves, depend simply on heat and moisture, as in a common poultice. The internal use of the infusion might be dispensed with.

IV. *Conclusion.*— Dr. Cormack has thus made out a good plea in favor of warmth and irritation of the mammæ being regarded as powerful galactagogue and emmenagogue agencies; and he has also shown that the interesting facts recorded by Drs. M'William and Tyler Smith are not examples of specific action but illustrations of a general principle, which may be rendered available in rational therapeutics.

Injurious affects may so readily be produced by *excessive irritation of the mammæ* upon themselves, upon the ovaries and uterus. and (as a consequence of the undue excitement of any of these organs) upon the whole system, that in following the practice recommended in this paper, it is necessary to proceed with caution.

First, as regards the *mammæ* themselves, care must be taken not to produce too much irritation, lest troublesome inflammation be excited in them, and in the glands of the axilla;—consequences which he has seen produced in such a degree as to require, for several days, cooling lotions and general antiphlogistic measures.

In irritatble subjects, or when the effects of the treatment cannot be daily ascertained, stimulating embrocations ought to be preferred to sinapisms. When sinapisms are applied every eight or twelve hours, for some days continuously—as is sometimes necessary—they ought to be compounded of two or three parts of bread to one of mustard; and a fold of soft linen ought to intervene between them and the skin. By attending to these conditions, patients will generally endure the poultice without injury for half an hour or an hour; and a greater amount of benefit will be obtained than by causing violent stimulation for a short period. It is always essential to maintain, during the intervals, great local warmth, by means of abundance of cotton wadding. If mammary irritation have been carried so far, through mistake or accident, as to necessitate recourse to refrigerating lotions and lowering treatment, it need hardly be remarked that the object for which it was used is not likely to be accomplished.

Secondly, as regards the *ovaries* and *uterus*, the effects produced upon these organs must be attentively watched; for the very greatness of the power which irritation of the mammæ exerts over these organs may constitute an element of danger. In endeavoring to excite menstruation, we must take care that we do not excite inflammation of the ovaries of the womb. When we find the patient complaing of severe pain in the loins, and suffering from general fever, we ought at once to discontinue mammary irritation, and prescribe rest in bed, abdominal fomentations, and the frequent use of the hip-bath. In cases of this description, as in ordinary attacks of dysmenorrhœa, we may often not only relieve pain, but accelerate a resolution of the inflammation, by administering opiate enemata.

Caution on the part of the practitioner will generally enable him to prevent or speedily remove the evils and inconveniences to which reference has been made. They may however, so easily occur through the want of it, and lead to so much discredit and embarrassment, that the author has been anxious to give them the prominence which they deserve.

Extraordinary operation on the Subclavian Vein. By the MATE OF A VESSEL; Recovery.

The following narrative is given with three objects: Firstly, to show the value of self-control and common sense in scenes of danger; secondly, the resources of nature under the most desperate circumstances; and thirdly, to correct the boastful surgeon, when he feels inclined to convince the world that all that is excellent and skilful centers in himself. The merest chance in the world elicited the simple and child-like narrative from the operator, and he seemed as much astonished as ourself, when the almost certain character of his performance was pointed out to him on a preparation of the heart and blood-vessels. Edward T. Hinckley, of Wareham, Mass., then mate of the bark Andrews, commanded by James L. Nye, of Sandwich, Mass., sailed some two years and a half since (we find the date omitted in our minutes) from New Bedford, Mass, on a whaling voyage. When off the Gallipagos Islands, one of the hands, who had shown a mutinous disposition, attacked Captain Nye with some violence, in consequence of a reproof given him for disobedience. In the scuffle which ensued, a wound was inflicted with a knife, commencing at the angle of the jaw, and dividing the skin and superficial tissues of the left side of the neck, down to the middle of the clavicle, under which the point of the knife went. It was done in broad day, in presence of the greater part of the crew; and Mr. Hinckley, the mate, being so near, that he was at that moment rushing to the captain's assistance. Instantly seizing the villain and handing him over to the crew, the knife either fell or was drawn by some one present, and a frightful gush of *dark* blood welled up from the wound, as the captain fell upon the deck. Mr. Hinckley immediately thurst his fingers into the wound, and endeavored to catch the bleeding vessel; with the thumb against the clavicle, as a point of action, and gripping, as he expressed it to me, "all between," he found the bleeding nearly cease. The whole affair was so sudden, that Mr. Hicnkley stated to me, he was completely at a loss what step to take. Such had been the voilence of the hæmorrhage, a space on the deck fully as large as a barrel head, being covered with blood in a few seconds, that it was evident from that and the consequent faintness, that the captain would instantly die, should he remove his fingers from the bleeding vessel. As Mr. H. said to me, with the simplicity and straightforward style of a seaman, "I brought to" for a minute, to think over the matter, The bleeding coming upwards from under the collar-bone, and being completely concealed by it, it was plain enough that I couldn't get at the blood-vessel without sawing the bone in two; and this I would not like to have tried, even if I had dared to remove my fingers. Feeling that my fingers' ends were so deep as to be below the bone, and yet the bleeding having stopped, I passed them a little further downwards, still keeping up the pressure against the bone with the middle joints. I then found my fingers passed under something running in the same course with the bone; this I slowly endeavored to draw up out of the wound, so as to see if it was not the blood vessel. Finding it give a little, I slowly pulled it up with one finger; *when I was pulling it up, the captain groaned terribly,* but I went on, because I knew I could do nothing else. As soon as I could see it, I washed away the blood, and was astonished and very glad to see there were two vessels, as I supposed them to be, one behind the other: *the cut was in the front one.* It was the full breadth of the knife, or about half an inch, and neither across nor lengthways, but about between the two, and went about half its thickness through the blood-vessel: *it was smooth and blue* in appearance, and the cut had stopped bleeding, as I supposed at the time, because the vessel was pressed together by being stretched across my finger. As I had often sewed up cuts in the flesh and knew nothing about tying blood-vessels, and supposed that was only done when they were cut in two, as in amputated limbs, I concluded to try my hand at sewing it up; so I took five little stitches; they were very near together, for the wound was certainly not half an inch wide, if so much." On inquiry of Mr. Hinckley, if he cut off the thread each time and threaded the needle again, he said Yes; but "I only cut off one end, and left the other hanging out." This he had learned from a little book, prepared for the use of sea captains and others, when no surgeon was on board. Mr. H. continued: "I twisted the ends together loosely, so as to make one large one, and let it hang out of the wound over the bone; then I closed all up with stitches and plasters. On the fourteenth day I found the strings loose in the wound, from which matter had freely come: it healed up like any other cut." Poor Captain Nye finally met a sad fate; he was drowned on the destruction of his boat by an enraged whale.

The practical anatomist and surgeon will at once see the internal evidence of the entire truthfulness of this extraordinary narrative, and the certainty that Mr. Hinckley must have closed up a wound in [the subclavian vein. Aside from the position of the wound rendering any other explanation impossible, and the color and amount of blood instantly lost, the fact that a wound of the subclavian artery must have been followed by aneurism, if not instant death, renders the conviction unavoidable that it must have been the vein. When the Captain "groaned terribly," as Mr. Hinckley was drawing up the vessel with his finger, the brachial plexus of nerves was evidently put on the stretch. Indeed, it is impossible to suppose, aside from Mr. Hinckley's high character and the corroboration of the log-book, that such a story could have been devised by any but a surgeon of decided practical ability. We may be mistaken in our views of its importance, but we think that in the estimation of our professional readers we have placed upon record one of the most extraordinary circumstances in the whole history of Surgery.

If the case be not worth an ordinary surgeon's eye and going the rounds of every journal in the land, we are mistaken; every student should commit it to memory: it will teach him modesty and self-possession.

From the Iowa Medical Journal.

Professor Armor's Prize Essay.

We regret very much our inability to publish entire this valuable essay. In accordance with our design, we will proceed to give a con-

densed abstract from it, in order that our readers may see the design
and the importance of this treatise,—the result of so much investigation
and research.

Waiving all discussion with regard to the independent vitality of the
blood, the manner of its development, growth or decay, its purposes and
its uses, whether for nutrition, or to supply the wants and demands
of the various structures by the elaboration of fibrine; the author avoids
these discussions, we say, and proceeds to the investigation into the presence of foreign matters in that fluid, in our essential or Idiopathic forms
of fever. That there is an admixture of deleterious properties, he proves
by the following facts: 1st. That diseases analogous to those fevers
have been induced by injecting putrid matters into the veins of animals:
2d. Animal poisons introduced into the blood easily produce these
fevers, also in small pox, measles; and 3d. These poisons gain access to
the blood through the medium of the air, and by the lungs: 4th. The
non-contageous fevers, as Remittents, and Intermittents depend upon a
poisoned or changed state of the atmosphere: 5th. Observation shows
that, in Essential or Idiopathic fevers, the blood is altered.

Not only is there toxœmia or blood poisoning, but that it is primarily
so, the difference in the phenomena is owing to the difference in the
character of that poison that each specific miasm has its specific effects.
Urea in the blood has its legitimate uramic developments because it
poisons the nervous centres, the virus of Small Pox attacks the skin and
the mucous tissue, and yet the peculiar nature of each poison is not yet
understood. Experience has perceived the legitimate action of each, and
a uniformity in the results show a similarity in the causes of producing
them. And yet, although these general relations obtain, there is not
always an identity, for in Typhoid fever and in Small Pox the fibrine of
the blood is defective.

As we have no certainty as to the nature of the impression, neither
have we an assurance as to the peculiar therapeutic action of remedies.
Mercury produces inflammation of the salivary glands. Arsenic the
mucous tissues, Beladonna the skin, Ergot the uterus, &c.

Zymosis or fermentation of the blood, has recently received much
attention, particularly at the hands of the illustrious Liebig. It is made
the basis of a plausible hypothesis, long since advocated, but subsequently
discarded. Its connection with Humoral Pathology attainted it, and it
fell into disrepute and neglect. Liebig, in his work on " Animal Chemistry," advances the following position, which is quoted and highly commended by the author of the Essay.

" The Chemical force and the vital principle hold each other in such
perfect equilibrium, that every disturbance, however trifling, or from
whatever cause it may proceed, effects a change in the blood." The
Zymotic change then is due to a molecule in a state of dissolution within
the body; this by contact diseases another, and so on, until the whole
may be diseased, and this act of dissolution is termed " decomposition
by contact." or the " action of presence."

Those bodies which contain *nitrogen* suffer most, and suffer first, and
as a large share of this element is formed in the blood, therefore, dissolution once commenced, unless arrested, will speedily and certainly pervade

the whole fluid mass. When this is not the case, then we must look for some sustaining principle, and this is found in the vital forces. Here, then, is the struggle. On the one hand is the vital law, asserting its powers and prerogatives; while on the other, is this Zymotic distemper, going on from molecule to molecule. Which shall triumph, will determine the fortunate or unfortunate result of the case.

But what proofs of this law of Zymosis? What are the proofs to show that putrefactive matters, by the entering into the blood, will produce the phenomena of fever? The answer is, that the putrid particles in the air of the dissecting room, communicated to the living body through the lungs, and putrid blood, brain and eggs, laid upon recent wounds with an abrasion of surface have caused vomiting, and even death. Putrid matter injected into the blood of healthy animals, and a small portion accidentally introduced during dissection, will produce symptoms of Typhus. Yeast or sugar thrown into the circulation, will also produce typhoid symptoms with ecchymosis of the skin, and the decomposition of animal and vegetable matters in quantities, will produce epidemic diseases. The case of the Sexton, while in the act of lowering a coffin let it fall, and the corpse being in a state of active decomposition, a large amount of sanies, highly offensive, was exposed and flowed out. One hundred and fourteen persons present fell dangerously ill of a putrid disease. It spread subsequently to some sixty others with like results. The case of the man who became diseased by skinning a diseased animal, sickened, and some of his blood injected into the groin among the lymphatics of a cat, produced fatal symptoms and it died in seven hours. These proofs are given to show that a poison may be introduced into the system, producing its legitimate phenomena, and when introduced into others and perpetuated carries with it, as resulting phenomena, similar manifestations and symptoms. The proofs we regard as conclusive of the position taken and are familiar to every physician of experience.

The blood then is a great pool, a cesspool oftimes in certain forms of malignant diseases, in whatever way or manner generated.

The blood has been found in a partial state of dissolution in putrid diseases, is a fact made notorious by clinical observation, and we find under this condition the fibrine suffers.

The essayist accounts for the alkaline reaction in the urine, as the result of the presence of hydro-sulphate of ammonia in malignant diseases, and is the product of decomposition.

The importance of the depuraors, from the skin; the bowels, from the kidneys, is strongly urged and yet not *too* much enforced. In a practical piont of view, we think this one of the most interesting and useful aspects of this essay. One reason the author assigns, and which has been repeatedly maintained, why these functions shoud be stimulated to increased activity, is that if the morbific matters be not thrown off a " backward movement " obtains, the poison accumulates, and all the symptoms are aggravated. The experiments of Orfila and of Golding Bird are referred to in order to show the importance of awakening the kidneys particularly, to increase depurative action.

He takes a conservative position with regard to the Humoralists and the Solidists. He adopts neither system wholly, nor yet does he entirely discard either. So long as the tissues look to the blood for life, and as long as the tissues undergo changes as a sequence of an altered condition of the blood, *so long* both are right. The one is a cause, and the other the effect of that cause.

The febrile state is the result of the alteration; the biotic forces are awakened because the nervous centres depend for their powers upon the integrity of the blood. This accounts for the great depression of animal and organic functions; to this state congestions follow, either with suspended or imperfect secretions, and there is a general languor of all the functions in these fevers.

The following important indications follow: 1st. To counteract the injurious operation of the poisons. 2d. To expel them from the system. The first is by the administration of salines, as Chloride of Sodium and the Cholorate of Potass, and by acids, as the hydrochloric, &c., &c. 2d. Tonics, stimulants, and depurants, alcohol and arsenic, are valuable antiseptics, because of the dissolved condition of the blood. (In the low putrescent forms creasote with chlorines?)

Fever is but the evidence that nature is endeavoring to effect a cure by throwing off the offending matters. This act is called an effort of the "vis medicatrix," and in the successful recuperative act, nature becomes the best and wisest physician.

This pathology reconciles the different modifications of diseased conditions under *epidemic influences.* We recognise two elements: *first,* the depressing poison of Zymotic state, and *second,* the inflammatory or functual derangements of local organs. This is nothing else than those conditions termed *sthenic* and *asthenic.* The treatment would be more rational. Blood letting and the antiphlogistic remedies in the latter must be used, if resorted to at all, most sparingly and with caution. The closing remark of the author we quote in his own language:

" *The great success in the treatment of disease is to be found in a broad, comprehensive, and rational pathology—a pathology that weighs every element of disease, whether of fluids or solids, that is capable of exciting, depressing or perverting vital actions.*"

We have at some length endeavored, but imperfectly however, to give the main leading points of this invaluable essay, that the reader may be able to understand somewhat its design and appreciate the importance of this contribution to medical science. We are aware that any attempt at a synopsis would be likely to detract from its true merits, and yet we hope it will be well received by all. The motive was just, and if we have failed, it was because we had not room to publish it entire. In the condensed extract we have occupied some pages to the exclusion of other matter, bnt we think not of more importance.

Our time cannot be better or more profitably employed than in the discussion of these grave questions connected with pathological science.

The physiologist, aided by the microscope, and the chemist with his laboratory, are astounding the medical world with their discoveries, and making medical science radiant with new and brilliant revelations. It makes the soul within us leap for joy, with the prospects of a still brighter and more glorious future in medicine, and that humanity will proudly exult in its increased attributes and triumphs. Every year adds fresh laurels to those which now bedeck her brow, and new jewels are being added to glitter in her coronet and crown. Within a few short years the untiring efforts of the medical philosopher have resulted in glorious and enduring results. Enduring, we say, because, in the main, the discoveries are *facts*, not suppositions; *truths*, not doubtful hypotheses. Microscopic investigations and chemical analyses, when successful in their experiments, produce results invariable and uniform, because the discovery of carb. ammonia, of urea, &c., in the blood, and albumen in the urine, are products of which there exists not any longer doubt. These are refinements, it is true, upon former investigations, and yet they are mathematical results. The particular mode by which these abnormal changes are effected may remain obscured, as they are now measurably hidden from us, but doubtless we shall be able hereafter to detect other mal-products and trace out certain phenomena as the result of their presence with comparative certainty. The present age in medicine is not engaged in inventing new hypotheses or false theories, but it is proceeding practically into things substantial, tangible and real. Hereafter there will be less mist or fog found enveloping medical science; no longer expansive systems or dogmas invented by visonary speculators, to confuse and bewilder; and to which their followers, as in olden time, will cling as to a confession of faith; but the scalpel, the microscope, and the laboratory are active in a utilitarian search after tangible objects and materials.

We shall at some future time call the attention of readers to the consideration of some features of this valuable treatise, with the view of keeping the subject before the medical public. Here where we have yearly visitations of the enieric forms of fever, the discussion of these subjects is of grave importance. The pathology of these fevers cannot be too much studied and examined in order to arrive at the most rational and effective treatment.   EDITORS.

On Ergot of Rye in Retention of Urine.   By M. Passot, of Lyons.

Ergot of rye has not only the property of exciting the uterine contractions in cases of inactivity of the uterus, but is also very efficacious in the retention of the urine which is caused by atony and paralysis of the bladder. M. M. Baudin and Payan were the first who endeavored to demonstrate that this agent does not act on the uterus alone, but rather on the lower part of the spinal cords. They also speak very highly of it as well in the affection which we have now under consideration as in weakness or paralysis of the lower extremities.

Drs. Kinsley, Canuto-Canuti, Sainmont, and Allier have also recorded cases which bear favorable testimony to the utility of ergot in paralysis of the bladder. I will now briefly mention some of them:

Capt. B., aged 60, suffered from dysuria, which had increased greatly during the last three months, until it suddenly turned to a complete retention, which necessitated the employment of the catheter several times a day. For two months a host of remedies were used without avail; there was not the slightest improvement. The prostate became enlarged, and the patient suffered much from the use of the catheter, which had to be passed twice every day.·

About eight grains of ergot of rye, infused in a cupful of boiling water, was administered three times a day. At the expiration of six hours, the patient passed a small quantity of urine, and required the use of the catheter only once in the day. Afterwards it was only passed once in the forty-eight hours, and after ten days the bladder was left to itself.

A lady, aged about 75, was affected with paralysis of the bladder, which for a time required the use of the catheter. Ergot was prescribed in doses of about twenty-eight grains in infusion. On the sixth day of this treatment, it was no longer neccessary to pass the instrument, the patient being able to pass water spontaneously.

A man, named Rousseau, aged 53, of a nervous temperament, was, in a fit of passion, attacked with a complete inability to urinate. The bladder was obliged to be emptied by the catheter. The inertia of this organ continued in spite of cold injection to it, cold enemata, the application of ice, also a blister to the hypogastrium.

Strychnine, applied by means of ointment as a dressing to the blister, also by frictions in the axillæ, on the following day produced cramps in the legs and arms, and was presently accompanied by stiffness, so that it became necessary to discontinue the use of this remedy. There was not the slightest action on the bladder. It was at this stage that the author conceived the idea of giving ergot of rye. He prescribed about ninety-two grains coarsely powdered, to be put into about thirty-four ounces of water, macerate for two days, filtered and injected cold into the bladder. Seven minutes afterwards the patient experienced a desire to urinate, which, however he could not then satisfy. The next morning the injection was again administered. Eight minutes after he had vesical tenesmus, and then spontaneous emission of urine. The injections were continued for some days. The cure was complete.

In 1848, Dr. Allier of Mareigny, sent a letter to the National Academy of Medicine, in which he gives as the result of his observations, that in only one out of fourteen cases ergot proved of no use.

I also am in possession of some cases which, in an incontestible manner, prove that ergot is capable of restoring the contractility of the bladder. The following is the most remarkable:—In the month of July, 1846, I was consulted by M. H., aged 60, of a dry constitution, and a very well-marked nervous temperament. Mr. H., admits having indulged in venereal excesses, and in the excess of the table, and it is these that he blames for the vesical paralysis from which he is now suffering, and which requires the catheter twice a day: otherwise there is no symptom of organic alteration, no fever, no enlarged prostate The canal of the urethra is free, through its entire length, and the urine when drawn off is perfectly clear. After having experienced the uselessness of tincture of cantharides and blistering the hypogastrium, I used the following prescription:

Freshly Powdered Ergot. 40 grains   Mucilage, 4 ounces.
A teaspoonful every half hour.
Ergot of Rye, powdered, 30 grains.   Cocoa butter. A sufficiency.
To be made into two suppositories ; one of them to be introduced night and morning.

On the same day, at the expiration of some hours, M. H. felt a desire to micturate. At my evening visit I ordered a bath. The patient was scarcely in it before micturation took place spontaneously and with force. From this time to his death, M. H. has always passed water freely and without the assistance of the instrument. I should add, that to make certain of the cure, I continued the remedy for three or four days, but in a decreasing dose. M. H. died on the 30th of January, 1848, of an acute pleuro-pneumonia, during the course of which not a single morbid symptom appeared in the bladder. But with regard to paralysis consecutive to apoplexy, or depending on other affections of the nervous centres, it is well known that they are unaffected by the remedy we are treating of.—*Medical Times and Gazette.*, from French Medical Journals.

~~~~~~~~~~~~~~~~

EDITORIAL AND MISCELLANEOUS.

———

The Pacific side of our continent presents a noble field of scientific inquiry, and among the objects of research, not the least interesting is the distribution and origin of the aboriginal races there found. The derivation of population from Polynesia and the Asiatic coast form interesting subjects of speculation and inquiry, which have already been to some extent devoloped; and the physiological effects of the climate, up and down that long coast, will yet be studied in a manner to yield rich returns for science in general, and for the healing art in particular. We take the liberty of making some extracts from a letter, which, though not designed for publication, glances so earnestly upon the scientific riches of that region, that it may stimulate some traveller thitherward, to bring back the gold of truth, as well as "yellow dust" of earth :

<div style="text-align: right">" San Diego, California.</div>

" Dear Doctor,

<div style="text-align: center">*   *   *   *   *   *   *   *</div>

" My business in this part of the world is to make a magnetical survey and a system of tidal observations between San Diego and our northern boundary along the coast, and this is what brings me now to San Diego.

" I have often wished for your company this summer, knowing your taste for scientific researches, for here there is much (almost too much) that is new and interesting presented to the senses every hour of the day, in whatever part of the country you may be.

" I made a visit to Puget Sound, during the month of August, and travelled on an Indian canoe, from Olympia, at the head of the sound, to Billingham Bay, a distance of one hundred and fifty miles. The journey from the Columbia river across the Sound is in itself worth a thousand miles of travel, and the voyage on the beautiful waters of the Sound can hardly be compared to any travelling that I have ever done—indeed, as I said before, it is too interesting to be made profitable. Geology, Natural History, Mineralogy, and every other ' ology,' worth mentioning, seem to stare with their treasures of knowledge invitingly spread before you, and it is a sort of self-denial to pay more attention to one than the other.

" The Indians of Puget Sound alone present the most interesting subject of study and observation. The beautiful faces of some of the children, and the forms and features of some of the men and women, give evidences of origin from a highly intelligent and peculiar race of men. And in many of their qalities too, they show a striking contrast to some of the other Indians of the coast. Their amiable gentle manners and musical tastes, make them, in comparison with the other tribes, what the Italians are to the Germans or Russians. A thousand interesting questions arise in relation to them which can only be answered by patient investigation.

. " In Geology, what a field of untrodden ground! the strange and peculiar character of the whole coast, forming for several thousands of miles an abrupt mountain wall, against which the sea is battling, with its everlasting solemn war, here and there breaking through and forming islands, or gradually washing away salient points, leaving but a dangerous ledge of hidden rocks; and the outlets of the large rivers, too, particularly the Sacramento and Columbia, following now new channels, produced by the combined action of the sea and volcanoes. presents another subject which would give work for all the geogolists of the world; and then, Natural History :—here is indeed an unknown field! The Rocky Mountains seem to present an insurmountable barrier to the propagation of species, for here you find everything different from similiar species on the eastern side, and thousands of species entirely new. All these things I would enjoy more if there were only some one here to enjoy them with me, but, with rare exceptions, nothing is interesting to men here unless it brings gold to the purse.

" I learn that you are starting a Medical Journal at Ann Arbor. I wish you much success, and am sure that you, as well as your readers, will receive much benefit from it. Please enter my name on your subscription books, and address the papers to Lieut. W. P. T————, U. S. Army, San Francisco, California.

" I found a curiosity, which I wish I could send you, while I was at Bellingham Bay, Straights of Fuca. It is the skeleton of a man, which I found under circumstances which justify me in conjecturing that it is the remains of one of the early navigators of that unexplored region. It was taken from a mound in the vicinity of an angular breast work, and although the works appeared to be very old, yet the soil was so dry that the skeleton was perfectly preserved. It had a fracture in the skull, as if done by a war club, and is, no doubt, the only relic of the little party who here attempted to defend themselves against the Indians. I am quite certain that it is not an Indian skeleton from the manner in which it was buried, and when I get it I will write a history of the manner in which it was found, and, if possible, send you the skeleton.

" How would you like the skull of a Flat-Head? They are quite abundant on the Columbia.

" Don't forget to send me your paper. It will be good company for me in, my wanderings.

" Yours truly,

" W. P. T————."

THE

PENINSULAR
JOURNAL OF MEDICINE
AND THE COLLATERAL SCIENCES.

| VOL. I. | JANUARY, 1854. | NO. VII. |

ORIGINAL COMMUNICATIONS.

Art. I.—*Practical Observations upon Polypus of the Uterus.* By Dr. Helfft. Translated from the German, by Professor A. Sager.

It is well known that pregnancy occurring during the existence of uterine polypi is not an unfrequent event. When the polypus is attached to the os uteri, and occupies the upper part of the vagina, it may give rise to hæmorrhage during pregnancy, and excite the premature expulsion of the ovum, or, if gestation proceeds to full term, it may seriously impede parturition. In this latter relation, especially, it forms a subject of consideration in most of the works upon obstetrics. When, however, the polypus occupies the cavity of the uterus, danger is rarely threatened until after the expulsion of the ovum, when it may immediately give rise to a dangerous hæmorrhage, or cause a retroversion of the organ. Not unfrequently, also, the projecting tumor is mistaken for an inverted uterus, and the indications of treatment derived from this erroneous diagnosis.

When a female afflicted with uterine polypus becomes pregnant, whatever may be the structure of the morbid growth, or wherever it may be attached, it rapidly acquires a considerable size, resulting from great development of its own vessels, in common with the tissues and vessels of the uterus itself. This fact is observable even when the polypus is of a fibroid character, and covered with merely a thin lamina of the muscular tissue of the uterus, which also constitutes the pediculated attachment of the morbid growth; but it attains a much greater size when its development takes place in, and is enveloped by, the proper tissues of the uterus.

This rapid growth of polypi, together with the circumstance that they always constitute a highly dangerous complication of pregnancy, should dmonish us of the necessity of removing small polypi as soon as they are discovered, and not to wait until after delivery, even when neither hæmorrhage nor symptoms of pressure of adjacent organs present themselves.

In the treatment of uterine polypi which, during pregnancy, pass out of the uterus into the vagina, we must be guided in the selection of means to be employed by the size of the tumor, and the accidents that accompany its growth. If it be discovered in the early months of gestation, when its size is yet moderate, and the pedicle thin, and hæmorrhage, with muco-purulent discharge, takes place, it may be removed by torsion. Generally, its influence upon the uterus is so insignificant as scarcely to attract attention, and furnishes no intimation of its formidable nature, and the ever-increasing danger of the disease.

A case of this character is described by Dr. Oldham. He was called to a lady who had been married five months. As the menses appeared but once after her marriage, she was now in the third or fourth month of pregnancy. From that time she experienced a frequently-returning and moderate hæmorrhage, that was seldom absent more than two days, and at last sexual commerce, or any active exertion, always produced a return of the discharge. From the frequency of this occurrence, the lady was led to doubt the fact of her pregnancy. The general condition of the lady was good, and the signs of pregnancy were unmistakeable. Upon examination, there was a very vascular polypus situated upon the anterior wall of the cervix uteri of about the size of a plum. She was directed to recline upon the back for two days, and an aperient was ordered. A speculum introduced embraced the polypus, which was easily twisted off with a forceps. An insignificant hæmorrhage followed, which spontaneously ceased. Perfect recovery took place, and the lady was fortunately delivered at term.

Now, although such polypi may be removed without inducing abortion or other dangerous accident, it cannot be denied that a less fortunate result may sometimes develop itself when, as the only practicable method, a ligature has been applied around the thick pedicle of a large polypus. In consequence of the great development and intimate union of the venous system of the uterus with that of the tumor, the violent separation of the latter may give rise to phlebitis, or direct absorption of the putrescent matter, arising from its decay, may take place. In either event, a fatal termination is justly to be apprehended. To this, moreover, may be added the danger of an abortion. The following unfortunate case furnishes evidence of the correctness of these views:

Dr. Oldham was called to a lady twenty-six years old, who was dangerously ill, in consequence of an early abortion. He found all the symptoms of a wide-spread metroperitonitis, with phlebitis, under which the patient succumbed in thirty hours.

He now learned that about five weeks previous she was attacked with a profuse metrorhagia, the cause of which was not at first detected. After the continuance of the discharge for eight or ten days, the attending physician directed her to take acid, and enjoined strict rest. The hæmorrhage, however, did not cease, and, upon making an examination, he discovered a polypus, of the size of an apple, attached by a thick pedicle to the anterior lip of the os uteri. Up to this time neither the physician nor the patient had the least suspicion of the existence of pregnancy. A ligature was applied with considerable difficulty, and, after two days, the tumor dropped off. The patient very imprudently left her bed immediately, and walked about the chamber. Pains supervened, and terminated only with the expulsion of a six weeks' fœtus. The hypogastrium remained quite sensitive, and pains of a severe character returned; chills occurred; vomiting of a green fluid supervened; the abdomen became tympanitic; and, although the usual remedies were had recourse to, the patient sank under symptoms of collapse, and soon expired.

Yet polypi of a large size have sometimes been removed, both in the early and advanced periods of gestation, as when the operation has been performed to remove an obstacle to parturition, or to check an excessive hæmorrhage, with a fortunate-result. In others, as in the case cited above, the termination has been an unhappy one. And the fortunate results attending operations, under these circumstances, are quite too exceptional to justify a resort to such measures, except in cases of the greatest emergency, and should, even then, be undertaken with the greatest caution and circumspection.

In those cases in which the polypus occupies the cavity of the uterus, and, in its development, corresponds with the progress of gestation, numerous considerations require especial attention.

Polypi of this character, by a rapid growth during gestation, not unfrequently attain the size of a melon. Yet their development is not attended with the slightest accident, nor does the uterus attain a greater

size or firmer consistency than when pregnancy is uncomplicated with
this anormality.   In a case related by Vidal there existed a transverse
presentation of the fœtus, which may have been caused by the tumor;
yet, inasmuch as in other published cases this presentation was not observed, the connection should, probably, be regarded as rather accidental
than necessary.

But, immediately after the expulsion of the fœtus, and while the placenta yet remains, the attention of the obstetrician will be attracted by
the unusual size of the uterus, and a suspicion excited of the existence
of twin pregnancy, although the size is less than usual in that condition.
After the completion of the parturient act, the uterine parieties contract
firmly about the polypus, and a hard and tense tumor is readily perceived upon examination of the hypogastrium.   In the absence of a
more thorough exploration, we may anticipate that, sooner or later, depending upon the size of the polypus, and the mobility of its pedicle,
it will be extruded into the vagina.   A profuse hæmorrhage and severe
pains sometimes accompanies the extrusion, which, in other instances,
takes place without either.

Having satisfied ones self, by the absence of the fœtal membranes and
the fœtal heart sounds, that the tumor which appears under such circumstances is not another ovum, but a solid tumor, it is better to leave
the uterus quite unmolested, than to introduce the hand for the purpose
of removing its contents, or to attempt its expulsion by the exhibition
of ergot.   So long as the uterine contraction remains firm, a very notable increase of volume may be experienced, without the occurrence of
hæmorrhage; and, if no attempt be made to remove the polypus, there
exists far less proportional danger, as the shrivelling of the tumor results
from the hæmorrhagic discharge.

Every operative procedure will excite an irritation, and may induce a
hæmorrhage, from the partial separation of the pedicle of the polypus.
There is, moreover, reason to apprehend the retroversion of the organ.
Such patients are, therefore, enjoined to observe the strictest rest, to employ mild aperient medicines, and avoid all causes of local irritation.
Nevertheless, we can never be certain that, in the extrusion of the polypus into the vagina, an exhausting hæmorrhage, with severe suffering,
will not take place, rendering the removal of the tumor a matter of urgent necessity.   With this object, we may employ torsion, when the
pedicle of the polypus is thin; and in those in which the thickness of
the pedicle precludes any other operation, a ligature should first be applied, to prevent hæmorrhage, and it may then be safely excised.

Art. II.—*To the Editor of the Peninsular Journal of Medicine.*

Mr. Editor:—If you consider the following worthy of a place in your journal, you are at liberty to insert it. The history of the case I am about to relate, perhaps, possesses nothing remarkable or unparalleled. Notwithstanding, I consider it one of much interest, as it illustrates, in a marked degree, the wonderful powers of adaptation inherent in the human system. The case occurred at the Aims-House in the city of Buffalo, No. 3, in the spring of 1853, and was under my immediate charge, I being interne at the time in that institution.

Phebe L—— was admitted March 15, aged *twelve years, lacking a few days.* She was below medium size, and possessed a nervo-sanguine temperament. She was pregnant, and at, or a little passed eight months. She had slight pains when she entered, similating the early stage of parturition. The pains increased, and in about six hours after admittance she was seized with a puerperal epileptic convulsion, which was protracted, and uncommonly severe. She was immediately copiously bled; cold was applied to the head, etc. As soon as the paroxysms subsided, an active cathartic was prescribed. On examination, the os uteri dilated. We then commenced giving nauseating doses of antimony, combined with a little opium. About half an hour from the first attack she had a second paroxysm, but not as severe as the preceding. She was again bled moderately, and the usual measures resorted to. After passing off, the antimony et opii was again given, and continued till the patient went to sleep, which was very soon after the second convulsion. She was very easy, having no pain or convulsions till the next evening, at the same time as the preceding, she had another convulsion, not quite as severe as the former. Nothing was done at this time, except wedging the teeth. After it passed off, there followed several labor pains in rapid succession, and then she was easy again, and soon went to sleep, without any anodyne. There was still no perceptible progress in the labor. Strange as it may seem, for the twelve days following she went through this routine every morning. First a convulsion, followed by about half a dozen pains, and then she would be perfectly easy till next day at the same time. At the fourth or fifth day there was a perceptible change in the os uteri and vagina, and at the end of the twelve days these parts presented a much more soft, relaxed, and yielding feel than at first, and the os uteri was dilated sufficiently to admit the point of the finger, the fœtal head being at this time distinctly felt.

The pains now ceased almost entirely. The bladder and rectum at this time became evidently paralyzed. We were obliged to evacuate the former regularly by the catheter, and the latter by enemata. She remained in this quiescent condition for a week, during which time she took some stimulus, as she was much exhausted.

After remaining in this state, as stated, for a week, more violent regular pains came on, following each other in rapid succession, which, in a short time, propelled the head into the cavity of the pelvis; but the uterine effort appeared unable to complete the labor. A dose of secale cornutum was accordingly given, and soon after she was delivered of a healthy boy, weighing eight pounds. After parturition, though very feeble, she got along without difficulty; and, after a protracted convalescence, she departed with her prize for Michigan, her former home. I have no comments in particular to make on this case. It is my opinion that the long-continued parturient efforts were a wise provision of Nature, instituted, in this case, as a preparatory process to true parturition.

E. T. DORLAND,

Medical Student, University of Mich.

ART. III. — *Review of Paget's Surgical Pathology; or, Lectures on Surgical Pathology. Delivered at the Royal College of Surgeons of England, by* JAMES PAGET, F.R.S.

The splendid generalizations of the beginning of this work, and the solid facts of the latter portions, especially on the subject of cancer, render it a prize both to daring theoretical minds, and to the lovers of sound practical knowledge.

Of all theories, not actually demonstrated, we have seen nothing more beautiful than the one involved in his philosophy of Nutrition. Starting with the fact that known chemical alterations in the composition of the blood determine changes in the action of certain organs, *symmetrically on the two sides of the body*, he deduces the probable conclusion that the other symmetrical changes, whether in symmetrical diseases, or in the first growth and formation of new organs in the foetus, are likewise dependent on certain changes in the composition of the blood. He thinks that there are subtle differences in the same tissue in different parts of the body, so that while homologous parts are identical in their composition, other parts differ. Thus, the skin of one arm is like the-skin of the other arm, but not like the skin of the leg or back. Hence, as a certain composition of the blood may disease the kidney on each side of the body alike, so, by still nicer selection, may some other blood changes cause diseases on certain portions of skin or bone precisely alike on the two sides. "The researches of modern chemistry have detected some of these changes, finding excesses or deficiences of some of the chief constituents of the blood, and detecting in it some of the material introduced from without. But a far greater number of the morbid conditions of the blood consist in changes, from the discovery of which the acutest chemistry seems far distant."

Thus far he states no new truth, but simply lays down his foundations, as others have done before him, and from reasonings like the above, he draws the conclusion that, from the embryo to gray hairs, a great portion of all physical changes, normal and abnormal, growth, development, nutrition, disease and decay, are determined by the qualities of the blood.

Of this old sweeping conclusion however, he makes a new use, by the help of one additional premise. That premise is this. As every exertion takes some peculiar product from the blood, and leaves it purified and fitted to act in a different manner on the system, so every organ, by its nutrition, takes, or "excretes" some peculiar element from the blood, and leaves it depurated and qualified for the nutrition of the rest of the system, and this "excretion" of nutrition is no less necessary for the qualities of the blood than the excretions which are more directly cast out of the body. "The hair, for example, in its constant growth serves not only local purposes, but for the advantage of the whole body, in that as it grows it removes from the body the various constituents of its substance, which are thus excreted from the blood." And the absence of these constituents from the blood is necessary to the proper nutrition to the rest of the body, just as much as the absence of the elements the renal secretion is necessary to the nutrition and functions of the brain.

There is thus established a sort of "complimental nutrition," whereby the abstraction of the material of one organ from the circulating fluid leaves it in the proper condition to nourish some other. A large and interesting class of facts in the sympathy between distant and unconnected organs is so beautifully explained by this theory, that the clearness with which it accounts for them may be taken as some evidence of its truth, albeit, the direct testimony of chemical analysis, it is acknowledged, cannot be had in the case.

Taking this principle, which was before announced by Treviranus, as the starting point, viz.: " *Each single part of the body, in respect to its nutrition, stands to the whole body in the relation of an excreted substance;*" for, although it is retained as a part of the body, it is just as much excreted from the blood as if it were cast off, or washed away. Thus, the phosphates in the bones are just as effectually removed from the blood as those in the urine. Taking this principle, I say, as a starting point, he maintains that when an organ takes its own peculiar elements from the blood for its own nutrition, it takes that which would be injurious to the nutrition of the rest of the body, were it not thus excreted. " The influence of this principle says the author, " may be considered in a large class of outgrowing tissues. The hair, for example, in its constant growth serves not only local purposes, but for the advantage of the whole body, in that, as it grows it removes from the blood the various constituents of its substance, which are thus excreted from the body. And this excretory office appears, in some instances, to be the only one by which the hair serves the purposes of the individual; as, for example, in the fœtus. Thus, in the fœtus of the seals that take the water as soon as they are born, and, I believe, in those of many other mammals, though they are removed from all those conditions against which hair protects, yet a perfect coat of hair is formed within the uterus, and before, or very shortly after birth, this is shed; and is replaced by another coat of wholly different color, the growth of which began within the uterus. Surely, in these cases, it is only as an excretion, or chiefly as such, that this first growth of hair serves to the advantage of the individual. The *lanugo* of the human fœtus is a homologous production, and must, I think, similarly serve in the economy by removing from the blood, as so much excreted matter, the materials of which it is composed.

" Further, I think, we may carry this principle to the apprehension of the true import of the hair which exists, in a kind of rudimental state, on the general surface of our bodies, and to that of many other permanent rudimental organs, such as the mammary glands of the male, and others. For these rudimental organs certainly do not serve, in a lower degree, the same purposes as are served by the homologous parts which are completely developed in other species, or in the other sex. To say they are useless, is contrary to all we know of the absolute perfection and all-pervading purpose of Creation; to say they exist merely for the sake of conformity with a general type of structure, seems unphilosophical, while the law of the unity of organic types is, in larger instances, not observed, except when its observance contributed to the advantage of the individual. Rather all these rudimental organs must, as they grow, be as excretions, serving a definite purpose in the economy by removing their appropriate materials from the blood, and leaving it fitter for the nutrition of other parts, or by adjusting the balance, which might else be disturbed by the formation of some other part. Thus they minister to the self-interest of the individual, while, as if for the sake of wonder, beauty, and perfect order, they are conformed with the great law of the unity of organic types, and concur with the universal plan observed in the construction of organic beings."

This view of the subject, whether true or not, is certainly very much more rational and logical than that great shadowy, spectral idea of some writers which attribute the male mammæ, the rudimentary feet of serpents, and the whole great class of rudimentary homologues, to the *disposition of nature to conform to the archetype.* The author's idea, so far as we know, is unique and original; certainly, it is put forth with freshness and power.

Another application of the principle is to the order of development in the fœtal state. The reason why the organs are so uniform in the order of their appearance, is because the formation of one part is a necessary excretion, without which the blood cannot be in a proper condition to develope the succeeding one, and hence an arrest of development in one part involves an arrest in the next part, whose nutrition is "complimentory" to it. Hence it is that the absence of one part in a mal-formed fœtus, is usually accompanied by the absence of some other part, and that in a fixed relation; as, for instance, it is a common or even general thing that fissure of the superior maxilla is accompanied by hare lip and absence of the brain, by deficiency of the neural arches of the vertebræ, and extreme shortness of the neck.

The author however will find it impossible to establish this as an universal law, unless he can show that there is *vicarious nutrition,* as well as vicarious secretions, and excretions, for we find that the non-development of one organ does not always cause a suppression of all the succeeding ones; and a fœtus from whom the brain is absent, or the heart missing, should, by that law, never arrive at the solid and rotund proportions of limb and chest, which we frequently see in such monstrosities.

However, he does not claim universality to this relation of organs. " *Certain organs,*" he says, "stand in their nutrition in a complimental relation to each other, so that neither of them can be duly formed or maintained in healthy structure unless the right condition of the blood be induced and preserved by the formation of the other. In man, the growth of the beard, and the development of the larynx both depend on the development of the testes, and castration prevents both from being perfected. In birds, too, a parallel phenomenon is observed. The height of beauty and completeness in the plumage and development in thé larynx is only attained by the male bird, the males only are birds of song, and in respect to plumage even, they reach its full beauty only at that season of the year when the testes undergo their annual enlargement, viz., the breeding season. If a buck be castrated, the next pair of antlers that is produced is stunted in size, and the second pair dwindles to a mere stump. Innumerable other instances might be given to illustrate complimental nutrition.

Respecting the theory, we must say, that we do not consider it proved, but we believe it to be one worthy of the closest investigation, for not only may brilliant truths be elicited, but the modifications of nutrition by changes in the composition of the blood, will probably be yet a most important element in therapeutics, notwithstanding Tully's theory of nervous influence.

The last two hundred pages are devoted to the discussion of malignant growths, and the treatment of the subject is full and masterly, and worth enough to make the work a valuable one were there nothing else in it. The engravings add much to its usefulness, and the whole work is worthy of its learned author.

E. A.

Art. IV.—*Reid's Method of reducing Dislocation of the Femur.*

Dear Doctor:—It may surprise some that we should be willing to expose our blunders, when they are known only to ourselves.

But if the following relation of accidents, which occurred to us in process of reducing a dislocated femur, by Dr. Reid's valuable method, can prevent their falling to the lot of others, we have no right to pocket our wit, if we did buy it. It must be some time before all the items of Dr. Reid's method will be universally known, unless practical facts are collated by the profession. We give below a true statement of our indirect route to success, leaving deductions to the reader.

Margaret Murry, aged about 30, robust and stout, slipped upon a wet platform about four o'clock, P.M. Felt severely hurt in the right hip and leg by the fall; was unable to rise without help. The slightest motion of the limb aggravated the intense pain, which extended through the thigh and knee; being, when at rest, most severe in the knee.

Domestic remedies having produced no alleviation, I was called five hours after the accident, and found the patient lying on the floor; left leg 1½ inches shorter than the right; toe turned inward. Such was the bulk of the thighs, that comparison, by the hands operating under a sheet, could not give any positive indication. A hollow was perceptible on the right side, near the situation of the trochanter major. Measurement, from the trochanter major to the external molleolus, was equal to sound side. Ditto from ant. spin. process of illium to external malleolus was near two inches shorter than sound side. No crepitation. What should the diagnosis be but dislocation of caput femoirs to dorsum illii? Grasping the foot with my right hand, and directing the knee with my left, we flexed the leg upon the thigh, and the thigh upon the body, bringing the knee across the other limb, until it was raised as high as the top of the pelvis. We then carried the knee outward, and still closer to the body, until the knee was near the axilla.

The patient now said that the first pain was relieved, and we brought the limb straight, causing severe pain, but no greater than slight motion had previously produced. The limb was not as short by measure as before manipulation; but the toe turned *outwards*, and the caput femoris could now be felt in the groin. When at rest, the pain in the knee was far less; and, when the thigh was slightly flexed, was, she said, "not worth minding." So that we received credit from the patient and attendants, but felt ashamed of having only changed the dislocation. The cause of our failure had been, neglect to bear the knee close enough to the body, and carry the foot out so far that the caput femoris should be lifted over the edge of the acetabulum.

I now placed myself on the left side, grasped the foot with the left hand, guiding the knee with the right ; flexed the leg and thigh, but kept the toe turned outward, and the knee on a line with the same side of the body till completely flexed, as we supposed (the patient being covered with a sheet).

The knee was now carried across the body, the toe turned inwards, and then brought down. The pain was less than before, but the position was not altered. And why? Not because the plan of operation was wrong, but because it had not been thoroughly carried out. We now directed the strongest attendant to *place a hand firmly upon the crest of the illii* of either side, with the thumb resting on the ant. sup. spin. processes, and keep the pelvis still, or inform me when it was moved. I then took hold as before, kept the knee and foot well out whilst flexing, until the thigh formed less than a right angle with the body, and then carried the knee inwards, still continuing the flexion forcibly, till motion of the head of the bone was perceptible. The toe was now turned inwards, and a slip, which was distinctly audible, with the patient's remark, "there, Doctor, something snapped, indade I'm betther now," told of our success. The limb was carefully straightened, with but little pain, and measured like the other. The patient was helped into a rocking-chair, and sat with ease till a bed was prepared. No unfavorable symptoms occurred. Passive motion was commenced in ten days. As a comparison of the power used with the old method by pullies, etc., I may state that but one assistant placed a hand upon the patient, and neither of us were a match for her in physical power.

J. H. B.

Coldwater, Mich., Dec. 17th, 1853.

Art. V. — *Observations upon the Longevity and Reproduction of Leeches.* By M. Bouniceau. Translated from the Annales des Sciences Naturelles, by E. Andrews, M.D.

On the fifth day of June, 1848, I uncovered a vessel into which I had put one middle-sized cow-leech, and four young ones, which another very fine cow-leech had produced on the 30th of September, 1846; which was the first from which I had unexpectedly obtained a coccoon, with the whole curious history of which I have often had occasion to entertain gentlemen interested in natural history. To be brief, in penetrating into the interior of the vase in question, and in tracing out the various galleries which that middle-sized leech and the four small ones in question had made through the earth in the vessel, guided somewhat by one of the small ones, which lay stretched at the entrance like a sentinel, and which escaped towards the bottom when it saw or felt me commencing to remove the earth, I found, at the bottom of the aforesaid vessel, the three other small ones, and the aforesaid middle-sized leech, which seemed to me to be actively alive. I immediately decided to separate the middle-sized leech, by putting it alone in a vessel, from the four young ones, who had the size and development of leeches about half way between small and moderately large ones, being about ten or twelve centimetres in length.

On the 17th of July following the cow-leech produced a coccoon, and thus proved that it had been fecundated by the young bloodsuckers. And so it proved of the young ones, for, having visited, on the same day, the vessel where I had put the four small leeches, aged twenty-one and twenty-two months—for they were only hatched, as I said, on the 30th of September, 1846—I perceived also a coccoon, which could only have been fecundated by the young leech which fecundated the old one.* Subsequently another coccoon was found in the same vessel with the four young bloodsuckers, and successively as many as eight, of which it is reasonable to suppose that two were produced by each individual, which was doing pretty well for the first time, since the old one only produced four. I proceeded to ascertain if these coccoons contained in their capsule ovules, or fecundated germs. This question was solved after about four days of a sort of incubation, occupied by some special from the parent, when I saw young ones come out full of life.

If you ask me, however, what became of the leech which produced those young ones, September 30th, 1846, I will say, sir, that I kept it until as late as May last, the time of its death, about eight years, during which time it became a mother, grandmother, great-grandmother, great-great-grandmother, great-great-grandmother's mother, and great-great-grandmother's grandmother; and the four young ones of which I spoke, and which it produced me in 1846, have produced, since the age of twenty-two months till about the time of their death, which took place long before that of their mother, four generations of young ones. It was at the age of five or six years that the last of the four young leeches of which I spoke acquired nearly the volume and development of the old grandmother whom I just mentioned. At this point I could decide exactly the age, and rate or growth, or duration of life which the medicinal or officinal leech can acquire, were I sure that the old grandmother in question died of old age; but she was in a state of emptiness or anæmia too complete for me not to think that she died of inanition, rather than of old age; and I am the more confirmed in this opinion, because she was the mother of several young leeches in August, 1852. I have, better than any of those who have spoken of the rate of growth of leeches in a given time, and of the length of their lives, been able to settle an opinion on the subject, having been able to preserve one of the first young ones which my very old dead leech produced, so long that, in size and development, it equalled the mother, and in length exceeded her. This was at the age of about six years. I conclude, therefore, that she herself was about six years of age in September, 1846, the period when she produced the young leeches in question. And I give, as a further proof, that in its empty condition it appeared more fleshy

* The reader will remember that leeches are hermaphrodite, each individual possessing the organs of both sexes. (*Trans.*)

more plump, and more solid than its offspring did at six years; which superiority seemed to me to be due to a couple more years of age, in all probability, which would make her eight years of age in September, 1846, and fourteen years of age at the time of the death of the last of the four young ones, which took place in March, 1852. And I can say that in May last, the time of the death of my old leech, it was fifteen years and some months in age, and had given proof in 1852 that it was still apt for reproduction, for I had given it only one companion, and I found in their cell several coccoons and young ones. As that last one was not recovered from its sufferings, which were due to my negligence, in leaving it to lack for water and nourishment, I continue to think that the old grandmother's death was owing more to that cause than to old age, and, consequently, that, except for my carelessness, the old leech would have had one or two years more of reproductive life, followed by three or four of old age, or repose, or unproductive time. It seems to me, therefore, reasonable to suppose, from the positive data which I have brought torward, that the common life of the *Hirudo sangnisuga*, or official leech, is twenty or twenty-one years.

To give you, sir, a just idea of the errors which have been circulated by the authors who have written on this point, I refer you to the work of M. Moquin–Taudan, edition of 1846, pages 208 and '209. I cite that work, because I think it is the most complete treatise which has been issued upon the family of Hirudines. In the place cited it may be seen—1st. That, according to my data, Achard is not correct in saying that medical leeches can be employed only at one year of age. I have ascertained and proved that they can be employed before that age. 2nd. Rejou is nearer to the truth when he says that they acquire a tolerable size in eighteen months. I am not certain about them in the wild state; but the domesticated ones, according to my experiment, acquire, in a year or fifteen months, the length of nine or ten centimetres, and a proportional diameter, which gives them the appearance of being moderately large, or holding a grade between moderately large and somewhat small. 3rd. You see very plainly how far from the truth Chatalain is in saying that the young leeches are only fit for suction at the age of four or five years. 4th. Fleury and Faber are evidently, after what I have had the honor to remark to you, altogether out of the way of truth. 5th. Derheims, who passes for an expert connoisseur in these matters, has committed the error of assigning to these annalides only five years of life; whereas, I have, in my collection, several subjects which are some centimetres longer than the old leech, whose biography I have just given you. 6th. M. Moquin–Taudon says that Audouin is of his opinion in assigning eight or ten years as the lifetime of the leech. 7th. Johnson has made a supposition which accords pretty well with my data, which I obtained from the book of nature, to which I see, with regret, that the greater part of the authors who have written upon the annalides in question pay little attention. 8th. It is very certain that Vilet could only have observed the death of leeches contained in jars of clear water. The leech cannot live many years without nourishment, and the clear water does not present any. When it is fed, its reproduction is far from exhausting it. It can, on the contrary, contribute to its longevity.

SELECTIONS.

From the New York Medical Times.

Opium and Charcoal—Their Comparative Effects on the System, described by one who experienced them in his own case.

[The writer of the following article, who describes so graphically the effects of both opium and alcohol in his own case, was received into the New York Hospital in 1849, suffering from a slight attack of dysentery. It was soon noticed that unusual symptoms complicated his case. On inquiry, he was found to be an opium-eater; and after his recovery, and during the period he was allowed to remain in the house, to enable him to recover, somewhat at least, from the pernicious effects of the habit which he had contracted, he furnished the Editor, (then on duty there,) by his request, with a history of the case, which is thought of sufficient interest to entitle it to publication. It has been somewhat abridged; but the language is, with but trifling exceptions, that of the writer himself.—*Editor N. Y. Medical Times.*]

The difference between opium and alcohol, in their effects on body and mind, is (judging from my own experience) very great. Alcohol, pushed to a certain extent, overthrows the balance of the faculties, and brings some one or more into undue prominence and activity; and (sad, indeed!) *these* are most commonly our *inferior*, and perhaps *lowest*, faculties. A man who, *sober*, is a demi-god, is, when drunk, below even a beast. With opium *(me judice)* it is the reverse. Opium takes a man's mind *where it finds it*, and lifts it *en masse* on to a far higher platform of existence, the faculties all retaining their former relative positions—that is, taking the mind as it is, it intensifies and exalts all its capacities of thought and susceptibilities of emotion. Not even this, however, extravagant as it may sound, conveys the whole truth. Opium weakens or utterly paralyzes the lower propensities, while it invigorates and elevates the superior faculties, both intellectual and affectional. The opium-eater is without sexual appetite; anger, envy, malice, and the entire hell-brood claiming kin to these, seem dead within him, or, at least, asleep; while gentleness, kindness, benevolence, together with a sort of sentimental religionism, constitute his habitual frame of mind. If a man has a poetical gift, opium almost irresistibly stirs it into utterance. If his vocation be to write, it matters not how profound, how difficult, how knotty the theme to be handled, opium imparts a *before unknown* power of dealing with such a theme; and, after completing his task, a man reads his own composition with utter amazement at its depth, its grasp, its beauty, and force of expression, and wonders *whence came the* thoughts that stand on the page before him. If called to speak in public, opium gives him a copiousness of thought, a fluency of utterance, a fruitfulness of illustration, and a penetrating, thrilling eloquence, which often astounds and over-masters himself, not less than it kindles, melts, and sways the audience he addresses. I might dilate largely on this topic, but space and strength are alike lacking.

Let no one, however, fancy, from these remarks, that the opium-eater *is blessed*. There is another side of the picture, dark, gloomy, and fraught with doom, to which I shall allude by-and-bye.

How became I an opium-eater? A lengthened train of causes (as I judge) led to this result. I can but touch on a few of them.

Exhausted nervous energy was the *fountain-head*. But whence this exhaustion?

1st. The accursed habit of nervous abuse, which *little* innocent school boys are taught by their depraved elders in school, and which, with no thought of its physical and moral harmfulness, is usually continued till unfolding reason and conscience open the victim's eyes to the real nature of his habit. It is usually, however, long enough protracted to have wrought no slight degree of nervous exhaustion.

2d. Tobacco chewing. In my sophomore year at Cambridge (being then 16 years old), a pipe-smoking grandam gave me a piece of tobacco to put in my mouth for a raging toothache. It quelled the pain; and from that moment I chewed nine or ten years without cessation. I chewed, too, immoderately, and spat incessantly, throwing out saliva in quantities perfectly suicidal.

Close application to study, with neglect of the rules of health, during my collegiate life, and during three subsequent years, while pursuing my studies at a theological school, where I pursued the same tobacco-chewing, unexercising life as at college, and still later, when settled as a clergyman, brought on a severe attack of dyspepsia, attended with great languor of body, and depression of mind, especially during the warm, weather.

In consequence of these feelings, I occasionally took a glass of wine or brandy and water, to supply the lacking *physical* basis for mental action. Thus passed three and a-half years; and by this time some portion of alcoholic stimulus had become almost a daily necessity, in order that the mind might execute its appointed tasks. If I omitted such stimulation, not only did I suffer languor and pain of body, but my thinking powers were inert and impotent. But I found, after a time, that alcohol was perilous to me, since I could not always calculate on its effects, so as to avoid being partially mastered by it. I abandoned alcohol, and substituted laudanum in its place. I cannot recall the precise quantity I at first used, though I think it was some twenty drops, taken two or three times a-day, or often enough to keep up the same level of sensation. The first feeling on swallowing the laudanum was a compound of pleasure and pain. The *pleasure* consisted in an agreeable warmth pervading the system, and a pleasant, gentle thrill passing along the nerves. The *pain* was a sort of *constriction*, or corrugation, by which the stomach seemed to be *drawn together* or *strongly compressed,* while a similar sensation ran along the nervous threads. However, both these species of sensation were of short duration, and then there remained only a painless, comfortless state of body, together with a clear, calm mood of mind, especially apt for all required mental tasks. When a propensity to gape and a sensation of languor indicated the *expenditure* of the stimulus, the dose was renewed; and so the days went by. After a considerable time, I substituted the opium pill for the laudanum. I think the pill, while producing all the *desirable* effects of the laudanum, produced less of the *pinching, unpleasant* sensation above mentioned, than did the laudanum. In other respects, there is little difference in their actions. I cannot tell precisely how long I was in reaching half an ounce per week; but that point I did finally attain. And at that point I for the most part remained during the three years I used opium in this vicinity. But I became greatly disordered in body, not *merely* through the opium, but also through the baneful habits connected therewith. I took no exercise; I sat at my books and papers, day after day, from breakfast time till 12 and 2 o'clock at night, in a hot study, filled with smoke from a cigar kept perpetually alight. I took a *hot bath once a fortnight*, instead of a *cold* bath *every morning;* in a word, *all* my habits (as I have since learned to understand) were the worst in the world for corporeal health. I suffered martyrdom from *costiveness*, often going a week, or nearly that, without a passage. Sometimes, too, I got into a physical state, which opium *would not* stimulate; and then I was compelled to employ alcohol. But alcohol, acting on opium-drugged nerves, is exceeding apt to produce maniacal intoxication.

After some ineffectual attempts, I determined to achieve freedom, were it possible, be the cost or the consequences what they might. I cast everything aside, and laid down upon my rack. And a rack it indeed was! For ten days and nights I had not, to my knowledge, one instant of sleep, or suspended consciousness. I was, for several days, half delirious; the blood in my veins felt like boiling water, and it rushed to my head in torrents, which seemed, every moment, as if they *must* burst asunder its bony enclosure. In a word, I believe that I was in a raging brain fever. In four weeks I was out, but I was shattered to pieces; and for a whole year I was feeble as a child, and one walking repository of aches and distressing sensations. At the close of that year I relinquished my profession, went to a brother's in the country in search of health, and, at first, simply for occupation, commenced in his office the study of law. For some time I remained weak, and, to complete the case, was finally attacked with neuralgia in the face and head. After bearing this as long as seemed possible, I consulted two physicians, and both ordered me *morphine* and quinine. Need I state the result? I was again brought under the power of opium, and the *habit* became fixed firmly as ever! For two years, while remaining there, I made no strenuous attempt to get free again.; but, using morphine regularly, and feeling well, I gave myself laboriously up to my legal studies. At the end of that period I came to New York, and went voluntarily into Bloomingdale Asylum for thirteen weeks, for the purpose of gaining my freedom. They were awful weeks; for, although, *per force,* I used no opium during such intervals, and so, *after a sort,* was rescued from the habit: yet I suffered inexpressibly from all kinds of ailments while there, and on leaving was extremely debilitated, and never for an instant free from pains and uneasiness.

I then completed my law studies, and opened a law office, at the same time assuming the editorship of a newspaper of extensive circulation, being put up for Congress, &c. &c. During these thirteen or fourteen months, I was almost entirely a stranger to opium; but I never felt well, free from pain, vigorous with my pristine strength, for one remembered day. It was with but a portion of my original self that I went through these *preparatory* processes. But when, through a series of events, in which I was rather passive than active, I found myself with the responsibilities of lawyer, justice, editor, and Congressional candidate, lying upon me all at once, at the same time that, from being a husband, and the father of three fair and noble boys, I was, by a sudden stroke, left a *solitary, homeless* being; my debilitated frame and unstrung nerves gave way, and I felt that, *as I was,* I *could not* sustain the burdens pressing upon me. I resumed morphine again; and, by its upholding and calming power, I managed to fulfil my multifarious tasks— all of them passably, and some of them with no small measure of success. So passed about two years, in the latter portion of which time I had reached a quarter-ounce bottle of sulphate of morphine per week.

I was then living with friends who were hydropathists and vegetable livers, and was influenced by them to leave off the use of tobacco, opium, tea, coffee, and meat, all at once, and to submit to the routine of cold-water drenching. At the end of twenty-seven days I got abroad, freed from opium, exempt from pain, but yet with the debilitated feeling of an invalid rising from a long and prostrating malady, and needing rest, good nursing, and a generous diet (and *only* these) to regain my full original strength; but these I could not command.

The time came at last when I *must* work, be the consequences what they would, and work, too, with my *brain,* my only implement; and that time found my brain *impotent* from a yet uninvigorated nervous system. If I *would work,* I *must stimulate,* and morphine, bad as it was, was better than alcohol. I took morphine once more, and lectured on literary topics for some months with triumphant success. While so lecturing in a country town, I was solicited to take a parish in the neighborhood. I did so, and there continued two years and a quarter, performing in that time as much literary labor as ever in three times the interval in any prior period of my life. In short, I had three happy, intellectually-vigorous, outpouring years, with bodily health uniformly sound and complete, with the exceptions hereafter to be mentioned. And yet, through those years I never used less than a quarter ot an ounce of morphine per week, and sometimes more. I attribute my retaining so much health, in spite of the morphine, to the rigorous salubrity of my habits, bodily and mental, in *other respects.* Once, and often twice a-day, the year round, I laved the whole person in cold water with soap; I slept with open window, the year through, excepting *stormy* winter nights; I lay upon a hard bed, guiltless of feathers; I used a simple diet; and, finally, I cherished all *gently* and *kindly*, while rigidly excluding from my mind all bitter and perturbing feelings. But, not to dilate further on mere *narrative*, let me say that I have continued to use opium, for the most part *habitually*, from my last assumption of it, up to the period of my admission into this hospital. A year since, however, I dropped morphine, and have since used the opium pill in its stead, sometimes taking an ounce per week; but generalty not over-passing a half ounce per week.

And here I may make the general remark, proved true from my own experience, that, for all the *desirable* effects sought from this species of stimulus, a half ounce of gum opium is about the same as an ounce or any larger quantity of said gum, and nearly the same as a quarter ounce of morphine or more—that is, half an ounce of opium stimulates and braces *me*, at least, *nearly*, if not *entirely*, as much as I *can* be stimu-lated and braced by this drug. All that is taken over this tends rather to clog, to stupify, to nauseate, than to stimulate.

Another point in my own experience is, that in a few weeks only after commencing or re-commencing the use of opium, I always reached the full amount, which, as a *habit*, I *ever* used, that is, either a half ounce of opium or a quarter ounce of morphine. I never went on in-creasing the dose in order to get the required amount of stimulation; but at one or the other of these two points I would remain for years successively. A third remark I would make is, that it is only for the first few weeks after commencing the use of opium that one feels *pal-pably* and *distinctly* the thrilling of the nerves, the sensation of being stimulated and raised above the *previously existing* physical tone, for which the drug was first taken. All the effects produced *after that* by the opium are to keep the body *at that level* of sensation in which one feels *positively alive* and *capable* to *act*, without being impeded or weighed down by physical languor and impotence. Such languor and impotence one feels from abstaining merely a few hours beyond the wonted time of taking the dose. It is not *pleasure*, then, that drives onward the confirmed opium-eater, but a *necessity* scarce less resistible than that Fate to which the pagan mythology subjected gods not less than men.

Let me now, before closing, attempt briefly to describe the effects of opium upon the body and mind of the user, as also the principal sensa-tions accompanying the breaking of the habit.

The opium-eater is prevailingly *disinclined* to, and in some sort *inca-pacitated* for, bodily exertion or locomotion. A considerable part of the time he feels something like a sense, not very distinctly defined, of bodily fatigue; and to sit continuously in a rocking or an easy chair, or to recline on a sofa or bed, is his preference above all modes of disposing of himself. To walk up a flight of stairs often palpably tires the legs, and makes him pant almost as much as a well person does after pretty rapid motion. His lungs manifestly are somehow *obstructed*, and do not play with perfect freedom. His liver, too, is torpid, or else but partially active; for, if using laudanum or the opium pill, he is constantly more or less costive, the fæces being hard and painful to expel; and, if using morphine, though he may have a daily movement, yet the fæces are dry and harder than in health. One other morbid physical symptom I remember to have experienced for a considerable time, while using a quarter of an ounce of morphine per week; and this was, an annoying palpitation of the heart. I was once told, too, by a keen observer, who knew my habit, that my color was apt to change frequently from red to pale.

These are substantially all the physical peculiarities I experienced during my opium-using years. It is still true, however, that the years of my using opium (or, in perfect strictness, *morphine*) were as healthy as any, if not the very healthiest, of the years of my life.

But what of the effects of opium-eating on the *mind?* The one great *injury* it works is (I think) to the *will*, that force whereby a man executes the *work* he was sent here to do, and *breasts and overcomes* the *obstacles and difficulties* he is appointed to encounter, and bears himself unflinchingly amid the tempests of calamity snd sorrow which pertain to the mortal lot. Hardihood, manliness, resolution, enterprise, ambition, whatever the original degree of these qualities, become grievously debilitated, if not wholly extinct. Reverie, the perusal of poetry and fiction, become the darling occupation of the opium-user; and he hates every call that summons him from it. *Give* him an intellectual task to accomplish; *place* him in a position where a mental effort is to be made, and, most probably, he will acquit himself with unusual brilliancy and power, supposing his native ability to be good. But he *cannot*, or will *not seek and find* for himself such work and such position. He feels helpless, and incompetent to stir about and hold himself upright amid the jostling, competitive throngs that crowd the world's paths, and *there* seek life's prizes by performing life's duties, and executing its requisitions. Solitude, with his books, his dreams and imaginings, and the excited sensibilities that lead to no external action, constitute his chosen world and favorite life. In one word, he is a *species* of maniac; since, I believe, his views, his feelings, and his desires, in relation to most things, are peculiar, eccentric, and unlike those of other men, or of himself, in a state of soundness. There is, however, as complete a "method in this madness," as in the *sanity* of other men. He is in a *different sphere* from other men, and *in that* sphere he is sane.

The first symptoms attendant on breaking off the habit, coming on some hours after omitting the wonted dose, are a constant propensity to yawn, gape, and stretch, together with somewhat of languor, and a general uneasiness. Time passes, and there follows a sensation as if the stomach was drawn together or compressed, as if with a slight degree of cramp, coupled with a total extinction of appetite. The mouth and throat become dry and irritated, and there is an incessant disposition to clear the throat by "hemming" and swallowing; and there is a tickling in the nose which necessitates frequent sneezing, sometimes a dozen, or even twenty times in succession. As the hours go on, shudders run hrough the frame, with alternate fever heats and icy chills, hot sweats, and cold clammy sweats; while a dull, incessant ache pervades the bones, especially at the joints, alternated by an occasional sharp, intolerable pang, like tic douleureux. Then follow a host of indescribable sensations, as of burning, tinglings, and twitchings, seeming to run along just beneath the surface of the skin over the whole body; and so strange are these sensations, that one is prompted to scream, and strike the wall, the bed, or himself, to vary them. By this time the liver commences a most energetic action, and a violent diarrhœa sets in. The discharges are not very watery or mucous, but, save in *thinness*, not very unlike healthy stools, for the most part. Not long, however, after the commencement of the diarrhœa, so copious is the effusion of bile from the liver, that one will sometimes pass, for a dozen stools in succession, what seems to be merely a *blackish bile*, without a particle of fæces mingled with it. But this lasts not many days, and is followed by the thin, not altogether unhealthy-looking discharges above mentioned, repeated often an incredible number of times per day. Whether from the quality of these discharges, or from whatever cause, the interior surface of the bowels feels intolerably hot, as though excoriated; and it seems as, if boiling water or aquafortis running through the intestines would scarce torture one more than these stools. In fact, all the internal surfaces of the body are in this same burning, raw-feeling state. The brain, too, is in a highly excited, irritable condition; the head sometimes aching and throbbing, as though it *must* burst into fragments; and a humming, washing, simmering noise going on incessantly for days together. Of course, there can be no sleep; and one will go on for ten days and nights consecutively, without one moment's loss of intensest consciousness, so far as he can judge! Strange to say, notwithstanding this excessive irritation of the entire system, one feels so feeble and strengthless, that he can scarce drag one foot after the other; and to walk a few rods, or up a flight of stairs, is so terribly fatiguing, that one must needs sit down and *pant*. (Let it be noted that these symptoms belong to the case where one is simply deprived at once and wholly of opium, without any medical help, unless the use of cold water be considered as such.) These symptoms (unaided by medicine) last, with gradual abatements of virulence, from twenty to thirty days, and then mostly die away. Not well and right, however, does one feel even then. Though, for the most part, free from pain, he is yet physically weak, and all corporeal exertion is a distressing effort. He must needs sleep, too, enormously, going to bed often at sunset in a July day, and sleeping, log-like, until six or seven next morning, and then sleeping, with like soundness, two or three hours after dinner. How long it would be before the recovery of his complete original strength and natural physical tone, personal experience does not enable me to say. His condition, both in itself and as relates to others, is, meanwhile, most strange and anomalous. He *looks*, probably, better than ever in his life before. In sufficiently full flesh, with ruddy cheeks, and skin clear as a healthy child's, the beholder would pronounce him in the height of health and vigor, and would glow with indignation at seeing him loitering about day after day doing little save sleep, in a world where so much work needs to be done. And yet he feels all but impotent for enterprise, or any active physical efforts; for there is scarce enough nervous force in him to move his frame to a lingering walk; and sometimes it seems as if the nervous fibres were actually *pulled out*, and he must move, if at all, by pure *force of voltition*.

Most singular, too, the while, is the state of his *mind*. His power of thought is keen, bright, and *fertile* beyond example, and his imagination swarms with pictures of beauty, while his sensitiveness to impressions and emotions of every kind is so excessively keen, that the tears spring to his eyes on the slightest occasion. He is a child in sensibility, while a youth in the *vividness*, and a man in the *grasp*, the *piercingness*, and the *copiousness* of his thoughts. He cannot *write down* his thoughts, for his arm and hand are *unnerved;* but in conversation, or before an audience, he can utter himself as if filled with the breath of inspiration itself.

From the Southern Medical and Surgical Journal.

Letters upon Syphilis. Addressed to the Editor of L'Union Medicale, by P. RICORD. Translated from the French, by W. P LATTIMORE, M. D.

TWENTY-FIRST LETTER.

My dear Friend,—*How do chancres cicatrize?* Allow me to say a few words on this important subject.

The period of reparation is indicated by the disappearance of the areola of the ulcer. Its edges become *degorges*, sinking and resting on the bottom; and the undermining ceases, if it existed. The margin becomes of a pale, grayish, pearly tint, and finally assumes the normal color of the surrounding tissues. The bottom cleans off; the gray, lardaceous, diphtheritic layer is at first pierced, as it were, by granulations which, finally occupying the place of the layer, give to the ulceration a granular aspect, and a healthy, rosy tint. The pus becomes less abundant, and of a healthy, creamy character; and it may, in this case, justly be said to be *laudable*, for it ceases to be inoculable. In proportion as the parts fill up, the epidermis spreads from the circumference to the centre, and the citatrization is completed in the same way as in any wound which has suppurated.

The *cicatrix of chancres* may remain more prominent than the surrounding parts, sometimes being on a level with them, but most frequently depressed, according to the thickness of the tissues affected. In a great number of cases, it is indelible; while in others it completely disappears, as frequently occurs after indurated chancres, or when the chancre is seated upon a mucous membrane.

But, as those whose experience has been extensive well know, the period of reparation is subject to various irregularities. In *serpiginous chancre*, one extremity often cicatrizes, while the other becomes more diseased; sometimes one side heals, while the other continues to ulcerate. Finally, the cure often takes place at one or many points of the centre, while the circumference is constantly augmenting its vicious circle.

You know, in fine, that, in certain individuals, where a proper course of treatment has not been pursued, where the physician has been ignorant of the means of repressing [granulations by cauterizations, or where foolish prejudices have prevented the employment of this remedy, the granulations are said to become luxuriant and vegetating and to give to the ulceration certain aspects which have obtained for it the name of the *budding, fungous,* or *vegetating* chancre. True vegetations, of varied forms, may then be produced; but, as these vegetations may be considered an accidental, epigenic tissue, they are not of a sypilitic nature, as we shall hereafter see.

At this period, as I have already said, that is to say, when the chancre has infected the economy, it may itself undergo a transformation, *in situ,* and finally present the characters of mucous papules, and thus give some countenance to the opinion of those who, from failure to analyze the subject, are unacquainted with these matamorphoses—of those who have admitted, besides, that these accidents could be sometimes primitive and sometimes secondary, and that they were, in all cases, contagious; an opinion which I have already controverted.

But here a point of doctrine arises, on which I insist, and to which I must again call your attention. It is this: That form of chancre which may undergo relapses at different times *never returns when it has once cicratrized?* If a new inoculable chancre developes itself after cicratrization has become complete, we can afirm that the chancre is the result of a new infection.

From what I have stated, it is very certain that, as far as we can arrive at a knowledge of the facts from a due acquaintance with the conditions by which they are surrounded—when we take into consideration the seats which chancres seem to select for their development, as well as their usually limited number—when we likewise know how to appreciate the variations which different chancres present with respect to their period of progress and of specific *statu quo,* and with respect to their course and duration, and the different aspects which they may assume at the period of reparation, and even of subsequent cicatrization—when, finally, we consider the more or less marked influence of the mercurial treatment in certain cases, we can usually arrive at a rational diagnosis, which is almost absolute.

The physiognomy of the primitive ulcer is ordinarily so expressive (permit me to use the word), at the specific period, that we are able, by seeing it, to name it. It is even necessary to distrust this first impression, inasmuch as it may occasion indiscretions which can scarcely be repaired. You have allowed me to illustrate my remarks by pathological anecdotes, and I shall avail myself of your kindness, happy if I can relieve the aridity of my previous descriptions.

One of our distinguished *savans* entered my cabinet one day, and without any preamble showed me—a diseased member, saying, " What is that?" I immediately replied, "It is chancre." "Very well, sir, my wife gave it to me." "Then, sir, it is not a chancre." "And why not, if you please?" "Because," I replied, "that which distinguishes simple ulcerations resembling chancres from true chancres is the source whence they have been derived." My patient was not the dupe of an argument which would have been sufficient for certain physicians whom you know; and he contented himself with replying, with much dignity and resignation, "Cure me."

But is the diagnosis always so easy as some of our classical authorities have assumed it to be? I appeal to M. Lagneau, who is so worthy a representative of these authorities at the present time. Observe now, whether, despite all the care he exhibits, he succeeds in distinguishing the primitive chancre from what, with so many others, he still considers the secondary chancre. Glance again at his synoptical and comparative table of the ulcers which are liable to be confounded with those produced by the syphilitic virus, and tell me whether he is successful, and especially whether he enables others to be successful in establishing this difference with certainty.

Mercury, that infallible touchstone in the eyes of believers—a touchstone which, in England, has been the basis of the division of syphylis into the *true* and the *false*—is a deceptive re-agent. It often cures non-syphilitic accidents, while it aggravates those which are syphilitic, and which sometimes get well without treatment.

How many chancres exist which are unrecognized by skilful practitioners! How many errors are committed with respect to the different varieties of indurated chancre, the most dangerous form of all! Sometimes simple excoriations are mistaken for the disease. At others, the disease is supposed to be a true cancerous degeneration. My friend, M. Vitry, of Versailes, must recollect the case of a patient to whom I was called by a physician in Paris, not to judge of the nature of his disease, but to amputate his pœnis. I recognized the existence of an indurated chancre, with considerable development of the plastic exudation, and pills of the protoiodide superseded the knife.

One of our learned professors, belonging to the faculty of Paris, who excels in diagnosticating syphilis, as well as other diseases, cannot fail to recollect the case of a Russian nobleman whom we saw together at the house of our honored and regretted master, M. Marjolin, and in whom he was unwilling to recognize the existence of a primitive accident, because nothing was observed but the specific induration, and because the nobleman could not explain how he had contracted the accident; yet, a short time afterwards, as I had predicted, we obtained the most striking proofs of a constitutional affection.

If you will allow me, I will relate a short anecdote. Cullerier, the nephew, one day sent to me a popular writer, in order to obtain my opinion relative to an ulceration situated upon the corona of the glands—an ulceration with an indurated base, and not then presenting those characters at its edges and base which are authoritatively assumed to constitute chancre. Nevertheless, I recognised an ulceration with the specific characters of induration already described, and with the ganglionary prolongation which we are shortly to study. Cullerier was not of my opinion, because he had examined the two women accused of imparting the contagion, and had found them healthy. Admitting neither mediate contagion nor spontaneous syphilis, and placing confidence in the word of the patient, he could not admit the existence of a primitive ulcer. I, who admit all rational sources of contagion, and often doubt until I obtain the most certain proof, remained convinced either that the patient had been deceived, that he deceived himself, or that he deceived us. In fact, scarcely six weeks had elapsed when very marked constitutional accidents—so marked, indeed, as to be exceedingly difficult to cure—were manifested. But, while Cullerier was yet pondering the question how and why this patient had contracted the pox, I was called to the house of a great lady.

I arrived, knowing nothing of the purport of my visit. This lady was mysteriously seated in her boudoir; and, in spite of the softened light of the room, I could perceive on her face the evident tokens of a secondary affection. "Doctor," said she, "I have to speak to you on a very delicate matter." Wishing to cut short a painful avowal, "I see what it is, Madam," said I to her; "for your face tells me plainly enough why I have the honour to be here." "What do you say?" replied she, with astonishment. "That you are diseased, Madam, and for that purpose desire my attentions." "Not the least in the world; and I have sent for you in order that you may assist in curing M. X—— (the writer sent to me by Cullerier) not only of his disease, but also of his dangerous *liaisons*." And she then drew a portrait, which was but little flattering, of the two women whom Cullerier had examined, and found healthy, and who, according to this lady, were the cause of the whole trouble. I had much difficulty, as you may imagine, in making her understand that the source of our poor author's trouble was much closer to me, and in obtaining the avowal that the pressing interest she manifested relative to him was not altogether based on a purely platonic affection.

It is ever thus, my dear friend, and here is the moral of this anecdote—that people of the world never make you complete avowals. By reason of their relations with great ladies, or others in whom they have confidence, their mind is a thousand leagues from the truth; their thoughts are not fixed upon the true source of their disease, and they seek it where it is not.

You see, then, how difficult, frequently, is the diagnosis of chancre, and how wrong we should be in denying its existence when patients will not aid us in tracing it to its source.

I am acquainted with all the difficulties of diagnosis in many cases, and I have seen persons of the greatest skill commit frequent errors in relation to it; and, for this reason, I have said, and I still assert, in spite of contrary opinions, that the only positive, univocal, pathognomoic sign of chancre, at the period of progress, or of specific *statu quo*, is the inoculable character of the *pus which it secretes*. From this fact I have drawn the following conclusion:

Inoculation furnishes the most certain sign of the specific nature of u l c e r.

t

I stated, in the work which I published in 1838, that, if mercury must be given in all cases where a virulent, primitive accident exists, it is essential to be assured of the fact of virulence by artificial inoculation. But compose yourself, my dear friend; this operation, so repugnant to some persons, and even dangerous, if not properly managed, is unnecessary in practice; and I have never advised its performance, as a general rule. The prognosis and treatment of the affection depend on other indications. The induration of chancre, with its accompaniments, in relation to which inoculation furnishes us no assistance, form the conditions whence we deduce the state of the constitution, and point out to us the specific treatment which the disease requires. This fact, I trust, I shall be able to demonstrate.

From the Southern Medical and Surgical Journal.

Letters upon Syphilis. Addressed to the Editor of L'Union Medicale, by P. Ricord. Translated from the French, by W. P. Lattimore, M. D.

TWENTY-SECOND LETTER.

My Dear Friend—It would afford me much pleasure to say a word relative to the treatment of chancre; but you know that, according to the plan I have proposed to follow, I cannot, in this connection, enter into many details.

Perhaps you will permit me here to say something in relation to prophylaxis. Medical police has advanced much of late years, especially since I and others have made examinations with the speculum, in private hospitals and in public dispensaries.

It is very certain that, since this mode of investigation has been generally employed, a great amelioration in the health of public women has been observed. Thus, in 1800, according to Parent-Duchatelet, one woman in nine was found diseased; since 1834, the number has been reduced to one in sixty. The speculum has had a great share in this amelioration.

But, to be thoroughly successful, I have always insisted that women should be visited every three days, without distinction of rank; whether they be *en maison* or *en carte;* whether they dwell in Paris or at the *barrieres.* You remember that inoculable pus may be formed after the second day of an artificial inoculation. Swediaur admitted that chancre may be developed within twelve hours. Frequent examinations with the speculum are, therefore, indispensable, if we expect the surveillance of public women to furnish a certain guarantee of freedom from disease.

I write this word *guarantee* with special design; for there are some people who, after contracting an accident in their adventurous love, think they have the right of claiming indemnity from the government. Perhaps you think I am not serious. I will offer a fact in proof of my assertion. Some years since I received a visit from a merchant of Lyons, who was in a state of great exasperation against the prefect of police. He came to get a certificate setting forth the fact that he had contracted a chancre in a house of prostitution, the character of which he imagined to be *guaranteed* by the authorities. He did not know that *toleration*, like all commissions, receives no guarantee from the government.

I pass on to state that the ameliorations daily introduced in the surveillance of prostitution, and the zeal exhibited by the brethren, on whom devolves the painful service of the dispensary of public health, and of the Hospital of Saint Lazarre, will furnish yet more suspicious results.

Public women are a necessary evil; this fact is generally admitted. I do not wish to examine the reasons favorably or adverse to the proposition, for this is not the place to examine them. But, if the evil is necessary, it does not follow that its quantity, so to speak, should be extended, as a learned Belgian brother lately seemed to wish; but it is essentially necessary to inspect it well in relation to its quality.

In insisting that public women shall not communicate disease, it should be so arranged that they shall not be liable to contract it from those who have commerce with them. How is this result to be accomplished? Is it necessary to institute an examination of the persons who visit them, and to prevent these visits should they prove diseased! But, apart from the difficulties of such an institution, the danger which we should thus seek to prevent would be augmented; for, instead of falling into a sewer, which the police could cleanse, the unclean would go elsewhere.

The establishment of lazarets and of quarantines, suggested by my friend Diday, of Lyons, in a moment of laudable philanthropy, where a clear patent of immunity from the pox, along with a certificate of vaccination—a patent that should be as indispensable as a passport—a patent without which no one should be admitted to any public office—could be furnished, cannot be thought of at this day.

Whatever may have been said by the author of this ingenious proposition, the difficulties in the way of such an institution seem insurmountable.

There was a time, you know, when those affected with pox were banished from Paris, and condemned to the rope if they returned—a time when, at Bicetre, patients were scourged at their entrance and exit. All this did not diminish the number of the infected. On the contrary, the scourgers, perhaps, deserved, in their turn, to be punished. These barbarous measures have fallen into disuse.

It is, undoubtedly, necessary to subject to rigorous surveillance all persons whom we can reach—soldiers, for example—and to sequester every patient over whom we have control; but a certain degree of toleration, the pardon of a fault which is sufficiently often involuntary, and excellent hospitals, with such attendance as may at present be found there, and which time will still further improve, are the best means of general prophylaxis, or those, at least, which will tend to diminish the gravity of the disease.

Moreover, all who are acquainted with the conditions to which women are subjected in the present state of society, with respect to labor and its remuneration, have, for a long time, acknowledged the fact that herein lies one of the most fruitful sources of prostitution, and, consequently, of the propagation of syphilis. Therefore, to ameliorate the condition of women with respect to labor, is to do a kind office as well to humanity as to morals and public hygeine.

You remember what I said with respect to the manner in which chancres are produced. It is necessary to remember this fact, in order to shun the sources of contagion pointed out. The most important fact which science teaches us relative to prophylaxis is, the necessity of avoiding exposure. This remark, doubtless, appears a little *naive;* but let debauchees remember it, for it is the very truth. I am now about to touch upon a delicate subject, which is full of shoals. It is still an unsettled question, in morals and medical deontology, whether the physician ought to give advice, with respect to preservation from evil to those who voluntarily expose themselves to the liability of contracting disease from immoral persons. I do not pretend to be more severe than Parent-Duchatelet, who treated this subject with a purity of intention of which you are well aware. Besides, am I not encouraged by the very character of the journal which gives such liberal hospitality to my letters? I address the learned—those who are physicians; and was it not yourself, my dear friend, who said that science is chaste, even stark-naked? Be not alarmed; for, after all, I shall only glide over this ticklish subject.

There is no sure and absolute preservative against chancre. This is my declaration.

If, in spite of a knowledge of this fact, one is still willing to run his chance, some precautions may be taken. It is especially necessary to bear in mind the precept of Nicholas Massa, so energetically rendered by the elder Cullerier: "The connection should not voluntarily be prolonged." At this moment, indeed, it is necessary to be egotistical, as was remarked by Hunter, but not egotistical after the manner of Madam de Stael, who called love the egotism of two.

The most minute attention, on the part of suspected persons, ought to be required in houses of prostitution. A fact with which we have been for a long time familiar, namely, that a deposit of virulent pus may be held in reserve in the genital organs of women, demonstrates the necessity of this precaution. This is a means of always preventing mediate contagion. I have told you that numerous experiments have proved to me that, by decomposing the virulent pus, we can neutralize it. Alcohol in water; water mixed with one-fifth Labarraque's liquid; all the acids diluted in water, so as not to be caustic; wine; solutions of sulphate of zinc and acetate of lead, destroy the inoculable power of virulent pus; while, if this pus remains unaltered, excessively minute quantities of it—homœopathic quantities, if you please—retain their power to act. M. Puche informs us that, at the *Hospital du Midi,* the effects of inoculation have been obtained by him from one drop of pus mixed with half a glass of water.

Fatty substances are very useful, especially to medical men, who are obliged to practice the touch in dangerous localities. Astringent lotions, which slightly tan the tissues, have frequently prevented contagion.

But, if cleanliness is necessary before intercourse, on the part of the one who may impart the disease, it need be minute only subsequent to the act in the one who is simply exposed to infection.

There is another means which the moral sense repudiates, and in which the debauchee has great confidence: this, undoubtedly, often serves as a security against infection; but, as was observed by a woman of much *esprit*, it is a cuirass against pleasure, and a cobweb against danger. This mediate *process* is an article which is often porous, or may already have been used; it frequently becomes displaced; it fulfils the office of a bad umbrella, which the storm may rend, and which, protecting badly enough from the tempest, does not prevent the feet from getting wet. I have seen, in fact, numerous ulcerations of the root of the pœnis, of the pœno-scrotal angle, of the scrotum, &c., in those who had taken these useless precautions.

Many patients believe themselves safe from contagion when they do not terminate the venereal act. A lady who consulted me on her own account, was very much astonished when she found that she had communicated a disease to her lover; because, she said, *he did not conclude.*

Some syphilographs believe that the urethral infection, in particular, is effected after ejaculation, which creates a vacuum, and because nature abhors a vacuum. But numerous facts have taught me the reverse of that statement. Ejaculation, on the contrary, must be considered as a powerful injection, from behind forwards, thus cleaning the urethra; and if urethral affections, already so common, are not more frequent, we must, perhaps, attribute the fact to this condition. Thus, an old, excellent precept recommends a prompt emission of urine after every suspicious intercourse.

The circumcision of the prepuce, the excision of nymphæ that are too long, also constitute hygenic measures relative to the genital organs, inasmuch as these appendices greatly favor contagion.

I ask your pardon for this digression: but it is the duty of science to destroy the influence of charlatanism with respect to the dangerous employment of a deceptive prophylaxis.

It would be necessary, were it possible, to indicate all the measures that prevent contagion, and, therefore, the propagation of syphilis—not in order to protect or to encourage the libertinage, but to protect the virtue and the chastity which so often become its victims.

I am yet to speak of cauterization as an abortive remedy against chancre. But I will make this the subject of my next letter.

From the New York Journal of Medicine.

Glanders or Farcy in the Human subject, as illustrated by the case of the late Dr. Stoutenburg, *of* L. I.   By William W. Strew, M.D., Oyster Bay, L. I.

Dr. P. A. Stoutenburgh, whose death was recently announced as having occurred from glanders, contracted from his horse. was a warm professional friend and neighbor, residing about two miles from our village. He was a remarkably stout, robust-looking man, aged 42, of nervo-bilious temperament.   During the past winter, he had been treating a favorite and valuable horse for glanders, and was repeatedly admonished of the necessity of caution in such cases.

I was called to him on Monday, April 11th.   He had been complaining some days previously, with symptoms of common cold, affecting the general system; with headache, depression of spirits, prostration of strength, and pain in the joints, for which he was taking wine of colchicum, supposing it to be rheumatic gout, as he had formerly suffered from rheumatism.   His tongue was loaded with a thick, yellow coating in the centre, white around the edges; bowels constipated; increased temperature of the surface; pulse 90, moderately full.   I gave him submur. hydrarg., and pulv. jalap, aa grs. x., with mustard pediluvium at bed-time.

12th. . Medicine operated three times; still complains of stricture and pain about the chest; great anxiety, with hurried abdominal respiration; skin hot and dry; pulse 100, expectorating thick, tough, and tenacious mucus, with great thirst and internal heat; V. S. $\frac{3}{5}$ xx. with pulv. doveri, grs. xv. at bed-time.

13th.   Had a more comfortable night, with some mitigation of the most unpleasant symptoms; pulse 90, soft and free; still complains of great internal heat and thirst, and anxiety of mind.   My friend, Dr. Townsend, met me this morning in consultation; we ordered a warm bath, and a pill composed of cal. gr. i., pulv. opi. grs. $\frac{1}{3}$, pulv. camphor and James's powder, aa grs. ij., to be repeated every three hours.   I was called in the night to see him, on account of his increased restlessness, which was somewhat connected with anxiety of mind, succeeded in quiting his fears, and gave him an anodyne pill of camphor and opium.

14th.   Complains of increased pain and stricture about the chest, with a suffocating sensation, particularly in the recumbent posture; still great heat of the surface; pulse 94, moderately full; V. S. repeated $\frac{3}{5}$ xx., and continued the pill of cal. opium, &c., as above, every four hours.

15th.   Rested more comfortably; there is mitigation of the unpleasant congestive symptoms.   Continued the pill to-day, and an enema of soap and water to move the bowels.

16th.   Still more comfortable, and continues to improve.   Omit the pill to-day; no specific effect of the calomel observed.

17th.   Remains comfortable, with the exception of a sense of prostration, apparently of the vital powers; tongue has a thick, muddy-looking coating, with slight disposition to nausea.

18th. So much improved as to be able to sit up and leave his room; prescribed for himself a mild laxative, in the form of a seidlitz powder.

19th. Quite comfortable to what he has been, still complains of some uneasiness in the epigastric region; tongue remains much loaded; repeated the laxative in the form of ol. recini.

20th. More restlessness and disturbance, particularly about the epigastric region, with increased conststutional disturbance; stomach was well acted upon, by an emetic of ipecac and antimony.

21st. Restlessness and prostration of the vital powers increased, with a typhoid tendency, and disposition to congestion of the vital organs, particularly the brain. There is also an aggravation of the former unpleasant symptoms, such as an increased temperature of the surface; thick, muddy-looking coating of the tongue; urine scanty and bloody-looking; pulse 100. There appeared on different parts of the body, in the cellular substance, several elevated and indurated patches, which rapidly tended to suppuration; one appeared at the root of the nose, between the eyes. Dr. Rinelander, of Huntington, met us in consultation. We concluded to apply an epispatic to the nucha and calves of the legs, to be dressed with ung. hydrarg., put him again upon the cal., and James's powder every three hours, and ordered his bowels moved at evening, with an enema of turpentine, and nourishing broths and stimulants to be freely given.

22d. Passed a restless night; there was an increase and aggravation of all the former unpleasant symptoms; also, increased swelling of the tumors, with considerable perturbation and confusion of mind, with some spasmodic difficulty in swallowing. He is evidently sinking with all the attendant symptoms of putrid typohoid fever; small frequent and feeble pulse; a peculiar sensation of pungent burning heat of the surface; heavy cadaverous smell of the whole body, putrid odor of the breath, perspiration, and secretions in general. Omit the powder, and put him upon stimulants and specific treatment, as the carbonate of ammonia, creosote, turpentine, &c.

23d. Aggravation of every symptom in every form, with inability to swallow, from spasmodic action of the glottis, or swelling of the throat, great difficulty in respiration, with delirium.

There was increased swelling of the tumors with a collection of matter in some, also numerous pustules began to appear in different parts of the system, rapidly accumulating, and some nearly ready to discharge. There was a gradual sinking of all the vital powers, with a rapid tendency to organic dissolution. He expired about 4 p. m., almost without a struggle.

The inferences to be drawn from the foregoing melancholy case, are of deep interest to the non-professional as well as professional reader. Notwithstanding the repeated admonitions to be more cautious, the doctor was unwilling to admit the nature of the disease in his horse, until a short time before he began to complain himself, when he ordered the horse to be killed. About this time, or, two weeks previous to his being taken, he received a wound on the index finger, from the tooth of the horse, while bleeding him in the mouth, which caused him a little uneasiness, and which many of his friends believed to be the exciting cause in producing the disease in himself. But such, it seems, could not have been the case, for the wound on the finger healed kindly; while on the contrary, we should have seen more specific influence of the disease originating from that point, and extending up the limb along the absorbents and lymphatic glands of the part, as is the case in dissecting wounds and other malignant poison introduced into the system in that way.

It will be observed, that the development of the specific symptoms of this disease were only manifested a very short time before his death, and then only in the form of "farcy buds," as they are called, or small tumors, which, together with the pustular eruption which characterized the true nature of the disease, forms another lamentable evidence of the contagious influence of the disease, as communicated from the animal to man. It has long been a recorded fact, that wounds resulting from the posthumous examinations of glandered horses were of a dangerous, and almost always of a fatal character, attributed to some specific poison or infection, analogous to that of any specific action or particular virus. M. Leorin was the first to discover and prove the transmission of farcy from the horse to man, as recorded in the *Journal de Med. Veterinaire*, Feb., 1812. But it was not till 1821, that a veterinary surgeon of Berlin, by the name of Shilling, published the first detailed case of acute glanders in man; since that period we have had incontestible proof, that glanders and farcy are fundamentally the same disease, resulting from the same common cause, and differing from each other only in situation and circumstances. Also, that they are not confined, as was supposed, to the quadrumania or animals alone; but that they are transmitted by contagion as well as infection, not only from the horse, &c., to man, but from one person to another. We have a case recorded in the *London Medical Gazette* for April, 1840, of a man who died in St. Bartholomew's Hospital of glanders, and the nurse who attended, took the disease from him and died also. We are to understand that glanders or farcy are never developed spontaneously in the human subject, but that they originate in quadrumania; and where they do occur in man, they have been transmitted to him from the lower animals; but, as we have seen, they may be propagated from one human being to another.

This contagious principle may be transmitted through the medium of the atmosphere, as well as by actual contact, from one animal to another. We have instances in which there was no possibility of contact with glanderous matters, and yet the disease was developed in healthy horses; and it appears that this contagious principle remains sometimes for years, where glanders or farcy may happen to have been developed. Persons have been known to have taken the disease without coming in contact with the animal, but merely sleeping over the stable where the disease existed; or from driving horses affected with it.

Are the subjects of Convulsions and of Anasthesia Conscious?

Hypocrates, in one of his aphorisms, says that a person suffering pain without realizing it, is in very great danger. This assertion of the great observer should not be permitted to pass without attention, or with that smile of complacency with which the remark has been met by some, in whose presence it has been repeated. There may be simplicity in the affirmation, that pain exists without the knowledge or consciousness of the affected individual; but it is believed, nevertheless, to be an actual fact, by more than a moiety of the correct observers of animal functions, and human sufferings.

The question has been discussed, indeed the ground has been assumed, that the individual subject of surgical manipulation, and under the influence of ether, chloroform, or any of the analogous agents, is not actually void of pain, or destitute of consciousness of its existence; but, like the inebriated man, who acts consciously from the impulse of the moment, yet, when free from the agent which has produced the impression, all recollection—memory—is dead, the same as if the pain had not existed, the act had never been committed.

So, too, in convulsions, the practitioner has often, from the stimulus of his own desire to know, as well as the sympathy or curiosity of bystanders or friends, to speculate as to the positive experience of suffering by his patient. For the most part, from the fact, that after the convulsive seizure has passed off, the patient has no knowledge, no remembrance of the circumstances which had given to others so much cause for uneasiness, the question has been summarily answered that, though rigid and relaxed, spasmed and distorted, contorted, and awfully tossed by the convulsive power, yet the patient did not positively suffer—had no knowledge of the agony endured, as evidenced during the continuance of active eclamptive. Such an opinion has been the comfort of the writer, who believes that it has been his misfortune to see more of convulsion than any one of his age in practice, until he was forced to entertain doubt.

The man with his senses bewildered, mind clouded, and sentiments debased by the influence of alcoholic drinks, may receive a castigation, or a serious personal or physical wound, and cry out with lamentations and groans, and yet not be able, after the poisonous influence has died away, to tell when or how it was received—indeed, may never know, unless informed by others, that he has submitted to an indignity, or by the blood and wound, that he has met with an accident, or received an injury. And again, these things may occur, and the memory, when the individual is first passing into a normal condition, will preserve very faintly the impression made at the moment of occurrence. This has been observed very frequently, though possibly not reflected upon by every one in this country, where, unfortunately, the opportunity is so often presented, by the unwise and illiberal perversions of the use of alcohol.

The same has been observed by every one who has employed the anæsthetic agents to any extent. Patients have, during operations, given

every evidence that they suffered all the torment known to be insepar-
able from the particular operation, and yet, after all has been accomplished, and the mind permitted to resume its throne, have no remembrance of anything during the moments passed under anæsthetic influence; while others have a dim recollection of circumstances as they occurred, or of the circumstances somewhat perverted.

Is this not the case with persons under convulsive attacks? A case
was presented to the writer's observation, which impressed him with
peculiar force.

An interesting boy, aged about three years, was observed by his parents to be unwell. Having lost two or three children by very sudden
spasms, their fears were active, and the physician was promptly summoned. On examination, no wireness, or tension of the pulse, or nervous twitchings of the tendons could be discovered, and the apprehensions
were attempted to be allayed. After a few moments he was observed
to bend his head to one side, and down towards a shoulder. His mother
asked him "what's the matter?" to which he very faintly replied, "nothing." This was repeated three times, the same answer given twice,
but no notice whatever the third time. But a very few moments elapsed
when he was seized with a most violent and general convulsion, dis-
torting his countenance, and affecting the muscles of his whole body and
limbs, lasting for full fifteen minutes actively, when it passed off, leaving him in a listless and apparently unconscious state for full half an
hour longer. At the end of this period he opened his eyes, looked round,
threw himself his full length, and very languidly exclaimed, " *What a
hard ride that was I had on the wagon!*" It was, indeed, a hard ride,
in a rough wagon, over a rough road; for, I believe, though I have seen
them of a longer duration, I have never seen a more violent action than
that convulsion; and I am sorry to believe that the little fellow knew his
sufferings, during their continuance, though he remembered them but
for a few moments immediately after their subsidence.

The case I have thought to be worthy of record, as a fact which may,
with others, establish a conclusion something like positive, if it will not
in itself settle a principle.   F. A. RAMSEY.

---

*Prize Essay, on the Zymotic Theory of Essential Fevers and other
Disordered Conditions of the Blood; Together with an Appendix
on Medical Theories and Vital Statistics.* By SAMUEL G. ARMOR,
M. D., of Cleveland, Ohio.

[We gave in last number a long extract from this Essay, but as the
subject is exciting much interest we commence at the beginning, and
will continue until it is finished.—*Ed.*]

"I profess a liberal medicine: I am neither of the old sects nor new, but follow where-
ever they cultivate truth."--*Klenius.*

There are few inquiries in pathological science of more interest than
those which relate to changed conditions of the Blood; for whether we

regard it as endowed with a distinct vitality, and obedient to the general laws of cellular growth, development and decay; or as ministering to-
the nutritive and textural wants of the system in the elaboration of fibrin
from elements furnished by primary assimilation; or as connected with
important chemical changes essential to a healthy action of the system;
whether we regard the blood as contributing to one or more of these
purposes in the animal economy, it becomes at once evident that destruction of its vitality, or change in any of its constituent elements, must
be followed by serious constitutional disturbances. Hence the interest.
with which its diseases should be studied, and the importance of understanding, in a curative point of view, the primary or secondary impression of disease upon this fluid.

It must be confessed, however, that the question of *priority* or *sequence* although of much interest to him who thinks or reasons about
the nature, origin and phenomena of disease, is often one of difficult solution. But to arrive at greater certainty on this point, if possible, so
far at least as relates to the Essential Fevers, is the object of this Essay:
and if I shall succeed in any degree in pointing out the distinction between *symptoms* of diseased action and *diseased action itself*, I will have,
to some extent at least, accomplished my object.

In M. Andral's classification of Lesions, in which he makes *all* disease to exist, he embraces some in which no *notable* change of either
organization or *composition* can be detected. Yet it is worthy of inquiry as to whether this eminent pathologist has not included in his
lesions, some which are but *symptoms*, not properly diseases—*actions*
and not *states*.

It is not my purpose, however, at present, to enter this field of inquiry.
I desire to call attention to another question in which no such controversy
can arise.

In the Essential or Idiopathic forms of fever it is evident that change
has been induced in the blood by the admixture of *foreign matters.*
The proof of this consists in the fact: 1st, That diseases analagous
to those fevers have been induced by injecting putrid matter into the
veins of animals: 2nd, These fevers are readily produced by the introduction of animal poisons into the blood, as in the case of small pox,
measles, &c.: 3d, These poisons are known to operate through the medium of the air, by thus gaining access to the blood through the lungs:
4th, The non-contagious fevers, such as Intermittents and Remittents,
are universally admitted to depend upon a poisoned or changed condition of the atmosphere: 5th. Actual observation establishes the fact that
the blood *is* altered in all Essential or Idiopathic fevers.

The best point of departure, therefore, is the general fact (for it should
be regarded as such,) that all Essential fevers depend *primarily* on a
poisoning of the Blood, and the proof as to primary impression will be
given in illustration of the facts already cited.

It must not be inferred, however, that I am laboring to establish the
identity of fevers. No such inference can be legitimately drawn from
any fact or reason which I shall present. True, so far as the general
fact is concerned that all foreign matters, when introduced into the

blood, change either its physical, chemical, or vital properties, all Essential fevers may be regarded as a *unit:* Yet observation abundantly establishes the fact that different poisons act differently on the human constitution, and upon the peculiar and specific character of each depends not only the destructive effect on the blood, but the local lesions that will ensue. Urea and its compounds, if retained in the blood, affect the brain and nervous system, and are apt to give rise to a low grade of inflammation in serous and sero-fibrous tissues; while mucous structures will suffer but little. But the small pox virus spends its force upon mucous and cutaneous structures, and leaves, unharmed, the serous and fibrous structures.

There can be no explanation given of this other than the general fact that the tissue or viscus affected seems to be that which has an affinity for the poison which has to be eliminated from the blood. In this process of elimination, inflammation and its sequela are excited, and local disease becomes manifest. Hence all Essential fevers should be regarded as distinct in species *according to the circumstance of the primary sedative impression.* This is the only true and rational classification of fevers.

We feel authorised in asserting, then, as a starting point in our reasonings,—what observation abundantly establishes,—that each specific miasm has its own peculiar and distinct law of development. But in the absence of reliable information as to the *essential nature* of these miasms it would be idle to speculate. Our knowledge on this point, must, at least for the present, rest on observation.

But it will be at once perceived that our knowledge of the action of remedial agents is not more certain. Indeed the perfect analogue of one is found in the other, and the reasoning applied to one applies with equal force to the other. Thus, that Mercury will excite inflammation of the salivary glands; Arsenic, the mucous structures; Belladonna, the skin: Ergot, the uterus; &c., has long been a matter of observation. But *why* they should do so is just as obscure as why the Typhoid poison should select for its destructive action the glands of Peyer, or the Small Pox poison should spend its influence upon the dermoid structures. The articles of the Materia Medica furnish a just illustration of the action of all foreign substances in the production of disease. Mercury, Arsenic or Croton oil, if uncontrolled by the judicious skill of the physician, is capable of giving rise to diseased action with as much certainty and as varied in its manifestations, as either of the animal poisons to which I have alluded; and analogy would lead us to suppose that if we could *control* the one, as we can the other, miasmatic poisons might be used as therapeutic agents. That all agents that affect the vitality or composition of the blood, bear certain general pathological relations, cannot be doubted: but that by no means proves the doctrine of identity. As well might we assert the identity of Small Pox and Typhus fever from the fact that the fibrin of the blood is found defective in both.

An important point, however, to be established, before conclusions, are drawn, is the fact that the blood does undergo change in disease, and from medication, diet, &c.; for if this be denied, our conclusions will be without a predicate and therefore unsound. But the chemists, have happily settled this point by furnishing us accurate analysis of the blood both in health and disease. In the condition of health the venous blood of a man, as represented by the number 1000, is composed of

Serum - - -	869,1547
Globules (fibrine included)	130,8453
	1000

This varies, however, according to sex, age, temperament, kinds of food, evacuations, &c. The rapidity with which some of the solid constituents of the blood are diminished by blood-letting, for example, is very remarkable. Thus, according to the researches of Dumas, the blood of a robust young man of 23 years of age gave:

At the first venesection,

Water, - - - - -	780,210
Globules, - - - -	139,129
Albumen, Salts, Fatty and extractive matters,	80,661
	1000

At the third venesection,

Water, - - - - -	853,46
Globules, - - - - -	76,19
Albumen, Salts, Fatty and extractive matters,	70,35
	1000

The more solid constituents of the blood, it will be seen, are rapidly supplied by a compensating quantity of non-sanguinous fluid; and hence the value of blood-letting when it is desirable to promote absorption.

Diet and drinks also very readily affect the constitution of the blood. According to M. Dennis, in the blood of a young man of 21 years of age, were found:

Water, - - - - -	770
Globules, - - - - -	154
Albumen, &c., - - - -	76
	1000

And after 40 days use of watery drinks:

Water, . .	804
Globules, . .	111.9
Albumen, .	84.1
	1000

It will be thus seen that the blood is very readily changed in its constitution by blood-letting, diet, and exercise. It sustains direct relations also to the air we breathe, to the water we drink, to the food we eat, and to the excretions of the body, by which it is purified; and that a fluid which is presented to us in such a compound and complicated form, and sustaining so many relations to the various modifying influences which surround it, should not become a frequent seat of *disease*, would be, indeed, an anomaly in nature.

Among the various hypotheses to account for fever, a Zymosis, or fermentation of the blood, has prevailed, under one form or other, from a remote antiquity. But it has been so inseparably connected with the old Humoral pathology, that it has received little consideration. Recently this hypothesis (for I shall regard it as such at present) has been rendered, to say the least of it, very plausible by the researches of the distinguished Liebig.

In his "Animal Chemistry" he calls attention to the fact that no other component part of the organism can be compared to the blood in respect of the feeble resistance it offers to exterior influences, and the reason assigned is, that "it is not an organ which is formed, but an organ in a state of formation." The following quotation embodies in a few words, the main leading thought of the author on this subject:—

"*The chemical force and the vital principle hold each other in such perfect equilibrium, that every disturbance, however trifling, or from whatever cause it may proceed, effects a change in the blood.*"

This, then, is an important starting point in our reasoning process; for, if it be really possessed of a low vitality, we may logically arrive at the conclusion, by an *a priori* argument, if we knew nothing of the facts, in confirmation of it, that all fevers, produced by endemic, epidemic, or infectious causes, have their origin in a primary diseased condition of the blood.

A Zymotic change of the blood is due, according to Liebig, to a decomposing organic molecule in the interior of the human body. This molecule, by a law of catalysis, induction, or contact, has the power of imparting its own motion to another molecule, with which it may be in contact. Hence chemists have defined it to be "decomposition by contact," or the "action of presence." We have illustrations of this law in the power which small quantities of substances, in a state of change, possess of causing unlimited quantities to pass into the same state; and it is an interesting fact, worthy of note in this connection, that all substances which readily suffer this transformation are, without exception, bodies which contain *nitrogen*. A large portion of the blood being composed of this element, we might readily conclude that it is the vital principle alone that keeps it from spontaneously passing into this condition of transformation. If the catalytic force be greater than the resistance offered by the vital principle, the blood must pass into a condition of decomposition.

It may be asked, however, with reference to this law of Zymosis, or induction, is there any evidence to show that the introduction of putrid matter into the animal system does give rise to effects which are at all comparable with those of fever? If not, the law which has been announced is but a speculation, and, at best, an hypothesis. But let us see. "It is a fact," says Liebig, "that subjects in anatomical theatres frequently pass into a state of decomposition, which is communicated to the blood of the living body." And the fact observed by Magendie, that putrifying blood, brain, eggs, &c., laid on recent wounds, cause vomiting, lassitude and death, after a longer or shorter interval, has never, as yet, been contradicted. Numerous experiments have demonstrated that putrid matter injected into the blood of healthy animals, will give rise to a set of symptoms which are very analogous to typhus. "If a small portion of putrid matter," says Dr. Armstrong, "be accidentally introduced into the blood during dissection, or if the experiment be made upon the lower animals, it produces fever, having exactly the characters of typhus under its continued form, and *no individual could confidently pronounce that it differed from it.*" Bernard has also shown that, by injecting yeast or sugar into the circulation, many of the ordinary kinds of fermentation are excited, giving rise to a disease very analagous to typhoid fever, accompanied by prostration of strength, bloody fluxes, ecchymosis, and a black and uncoagulated condition of the blood. "Lastly, it is," says Liebig, quoting from Henle, "a universal observation that the origin of epidemic diseases is often to be traced to the putrefaction of large quantities of animal and vegetable matters; that miasmatic diseases are endemic in places where the decomposition of organic matter is constantly taking place, as in marshy and moist localities; that they are developed epidemically under the same circumstances after inundations; also in places where a large number of people are crowded together, with insufficient ventilation, as in ships, prisons, and besieged places."

It is also worthy of note that these factitious fevers, produced by the introduction of deleterious substances directly into the blood are analagous, both in their symptoms and pathological lesions, to those produced by the sting or bite of certain animals; they present, also, the same general class of symptoms that are present in small pox, malignant scarlatina, and other eruptive diseases.

In Mr. Walker's work on Grave Yards, he also presents an array of facts, which prove, beyond all controversy, that putrid animal exhalations have given rise to diseases that have raged like a pestilence or epidemic. He cites an instructive instance, which occurred in 1733, at the parish of St. Saturnine, in Burgundy. A sexton, while letting down a corpse into the vault, accidentally broke a coffin which contained the body of a fat man that had been buried twenty-three days. A discharge of sanies followed, which greatly annoyed the assistants; and, "of one hundred and twenty young persons, of both sexes, who assembled to receive their first communion, all but six fell dangerously ill, together with the *Cure*, the grave-digger, and sixty other persons." The disease is described as a putrid, verminous fever, accompanied with hæmorrhage, eruption, and inflammation.

Facts in support of these views might be accumulated at great length. Dr. Francis Home communicated measles by means of a drop of blood from a patient affected with the disease. And the experiments of M. Gendrin, as given in Williams' Principles of Medicine, is a striking one in point:—"A man who had been skinning a diseased animal was seized with a putrid fever, attended with an eruption of sloughing pustules. Some blood taken from this man was injected with the cellular texture of the groin of a cat; the animal was soon after affected with vomiting of bile, dyspnœa, frequent, small, and irregular pulse, dry, brown tongue, slight convulsions, and died seven hours after the injection." The same pathologist induced in animals various and severe symptoms, followed by death, by injecting inro their veins the blood of persons laboring under small pox. M. Dupuy and Lauret also communicated the malignant pustular disease known as " Charbon," by injecting into the veins of the healthy horse a minute quantity of blood of the diseased animal. Andral relates an extraordinary case in which a malignant fever, followed with pustular eruption and death, was occasioned by the mere contact of the lips with the diseased blood of an animal.

May we not, then, infer, from these facts, that the blood is the hot-bed in which many malignant diseases are propagated, whether by ova, parasites, cellgerms, or zymotic action.

But our proof does not rest here. Clinical observation has long since established the alteration of the blood in diseases which are termed *putrid:* the blood appears to be in a partial state of *dissolution;* its vitality is destroyed, and its fibrine either not elaborated, or dissolved in the process of putrefaction. As a result of this decomposition, an increased quantity of hydro-sulphate of ammonia has been found in the blood of patients suffering from typhus and other malignant diseases; and hence the *alkaline* reaction of the urine that is so often observed to be present in these fevers.

These observations have been made the basis for the support of a great group of maladies which go by the name of Zymotic diseases, and include, according to the statistical nosology of Mr. Farr, small pox, chicken pox, all eruptive diseases, influenza, scurvy, purpura, ague, remittent fever, yellow fever, tpphus, puerperal, plague, hospital gangrene, &c. And, in proof of their Zymotic origin, the fact has been offered— 1st, that the vitality of the blood is low, and that it, therefore, readily suffers transformations; 2nd, that we can produce in animals and man factitious diseases, by inoculations or injections of putrid or contagious matter, having all the characteristics of the essential fevers; and 3rd, that clinical observation establishes the fact that the blood is changed. And that the febrile phenomena present in these fevers indicate a condition of the system, independent of inflammatory action, I infer from the fact—1st, that, in the absence of complication during the progress of the disease, there is no evidence of inflammation revealed by post mortem inspection; and 2nd, that the symptoms co-exist with a diminution of the fibrin of the blood, and diminished tolerance of the loss of blood. In some of the most malignant forms of fever—those in which the fibrin of the blood is at its minimum—there is often not much heat of body, and but little increase of pulse. The patient often dies in the cold stage of such fevers, without, in fact, having any fever! Evidently, therefore, the term *fever* may be used in two very different senses—in one, signifying a collection of symptoms depending on local inflammation; and, in the other, a *condition* of the system entirely independent of such inflammation. In one the term indicates the name of a *disease,* and in the other the name of a *symptom*. Hence the distinction between essential and symptomatic fevers; and hence the inference, also, that the essential fevers have their origin in certain qualitative changes of the blood, caused by the introduction of foreign matters.

Further proof that the general class of diseases which have been termed Zymotic have their origin in the blood, is drawn from the symptoms usually present. These will be found accurately detailed by all standard writers on General Pathology, under the head of " *Necraemia,* or *death beginning with the blood,*" such as petechiæ and vibices on the external surface, the occurrence of hæmorrhage in internal parts, the general fluidity of the blood, its frequently dark and otherwise altered aspect, its proneness to pass into decomposition, the general prostration of all the vital powers, the dark tongue, sordes on the teeth, suspended secretion, and the general arrest of molecular nutrition. Indeed, the very *universality* of diseased action points to a cause more general than can be found in any individual function.

I have thus far spoken of admixture of foreign elements in the blood from *without*. There are causes, however, which operate upon it *intrinsically*, as well as *extrinsically*. Thus, defective excretion is followed by a direct *backward* action on the blood, resulting in changes of its chemical or vital properties. The excretory organs are the natural emunctories, through which effete matters, generated within the organism, are expelled from the blood. The product of the various excretions may be regarded, therefore, as the correct expression of the numerous changes that are taking place both in the healthy and diseased animal fabric. In febrile diseases these organs are generally suspended in the exercise of their healthy function, an increase of perspiration, or in the flow of urine, or a spontaneous diarrhœa, being generally accompanied with a subsidence of the febrile phenomena.

Relatively considered, the *kidneys* may be regarded as the most important emunctories through which morbid matter is expelled from the blood. The experiments of Orfilla on this subject are highly satisfactory. He found that the pernicious effects of small and repeated doses of arsenic could be readily averted in animals, by giving them, at the same time, a dieuretic medicine; and the converse fact has been frequently observed—namely, that persons who suffer from disease of the kidney, by which its function is impaired, very readily contract infectious diseases, and are apt to suffer from their effects. It has also been observed that opium, arsenic, mercury, &c., operate with dangerous energy on such patients.

The experiments of Dr. Golding Bird are very conclusive on this subject. His observations have been extensive and accurate. Two, of many, cases are here given. In the first, a case of ague, the patient was kept in the hospital from the 23rd of May to the 16th of June following.

The following is his table of analysis:

May 23rd. Passed 12 ozs. urine and 352 grs. solid constituent.

"	26th.	"	40	"	828	"
"	28th.	"	35	"	725	"
"	30th.	"	48	"	1054	
"	31st.	"	45	"	743	
June	2nd.	"	35	"	514	
"	4th.	"	30	"	879	
"	6th.	"	27	"	1036	
"	7th.	"	36	"	436	
"	9th.	"	40	"	1172	"
"	11th.	"	45	"	742	
"	13th.	"	40	"	916	"
"	14th.	"	43	"	984	
"	16th.	"	37	"	1044	"

There was a decided improvement, says Dr. Bird, on the 30th, severe paroxysm on the 3rd, better again on the 6th, and no return of the ague after the 9th.

In the second case of ague—girl, aged 19—patient was kept in hospital from 23rd of May to June 7th. On the 23rd of May there was a severe paroxysm, and the amount of solids excreted was 280 grs. On the 27th she had a return of paroxysm, and there was 280 grs. solid constituents in the urine. On the 28th she was better, and the solid constituents in the urine. On the 28th she was better, and the solid constituents amounted to 538 grs. On the 30th they amounted to 625 grs.; and from this time the patient rapidly got well.

In this, also, it will be observed that *pari passu* with the patient's improvement there was an increase of the solid constituents of the urine. In Typhus and other adynamic forms of fever, the same facts have been observed.

Are we to infer, however, from these observations, the defective excretion is the primary *cause* of the fever? By no means. That would be an imperfect view of the pathology of these fevers. I can conceive of no instance in which a lesion of secretion can be properly classified among the *primary* elements of disease. Some change must precede it, either of structure, of innervation, or of the blood from which the secretion is formed. The examples cited simply show the curative effects of the removal of foreign matters from the blood by means of depurating organs and at the same time go far towards establishing the ancient doctrine of *critical discharges*.

They also serve to point out the two causes of disease which constantly present themselves for our consideration—causes *extrinsic* and causes *intrinsic*. Of these one or both may be in active operation. It is an erroneous dogma to suppose that but one poison can act on the system at a time. As rational would it be to suppose that but one medicinal agent can produce its effects upon the constitution at a time.

I have already alluded to the fact, demonstrated by observation, that different poisons spend their influence upon different tissues of the body. Is it an unwarrantable speculation to transfer this law of *specific contamination* to the structure of the blood, and thus explain the action of different foreign bodies upon that fluid? Some poisons may be regarded as comparatively innoxious; they emerge from the body unaltered, with one or more of the ordinary secretions: others destroy some element of the blood (or its corpuscular element in the lymphatic glandular system,) so that it is never again susceptible to the action of the same poison, as in the case of some of the eruptive and contagious diseases; while others, by entering into chemical union with one or more elements of the blood essential to life, destroy its vitality and general necræmia and molecular death soon follow.

This will be recognized as an unproven speculation of the old fashioned Humoral Pathology. And, in the absence of positive proof, I do not, of course, offer it as one of the "fixed facts" in Medical Science. Yet observation, reason and analogy throw around it a *plausibility* that entitles it to still further investigation.

In submitting these views I would not be understood as attempting to sustain an exclusive Humoral Pathology; nor would I underrate the importance of pathological changes in the solids. With Bichat, I regard "every exclusive theory, whether of Humoralism or Solidism, as a pathological absurdity." The relation between them is too direct and intimate to be ever separated; neither can the one or the other ever be regarded as an "exploded" system. Humoralism will never be exploded as long as the blood is the source of life to the tissues of the body; nor will Solidism be disregarded as long as the tissues continue to undergo change from altered conditions of the blood. My object is rather to fix the mind upon what I regard as an important truth, viz., that in all Essential or Idiopathic fevers, changes of the solids depend on previous alterations (quantitative and qualitative) of the blood.

This altered condition of the blood is soon made manifest by general febrile phenomena. The nervous centres, depending for their powers directly upon the state of integrity of this fluid, become perverted and weakened in action; the functions of animal and organic life are depressed; passive congestion, induced by depression of nervous power, follows; and hence the torpor and arrest of glandular action, and the sluggish and languid state of all the functions so characteristic of these fevers. **TO BE CONTINUED.**

Physicians in Iceland.

Madame Pfeiffer, in her "Journey to Iceland," gives the following not very flattering account of the condition and rewards of the profession in that country. She says: "Among the salaried offices, the most laborious are those of the physicians and clergy. Their circuits often embrace a distance of over a hundred miles. When the doctor is sent for in winter, the country people turn out with shovels and pickaxes to clear the road. They bring several horses with them, so that he may change from one exhausted animal to another during his long rides through the fog and darkness, the snowdrifts and storms. Often as he returns to his own fireside, worn out with cold and fatigue, he finds another summons. He must leave his family and face new dangers, before he has had time to relate the perils he has just experienced. The physicians receive but a small salary, the priests still less."

EDITORIAL AND MISCELLANEOUS.

The Serapion.

We had the pleasure, in December, of attending a public meeting of the Serapion. The exercises of the evening consisted of an address from Dr. Tappan, the President of the University, and the reading of the " Mint," a manuscript periodical issued by the society. The exercises of the evening were of a high order, both in taste and talent. To those who are not acquainted with the Serapion, we would say that it is a medical society, which meets weekly for the reading of original papers and selections, and for the oral discussion of scientific questions. Its weekly meeting are carried on by the students of the Medical College, but its annual meetings includes medical men from all parts of the State, some of them alumni of the institution, and others elected to the honor of membership. There are also monthly meetings in which public addresses are delivered by gentlemen invited for that purpose.

The elevating influence of such associations on the profession is direct and mighty. The exercises carried on in them tend directly to the development of the arts of communication, on which depends *organization*, the great want of the present time. We have power enough, but we have not discipline enough to render the profession's power avilable to its higest extent. When the arts of speech and writing shall be fully cultivated, so that thought shall flash to thought along the ranks of the profession, with ease and yet with fire, the elements of strength will rush spontaneously to their appropriate combinations and organized power do a new work in the world.

Schieffelin's Medicines.

We were shown, the other day, a splendid suite of specimens illustrating Materia Medica, prepared by P. Schieffelin, Haines & Co. The series consisted of nearly three hundred samples, illustrating both the pure and the adultrated articles ; and to medical students, especially those who are to practice in the country and must be their own apothecaries, the information derived from the study of such a suite of specimens is invaluable. The series is to be seen in the cabinet of the University of Michigan.

Correction.

The article on the sewing up of the subclavian vein by the mate of a vessel, which appeared among our selections of last month, was taken from the " Scalpel." The credit was accidently omitted, much to our regret, for we intend in every case to give full credit for all selected articles. There is nothing which we despise more than grudging other journals their merited dues.

Medical Books and Surgical Instruments.

We are often inquired of for the places where various Medical Works or Surgical Instruments can be procured. We take this opportunity to say that

A. B. Wood. of Ann Arbor, has, we believe, by far the most extensive assort-
ment of Medical Books in the State. He attends to orders from abroad
promptly, and will procure, at the shortest notice, from New York, Boston
or Philadelphia, any rare or new work which may be ordered, if it is not
already on his shelves.

Maynards', of Ann Arbor, and Higby & Dickinson, of Detroit, have arrangements to furnish Surgical Instruments of any kind or description to order.

New Truss.

So many Trusses have been invented that new ones meet with but little
favor, but we sometimes meet those which combine, in a marked manner, various excellencies. We have seen one lately composed of an elastic band and
a spring pad, which, simple as its construction appears, has been worn with
signal relief by several patients in this place. It was invented by Mr. Silas
Pratt, who has patented it, and intends to bring it effectually before the public. We think it will work its way to favor, and we make these remarks
because we believe that men possessing mechanical tact and ingenuity should
always be encouraged to exert their skill in producing instruments to answer
the demands of the Surgeon.

NOTICES OF WORKS RECEIVED.

A Practical Treatise on the Diseases of Children. By FRANCIS CONDIE,
M.D., Sect. Coll. Physicians. Phil:

To call the attention of the medical fraternity to a new edition of this American medical classic seems almost a work of superrogation. The name of Dr.
Condie is too well known and his influence too generally felt and acknowledged
in the department of Pathology to which the present work refers to require
other than a very brief notice of this new edition.

Preserving in the arrrangement and classification of subjects the same order
as in former editions, he has embodied in the discussion of the several diseases
many uew facts and important views on their pathology and treatment:
Among these, we are pleased to notice a summary of the opinions of Drs.
Fuchs, Gairdner and Rees, on that condition of the pulmonary air-cells denominated Atelectasis Pulmonum, and which for a long period has been, and
even still continues to be confounded by some writers with the consolidation
resulting from Pneumonia. We need scarcely to remark that so important
an error in the anatomical results of disease leads directly to the most injurious practical consequences.

While every other part of the work bears ample evidence of the research of
the learned author, we are happy to observe that the confusion and uncertainty arising from the adoption of views too often immature and crude, which
are put forth in all manner of forms, has been avoided; that he has subjected them to a careful scrutiny, and adopted them only when they have
been found to abide the test of true experience.

If long years and mature thought, devoted to the diseases of infancy and
childhood, can furnish a just claim to consideration, few men of this or any

·other country are better entitled to speak with authority than the author of the present treatise. We regret however to find that the rare, yet interesting disease, denominated by the French writers. *Contractures essentielles*, has been overlooked, end hope to see the defect supplied in the next edition, which will undoubtedly soon be demanded.

With respect to the style of the getting up, we need only state that is is issued by the enterprising Philadelphia publishers, Blanchard & Lea.

For sale by A: B. Wood, Ann Arbor. A. S.

Paget's Surgical Pathology.

This capital work is a volume of about seven hundred pages, published by Lindsay and Blakistone, Philadelphia. For a fuller account see the review of it on another page. We esteem it a valuable addition to our stock of reading matter: For sale by A. B. Wood, Ann Arbor.

Ricord and Hunter on Venereal ; *or, a Treatise on the Venereal Disease.* By JOHN HUNTER, F. R. S., *with Copious Additions*, by DR. PHILIP RICORD, Surgeon to the Hospital du Midi, Paris, &c. *Edited, with Notes,* by FREEMAN J. BUNISTEAD, M.D;, Physician to the North West Dispensatory, New York,

This work, appearing in this country for the first time in this form, is of high value, bringing down to us the work of the immortal Hunter, in combination with the teachings of the distinguished Ricord. It contains eight beautiful lithographic plates, illustrating venereal diseases and the instruments used in treating them. The whole makes a volume of a little over five hundred pages, covering the whole ground of the venereal poison, gonorrhœa and syphilis, with the consequences, direct and remote, and the [modes of of treatment. It is published by Blanchard and Lea, Philadelphia. For sale by A. B. Wood, Ann Arbor.

Dr. Armor's Prize Essay.

This is a brief essay on the zymotic, or fermentive theory of fevers. Those who would read, will find it among our selections.

Introductory Lecture addressed to the Class of the Kentucky School of Medicine. By H. M. BULLITT, M, D., Professor of Pathology and Physiology.

The Kentucky *bullets* were always swift on the field of battle, and we see that they are also ready and keen on the field of science.

The Transactions of the New York Academy of Medicine. Vol. 1, Part 2. Containing Hospital Hygiene, illustrated.

This is a report of some striking facts respecting the propagation and treatment of Typhus Fever. We shall treat our readers to some of its contents at another time.

The Legitimate Goal of Professional Ambition. Address introductory to the Course of Lectures in the Medical Department of the St. Louis University, by W. M. McPHEETERS, M, D,. Professor of Materia Medica and Therapeutics,

A most useful topic, and well suited to present before a class of candidates for the profession, for there is no principle more wild and lawless, while yet sublime and indispensable, than ambition, and an attempt to guide the arrow to its mark is worthy of praise. The high moral and religious tone of the close is admirable.

Treatment of Vesico-Vaginal Fistula. By MARION SIMS, M. D., of New York. Published by Blanchard & Lea, Philadelphia.

A valuable monograph on this most difficult and perplexing surgical operation. Its circulation among surgeons generally would be of great use.

Seventeenth Annual Report of the Trustees and Superintendent of the Vermont Asylum for the Insane.

From this report we clip the following summary:

"The number of patients remaining Aug. 1, 1852—

Males,	175	
Females,	176	
		351

There have been admitted during the year—

Males,	70	
Females.	89	
		159

Total enjoying the benefits of the Asylum,	510	

There have been discharged during the year—

Males,	62	
Females,	76	
		138

Remaining Aug. 1, 1853,	372	

Of the 138 discharged, there have

Recovered,	72	
Improved,	10	
Not improved,	13	
Died,	43	
		138

"Since the opening of the Asylum 2066 patients have been admitted, 1694 have been discharged, and 372 remain in the Institution. Of the 1694 who have been discharged, 968 have recovered, equal to 57.14 per cent. Of those placed in the Asylum within six months from the attack, nearly nine-tenths have recovered.

"TERMS OF ADMISSION.—For those of this State, two dollars per week for the first six months, and one dollar and seventy-five cents per week thereafter.

"For those of other States, two dollars per week, or $100 per year, if the patient remain such a length of time.

"When the insanity is connected with epilepsy or paralysis, the terms are two dollars and fifty cents per week.

"No charge is made for damages in any case.

"Applications may be made to Dr. W. H. Rockwell, Brattleboro, Vt."

THE

PENINSULAR

JOURNAL OF MEDICINE

AND THE COLLATERAL SCIENCES.

| VOL. L | FEBRUARY, 1854. | NO. VIII. |

ORIGINAL COMMUNICATIONS.

Art. I.—*Observations on the Cause, Nature, and Treatment of Epidemic Cholera.* By A. B. Palmer, M.D., Prof. of Anatomy in the University of Michigan.

From the year 1817, when this terrible scourge first assumed a distinct epidemic form in the marshy district of Jessora, in the Delta of the Ganges, and particularly since it made its appearance in Europe, in 1829, it has justly received a large share of the attention of the profession. Men of the highest order of intellect, and of the most profound attainments, with all the advantages of the present advanced state of the physical sciences—with all the appliances for measuring the temperature, the pressure, the moisture, and the electrical state of the atmosphere, by their sides, and with scalpel, and test-glass, and microscope in hand—in the crowded lanes of cities, and on the open plains—upon the hill-tops, and in the valleys—amid the frost and gloom of Russian winters, and in the fiery heat of tropical summers—by the bed-side, and in the dead-house—they have plied the principles of all these sciences— now assisted, and now, perhaps, retarded, by the most ingenious speculations; and the results of these investigations have been spread before the medical world in elaborate reports; and the most profound and erudite minds have been engaged in arranging, generalizing, and comparing these accumulated facts, and drawing couclusions from them:— still, it must be confessed, that far fewer principles are fully and demonstrably established than would be desirable; either as to the essential cause of the disease, its mode of propagation, the organs primarily and principally involved—the specific manner in which these organs are affected—the essential changes which are left behind—or, even, after so much experience, as to the best mode of treating it.

After all that has been written upon cholera, an experience in it, though not small, yet presenting no striking peculiarities, the same, or nearly the same successive features of the disease ever presenting themselves, it is hardly to be expected that I should be able to throw much new light upon it; but the subject is so interesting in itself, the re-appearance of the scourge among us so probable, it is so alarming to the community, and really so terrible in its ravages, and, in my estimation, so capable of being influenced by preventive and curative measures, that I feel justified in presenting it to the readers of the journal.

In what is to follow, I shall not attempt a complete treatise on the disease, or indulge in any extended references to its literature; giving rather such views as may seem most important to be presented, and such as are the results mainly of my own experience and reflection; neither attempting to follow any particular leadings, or to avoid any path that may have been pursued by others.

The subject is naturally divided into—

1st. The cause—essential and predisposing.

2ndly. Its nature, symptomatology, and pathology; and,

3rdly. Treatment—prophylactic and curative.

1. The essential *cause* of cholera is involved in obscurity. An effect cannot exist without a cause; there can be no disease without an antecedent producing it—an antecedent consisting either in a distinct and special agency, operating upon the organism from without, or in combination of various and, sometimes, varying circumstances, either without or within itself. A disease like the one under consideration, distinct and specified in its character, far-spread and migratory, affecting alike a great variety of persons, of different conditions, and under divers circumstances, must be produced by some special agency, capable of spreading and operating from without.

As no agent of this kind can act where it is not, it has locality; surrounds and pervades the bodies of those affected by it.

It either arises from earth, comes down from the heavens, or has its habitation in the atmosphere, or other substances where its influence prevails. What is this agency? What is the particular thing, or the particular combination of known or unknown materials existing in or constituting the atmosphere we breathe, the aliment we imbibe, or in the condition of the caloric or electricity which surrounds and pervades it?

This question has been long asked, but has not been definitely and positively answered, though attempts have not been wanting to supply the deficiencies of knowledge by an abundance of hypothesis.

If, in the searches after this subtle cause, no *positive* conclusions have been arrived at, if science has not been able to say what the cause of cholera is, some *negative* conclusions have been pretty clearly established. Science is able to say, to a considerable extent, and with a degree of certainty, what it is not.

Though the disease had its origin in a hot and moist climate, no particular condition, as to temperature or humidity, can be considered as the cause, as it has prevailed in every climate, and at all seasons—in every state of the atmosphere, as to dryness or humidity, density or rarity. Neither does it depend upon any appreciable electrical state, as it has been found, by experiment, that the most opposite electrical conditions do exist where the disease prevails. Though some connexion or certain relations seem to exist between this cause and malaria or marsh-miasmata, intermittent fevers in some instances being supplanted by the cholera, and re-appearing again when the latter had gone by; yet the cause of cholera cannot be common malaria, as it has prevailed where intermittents were never known, and has avoided, in its progress, many districts where intermittents most prevail.

From all these facts—from the disease pursuing general and most extensive courses, passing from point to point, preserving its identity under the greatest variety of circumstances—thousands of miles and long periods of time producing no materially modifying influence upon it—from all the facts of the case, we can but conclude that there is a *specific virus*—a particular poisonous substance —a *materia morbi* which is the essential cause of cholera. Beyond a doubt, the facts which have been observed can be best, and, indeed, alone satisfactorily accounted for by this supposition.

In regard to what this *materia morbi* is, speculation has been busy; and the following *hypotheses* on this point, embracing, as they do, all the known forms of matter, chemical or organic, dead or living, which at all consist with the facts, though none of them are claimed as anything more than theories, are each more or less plausible, and, it would seem, among them must contain the truth.

This poison may be supposed a peculiar emanation from the air—a particular combination of some occult gaseous or chemical agents, too subtle for our instruments—or it may be supposed a series of organized nucleated cells, similar to the poison of small pox, and other strictly contagious diseases; or an insect or animalcule too minute for our glasses; or, with quite-as much plausibility as-any of the preceding, it may be supposed to be a vegetable fungus, by its minuteness equally beyond the power of detection.

This poison, whatever it is, by being either inhaled with the air, absorbed by the surface, or swallowed with the aliment, circulates throughout the system, impressing the solids or changing the fluids in such a manner as to give rise to the morbid condition and action which constitute the disease.

On the assumption of this specific character of the cause, what is its mode of propagation?

Whatever be this cause, or however it may be propagated, it is certainly progressive. It travels, it comes, it acts, it goes away, or becomes inert. But how does it come? By what means does it travel from point to point? It was either inexhaustible in its amount and force in its original source—an idea not to be ontertained, when we consider the immense extent of its prevalence—or it is reinforced, as it progresses, by additions to its mass. How is it reinforced? By what means does it obtain—from what source does it derive these additions? " Soil, climate, subjects, locality, time, are all changed; but, nevertheless, the *same agent* is generated and regenerated—the *same*, for the effects of its causative action are identical—precisely the same amidst the snows of Russia and under the burning line."*

At this point the contagionists and non-contagionists are brought in collision; or, rather, here is the point where they should meet each other with their facts and arguments; while, in reality, they have, for the most part, been engaged in a general war of words, scarcely having arrived at any precise point; neither fully understanding the other, or possibly themselves; and each embracing both truth and error.

In this, as in many other controversies, much of the difference has arisen from not understanding alike the precise meaning of terms. It has been said, with much truth, that words are fissures, into which each person pours his own thoughts; and this remark will apply with great force to the word contagion.

If by a contagious disease is meant one which is capable of being communicated from the sick directly to the healthy, by means of an agent generated in the body of the former, and is ordinarily propagated in no other way, then the facts certainly will not encourage the idea that cholera is contagious; for it is evidently communicated in other modes; or if it follows, from this admission of its being contagious, that, when the disease is prevailing in a particular locality, those who are

* Prof. S. H. Dickson.

brought in immediate proximity to the sick are perceptibly more liable to take the disease than those who avoid such proximity, then we are surely unwilling to admit that it is contagious to any considerable extent, at least; for this is found not to be the fact. If, however, the term contagion is made to embrace what is more properly understood by *infection*—that is, a morbific agent, capable of being imparted and communicated to the atmosphere of a locality, in consequence of which the place previously free from this form of disease becomes specially liable to it; as, for instance, a vessel arriving in a port, or a caravan in a town, coming from a locality where a special disease prevails, bringing articles impregnated with effluvia from the air of the region infected, (and whether having persons in the company or crew laboring under the disease or not,) so affecting the locality where they arrive as to cause the disease to prevail there, whether the inhabitants of the port or town come in proximity with persons diseased or not. If the word contagion is meant to embrace this state of things, in this sense the facts would warrant us in regarding the cholera contagious—not, by any means, admitting that it is propagated exclusively, or even principally in this manner; but that it may be, and, at least, occasionally, is thus propagated.

But it is quite time that the profession attach a precise and invariable meaning to the term contagion, and thereby avoid much loose controversy. The most usual ideas of contagion, or of a contagious disease, is one in which a morbid material is generated in the body of a person laboring under the disease; which material, when communicated to another, whether by actual contact, by fomites, or through the medium of the air, produces the same disease in the latter; and it would be much better if the term were restricted to this definite meaning. This generation of a poison in the body of the sick, and its communication to another, is certainly the essential idea of contagion; and those diseases alone should be called contagious which have this character. All contagious diseases have a poisonous material—a *materia morbi;* but all *materiæ morbi* are not generated within the bodies of the sick, and, when generated and multiplied exterior to those bodies and independent of them, the essential character of contagion is lost. A disease produced by such a cause may be called *infectious;* but it is not contagious, and should not be so called.

With this view of the subject, it is by no means absurd, as has been alleged, to say that a disease is portable, may be transported from place to place, and yet not contagious. In these remarks, no new distinction is attempted in the signification of words. Not to refer to medical writers, (many of whom are by no means clear on this subject,) Noah Webster says, " The words *contagion* and *infection* are frequently confounded. The proper distinction between them is this: *contagion* is the virus or effluvia generated in a diseased body, and capable of producing the specific disease in a healthy body, by contact or otherwise; *infection* is anything that taints or corrupts; hence, it includes contagion, and any other morbid, noxious matter which may excite disease in a healthy body."

He who contends for the contagiousness of cholera, must insist that the poison which produces it is formed in the bodies of those laboring under the disease, and is communicated from them to the well. Has the history of the spread of the disease justified this conclusion? We think that the ultimate deliberate opinion of the profession will be that it has not. Our ideas can be better understood on these points by definitely stating how we suppose the morbid material is reproduced and extended; and here we shall have occasion to refer to the several theories of the nature of the poison.

If it be a gaseous or chemical body formed in, and of the elements of the atmosphere, it was originally generated in the malarious and heated atmosphere of India; and we may suppose that it has multiplied and extended, by a process similar to fermentation, in farinacious or saccharine matter from yeast; a change is effected in the material, a new combination takes place in its elements wherever the yeast is introduced; and the circumstances of warmth, moisture, &c., are favorable: so we suppose the new morbid product is formed wherever the elements and other conditions for its formation exist; that it is carried on by a continuous propagation, as " a little leaven leaveneth the whole lump;" and it would not be unreasonable farther to suppose that this morbid fermentation might be hastened on by some of the material being carried by fomition, by confined air in the hold of a ship, by the bodies and clothing of persons affected by the disease; and possibly it may be multiplied in the bodies of those persons; and this material, thus transported, may serve as the starting point for a new propagation, when deposited in the place where the necessary elements exist, and the circumstances for the process are favorable. In the same manner, a quantity of leaven deposited in one point of a mass, in a fit condition for its action, may, in time, pervade the whole; but the process will be hastened by placing this leaven successively at different points; and, in case of a deposit in a single point only, some parts of the mass might escape, which would have been effected if the distribution had taken place.

Again, if leaven be deposited in a place where the elements for action are deficient, or the circumstance which best favor that action do not exist, some slight local evidence of the ferment may be observed, but no extensive action will result. Now, do not the facts with regard to the spread of cholera precisely correspond to this analogy?

From India to the western borders of Europe it took a general pro gressive north-western course, because the circumstances in this direction were favorable to its spread. It took this direction in a degree inde pendent of intercommunication; but still, it usually followed thorough fares, and was often apparently hurried on from point to point, by the passage of vessels and caravans. If, as was often the case, it was carried out of its route by travellers—carried into a region not favorable to its extension, a few isolated cases occurred, but it soon died away.

The same essentially have been the facts of its spread every where. Again and again has it been apparently (may we not say certainly?) brought to a place by the arrival of a vessel, or of persons coming from a district where it prevails; and it has as certainly made its ap pearance in places far distant from where it has appeared before, in the general direction of its progress, but where spaces of country uninhab ited have intervened, and where no communication had taken place.

On the hypothesis that the poison of cholera is a nucleated cell, the mode of its spread can be conceived without difficulty. Nucleated cells are organized bodies of animal origin. They consist of minute cell walls or sacks, usually filled with a fluid; and within the sack, adhering to its surface, are small dots, or nuclei. These nuclei when the cell is active, and placed in a situation where it can assimilate *to* itself appro priate materials, are developed into other cells of a similar character, often in considerable numbers within the original. These, on their in crease, burst the parent cell, each of them, in turn, producing numerous others, often in rapid succession, and in indefinite progression.

The strict contagionists, embracing these notions of the cause of cholera, would contend that the cells can be produced only in the bodies of those affected by the disease, while others would believe that they may be reproduced in the atmosphere where the circumstances are favorable, and may spread, by continuous multiplication, with the great est rapidity, and to the largest extent, being sometimes aided by trans portation, precisely as in the case of the supposed gaseous ferment; and with this supposition the cell theory will account for the facts of the spread of cholera, as fully, and on the same principles, as the gaseous hypothesis.

The animalcular theory of the cause of cholera, equally well accounts for its spread, and in a similar manner, with the exception of the parti-

cular law of increase, which, in this case, is generation, or animal procreation. These animalculæ, it may be supposed, would spread themselves more readily wherever the circumstances most favorable to their
subsistence and development exist, are capable of multiplying with astonishing rapidity in the atmosphere—(as is known to be the case with
some animalculæ)—may be transported in the same manner as other
supposed agents; and it has been thought by some (rather fancifully,
perhaps) that the existence of animals possessed of will more satisfactorily accounts for the singularly erratic course which, in particular localities, the disease has been observed to take. This animalcular theory
is not without much plausibility; it receives great support from analogy
to facts well ascertained; and numbers among its advocates some of the
most profound medical philosophers.

In a precisely similar manner, with the exception of the particular law
of propagation, is the spread of this poisonous material accounted for,
on the hypothesis of its being a vegetable fungus.

This is a theory first distinctly advanced a few years ago by Dr. Codwell, a distinguished European writer. Among a variety of arguments
which support his theory, he shows that *fungi* exist and propagate in
the atmosphere, are of Protean composition, and have an affinity for the
body; and that they are often found in insects and animals, and in the
human system. He shows, from authority, that a single fungus of one
of the varieties has produced 10,000,000 of sporules in a short period,
and is, therefore, capable of the most rapid spread and multiplication.

Since the appearance of Dr. Codwell's views, Prof. J. R. Mitchell, of
Philadelphia, has issued a small volume, containing six lectures, first
delivered in the winters of 1845–6, and previous to Dr. Codwell's published articles, in which he—Professor M.—advances the theory that
malarial and epidemic fevers are produced by vegetable fungi, and is
disposed to contest with Dr. Codwell the originality of the ideas, that
fungi are an extensive cause of epidemic diseases. Professor Mitchell
seems to apply his theory to cholera, and urges, in support of it, the alleged fact that the *potato rot* is produced by a fungus; that fungi retain their vitality in a heat sufficient to boil water, and in cold which
will congeal carbonic acid gas; that some of the fungi, of perceptible
size, are known to be poisonous; that the microscope has detected,
mingled with blood, sporules fourteen times smaller than a blood globule;
that aptha is produced by fungi, &c. &c. This work manifests a great
amount of research, is arranged with much ingenuity and ability, is certainly plausible, and well worthy of attention.

It may be objected to all these theories* of the cause of cholera that no positive morbid material has actually been discovered; and this objection is good, and sufficient to prevent the assumption of its existence as an ascertained and demonstrable fact; but it does not destroy the value of the inferential truth. The fact that we cannot perceive a thing by our gross senses, is no proof of its non-existence. With all our boasted faculties, we are beings of very limited perceptions. We are placed in a universe between the extremes of infinite magnitude and infinite minutiæ. We can perceive but a few links in that chain of existence, which extends from the infinite to us, and from us to nothing. The appliances of art, it is true, have greatly aided our natural senses— have vastly extended the range of our perceptions. The telescope has brought near the distant, and enabled us to grasp the dimensions of the vast; while the microscope has equally extended the sphere of our observations in the other direction, and enabled us to perceive the existence of the minute: still, there is an infinity of magnitude beyond the powers of the telescope, and an infinity of minuteness which no microscope can reveal.

Circumstantial evidence in law is often as strong as positive testimony; and inferential proof may carry as clear conviction as an alleged fact; and the inferential proof, in this case, has left upon the minds of many not a reasonable doubt of the existence of a specific poison—a material substance as the cause of cholera. It should be remembered that *marsh miasmata* has never been detected by any sensible test; yet what intelligent physician doubts its existence? The evidence is entirely inferential; we believe in its existence, because certain effects which we observe cannot be as well accounted for by any other supposition. In the same manner, and about as clearly, we come to the conclusion that cholera has a specific and material substance as its essential cause. If this be admitted, it is difficult to see how, in the present state of our knowledge, we can avoid the conclusion that this material must have the form of one or other of the substances before enumerated. They embrace the whole inorganic world, capable of such free movement and wide-spread activity, and all the known forms of organized existences, capable of the same subtle extension.

This speculative part of the subject has been dwelt upon at such

---

* The term *zymotic* has come now by a pretty general consent, particularly in England, to be applied to all epidemic diseases, and signifies that material specific poisons are the essential causes of these diseases; but the term is restricted in its meaning beyond this, and made to imply that these poisons act on the blood in the manner of a *ferment;* but, as I am not prepared to adopt this view, to the exclusion of all others, I have not used the term.

length, because it is believed to contain essential truth, and because, in the absence of positive knowledge upon a subject of so much interest, plausible theories have their uses. They often lead to the full discovery of truth; and, besides, give some definite and precise ideas, which, though they be hypothetical, have a more satisfactory and salutary effect on the mind than no ideas at all, or than those that are vague and undefined, floating loosely beyond the verge of distinct conceptions.

But we proceed to a branch of the subject less doubtful in its nature, and more practical in its character; viz: The *predisposing causes* of Cholera,—or the circumstances and conditions, as it regards localities and persons, which favor the spread of the essential Cholera-cause, and render it more effectual and fatal. Whatever view may be taken respecting the nature, or even the existence of the specific poison, it is certain that in order to give it a potency and effect, certain other conditions must exist. These have been much dwelt upon, and their general features pretty well established in the opinion of the profession. It should be confessed, however, that in particular cases, general rules have been set at defiance,—the facts, however, are sufficiently uniform to establish the general rules. Briefly, and generally stated, the localities most liable to its spread, other things being equal, are low, moist, and particularly filthy situations. Warm climates and seasons rather more favorable than cold, and a densely populated region more than one scarcely settled.— It is more liable to follow water-courses and thoroughfares, partly because these are usually more low, filthy, and densely populated, and partly, we believe, because the morbid matter is conveyed by intercommunication. Still, it takes general, and sometimes particular causes in obedience to laws we do not understand.

With regard to classes of persons most liable to be attacked and to become its victims,—the intemperate, the destitute, the filthy, the vicious, the enfeebled, the terrified, and the degraded, are immeasurably more subject to its ravages than those in opposite conditions. Yet, when the poison is in abundance, and possessing great activity, no class or condition can claim an exemption, and none can boast a complete immunity from danger. Yet the cases are so rare in which the poison is sufficiently intense to effect perfectly healthy persons, who place themselves under the most favorable circumstances, avoid all predisposing causes, and, in short, obey all the Hygienic laws, that the violation of these laws,—or, in other words, these *predisposing causes*, in a vast majority of cases at least, become necessary antecedently to the production of the disease. So much have the habits and state of individuals to do with the prevalence, or suppression of this scourge, that, as a general proposition, it may be stated that "the Cholera poison owes its potentiality to the conditions in which it finds the subjects of its invasion." If this be so, these particular predisposing causes possess the deepest interest, and are worthy of a more particular consideration. Dr. Wm. B. Carpenter, in a very able article in a recent number of the British and Foreign Medico Chirugical Review, advances the doctrine that the essential, or at least most important condition predisposing to all epidemic diseases, consists in the existence in the blood of decomposing matter, and shows that those influences which have generally been regarded as predisposing causes, and which he proves are such, all, or nearly all, tend to produce that condition of the vital fluid. And he argues that in this disease, the Cholera poison is rendered potent in the system, by operating through decomposing materials. He arranges the generally-recognised predispositions, causes of these diseases, Cholera, &c., under three heads, viz: 1. Those which tend to introduce into the system decomposing matter that has been generated in some external source. 2. Those which occasion an increased production of decomposing matter in the system itself; and, 3. Those which obstruct the elimination of the decomposing matter naturally or excessively generated within the system, or abnormally introduced into it from without.

1. Under the first head he ranks the ingestion of putrescent food, water, contaminated by sewerage or other decomposing matter, and the inspiration of air charged with putrescent or miasmatic emanations.

2. Under the second, any unusual source of degeneration of tissues within the body, such as excessive muscular exercise, injuries, &c.; and I would add, fear, dependency, and other depressing passions, and the derangement of secretions.

3. Under the third, an insufficient supply of air, a high external temperature, (which slackens the respiratory process) and the ingestion of alcohol; to which I would add, the sudden occurrence of a cooler and moister atmosphere, as a rain-storm after unusual heat.

Whatever may be thought of Dr. Carpenter's theory, if we add to this category insufficient food, and whatever cause not enumerated, which will depress the vital energies, and add particularly, all those substances, whether in the shape of indigestible food or of medicines, which will irritate the mucous membrane of the stomach and bowels, and we have embraced the predisposing causes of Cholera.

The Cholera, as it appeared under my observation in Chicago, during the summers of 1851 and '52, corroborate the views which have been taken, respecting the etiology of the disease. In 1852, as City Physician, I gave it more especial attention, seeing a large proportion of the cases which occurred. The disease commenced on the 18th of May. It had prevailed for some time before at New Orleans, St. Louis, and on the Mississippi and Illinois rivers at various points. The first four cases in Chicago, occurred in persons who were residents of the city, and had not left it for several months. The very first case occurred in a mechanic, who had been making some repairs upon a canal-boat which had come over the canal from La Salle, a town about one hundred miles distant, at the head of navigation of the Illinois river, and where there had been a few cases of the disease. It proved fatal. No case nearer than La Salle, had previously been known. The next well-marked case occurred on the 21st of May, three days after. It was in a man who had spent the winter in the county poor-house, several miles from the city, but who had been in town at labor since the opening of spring,— was in a distant part of the city from the first, and had had no connection with him. This man was of a feeble constitution, and rather irregular habits,—was lodging in a low boarding-house in a filthly lane, where large numbers were crowded together in small apartments, illy-ventilated, and where personal and domestic cleanliness were neglected. He was in an advanced stage when first seen and soon died. The next case was in another part of the city, occurring about the same date, and in a man of decided intemperate habits, and was fatal. I did not see this case, but a report of it was received from a reliable source. The fourth case occurred three days after, in the same boarding house with the second, in a laborer of intemperate habits, but was seen before the full collapsed stages occurred, and recovered. The next two cases were attacked on canal-boats, between La Salle and Chicago, and were brought into the city early in the morning of the 26th. These were in an advanced stage, and were both fatal. No other cases were reported or came to my knowledge until June 1st. A case then occurred in an intemperate laboring man, in a part of the city rather remote from any of the others, and having no connection with them. On the 3d and 4th, several cases occurred in different parts of the city, no connection being traced between any of them and other previous cases; and from this time, evidence was daily afforded that the Cholera poison pervaded every part of the city, with only sufficient intensity, however, to become active upon those who were under the influence of the predisposing causes. The tide of emigration soon began to pour in, principally from Sweden and Germany, and the disease during the whole season, (it continued until the middle of November, attacking, in a population of 40,000, about 1,5-00, and reaching a mortality of six-hundred and twenty-nine) was confined almost exclusively to these emigrants, and to the lowest and most destitute class of foreign Irish, Dutch, and German residents. The Swedish emigrants suffered more severely than any other class. For most of the summer they were arriving almost daily, and often in large numbers. Driven from their sterile native hills by poverty and the severest necessity, they were huddled together in crowded emigrant-ships, where their destitution of means could obtain for them only the most scanty accommodations, and hurried immediately on from ship-board by the most speedy conveyance, most of them by railroad, in crowded emigrant-cars, with the filth, as well as the other morbid influences of their long sea voyage still upon them — this being their first stopping place after leaving their distant homes, and here their first opportunity for gratifying a ravenous appetite for green, acid, indigestible, and often putrid substances—already laboring, as many of them were, under severe diarrhœa, they were in the most susceptible condition possible for the action of the Cholera poison; and when exposed to it, where it existed in a degree insufficient to affect seriously, those who were in an ordinarily healthy condition were seized in great numbers, and unless the most prompt and efficient assistance was rendered, were swept off with the greatest rapidity. The almost total exemption of our regular, well-to-do citizens, amid such prevalence of the disease among the opposite class, shows very strikingly, the influence of personal habits and conditions upon the prevalence of the disease, and the particulars in which the habits and conditions of the respective classes differed, point out unmistakably what the predisposing causes are. They are such as have already been enumerated, and most of them need not be more particularly dwelt upon. From numerous facts which came within my observation, I am well persuaded that the quality of water drank, had an important influence upon the susceptibility to attacks of Cholera.

At the time to which reference is made, the whole of the city of Chicago was not supplied with pure water from the lake, by means of the hydraulic works as now. The city is situated upon a plain, varying not more than twenty feet, in the more inhabitable parts, from a level. It is separated into three divisions, South, North and West, by the Chicago river, which extends from lake Michigan, west, and divides into two branches at nearly right angles from the main trunk, about a mile from its mouth. The subsoil is clay, with a rich alluvium upon the surface mingled with sand. The south division was principally supplied with water from the old hydraulic works then in operation, while the west division was supplied only to a limited extent, and the north division was entirely destitute of such supply. In this division, and in most of the west, and also in the outskirts of the south, the inhabitants were supplied with water either from cart-men drawing it in barrels from the lake, or from wells in which the water was a short distance from the surface of the earth, and necessarily received much of the filth and decomposing matter from it. It was in fact surface water, not as a general thing receiving its supply from any other source than the rain that fell upon the surface, and found its way immediately through the soil into these superficial excavations. Nearly all of the inhabitants who were in comfortable circumstances, procured their water from the cartmen, while many of the poor used the surface water where it was not too intolerable to be thought of. There were very few cases of Cholera, almost literally none, in the south division where the hydrant water was used,—as little among the well-to-do inhabitants who procured water from the carts, while those who used the surface or well water, which doubtless contained a considerable portion of decomposing matter, were the persons who principally suffered. This might have been considered as due to other circumstances in their condition, had it not been for the following fact: In some parts of the city inhabited by a class of persons in quite as bad, and even worse hygienic condition in every other respect,—where the ground was so low that the water was almost at the surface, and was so filthy as absolutely to prevent its being used, the people being obliged to get water from the carts, the Cholera prevailed to a much less extent than in more elevated and more cleanly parts inhabited by the poor, but where the surface water was used. We had there the unusual phenomenon, the very reverse of what has occurred so generally elsewhere—of Cholera prevailing more in the localities where the altitude was greatest. But such was the case where no other recognised fact could account for it, than the use of the surface water.

I am constrained to mention one other circumstance in the history of Cholera in this city during the summer of 1852, over which, were it not for the cause of truth and humanity, I would gladly draw the veil of forgetfulness:

Soon after the outbreak of Cholera, the building which had been previously erected as a Cholera Hospital was burned down. A Small-Pox Hospital, or Pest-house, was located about two miles from the more densely inhabited portion of the city, and had a few inmates with Small-Pox. As Cholera cases were found by the Health Officers in the streets, and as admission into dwellings could not be obtained, there was a temporary necessity for taking them to the only building belonging to the city, and cases of Small-Pox and Cholera were put into the same building together, though not into the same room. The Cholera poison was thus conveyed there, and the circumstances seemed favorable for its multiplication. The effects were most disastrous upon those having Small-Pox, and the cases of Cholera which occurred in the house were of the severest possible grade. While cases of the Cholera were being brought to this place, a family of German emigrants, consisting of a father, mother, and five children, were found in a lumber yard by the Health Officers, the mother having Small-Pox, and two of the children a mild form of Varioloid. As the agents of the public conveyances refused to take them on to their destination in the interior, and as no house would receive them, or any part of them, the whole family were taken to the Pest-house. After being necessarily all together in one room for a few days, the father, a vigorous man of thirty-five or forty, slept as usual during the night, and awoke at six the next morning and started to go out of the house. He fell exhausted just outside the door, had a very slight evacuation from the bowels, was helped to his bed, and was seen by me a little after 7 A.M. With no other evacuations, he was then in the most profound collapse,—perfectly pulseless at the wrist, cold, shrivelled, intensely blue, and died at nine the next morning. Within two days, three of the children and the mother died, with fully developed Cholera symptoms, running their course in unusually short periods, some of them being dead, though due diligence was used, before I was able to see them. The two remaining children were immediately sent away, and escaped the disease. In justice to myself, I must say that I used all the influence I possessed, to prevent this mingling of these diseases, even under the pressure of the apparent necessity, and a Cholera Hospital was soon erected. How far the Small-Pox and Cholera poisons mutually influenced each other, or whether they had any effect, are questions of interest; but one thing is certain, that in an experience of twelve-hundred cases of Cholera, I have never witnessed such virulence of the disease, as occurred at this place within these few days.

With a reference to the following historical incident, I shall close the subject of the *cause* of Cholera, and then proceed to consider its nature and *treatment.*

Dr. Verrollot, Physician to the French Embassy, near the Sublime Porte, has written a minute history of the spread of the epidemic in 1847 through Asia and a part of Europe. In describing its general spread and terrible ravages, from the shores of the Caspian Sea, up the River Volga, among the semi-civilized Musselmen, and still more filthy and degraded Russians, he mentions with great, but reasonable enthusiasm, one place as a remarkable exception:

"There is a small Moravian colony called Sarepta, situated in a bend of the river, in the midst of the Kalmuck hordes, eulogised by all travelers for its remarkable industry and minute cleanliness; and for all other laudable and fortunate features of character. The Cholera seemed to respect this sacred spot, passing by in 1830 and in 1847, without inflicting on it the least evil." This fact, corroborated as it is by others of like character, speaks volumes on the subject of prevention, and leaves nothing farther necessary to be said. If the inhabited globe were a Sarepta this terrible scourge would disappear from it forever. The conditions for the multiplication and extension of the poison, would cease to exist, and there would be no subjects favorable to its attack.

(TO BE CONTINUED.)

CHICAGO, January 3d, 1853.

ART. II.—*The Birds of Michigan.* By CHARLES FOX.

Since the list of Michigan Birds was printed in the October number of this Journal, a skin of the bird supposed to be the common buzzard, (Buteo vulgaris) was sent to DR. CASSIN, the well known ornithologist, of Philadelphia, and by him decided to be the young of the red-breasted buzzard, (Buteo lineatus). This species has already caused much confusion, by its change of plumage. The young was described by Wilson as a distinct species, under the name of *Falco hyemalis;* and, again, as a third species by Nuttall, as *Falco buteoides.* It does not appear to be common on the Detroit river, in any stage of plumage; but the writer has occasionally observed one or two young birds for a short time in the autumn. This year it was uncommonly abundant, and was to be found in or near marshes. Three specimens, which were procured, had the stomach full of frogs; to which, in two instances, a small snake, apparently the young of *Eutainia Sirtalis* (Baird) was added; but in none of them was there a trace either of birds or quadrupeds.

To my former list, I am able to add the following, now in the museum of "the Flint Scientific Institute,"—a society formed in the beginning of this year, (1853) for the investigation of the Natural History, Meteorology, and Agriculture of that region. Though a beginning only has been made, some valuable works have already been purchased, and about ninety birds are stuffed, and deposited in the museum, together with specimens from other departments, including Botany. I am indebted to the politeness of the President, DR. DANIEL CLARK, for the catalogue in which I find the following:—

Cape May Wood-Warbler,	Sylvicola Maritima,
Canada Wood-Warbler,	———— Canadensis,
Black and Yellow Warblers.	———— Maculosa.
Ruby-Crowned Knight,	Regulus Calendula,
Golden-eye Duck,	Fuligula Clangula.

A fortnight since, a bird resembling this last was picked up in the Detroit river, recently dead; and a doubt has arisen whether it is the young of this common *eastern* species, or the *C. Barrovii*, discovered by Richardson in the Hudson Bay country. The two, in the adult state, very greatly resemble each other, but the young male of the latter has never been described. Audubon does not seem to have met with the young even of the *F. Clangula*. The most marked distinction, in the adult birds, is, that in the *common* species, the white patch at the base of the bill is oval, and in the northern species it is crescent shaped. The latter is also a larger bird. It were well for our naturalists to pay attention to this, for these lakes are the very place to find occasional specimens of the north-western birds, especially of the *Anatinae*. Dr Clark adds a list of birds " known to be in that section, but which have not as yet been secured." The following among the number mentioned are now in this State:—

White-winged Crossbill,	Loxia leucoptera,
Summer Red Bird, (of the Eastern States,)	Pyranga aestiva.

Art. III.—*To the Editor of the Peninsular Journal of Medicine:*

Sir:—During the past summer, I attended a *Post Mortem* examination held upon the body of Mrs. W. of this town, who died of disease of the stomach and liver. For a number of years before her death, she had been subject to attacks of vomiting, chills, spasmodic pain in the right hypochondriac and the precordial regions, which often lasted for several days. These attacks, as I had been informed by her former physician, had been relieved by anodynes, antispasmodics, the warm bottle and by the natural effort of vomiting; and she was able to perform her accustomed domestic labors till about two years since, when she was taken more severely ill than usual, and at the instance of an interested person sent for one of that class of physicians who style themselves Homœopathists. Dr. Small Pill was her medical adviser until about ten days before she died, when we were sent for.

What she had taken during this period, we are unable to say; except that she had been supplied at our office, with sulph. morphine, which she was advised to take by her homœopathic doctor, and which she had found to be the only medicine that afforded her any relief from the pain, &c., which she often suffered from.

For the last few days of her sickness, vomiting had been almost incessant, and all the means used to arrest it were ineffectual. At the autopsy, the mucous coat of the stomach was found thickened, softened, and of a dark color. The liver contained numerous cavities, in which were found calculi about the size and shape of the common *buckwheat* kernel. They were dark externally and yellowish within, and could be broken with but little force, when tried. There was also found, throughout its substance, a quantity of thick, yellowish matter, conveying to the fingers when rubbed between them, a gritty sensation. In the *gall bladder* were found a number of larger calculous concretions, but quite similar in shape to those found in the substance of the liver, and embedded in the same yellowish, soft, gritty matter.

These were quite too large to pass the duct into the duodenum, but many smaller ones had evidently passed, occasioning the attacks of spasmodic pain, chills, vomiting, &c. No other internal marks of disease were perceptible, but the skin was of the yellowish color usually seen in affections of the liver.

One thing further in regard to our homœopathic friend, and we have done. He seized one of the larger calculi, carefully laid it aside, and confidentially told Dr. C., that he *intended to prescribe it in proper doses, the next case of the kind he might be called to treat!* (Similia similibus, curantur).　　　　　　　　　　　　　　　　　　　**C.**

SELECTIONS.

Report of the Committee on Medical Education. Extracted from the Transactions of the American Medical Association.

The undersigned, members of a standing committee, being required by a rule of the National Medical Association to prepare a report on the general condition of medical education in the United States; to compare it with the state of medical education in other enlightened countries; to notice the courses of instruction; the requirements for graduation; the modes of examination for conferring degrees; the number of pupils and graduates at the several medical institutions in the United States; to notice, also, the prerequisites to appointment in the medical staff of the Army and Navy; the legal requirements exacted of medical practitioners in the several States; and all such measures, established or prospective, in reference to medical education, and the reputable standing of the profession, as may be deemed worthy of special consideration, beg leave to submit the following remarks, made in compliance therewith, as their Report.

On turning to the records of the Association, the Committee have had the gratification to find that the ground assigned them to occupy, has been so faithfully cultivated by their predecessors, that there remains but little for them to do. A brief analysis of the reports heretofore submitted to the Association, aiming, as they all do, to advance the dignity and augment the legitimate influence of the profession of medicine in the United States, might seem to be a sufficient compliance with the requirements of the rule under which the Committee are called to act; but as each of their predecessors, notwithstanding the unity of their purpose, have expressed opinions in some respects, distinctive, it has been thought best, by your Committee, even if the *Transactions* should appear tautological, to present their own views on some of the subjects referred to them, and leave to the Association the responsibility of their repetition.

In one or another of the reports on the general subject of medical education, ranging from 1847 to 1851, careful and accurate statements on the several subdivisions which follow have been made, to which we beg leave to refer, in order to save the necessity of recapitulation.

1. The number of medical schools in the United States.
2. The number of professors in each school.
3. The length of the lecture term in each.
4. The qualifications of prerequisites to admission.
5. The qualifications of candidates for degrees.
6. The number of students in attendance.
7. The ratio of practitioners to the population.

8. The names of those States which have and those which have no laws on the subject of medicine.

9. The effect of repealing the statute in those States where conservative laws once existed in relation to medical practitioners.

10. A comparative view of the colleges of medicine in the United States and in Europe; of the preparatory training to which medical students are subjected on the two continents and the islands of Great Britain; of the subjects they are required to study after matriculating; the relative length of their terms of pupilage; and the relative number and rigor of the examinations to which they are subjected after their course of instruction has terminated.

The latter topic was fully discussed by the Committee for 1849, and was presented to the Association in a manner well calculated to arouse the pride of the profession in the United States, and intended evidently to stimulate that sentiment, so as to bring its power to bear in such a manner as would erase the evidences of the disparity which confessedly exists between our own schools and those of the continent of Europe. A disparity which has no reference to the character of our public teachers, but grows out of the difference in the political organizations or governments of the different countries in which the schools are situated. A strongly conservative government, which exercises an attribute of sovereignty in restraining unqualified persons from assuming to exercise the functions of a physician, has a right also to require the highest order of qualifications from those to whom it accords that privilege, and the right of exacting a pecuniary *honorarium* therefor. Very different is the case where sovereignty resides in the masses, and where that sovereign is morbidly jealous of every thing to which the idea of monopoly can attach. Hence it is important to keep in mind that there is some relation between the government of a country and the practice of medicine therein, in all that we propose to do to increase its respectability.

Although the report just quoted, was drawn up with great care and ability, and was the result of laborious inquiry, and embodies a much greater amount of information than either of the others, it will be found that each one possesses merits peculiar to itself; some dwelling most upon the facts of history, whilst others have ventured more widely into the region of opinions, and the discussions necessary to their elucidation. All, however, tend to one point; the aim of all being, through the instrumentality of this Association, to arouse the profession of the country to such an effort as shall shake from itself the reproach of ignorance and of quackery, by which it has been humbled in its own estimation, and abased in that of its fellow-men.

Your Committee are pleased to bring, from the different sections of the country in which they reside, gratifying assurances, that the labors of this Association have thus far been fruitful of good results. The voluntary principle in its organization, and its representative character, increases from year to year its moral power and influence, which have been made manifest in the increase of State and County societies, and in the efforts which many of the medical schools have made to conform to its recommendations.

With a view to remedy the evils that are admitted to exist in our system of medical instruction, the following suggestions have been offered by previous committees:

1. That there should be made in all cases, by those designing to become medical students, a more extended and thorough preparation for entering upon professional studies than is usual in the United States.

2. That all candidates for the degree of M.D. shall have studied three years, including the time allotted to attendance upon lectures.

3. That they shall have devoted at least three months to dissections, one term to hospital practice, and

4. Shall have attended two full courses of lectures.

5. That the faculty of the several medical colleges insist upon the fulfillment of these requirements, and upon a faithful attendance by the students on the lectures of the professors.

6. That candidates for degrees be examined at the close of the first term in certain specified studies; the effect of which would be, practically, to divide the studies into those appertaining to a junior and a senior year.

7. That the number of professors be increased to seven, and the lecture term extended to six months.

8. That measures be adopted to prevent the multiplication of medical schools.

9. That the business of teaching be conducted by bodies distinct from those who may be authorized to grant licenses or diplomas.

The foregoing is an epitome of the subjects which the several committees, in whose footsteps we are compelled, in a great degree, to walk, have presented to the consideration of the Association from year to year, and, by it, has been laid before the profession of the United States.

Of the opinions that have been expressed, and not embodied in the form of distinct propositions, for the adoption of the Association, is not so easy to give an abstract.

In 1848, an invitation was given by the Association to all the Medical Institutions in the Union, to forward each year, to the Chairman of the Committee on Medical Education, a copy of their catalogue and the annual announcement of their plan of instruction for that year. It is to be regretted, that this invitation has not been so far complied with, as to enable the Committee to show what changes have been made by the medical schools, or what advances they have made towards the realization of the ideal of the National Association.

Enough, however, has been received to authorize the Committee to say, that there is a general desire, not only on the part of the schools, but in the great body of the profession, to come up to the national standard. This disposition has manifested itself in various ways. Some of the colleges have lengthened their regular term of lectures, or create d new professorships, and added new subjects to the curriculum of studies. Others have established preparatory or supplementary courses of lectures as a means of meeting the new demand made upon them, in consequence of the agitation of this subject, since the organization of the National Association. The private practitioner has taken new views of duty, and

refused to admit into his office the unqualified applicant, and the local
societies have voluntarily erected barriers to his taking the initial step in
that direction.

Yet, notwithstanding the vigorous efforts already made, and still in
action, judiciously designed to elevate the character of the alumni of
the various schools in the country, the number of those who fill the
ranks of the profession without education is not perceptibly diminished.
For this evil, in the present state of public sentiment, and in the absence
of laws, which are but organizations of public opinion, for the prohibit-
ion of quackery, there seems to be but one effective remedy. Although
the education of those who flock to the public schools may become more
general, and even more thorough than at present contemplated, so that
the professional character of the pupils may reflect honor upon their alma
mater, there will be found, in the same theatre of action, another set of
men, naturally as astute, perhaps, who, knowing the worth or pecuniary
value of a popular, in contradistinction to a professional reputation, successfully appeal to the prejudices of that public whose higher judicial
tribunals confirm in every man the right to assume the title of Doctor,
and his equal right to demand and receive the *honorarium* due to medical attainment and professional skill.

Your Committee, as they conceive, have sufficiently elevated ideas of
the mission which the medical colleges now in being are designed to
fulfil, and feel an honorable pride in tracing their professional paternity
to this source. They also feel, that one thing more is wanted as a remedy for the evil just referred to, and that is the establishment of free
colleges for the preparatory and professional education of the young men
now scattered over the wide and half-cultivated domain of the West.

To show that such a measure can be carried into effect, notwithstanding the popular character of our political institutions, the Committee take
the liberty of alluding very briefly to the organization of the University
of Michigan, which is the only institution in the country endowed by
Government and regulated by State authority. By the medical faculty
of the University, all candidates for the degree of M.D. are rigidly required to comply with the conditions of the National Medical Association,
except attendance upon hospital cliniques, and have been notified that,
in the future, it is in comtemplation to exact the same preparation for
admission to the medical as is now prescribed for membership of the
department of arts. As an incentive to the prosecution of classical
studies, one year will be deducted from the term of medical studies of all
students who graduate first in the department of arts.

The lecture term in the college of medicine of this university extends
from October to April—seven months. During this time, there are
five professors daily or continuously on duty, who are restricted to four
lectures each day. Daily examinations are made on the subjects of the
day preceding. The pupils are divided into two classes, seniors and juniors ; and the seniors into two sections, one of which reads essays on
medical subjects every Saturday. The juniors may engage in this exercise, and, being stimulated by the example of the seniors, many of
them do so, to their obvious advantage. At the close of the first term,

ical instruction, on which they propose to speak more freely than has been customary in this Association. We admit its great importance ; but we question its utility to the majority of students who annually throng the lecture-rooms of our metropolitan schools ; to which they are led, not for the sake of seeing practice in the hospitals, but by the attractive talent of the professors, and the intellectual charm of the lecture-room.

It is not our design to treat with disrespect any remark which may have been made heretofore on this subject, yet our sense of accountability to the great body of our constituency, compels us, in some measure, to dissent from former opinions, or, at least, to state the case in such a way, as shall lead to opposite conclusions, if not to reforms in practice.

To avoid misapprehension, we will reassert the expression of our faith in the value of bedside experience to the medical neophyte, and propose only in the remarks which follow, to show that this cannot be attained by young men passing in groups, and in all stages of preparation, through the wards of a hospital, at the heels of a professor. To suppose an example. An elegant and practical lecture has just been delivered on the subject of pleuro-pneumonia. The class is dismissed from the lecture-room and reassemble at the hospital. The surgeon leads them from ward to ward, in which they find varicose ulcers, chancres, buboes fistulas in ano, and such like affections, incident to men worn out by vice, and who are brought together by diseases, vice and want. Of course, the students see no particular relation between the theme of the professor and the cases in thehospital.

But having purchased the tickets of the professors, and paid for the privilege of visiting the hospital, in conformity to the requirements of the faculty, and in compliance with what he supposes to be the prevalent opinion of the profession, the student makes another visit, and by dint of effort, he gets within sight of the patient, and in hearing of the gentleman, who devotes a minute's attention to a case which may be one of obstructive disease of the mitral and tricuspid valves. The young man's preparation for this interview may have been a lecture, from his anatomical professor, on the osseous tissue, in which he had been shown its mode of developement and chemical composition, without ever having dreamed that the earthy material of bone, or the cartilaginous nidus, in which it is naturally deposited, could ever, by abnormal action or arrangement, be the occasion of the dyspnœa and the serious deposits, which he sees in the case before him. In the next bed, perhaps, is an idiopathic dropsy. He perceives that decumbitus is painful in both—that respiration is embarrassed in each, and that the cellular tissue in the two are alike filled with water. He hears just enough from the teacher to confound his own perceptions of the analogies in the two cases, gets a wrong impression of the value of clinical instruction, and soon discontinues his visits to the hospital. This is not a fancy sketch, but a scene of yearly occurrence.

If this sketch is not a fiction, it seems to the Committee, to teach the necessity of placing restrictions upon admission to the wards of a hospital, and an equal necessity of filling the minds of young men with a knowledge of the structure, functions, and chemistry of man's organi-

those who design to graduate at the University are examined in anatomy, physiology, materia medica, and chemistry. Their final examination takes place in presence of the Censors of the State Medical Society, and, as an incentive to excellence, at that time, the Board of Regents, by whom the degrees are conferred, authorize the Faculty to select one of the theses, if one be deemed worthy, for publication, by the Superintendent of Public Instruction in his annual report, which, being a public document, is printed by legislative authority.

We are aware that former committees have objected to an increase in the number of medical schools, so situated as not to give to their pupils the benefits of hospital practice, the reasons for which, at first sight, appeared entirely satisfactory, and may do so now to a large majority of this Association. We believe, that this subject should be examined from two distinct points of view, one of which exhibits the character and qualifications of those who graduate at the best schools, and the other, the character and influence in society of that other multitude, who choose to exclude themselves from all these advantages, but come, nevertheless, by some illegitimate entrance, into the great professional amphitheatre. If there was a necessity for studying this subject only from the first point of view—of looking only to the effects produced upon the pupil by his attendance upon the college lectures and the hospital clinique, and if we could leave out of sight and out of mind the great number of practitioners with which the country would be filled—if the elementary schools of medicine were any less accessible than they now are—there would be no division in sentiment ; no dissent from the opinions expressed by preceding committees, touching this matter. If there were in existence laws, which could be enforced, for restraining irregularities in practice, and if none dared exercise the functions of the physician except he were regularly invested with the baton of office, there would be great propriety in limiting the number of schools, and at the same time increasing their demand upon the mental energies of the pupil, as conditions precedent to receiving a degree.

In the absence of such laws, and for the want of any power to bear upon the profession, other than the power of opinion, the wisest course, in the judgment of your Committee, would be, to extend the hand of fellowship to all such schools as, having a competent faculty, shall give a course of lectures on general, comparative, and descriptive anatomy, physiology, and its application to pathology ; chemistry, with its relations to pharmacy and toxicology ; materia medica and therapeutics, the principles of surgery, obstetrics, including the doctrine of ovology ; and the principles and practice of medicine.

If such schools could be restricted in conferring degrees to the grade of Bachelor of Medicine, a practical and valuable distinction would be made between those which teach the elements of medical science, and that other class, having their seat in the great commercial cities, and whose propinquity to hospitals enable them, if their advantages are rightly improved, to combine the inculcation of principles with their practical application and elucidation.

By this remark, the Committee are led directly to the subject of clin-

zation, and all that relates to his normal condition as a psychic and physical existence, before they be allowed to take note of the abnormal deviations to which man is liable, or to think of prescribing a remedy for those deviations, when they have occurred.

An eminent professional writer, of the early part of the present century, in his letters on the education of a surgeon, makes some remarks so *germain* to the object we have in view, that of showing the futility of teaching clinical medicine to young men who have no knowledge of anatomy, that the Committee are tempted to incorporate them into this part of their report.

"If it were my wish to inspire a young man with professional enthusiasm, I should expect to accomplish it in no way so happily as by teaching him to study, night and day, the structure of the human body ; to witness no form of disease, without comparing the symptoms with the natural functions, the probable changes which cause disorder, with the natural and healthy condition ; to dissect and to meditate. The man thus prepared for practice, and pursuing through life those inquiries with diligence, would show himself in every professional act, a feeling and a thinking man ; for reasoning on the probable changes going on within the body, has a powerful effect on the manners and feelings of a physician ; and he will be most involved in serious thoughts and compassionate feelings, who connects every symptom with some probable change and that change with the sufferings and probable fate of his friend. He examines with unaffected anxiety the seat of internal disease, and is agitated by every alteration of countenance, and by every sensible change. He takes a double interest in the fate of his patient ; because, along with a malady painfully affecting a fellow-creature and a friend, he is occupied in watching certain phenomena in the animal machine, certain progressive disorders in its particular organs, which, from a long study of their structure, he foresees are likely to happen, and the signs of those changes are the presages of life or death." *(John Bell.)*

This is what, in the language of the botanist, may emphatically be called the "natural method" of showing that medicine may be exalted to the dignity of a science, though often reduced to the level of a trade. It is the method the Committee ask the Association to indorse. A thorough knowledge of the principles and elements of the science of medicine should precede any attempt at their practical application.

On the subject of clinical instruction, the Committee, from its intrinsic importance, have been induced to bestow a good deal of attention. Its Chairman, having for twenty years of his professional life been in charge of a hospital, either in the army or in civil life, feels authorized to ask the Association to revise its opinions heretofore expressed. He knows, and feels that everybody else should know, how improper it would be to allow a class of medical students, one after another, to auscultate a patient in the advanced stage of consumption, and how little they would learn from a clinical lecture without it. One object to be accomplished in bringing together the pupil and the patient is to train the perceptive faculties of the student ; to educate, in fact, his sense of touch, his eye, and his ear. How much progress is made in this process, except by the resident pupil of a hospital, is very well known by students and teachers.

Because the end has not yet been attained, we would by no means relinquish the pursuit. We would reconstruct our hospital organizations, and adapt them to the wants of the time. This could be done by erecting them into schools of practice, with a special faculty, whose plan of instruction should have a direct relation to the cases in their wards, so that each one should become an illustration of the text of the professor. Schools thus constituted, and authorized to confer some distinctive honor upon their graduates, would fill a hiatus in our system of medical teaching. A supplementary school of practice, conducted on the plan proposed, would obviate the objections now made to clinical instruction, and do away very much with the sentiment of feeling of jealousy entertained towards the medical schools in the country, which not only do great good, but prevent infinite evil. How they do this, is best understood by those members of the Association who come from sections of the country sparsely populated. They are best aware how many young men, without their instrumentality, would pass from the office of the private preceptor without the advantages these schools can give them, wanting in that professional *esprit de corps*, which the associations of the anatomical theatre and the lecture-room, do so much to foster the growth of in the breast of every graduate who recognizes the influence of a medical alma mater. This Committee, then, would not discourage the organization of medical schools in different sections of our country, but would foster them as places fitted and designed to teach the elements of the science of medicine, and trust to the influence and example of the private instructor, who is emphatically the true clinical teacher, and to the hospitals, as schools of practice, to teach the art of applying the principles, which the faculties of these schools have imparted. In this way, the number of uneducated young men, now permitted, by the absence of salutary laws in all the States of the Union, with only one exception, to exercise the functions of physicians, will annually diminish, and be replaced by those having a higher sense of professional honor, because a wider range of professional attainments.

Having achieved this, and so far added to the respectability of our profession, the Committee would urge the Association to take one more step, scarcely less important, as a means of augmenting its usefulness, on the supposition that its usefulness depends essentially upon its respectability, and to insist upon a more thorough and extended course of preparatory study before commencing that of medicine. In the existing state of public sentiment, we would give to preparatory scarcely less consequence than to professional education. The first, being more appreciable by the public, helps the physician to take that social position which furnishes to his colleagues the strongest guarantee that he will never sink to the level of the quack or the mountebank. When, as at the present time, by the establishment of schools of science and departments of agriculture in our colleges, the artisan is made familiar with the elementary forms of the matter to which his skill is to be applied, and the tiller of the soil is made acquainted with the geological structure of his farm, of the principles in chemistry by which he applies the elements of fertility to his fields, of the organization and habits of the plants best adapted to the soil, and of their relations to the meteorology of the climate in which he lives, there is an evident necessity for his medical friend having some general knowledge of these subjects, on account of their hygenic relations to his patrons, among whom may be individuals of the classes just described.

The necessity of a thorough preparation for professional study is not an idea of recent origin. The Father of Medicine held that, to be an eminent physician, it was necessary not only to be well acquainted with the structure of the human frame, but also to be skilled in logic, astronomy, and other sciences; and of him it may be truly said that he cultivated the art of medicine upon the strict principles of the inductive philosophy, more than two thousand years before the world gave Lord Bacon the credit of introducing this method of philosophizing. His devoted admirer, Galen, was skilled in all the sciences of the day—in logic, mathematics, rhetoric, and philosophy.

Aside from the influence of authority, or the obvious power it gives him of making an impression on the popular mind, there are other considerations which should induce the student to devote his early years to the study of the classics; to researches in metaphysics, mathematics, and the natural sciences. The light that they shed upon his professional path, shows that each of these departments of study has the quality of a lens, which concentrates its rays upon and gives brilliancy and distinctness to every medical subject on which they are brought to bear.

In our utilitarian age, the study of the classics is discouraged, because they do not obviously tend to increase the amount of " daily bread " in any given community. " That they conduce to mental vigor, and prepare the mind for professional pursuits, and lead to those refinements of thought, and delicacies in sentiment and action, so essential to the physician, is it not a matter of sufficient importance to counterbalance the loss of time expended in their pursuit? Polished language, delicate manners, and fastidious taste, and solitary studies, an indifference to common praise, or vulgar abuse, characterize the man devoted to learning. A classical education is found to exalt the generous affections, and, by examples of prudence, patience, and self-command, teaches at once a just contempt for the vexations of the world, and enthusiasm in behalf of humanity and of science, and purifies the mind from low pursuits."

Although the practical metaphysician has been styled the Jesuit of modern literature, and the study itself been treated with scorn, we would not have it omitted by the student of medicine.

It has been asked, what will a head filled with the categories of Aristotle, the forty Summa Genera of Bishop Wilkins, or even the refined and exquisite metaphysics of Dr. Gregory, do, in curing the maladies of the human body? This becomes a pertinent question at a time when the professional mind is directed to psychological studies, in connection with insanity, and especially as the eminent men whose laborors have shed lustre upon themselves and blessings upon humanity, find reason for arranging themselves into distinct schools, taking the name of Psychics, Somatics, or Psycho-somatics, according as they are led by their researches into the belief that insanity is a mental, physical, or physico-mental malady. They who look into the " Law of Lunacy," or examine the cases of those dispossessed by disease of the natural agency of the mind, who commit criminal acts, under the direction of a morbid or delusive idea, will cheerfully admit that even metaphysics has its practical uses. Aside from its direct application in professional life, it has been said by Bishop Barclay, that it is of the number of those preparatory studies, which may be compared with crops, raised not for the sake of the harvest, but to be ploughed in as a dressing to the land.

Botany, zoology, and meteorology are so obviously the allies of the physician, that no argument seems necessary to establish that relation.

Among the many interesting subjects of study which should arrest the attention and challenge the investigation of the medical student, there are few which can justly claim so large a share of his time as geology, and particularly that branch of it which treats of the structure and relations of mountain chains. Next to the division of the surface of the earth into land and water, the direction, height, and form of the elevated ridges which traverse the land, play the most important part in its physical history. Whilst the student of philology, ethnography, medicine, and physical geography, alike see the immense influence which the direction and position of mountain chains have exercised in the distribution of languages, in the migration of races of men, in giving form and outline to continents, in the modification of climate and origination of disease, the geologist acknowledges in them the grandest and most imperishable record of the great cycle of events, the study of which is his peculiar province.

As the medical student wanders from the strictly professional path of study into the domain of language, of metaphysics, of physical sciences, or the philosophy of nature, he will find that " the plan of the universe has proceeded from one All-comprehensive mind; and, as his circle of knowledge enlarges, that the unity of truth, and the consequent harmonious connection of knowledge, cause the boundaries of different sciences, and the possible subdivision of the general domain of knowledge, so to shade into each other, that it is sometimes difficult to determine them with precision."

When the young physician has attained eminence in social position, by moral character and reputation for intelligence, out of his profession, if he has not received the most practical kind of medical instruction, we have reason to believe that the instinct of self-respect will prompt him to an active cultivation of his profession, as a means of achieving equality with those who may be moving in the same sphere, lest he be thrown out of his orbit. Such an individual, by strengthening his feeling of self-reliance, will ride over all obstacles which lie in his way to professional distinction, and take a manly stand against all the forms of error, no matter in what guise hey make their appearance.

For the considerations already set forth, as well as for the additional reason that such studies furnish a dignified and rational relaxation to the physician in his moments of leisure, which would otherwise run to waste, we would urge an early and faithful devotion to them. They will prove also a happy and pleasing resource in the wane of life, when necessity no longer impels him to labor, and his great and active duties to society draw near to a close.

The Committee beg leave to conclude their Report by presenting the following resolutions:—

1. *Resolved*, That the Association re-affirm its formerly expressed opinions on the value and importance of general education to the student and practitioner of medicine, and that it would gladly enlarge its rule on this subject, so as to include the Humanities of the schools, and the natural sciences.

2. *Resolved*, That, in the opinion of this Association, a familiar knowledge of the elements of medical science, should precede clinical instruction.

3. *Resolved*, That, in order to accomplish the latter, the hospitals, when they shall be elevated to the rank of schools of practice, and the intelligent private preceptor, are the most effectual instrumentalities to be employed.

Z. PITCHER, *Chairman.*

Parsons and Doctors.

From the London Punch.

Many surgeons, doubtless, remarked an absurd letter from a clergyman, which appeared the other day in the *Times*, recommending charcoal, in combination with brandy and opium, as a cure for cholera. One of them has, fortunately, written an answer to that communication, pointing out that the quantity of the last-named drug prescribed by the parson would amount to 10 or 12 grains every half hour, and, of course, cure—by destroying the patient. This clergyman, no doubt, is a well meaning person; but he should confine himself to pointing the way to heaven, recollecting that the opposite place is paved with good intentions.

Possibly, he over-stated the quantity of opium, by what may be called a clerical error. A proper dose of it is well known to be beneficial in the complaint in question. Brandy is also found useful; and to these two ingredients of the mixture we should be disposed to ascribe any favorable results of its administration. The third is probably inert ;

otherwise it would be a convenient medicine, as anybody, in case of need,.might munch cinders.

Clergymen, in their anxiety to do good, are too often accustomed to add the treatment of bodies to the cure of souls. In order to minister to patients as well as penitents, they ought to possess the gift of healing, and that having ceased to be supernaturally imparted, they had better acquire it in the ordinary manner, by attending the hospitals. Some add HOMŒOPATHY to what the rubric prescribes in the Visitation of the Sick, and, by so doing, do the least harm that it is possible to do by empiricism, as the swallowers of their globules, at least, die of their diseases; but we would advise even the homœopathic divines to stick to theological mysticism, and not deal in " riddles," which will generally be "affairs of death."

Extract from Transactions of New York Academy of Medicine. By J. H. GRISCOM, M.D.

LETTER FROM MR. PARKER.

PERTH, AMBOY. NEW JERSEY, March 15, 1852,

DR. JOHN H. GRISCOM:

Dear Sir:—Having read your treatise on the " Uses and Abuses of Air," I send you an account of what occurred in this place some years since, and which proves the efficacy of fresh and pure air, not only in preventing, but curing disease.

In the month of August, 1837, a number of ships, with emigrant passengers, arrived at Perth Amboy from Liverpool, and other ports, on board of some of which ship fever prevailed. There was no hospital, or other accommodations in the town, in which the sick could be placed, and no person could admit them into private dwellings, fearing the infection of the fever. They could not be left on board the ships. An arrangement was made to land the sick passengers, and place them in an open wood, adjacent to a large spring of water, about a mile and a half from the town. Rough shanties, floored with boards, and covered with sails, were erected, and thirty-six patients were taken from on board ship with boats, landed as near to the spring as they could get, and carried in wagons to the encampment (as it was called), under the influence of a hot sun, in the month of August. Of the thirty-six first named, twelve were insensible, in the last stage of fever, and not expected to live twenty-four hours.

The day after landing there was a heavy rain; and the shanties affording no protection with their "sail" roofs, the sick were found the next morning wet, and their bedding, such as it was, drenched with the rain. It was replaced with such articles as could be collected from the charity of the inhabitants. The number at the encampment was increased by new subjects, to the amount of eighty-two in all.

On board the ship, which was cleansed after landing the passengers, *four* of the crew were taken with ship fever, and two of them died. Some of the nurses at the encampment were taken sick, but recovered. Of the whole number of eighty-two passengers removed from the ship, *not one died.* Pure air, good water, and, perhaps, the rain (though only the first thirty-six were affected by it), seem to have effected the cure.

No report has been made of these circumstances, and I send this from my recollection, and the information derived from the physician, Dr. Charles M. Smith, who still resides here, and to whom I refer you.

Yours respectfully,

JAMES PARKER.

A few further particulars of this case have since been derived from a statement of Dr. C. McKnight Smith, the gentleman referred to by Mr. Parker.

The ship was the Phœbe, with between three and four hundred passengers; a number of them had died on the passage. The shanties spoken of were two in number, thirty feet long, twenty feet wide, boarded on three sides about four feet up, and over them old sails were stretched. Of the twelve who were removed from the ship in a state of insensibility, such appeared the hopelessness of their condition, that the overseer (who is a carpenter) observed, "Well, Doctor, I think I shall have some boxes to make before many hours." "The night after their arrival at the encampment," says Dr. Smith, "we had a violent thunder-gust, accompanied by torrents of rain. On visiting them the next morning, the clothes of all were saturated with water; in other words, they had had a thorough ablution. This, doubtless, was a most fortunate circumstance. The medical treatment was exceedingly simple, consisting, in the main, of an occasional laxative or enema, vegetable acids, and bitters. Wine was liberally administered, together with the free use of cold water, buttermilk, and animal broths." The four sailors, who sickened after the arrival of the vessel, were removed to the room of an ordinary dwelling-house. The medical treatment in their case was precisely similar, yet two of them died. Two of the number suffered from carbuncle while convalescing. The Doctor adds "My opinion is, that, had the eighty-two treated at the encampment been placed in a common hospital, many of them would also have fallen victims. I do not attribute their recovery so much to the remedies administered, as to the circumstances in which they were placed; in other words, a good washing to begin with, and an abundance of fresh air."

The first of these cases I regard as presenting a type of the average hygienic character of hospitals in general, as *they are;* the last, a type of what they *should be,* in this respect, excepting, of course, the materials and style of structure. In making a few remarks upon them, I will ask attention to one fact, which contrasts them still further. Two of the most frequent troubles which the physician meets with in the treatment of typhus, under ordinary circumstances, are erysipelas and pneumonia, .which supervene in no inconsiderable number of cases. It is very generally believed that the former complication is a more or less direct result of the impure air, causing it, oftentimes, to become endemic in a ward or hospital; while pneumonia, on the other hand, is more commonly attributed to exposure of the patient to a draught of air, in some way or another, even when the manner or period of the exposure cannot be defined. In the last of the two cases I have presented, it does not appear that either of these complications occurred in a single instance, notwithstanding the unusual exposure of all the sick; while it is well known that in ordinary hospitals, as I have stated. both are frequently noticed.

In one of the shanties at the Ward's Island Emigration Hospital, then occupied by typhus cases, it was once remarked to me, by the physician on duty, that pneumonia seemed to run from patient to patient along the whole length of the ward, a circumstance which he attributed to the cold air from the windows impinging upon the patients' heads, although no windows were open; but which, to my mind, was rather caused by a *want* of pure air, the atmosphere of the ward being exceedingly foul, and there being no way by which the external could find access. And I respectfully submit the question whether, if erysipelas, as undoubtedly is the case, is caused by the action of a foul and infected atmosphere upon the patient, be such action indirectly through his general system, or directly upon his external tegument, pneumonia may not be regarded as an erysipelas of the pulmonary tissues, produced in the same manner, seeing that they are exposed, both directly and indirectly, to the influence of the same foul atmosphere.

Regarded in its general aspect as a source of life and health, an ample supply of pure air, in conjunction with the immediate removal of secreted and exhaled impurities, beyond the possibility of re-inhalation, is a subject of profound interest to all humanity; but to the practitioner of medicine it presents itself with increased force. There is imposed upon us a double obligation. The question should be constantly before our minds, whether we shall deny, or allow to be denied, to our patients, the use or oxygen, in the fullest measure in which it can be found in the atmosphere? Whether, while searching our Materia Medica for the most appropriate remedies, according to our theories of disease and treatment, we will continue to overlook the most potent of all restoratives, that derived from nature's own laboratory.

If we can believe and understand that, by the influence of the rays of the sun upon its different aspects, the towering pile of granite on Bunker Hill is caused continually to sway to and fro upon its base, with equal readiness may we comprehend that the refined and delicate living animal organism will vary in its phases of health, with the varying quality of the air upon which it depends, every moment, for its actual existence.

It was about the middle of the seventeenth century that Thomas Sydenham burst the trammels of prejudice in which both the medical and the popular mind of this country, and of the world, had long been bound, in reference to the innocuousness and availability of the operations of nature, and demonstrated the value, in the management of diseases, of the great medicament which he had furnished from the beginning of creation. When he tore away the bed-curtains, drove his patients from their sweltering beds, threw up their windows, or ordered them on horseback, the community thought him crazy; such kind of treatment was opposed to all their experience, and he had no authority for it from books. But, holding them in light estimation, when they contravened the obvious dictates of reason and nature, he consulted only the latter, and saved many from loathsome death by small-pox, and from premature graves by consumption.

One century later, the world was shocked by receiving from Calcutta a horrible lesson of the consequences of confining human beings in a close and unventilated atmosphere. Ten hours sufficed to produce intolerable thirst, intense fever, delirium, and death, in one hundred and twenty-three out of one hundred and forty-six persons, and a high putrid fever in those found alive at the end of that time. That "black hole" has ever since been a by-word and a reproach to humanity, while its lesson has been too little heeded.

And now, one century later still, and there comes from Perth Amboy, in the New World, a lesson of the omnipotent sanitary influence of that same subtle, invisible agent—a lesson which should be treasured in the memory of all upon whom rests the responsibility of administering to the relief of their fellow-men.

Let it never be forgotten for a moment that this agent, to procure which we have neither to dig into the earth, nor transport from foreign climes, nor distil from the alembic, nor refine in the crucible, but which is pressed upon us with a force, and in a measure, equalled only by the supreme benevolence which furnishes, and unceasingly renews it. This agent, when left free to act its part, removes the effete poison from the blood, and imbues it with continual health and freshness; but, when stifled and confined, whether intentionally or by accident, turns, like a viper, upon the arm that nourished it, and plants a deadly venom in its veins.

Prize Essay, on the Zymotic Theory of Essential Fevers and other Disordered Conditions of the blood; together with an Appendix on Medical Theories and Vital Statistics. By SAMUEL G. ARMOR, M.D., of Cleveland, Ohio.   [Concluded from page 332.]

The importance of all these conditions I would by no means underrate. They present to us, indeed, an exceedingly interesting field of

inquiry. From an impression first made upon the nutritive and assimilative functions, we are at once introduced to multiplied elements of disease. There is not a function, not a nerve, not a gland, not a capillary
vessel of the body but must feel the depressing effects of a contaminated
condition of the blood. And this sluggish and languid state of the excretory organs becomes the cause of a still more poisoned condition of
the blood, until this source of life becomes itself dead, and spreads death
instead of life throughout the body.

The admittance of the Zymotic theory into the field of pathology
would, doubtless, lead to greatly increased knowledge of the real nature
of diseased states. In a large class of fevers it points out the only two
modes of cure: 1st. To counteract the injurious operation of the poisons:
2nd. To expel them from the system. The first of these indications
is carried out in low typhus and adynamic forms of fever, by the administration of saline medicines, such as the chloride of sodium, the
chlorate of potash, hydro-chloric acid, &c. Arsenic, quinine, alcohol,
and other antiseptic remedies, are also valuable agents in arresting the
Zymotic condition of the blood.

The other indication is the one most usually pursued—viz.: to expel
the offending matters from the system. This may be said to be Nature's mode of cure; and, in the absence of reliable knowledge as to the
nature of the poison and its antidote, the physician can only aid Nature
in her work of elimination. This he attempts by the administration of
tonics, stimulants, supportants, and depurents. The powers of life must
be supported while Nature effects the cure. But, even in her own work
of depuration, Nature may be greatly aided. The kidneys, skin, and
alimentary canal are the principal channels through which foreign matters are expelled from the blood; and hence the utility of diuretics,
aperients, and the so-called *Water cure.* The latter, by a combination
of diuresis and diaphoresis, may be rendered a most powerful therapeutical agent in cutting short a fever in its premonitory stage, or at its
final accession. The absurdity of hydropathy, as a one-idead system of
cure, is its blind and indiscriminate application to every variety of disease; and it is to be regretted that a remedy of such valuable therapeutic
power is frequently brought into undeserved disrepute, by falling into
the hands of ignorant intermeddlers with Nature.

If the views of the pathology of essential fevers which I have presented be correct, it is almost impossible to avoid giving assent to the
doctrine that regards the fever as an effort of the "vis medicatrix," instituted for the purpose of expelling the poison from the system; and,
while it repudiates the doctrine of the boasting fever curer, as well as the
doctrine of non-interference, which has been aptly styled a "meditation
on death," it rests upon the great physiological truth, that Nature is
ever active in her recuperative powers, and is, after all, the best and
wisest of physicians.

This pathology also offers the most rational explanation of the modification of diseased action growing out of prevailing *epidemic influences.*
It fixes the mind upon two controlling elements of disease: *first,* upon
the depressing effects of a Zymotic poison, by inducing changes in the

blood; *second,* the local inflammatory or functional complication that may be engrafted upon and influenced by this.altered condition of the blood. It thus draws the line of demarcation between general and special pathology; by keeping in view *constitutional conditions as modifying local action,* and by this means enables us to comprehend the most important question, practically considered, within the wide range of medical inquiry—the distinction between *Sthenic and Asthenic* diseases, between depressed and exalted action. Its tendency is to give us broader views and clearer conceptions of the varied elements of disease, as they act and re-act, and insensibly shade into each other.

It modifies, moreover, and renders more rational, the *treatment* of disease. Does an inflammatory affection overtake one whose blood is contaminated by an epidemic influence, or by putrid emanations, vegetable or animal; or whose blood is only imperfectly or badly repaired by insufficient or unwholesome diet?—then, of course, the inflammation is *œsthenic* in character, and blood-letting and other antiphlogistic remedies must be resorted to, if at all, with great caution. If the blood has been "touched corruptibly" by an epidemic influence, or a typhoid poison, we must husband rather than depress the flagging powers of life. To adopt, in such cases (as we fear is too often done), the ordinary treatment for an acute pneumonia or dysentery, as the case may be, regardless of the evidence of *blood disease,* such as loss of tone and strength of the vascular system, sluggish functions, dull mental faculties, feeble and compressible pulse, and brown or dark tongue, would be to hasten the dissolution of the patient, and bring both doctor and medicine into disrepute. The great secret of success in the treatment of disease is to be found in a broad, comprehensive, and rational pathology—a pathology that weighs every element of disease, whether of fluids or of solids, that is capable of exciting, depressing, or perverting vital actions.

I have thus ventured to present a few facts, with the hope of calling attention to a subject which may not, as yet, have occupied the minds of some members of the profession; and, although I may have presented but a dim vision of the true light, yet "I TRUST I HAVE GOT HOLD OF MY PITCHER BY THE RIGHT HANDLE."

MEDICAL THEORIES.

The history of Medical Science is the history of Medical theories; and, although many of them appear to differ widely with each other, these differences will be found, on examination, to be more apparent than real, often more in words than things, and *incomplete* rather than *false.* The subject which I have presented, in the foregoing essay, is now attracting the attention of some of the best medical minds of Europe; and yet pathological changes of the blood is an *old* doctrine— old as the history of Medical Science. The Zymotic theory of disease has existed, under some form, since the days of HIPPOCRATES; and a lapse of two thousand years has but confirmed many of his views.

True, he was a Humoral pathologist, in the fullest sense of the term; yet his pathology of disease, although simple, was the result of close observation. He taught that disease consisted in a morbid state of the fluids, and that Nature cures by certain evacuations, as of sweat, urine, &c. Who doubts his doctrine at the present day? Who can gainsay his facts? But Hippocrates did not see the *whole truth*. He failed to estimate the importance of a healthy *equilibrium* of the blood. This was left for Themison, who, not taking an enlarged view of the varied elements of disease, made capillary congestion embrace almost the whole domain of pathology. One dealt with changed *qualities* of the blood, the other with its changed *quantities*, and each taught an important truth. So also Brown, the "child of genius and misfortune," was so enraptured with one or two truths, that he was never able to see any others; and, although simple *over-action* and *under-action* frequently attend disease, they constitute but fragments, as it were, of a more perfect pathology; and the lancet and the brandy bottle, although good in their place, constitute a very incomplete magazine of therapeutics.

Thus it has been from the days of Hippocrates to the present. The most brilliant lights that have gilded the skies of medical philosophy, have taken partial views of subjects in their nature and extent complex and vast. Yet one has contributed a truth in physiology, another in pathology, and still another in therapeutics. The accumulation of these has greatly enriched our medical literature, and enlarged the boundary of our knowledge. We now have spread out before us the ingenious and truthful inferences of a Laennec, and Andral and Gaveret: the patient and philosophical researches of a Golding Bird; the practical truths of a Williams and a Watson; and the clear and comprehensive conclusions of a Forrey, based upon the comparative statistics of more than three-fourths of the earth's surface.

The object of all research has been to arrive at the best, the true theory; and yet, amidst our vast accumulation of facts, we may well stop, and inquire—Has a true and complete theory of Medical Science been established? Surely no rational mind can so claim. If not complete, then, what is our relation to the past? In the rejection of old and the establishment of new theories, have we made progress, or have we not? If the world has not been benefitted by these inquiries, and the aggregate duration of human life has *not* been lengthened, then there has been really *no* progress, and the zealous medical inquirer might well turn, in despair, from any further investigations. But if it shall prove that, amidst all this conflict of opinion and theory, there has been a regular and steady progress in the establishment of those medical truths upon which the science at present rests, it will be an inducement for us to set out on a fresh voyage of discovery, with new hopes and energies. Haply *we* may return from our explorations the possessor of a new truth, as a contribution to our divine art.

The fact that many a speculative theory has fallen before the rigid test of *inductive truth*, should not discourage us from making renewed efforts. Does it not prove, on the contrary, that we to-day occupy an

advanced position in the healing art that we never before occupied?
Truths have been preserved, and errors have been discarded; the *chain
of authority has been broken*, and the medical philosopher inquires for
neither sect nor theory, but for TRUTH. Chemistry and the microscope
are at this moment making rapid acquisitions of new truths, and explaining old ones. It is a disingenuous and false charge, therefore, that
Medical Science is stationary. In no department of human inquiry has
there been greater progress; and, in confirmation of the proposition that
MEDICAL SCIENCE HAS MATERIALLY LENGTHENED HUMAN LIFE, I introduce, in conclusion, by way of appendix to my Essay, 'the following
statistics, bearing on this point, which I extract from the Annual Address recently delivered before the New York State Medical Society, and
the Legislature then assembled in Albany, by ALONZO CLARK, President of the Society, and the distinguished Professor of Physiology and
Pathology in the College of Physicians and Surgeons of the State of
New York.

It is seldom, indeed, that we have condensed such an array of facts
and figures bearing upon this point, and I am glad in this connection to
avail myself of his labors.

VITAL STATISTICS.

Professor Clark first introduces the testimony of the great English
historian, and proves, by an unanswerable array of testimony, that
medical science *has* greatly lengthened human life.

Macaulay, in his history of England, says: "The term of human life has
been lengthened in the whole kingdom, and especially in the towns. In
the year 1685, not accounted a sickly year, more than one in twenty of
the inhabitants of the capital died: at present only one in forty dies
annually. The difference between London of the 19th century, and the
London of the 17th century, is greater than the difference between London in ordinary years, and London in the cholera.'

Dr. Simpson, in his paper "On the Statistics in Surgery," states, that
in 1786 the yearly rate of mortality in the whole of England and Wales
was *one in forty-two;* in 1801, it was *one in forty-seven*, and in 1831,
it had diminished to *one in forty-eight*, showing a reduction of
annual deaths by 28 per cent. in the short period of half a century.—
[Dublin Rev. vol. 7, p. 97.]

These statements correspond with deductions from the English parish
registry returns, made by a careful student of statistics and distinguished
writer of our own country, published in the 13th vol. of the American
Journal of Medical Sciences. This registration, however, is incomplete,
and the American writer points out the sources of this defect. It is not
necessary to specify them here. They are believed to be constant, and
nearly equal for the whole period; so that while the proportion of deaths
to survivors is rated too low, the rating is equally too low for all portions
of the half century. The error therefore, does not materially invalidate
the great conclusion to which Dr. Simpson's figures would lead us. Marshall, in the publication of the bills of mortality, preserved in London

since 1629, has given us the fullest confirmation of this gratifying fact, so far as this largest of towns can furnish it. Finlaison recognises it as an important element in the construction of his celebrated Annuity Tables.

Mr. Milne, in making up his well known *Carlisle* Life Tables, ascertained with the greatest care the deaths in that town and its vicinity, for the nine years following 1778: they were in the proportion of 1 to 39.99 of the population of each year. It is ascertained with equal certainty (see 'Registrar General's Reports) that for the seven years, ending with 1844, the deaths in this same Carlisle and its vicinity were annually 1 in 52.6. The interval between these two periods is just 50 years, and the reduction of mortality is 22 per cent.

The deaths in the town of Northampton were carefully studied during the latter part of the last century, and compared with the population. Dr. Price made this comparison the basis of some of his life-tables. Here we have another unquestionable increase in the duration of life. The Registrar General, in his Report for 1847, says of this town: "In the last century, the people here lived about 30; now they live 37 years (37½). In earlier times their life must have been shorter. Then the community had no skillful physician, no surgeon—an infirmary, a dispensary, a lunatic asylum, and from 20 to 30 educated medical men, an evidence that more skill is now devoted to the preservation of life." Thus it appears that although this Northampton is even now one of the least healthful of all the smaller towns of England, yet that the decrement of deaths there is equal to 23 per cent.

These statements, I believe, exhaust the reliable statistics of England, bearing on the subject in which we are here interested, excepting only those that relate to annuitants and the insured.

The inquiry now naturally arises, is this the end? Can the life of man be still further prolonged. We would fain hope that its maximum duration is not yet attained, and this hope is not without encouragement. We learn from the Registrar General's Report, that the mortality of England was slowly but steadily diminishing, during the eight years from 1838 to 1846. The figures that represent its ratio to the living are for the several years respectively as follows, viz: 2.24, 2.187, 2.29, 2.160, 2.167, 2.12, and 2.082 per cent. But whatever view we are compelled to take of the future, who can doubt the cheering evidences of progress in the recent past?—substantial progress. I will adopt the suggestion of the Registrar General, and assume for the present, what I hope soon to prove, that what man desires most of all earthly things, is secured to him in fair measure, by the unobtrusive, unnoticed labors of our ill-rewarded profession. In the lapse of half a century, 28 persons, or if you prefer the lower estimate, 22 persons saved alive out of every hundred, all of whom must previously have perished! What are all the other improvements of the same period, compared with this? What, though we boast that steam has been made the day laborer for the nations: what, though the steamship equals in magnificence the fairy palace of fiction, and skims the water with its wooden wings, as does a bird the air; what, though the iron ways encircle the earth, and daily exhibit, as I believe they do, the highest reach of human power, a perpetual wonder; what, though the electric fluid has become our news-carrier; what, though the arts have improved so as to cheapen many of the necessaries of life to half their original cost! Neither of these, nay, all combined, can hardly single out the life that they have saved.!

Again, France exhibits to us very strikingly the great results of professional labors. M. Charles Dupin, whose name is a sufficient guarantee for his statements, lately read before the Institute a paper on the vital statistics of that country, showing that from 1776 to 1843, (67 years), the duration of life had been increasing at the average rate of 52 days annually, so that the total gain in $\frac{2}{3}$ of a century amounted to $9\frac{1}{2}$ years; and that in no year of that period, whether during the Republic, the Consulate, or the Empire, did the annual increase fall below 19 days. What a fact have we here! Even during that dread period of French history in which the death angel assumed the cap of liberty, and taxed the arts for new inventions to destroy life, and during the succeeding 13 years in which the war spirit reaped an almost unprecedented harvest when science and arts vied with each other in contributing to this work of slaughter, and the history of Europe is but little more than the history of battles: during all this period, medicine alone lent all its energies to the preservation of life. How striking the contrast! How proud the success! In France, that glutted the guillotine with the blood of her sons, and strewed every battle-field in Europe thick with their dead bodies: even in death-smitten France, medicine saved, in 20 years, more than war and the delirious spirit of freedom could destroy.

But we shall be told, doubtless, that we are claiming for our profession more than we have any fair right to; that society has improved in all its relations, and that to these improvements are due, in a fair proportion, the results which have been quoted. Let us consider for a little in what these improvements consist. Within 150 years, the arts have reduced the costs of many of the necessaries of life; but then the necessaries of life have been actually multiplied by this same process of reduction, and food, the first of necessaries, has not been cheapened: its money price is indeed less, but its labor cost is greater. The home condition of the laborer (I speak only of the countries from which I have drawn statistics) is more miserable than it was a century and a half ago. The rich have, it is true, become richer, but the poor have at the same time become poorer; in other words, wealth has greatly increased, but it is not distributed in other countries as it is in our own. Who that has visited the homes of labor in England or France, will believe that the over-crowded, half-clad, half-fed population of a manufacturing town can be compared in domestic comfort with the laboring classes of other times, when the honest housewife wrought out of the noisy wheel and loom the honest, warm, abundant homespun; when the labors of the field brought to a country, not over-populated, abundance of food; when labor had not yet destroyed its compensation by rivalry with itself; when the infirm poor were not yet so numerous that the benevolent rich could not look after them, and supply their wants. Who will believe that the crowded, hot, dusty, ill-ventilated manufactory can contribute to health like the open field where men once labored with its fresh breeze and its sunshine. The

better and middle classes have always been long-lived. *Their* home
condition may have been improved in the period referred to; but have
they gained as much as the many, the laborers, have lost! I confidently
believe that so far from their being a betterment in the social condition
of Europe within 150 years, when a fair balance is struck, it will be
found that things personal contribute less than formerly to prolong life.
Still, it cannot be denied, that in the general improvement of society has
been done for this great object. It is in cities chiefly that these important changes are seen; and even there they are confined mostly to the
rich, or at best are brought by the rich only to the doors of the poor, beyond which they rarely strive to pass. Staying as far as possible the
spread of pestilence; improved ventilation in the widening of streets, and
in the construction of dwellings and public buildings; diminishing the
causes of disease by the removal of filth, and by a judicious drainage;
and the encouragement of personal cleanliness, by making water abundant and bathing cheap; these, no one will deny, are benefits, solid benefits. But *all that is valuable in them is based on principles elaborated
and promulgated by the medical profession.* Even the details of the
plans by which the public have realized these benefits, have in many instances been prescribed by the profession. There is an implied recognition of this fact, in the name "medical police" which is given to the
department that governs most of these things, and still more in the fact
that their supervision is in a considerable degree entrusted to an "inspector"
chosen from the medical profession. These, then, are medical facts
popularized, as are a thousand other medical facts in hygiene and the
laws of regimen. May we not, then, freely imparting as we do to the
public the advantages derivable from these things; may we not ask to be
remembered as the authors of the doctrines from which these benefits
flow?

There is another view of this subject. We hear enumerated among
the causes of *tuburcular consumption,* imperfect protection either by
house or clothing, against the vicissitudes of weather; scanty and innu-
tritious food; imperfect ventilation; vitiated air; dwelling in dark, damp
places; indifference to personal cleanliness. When it is remembered
that these are important points among the particulars in which it is
claimed that society has so greatly improved, it will be expected that this
formidable malady must gradually recede before the advancing improvements. But Sir James Clarke assures us, (in his book on Consumption)
that this is not the case. He has carefully studied the London bills of
mortality, making annual averages for periods of ten years, to avoid the
influence of epidemics and accidental agencies; and he finds that from
1700 to about 1830 there was no diminution in the frequency and the
fatality of this disease, but rather that the *proportion of deaths from it
has been increasing during that whole period.* At the same time this
author fully confirms the statement already quoted from the history of
England, by showing that the mortality from all diseases, consumption
included, has diminished nearly one half; consumption excluded more
than one half. I need hardly add, that the profession has never claimed
great control over this affection; and that during all the period here re-

ferred to, it was held to be incurable. This statement favors a conviction that the advantages we have gained over disease are more in actual practice than in prevention and hygiene.

But we have facts more directly to my purpose: such as will show the physician's care of the sick, freed from all other agencies that are supposed to have influence in prolonging life; and comparing the results of that care, at different periods, our claims will be in no respect weakened.

Dr. Merriman deduces from the bills of mortality just referred to, the fullest evidence, that in the department in which he was so much distinguished, the most signal improvement has been made. In 1680, one in forty-four died while under the care of the medical attendant; within 50 years from that time, only one in seventy died under the same circumstances; in another term of 50 years, mortality was reduced to one in eighty-two; and in 40 years more, (the period ending with 1820) it had fallen as low as one in 107. Here is a condition in which knowledge and skill are left to work their way unhindered and unhelped. Hygiene has little to do with it; the improvements of society even less. It is nature and the doctor, and how has the doctor triumphed?—fifty-nine per cent. of such as must have died in the latter years of 1600, saved in the progress of above a century and a half! This is doing something to lift from the sex the heavy weight of the primal curse; and we challenge, in return for it, their kind regard.

Let us now bring our inquiry nearer home. The records of the New York Hospital, a medical charity supported from the treasury of the State, show the mortality, together with the number of patients treated annually since its foundation. The first 50 years of its existence end with 1842. If this term be divided into periods of ten years each, the progressive improvement is uninterrupted; so that while the relation of deaths to admissions in the first 15 years was one in 7 7-9ths, in the last 5 years it is one in $11\frac{1}{5}$. This is a gain of more than 30-100ths, or 31 saved alive out of every 100 that formerly would have died. Now here is little besides medical treatment. The growth of the city has not materially improved the site of this Institution. The same building is now used that was used when it was opened, though others have been added. The wards were no more crowded through their early years than they were in 1842; the comfort of the patient has been equally cared for at both periods; and it is proper to give emphasis to the statement, that in this important result, vaccination has had no part. This inestimable discovery was made, it is true, early in this period of 50 years, but it could in no way have affected this hospital, because small-pox has never been admitted into it since its foundation. What then have we here but improvement in the practice of medicine and surgery? And it cannot but be noticed, first, that the result here recorded equals, even exceeds, what is claimed in society at large, from all beneficial causes operating together; second, that this result gained without the aid of vaccination, shows that, great as is the amount of good done by this discovery, it is far from being the only life-saving agency by which the world has been blessed in the past half century.

The important deductions here made from the statistics of the New

York Hospital, are sustained by similar facts as collected from the records of the Pennsylvania Hospital, Philadelphia. That institution was opened for the reception of patients in 1752. Its first 90 years were completed, then, in 1842. During this period it received 39,290 patients, and lost of that number 4,100. I have not been able to obtain annual reports, but the deaths for the whole term of 90 years were one in $9\frac{1}{2}$ of all admitted, while in the last of these years it was only one in 11,87. This gives us the last year better than the whole by more than 19 per cent.; an improvement we could only have been prepared for, after learning the striking facts substantiated by the fullest details from the New York Hospital.

From the statistics of the last century it appears that the number of patients admitted into the Pennsylvania Hospital, in the ten years ending with April 1852, was 13,472; of whom 1056 died, making the deaths a little better than one in $12\frac{3}{4}$. Thus we have a gain in the last ten years, over the preceding 90, of more than 25 per cent.

In appreciating the value of these facts, it must be borne in mind that the physicians and surgeons to whom hospital duties are assigned, are but the representatives of their profession. They are the exponents, the public manifestation of its condition. What they do within the hospital walls, others are doing in private circles, each in his own proper sphere.

Is it not true, then, that medicine is the first of the progressive arts; and not first only, but incomparably above and beyond all others in the priceless benefits it has bestowed on man? Yet who has risen up to give it public thanks for its herculean labors? Who has proposed to commemorate the vast achievment of prolonging the years of the life of man more than one-fourth their former average, throughout civilized Europe and America, in the short period of half a century?

When a great canal or railroad is completed, the air is rent with clamors. Men's voices are inadequate to express their joy, and cannons thunder forth their glad congratulations. Orators speak of "the marriage of mighty waters;" and men, as they meet in the street, say, the great work is accomplished. Well, is it not better thus?—for what celebration can adequately commemorate these triumphs of medicine! What monument can typify their greatness? Yet we have a right to demand a fair estimate of the value of our profession to society, and an honest acknowledgment of what it has done for the well being of man. Grant us this, and, by the blessing of God, we will raise our own monument; it shall be the armies of living men our hands can rescue from the grave.

From the Western Lancet.

Non-fatal Accidents from Anæsthetics, with observations. Read before the Medico-Chirurgical Society of Cincinnati. By W. H. MUZZEY, M.D.

Recently, in one of the courts of justice in Paris, two surgeons were condemned to pay a fine (merely nominal) for allowing a patient to die under the effects of chloroform. The court sustained the following allegations, and hence its decision:

1st. That chloroform was unnecessarily administered, as the operation to be performed was not of sufficient magnitude to justify its employment.

2nd. That the room was not sufficiently ventilated.

3rd. That no provision had been made against accident.

In view of the last point, the very natural question arises, What precautions against accidents should be taken by those administering anæsthetic agents?

One answers, that no death has occurred from the use of sulphuric ether, and therefore there need be no apprehension from its administration; another has never *heard* of a death from chloric ether, and claims for *it* great advantages over other agents; whilst the advocates of chloroform attribute all accidents to the *impurity* of the article.

It is not my purpose to discuss the comparative merits of these agents, but I am persuaded that each, however pure it may be, will meet with idiosyncracies forbidding its administration.

In death from anæsthesia, there is suspension of respiration from paralysis of the nerves presiding over this function, and consequently, suspension of the heart's action. To re-animate, M. Jobert de Lambelle (of l'Hotel Dieu) counsels the use of irritants to the skin, currents of air passed over the body, excitants applied to the tongue, cauterization of the mouth and throat with ammonia and currents of electricity. M. Ricord remarked to me, that artificial respiration alone, if persevered in, would prevent fatal results, and instanced three cases in his own practice which were saved by that procedure.

The following case will illustrate the value of the suggestion; but first a word as to the agent employed, and means of its administration. We have used for four years the mixture of one part (by measure) of chloroform, and two parts of washed sulphuric ether, both of which are from the manufactory of Messrs Powers and Weightman, Philadelphia. The vehicle for administration is a large silk handkerchief (an old bandana) of very loose texture, which has been used for this purpose solely for four years. This is shaken out of its folds and gathered lightly in the hand, and usually a fluid drachm of this mixture is put upon it, and it is held lightly over the face, covering the nose and mouth. If there is much irritation of the lungs, the handkerchief is removed from time to time till it ceases, and when the patient is sufficiently quiet for the commencement of an operation, we not unfrequently add a little fresh material, and leave the handkerchief upon the face for a few minutes.

JUNE 6th, 1852.—Michael O'Hara, a native of Ireland, emigrated 7 years since; is 27 years of age, of sanguine temperament, full habit, capacious chest, has great muscular developement, and weighs 170 pounds. Once in two or three weeks drinks freely of whiskey for two days, and works steadily in the intermediate time. Had a "spree" for two days last week. Eight months since, was working under a bank of earth, which caved upon him and injured his back, since which, has had incessant pain in the lumbar portion of the spine, notwithstanding internal medication and the application of cups, blisters, and irritating ointments, now, pressure over the third lumbar vertebra produces pain.

15th.—Propose to apply the actual cautery over the spine.

16th, 8 o'clock, a.m.—At the patient's lodgings, an Irish lad of 16 years present with us. Patient has eaten nothing for 13 hours; is lying on his back in a room ten feet square; the head of the bed is under an open window, and at the foot, the door stands open. Circulation full and strong, with 80 pulsations per minute. Commenced the administration of the mixture of chloroform and ether. The first approach of the handkerchief to the face caused slight coughing, which soon subsided. In four minutes the patient became very loquacious, jabbering in Gaelic, and made great muscular exertion, (usually the case with Irish patients,) and muscles became rigid; pulse 70. The handkerchief was removed for 30 seconds; the muscles relaxed; the respiration became disembarrassed, and pulse 65. Inhalation was resumed and continued for one minute, when I considered the effect nearly sufficient. Putting half a fluid drachm of the mixture upon the handkerchief, I left it upon the face, and stepped below stairs for the heated iron, leaving the lad with the patient. (The iron was in a stove twenty-five yards from the bedside, and I found subsequently, on going over the ground with the same expedition, that I was absent from the room 40 seconds.) On my return the wrist was pulseless, and the action of the lungs and heart entirely suspended. I shook the patient, dashed water in his face, turned him upon his side, then upon the back again, gave various positions to the head, pressed upon the chest to expel the air from the lungs and allow fresh air to replace it. This was kept up for one minute. I then placed myself on the bed at one side of the body, and with my own mouth upon that of the subject, inflated the lungs, then expelled the air by pressure upon the chest, and allowed the pure air to take its place; this in turn was expelled, and the lungs again inflated by my own. In this manner I kept up artificial respiration for the space of three minutes, every alternate inflation being from the atmosphere. Suspending these efforts for a few seconds, and seeing no signs of life, I despatched the lad for a professional friend, and resumed artificial respiration. After one minute, I thrust my finger into the throat, and agitated the epiglottis, in hopes to provoke a spasm of the glottis, but without success. Continued artificial respiration for another minute, and a second time thrust my finger into the throat, with no better success. Artificial respiration for half a minute, and a third time thrusting my finger into the throat, but deeper than before, so as to penetrate between the cords of the glottis, I suddenly withdrew it, but immediately repeating the movement with greater violence, the much wished-for " spasm" grasped my finger, and there was a slight quivering motion of the chest. Artificial respiration resumed, and in two minutes the patient had no need of my assistance.

He was still insensible, but the application of the iron, which was reheated, partially aroused him. Five minutes after, he was perfectly sensible, complained of great weakness, but had no idea of the peril he had passed through. Half an hour later he seemed as well as patients ordinarily are after the use of chloroform, and subsequently there were no unusual symptoms.

The amount of the mixture used on this occasion was six fluid drachms —two of chloroform and four of ether.

There was no pulsation of the heart, or respiratory movement for seven minutes.

Re-animation is attributable to artificial respiration and irritation of the glottis.   .   .   .   .

My father, Dr. R. D. Muzzy, informs me, that a year since, on account of untoward symptoms similar to the above, he was obliged to postpone an operation which was subsequently performed without anæsthsia.

In March, 1849, we were near loosing a patient, from the unskillful management of chloroform by a non-professional bystander; and not long after, we tried the mixture of chloroform and ether, and have used no other anæsthetic agent since, under the opinion that the ether sustains the vital powers against the purely sedative effect of the chloroform.   Experience has taught us, however, that there is liability to accident from its use.

I am constrained to believe, that a frank avowal of the profession would create astonishment at the great number of non-fatal accidents that have occurred, and that the details would aid in the establishment of principles for conduct in its administration, and serve to throw around the sale and use of anæsthetic agents, such guards as would protect the community from their direful effects.   Even in Edinburgh, where it is claimed, that in a hundred thousand cases where chloroform has been used, not a single accident has occurred; *untoward symptoms have compelled the suspension of the use of the article,* (as I was informed by an assistant of Dr. Simpson,) which the operators profess to be able to trace to the *impurity* of the agent employed.

My attention has just been called to the researches of Prof. Hosford, Cambridge, Mass., *(Boston Med. and Surg. Jour., Oct.* 19,*)* and to a paper in the *Am. Jour. of Med. Science for Oct.,* from Dr. Bickersteth, of Liverpool, to which I refer as corroborative of the positions herein assumed, viz:

First, That accidents from anæsthesia are generally attributable to idiosyncracies in the subjects.

Second, That derangements of the circulation depend upon the disturbance of the function of respiration.

Third, That artificial respiration is the most valuable of all means for counteracting dangerous symptoms.

EDITORIAL AND MISCELLANEOUS.

The Uprising.

We have now reached our eighth number. Thanks to the high spirit and the liberal responses of the profession in this and adjoining States, we have fairly *established our Journal*, and by their farther help and good will, we mean to make it *one of the best in the United States*. We do not occupy this post from the mere petty aspiration of being an Editor of a Journal of Medicine. Our ambition grasps at nothing less than to be the trumpet of the profession, when organizing its scattered strength, and concentrating its immense, but undirected resources into proper combinations, it shall rise in its splendor and power to the confusion of its enemies, and the rejoicings of its friends. For this movement the veterans of the host have struggled long, and every young physician that has entered the ranks has sighed for it *Organization has been the want of the age*—it is the instinctive demand of the great medical army. And now at last, the movement has begun, and already is making its power felt. We have not created it ; our pen did not arouse it ; it swells spontaneous and irresistible from the entire body of men, of strong souls and deep hearts who love their profession, and thirst to see her honored and prosperous as she deserves. It is this movement whose exponent we are, and among whose champions we intend to stand ; and we look with confidence for the time when the profession organized and centralized, shall outdo even its present zeal in improving and making discoveries in the healing art, and add to them such measures as shall be efficient in protecting the minds of community, from the impositions of quackery.

Meeting of the State Society.

We take occasion, thus early, to remind our readers that the State Medical Society meets at Ann Arbor, on the last Thursday in March. The movement for a better discipline and more compact arrangement of the forces of the profession, is likely to render this a meeting of interest and importance. Those who were appointed our delegates at the last meeting, to the National Convention, represented the Society and the Profession of Michigan with honor in that body, and we now, in consequence of their appointment, occupy a higher and more dignified position among our sister organizations. Come up to the gathering therefore, one and all, and bring with you enthusiastic souls, and high hearts. The bond that must bind us, must not be a paper constitution, but living sympathy.

New Journals.

We have received the first number of the *American Medical Monthly*. This journal is edited by Edward H. Parker, M. D., and is conducted by the faculty of one of the New York Medical Schools. It contains eighty pages, and altogether, makes an appearance which promises to rank it high among our monthlies.

The Dental News-Letter.

Of this we have received the second number ; it contains much interesting matter, and we rejoice to see by it, that the Dental profession is exerting itself so successfully, to maintain a high standard. It is edited by J. D. White, M. D:, D. D. S. and J. R. McCurdy, Philadelphia.

The-Western Journal of Medicine and Surgery.

This journal has commenced a new series, and is very much improved in its appearance. We are glad to see it revive so fresh from its temporary sleep. The size is 'reduced to eighty pages, and the price to three dollars. It is edited by Lunsford P. Yandell, M. D., Professor of Pathology, Anatomy, and Dean of the Faculty of the University of Louisville.

Functional and Sympathetic Diseases of the Heart.

This is the title of a paper read before the Society of Statistical Medicine, in New•York, by John C. Corson, M. D., late physician to the Brooklyn City Hospital, and physician to the N. Y. Dispensary. We have not had time to read it thoroughly, but from a hasty glance he seems to us to have treated the subject in a sound, common sense manner. The first portion of the essay is devoted to the diagonisis between functional and organic diseases of the heart, and especially to those murmurs resulting from anæmia. A table in which he gives in parallel columns the diagnostic symptoms, contains so much practical information in a small space, that we clip it out for the benefit of our readers :

In Functional Heart Affections :

Præcordial *dulness* on percussion is not permanently *extended*, nor the *apex displaced.*

The *impulse* in *plethora* is strong *bounding ;* in *irritation*, smart *knocking ;* in both, widely jarring; in *debility*, small, soft *tapping.* sometimes *hurried.*

The whole *movement* of the heart is more *elastic, light,* or *easy.*

Functional murmurs are *soft blowing*, *aortic* and *systolic ;* are from *anæmia*, and usually with the venous hum in the neck.

Functional is more *paroxysmal.*

Active exercise is often well borne, and benefits.

The *causes* are mainly *dyspepsia, anæmia, plethora, nervous* or *generative disease.*

In Organic Heart Disease :

Præcordial *dulness* in enlargement is permanently *extended,* and the *apex crowded* to the left.

The *impulse* in *hypertrophy* is strong, broad *heaving;* in both together, strong, large *bulging;* in all with *extended dulness.*

The whole *movement* of the heart is more dead, clumsy, or 'bored.'

Organic murmurs are 'harsher, louder, often grating, aortic or mitral, systolic or diastolic, or both and very rarely with anæmia or venous hum.

Organic is more *uniform.*

Active exercise always *aggravates.*

The most common *causes* are, first, *rheumatism;* and next, Bright's disease.

Michigan Journal of Education and Teachers' Magazine.

This is a monthly of thirty-two pages, and is worthy of the patronage of all friends of education. It is jointly edited by Prof. Haven, of the University, Prof. Welch, of the Normal School, and Rev. J. M. Gregory, of the Commercial College, Detroit. It therefore represents the three great branches of the educational system of this state ; and, from the reputation and known ability of its conductors, it must be eminently successful and useful.

Tappan's Report to the Board of Regents.

This is a report drawn up at the request of the Board, and containing information respecting the celebrated Prussian system of schools, together with observations and recommendations respecting our own. The lugubrious howlings which have been made in certain quarters against this report have caused us to look at it more carefully than we otherwise should have done. Those who have noticed the squirmings of some two or three papers about this time, have, doubtless, remarked a curious want of proportion between the magnitude of the faults they pretend to find in the report, and the excess of their wrath over them: so that it is evident that the writers were not moved by their zeal for the subjects on which they scribbled, but had their eye on some other object. An examination of the Report shows that it is a masterly thing, that the even petty faults charged upon it are falsely charged, and are not to be found in it. At the same time, its depth of research, and comprehensiveness of thought, are such as ever distinguish the productions of master minds.

Medical Organization.

The following notice we insert with great pleasure. The movement of organization is onward.—Ed.

Dr. Andrews—Dear Sir—I hope that this may be received in time to enable you to publish in the February number of your Journal, notice of a Meeting of the Physicians of Oakland, Lapeer, St. Clair, and Macomb Counties, which has been called at Romeo, on Wednesday, the 8th day of March next. This call is made by the medical societies of Lapeer and Macomb conjointly, the only county organizations, I believe, in this part of the state.

The lack of numerical strength in these societies, has rendered them less efficient and useful than they would otherwise have been; and the object of this meeting is, if possible, to consolidate, in one organization, the members of the profession in the counties named. It is to be hoped that the medical men in this region will respond with zeal to the growing interest being manifested in the state and throughout the country in the importance of thorough medical organization.   I remain, Sir, yours truly,

                                     WILLIAM BROWNELL,
Utica, Feb. 3, 1854.   Secretary.

CORRECTION.

Dear Doctor—Through the carelessness of haste in myself, and some miss-deal of the printer, several inaccuracies appear in my communication on dislocation of the femur and reduction, by Dr. Reid's method, in your January number. Will you please to notice the following errata : page 298, fifth line from the bottom, for right, read *left;* page 299, fifth line from top, for right, read *left;* page 299, ninth line from top, for femoirs, read *femoris.* On the same line, [for illii, read *ili;* also, on sixth line from bottom, for illii, read *ilium.*

Hoping to be more cautious in future, I remain, very respectfully,
                                     Yours, &c.,
                                        J. H. B.
Jan. 21st, 1854.

THE

PENINSULAR

JOURNAL OF MEDICINE

AND THE COLLATERAL SCIENCES.

| VOL. I. | MARCH, 1854. | NO. IX. |

ORIGINAL COMMUNICATIONS.

Art. I.—*A Bomb for Buffalo, fired by* Bullhead, Corporal in the Army of Quack Killers.

I, Bullhead, have been perusing the Buffalo Medical Journal in great alarm, and distress of mind. I marvel much, Mr. Editor, that you allow that squib battery down at the other end of Lake Erie to go on for months firing slanders and false statements at the University of Michigan, without condescending to reply to them. Why don't you charge like a man, spike the guns, and silence the battery? I am astonished at your want of spirit, your apathy and your inactivity; yea, also, and I am alarmed for the terrible onslaught which is made against the glory of the profession in Michigan. Yet I am no coward, sir. I am willing to face all common foes, and to peril my life in defending our citadel from all *common* modes of attack; but to meet an army that has a *Buffalo Hunt* for a vanguard, this scares me. I feel like a sailor when he sees something *White* over the *Lee*, and knows that breakers are ahead.

See what ponderous shot are fired at us. For instance, the Buffalo Journal says a State institution cannot succeed because it "is not sustained by the good will of the profession." Now, sir, it is indeed true that the profession in this State loves and cherishes its institution, and the various local societies are continually sending up expressions of their pride and gratification at its success, but this is nothing, you must go down to Buffalo, sir, if you want to see a successful institution, you must mark the crowds of students there, and especially observe the *notorious* and very *remarkable* species of "good will" by which the profession of that city and region sustains that College. Again, Prof. Lee says that competent men for Professors cannot be had for a thousand dollars a year, *consequently* Professors in a State institution must always be a poor article. Assuredly logic hath its foundation in that man's brain, and I shall speedily go myself to Buffalo, to ascertain exactly *how much more than a thousand dollars* that institution yields him, and how much his talent exceeds that of the thousand dollar men.

And further, Editor Hunt states to the public that the Michigan University cannot possibly be supplied with dissecting *materiel.* Indeed, he says it is so destitute, that at the end of three months only one class had been formed, and the lecturer on Anatomy had not a single subject to illustrate his lectures with. Oh! woe to the College; this is very bad. But somehow, Mr. Editor, this buffalo does not bellow correctly. I, Bullhead, walk the rounds of our citadel frequently, to count the dead, and look after the welfare of the living, and I certainly know that at the very time Dr. Hunt was penning this false statement, *fifteen* dissecting classes had been supplied with subjects, and the Professor of Anatomy had been furnished with *three* for his lectures. I also know that three other classes were supplied shortly after, and that then a large surplus of *materiel* was left for which there was no demand. Yet I am frightened and sore amazed, for what if the world should hear the voice of Hunt, and believe his words; then, surely, though we have plenty of *materiel,* yet should we have none to cut it up.

Finally, the Buffalo Journal says that our institution is doomed, because its Regents once in six years are elected by the people, *ergo* all its appointments will be made by these Regents on political grounds, *ergo,* the abyss of ruin gapes for its downfall. This is a strongly democratic state. Now, Dr. Andrews, you poor unfortunate whig, how came *you* by an appointment in the institution, contrary to the verdict of the infallible Buffalo Journal? Don't you see in the light of this logic, first that you have never received any appointment, and secondly, that you will surely be turned out of it. Come to my quarters, old comrade, when you are expelled, and I will divide my last rations with you. Meanwhile, as prospects are evidently getting desperate, stand your ground bravely. Bring out your long *Gunn,* and call on *Abram* and *Moses* and *Samuel,* and all the prophets to help, and fight for life.

REMARKS BY THE EDITOR.

We think the Corporal's terror unfounded, and his zeal altogether uncalled for. We have watched for sometime the articles which the

Buffalo Journal has aimed at the University of Michigan, and so far from esteeming them dangerous, we have thought that they have actually served to bring the school into favor, and to increase its numbers. Instead of replying to them, therefore, we have thought it better to let them have free course, and would even recommend the Board of Regents to pay something, if necessary, to have them continued, as they are the best kind of an advertisement.

The only false statement which we care enough about to contradict, is, the assertion that the Michigan University is scantily supplied with anatomical *materiel*, and that at the present session there is " almost a total destitution."

The laws of this State protect the pursuit of practical anatomy, and provide the University with certain facilities in obtaining *materiel* which no private institution can have. In consequence of these and other advantages, a *larger proportion* of the students dissect at each session than is usual in medical colleges, and although brief delays have sometimes occurred, yet there has never been a session when there was not before the close a *full supply, and a surplus left*. The present session has been one of overflowing abundance. Eighteen dissecting classes have been supplied. The professor of Anatomy has had three for his lectures; two have been sent to private physicians in other parts of the State, and a very large surplus is left on hand. Indeed, such is the completeness of the arrangements, that had it been necessary, it would have been easy to supply not only Michigan University, but two such schools as Buffalo, besides.

We regret that the Editor of the Buffalo Journal descends so low as to prostitute his columns to the circulation of false and unmanly reports about rival schools. We, on our part, have heard a thousand disparaging statements respecting the Buffalo College, but we scorn to publish them. We hold her to be worthy of all courtesy and honor as a sister college, and believing that students who go there and attend to their duties will become good practical physicians, we bid her God speed on her course.

Yet, though there are facts in our possession which would make her ears tingle were we to give them publicity, we scorn to do so mean a thing. To taunt the Buffalo school with her misfortunes, and to flay her alive for faults which perhaps were only induced by these misfortunes, shall never be the work of the Peninsular Journal, while we hold its Editorial pen. On the contrary, we say to all institutions whose object is to give to the world educated physicians, ye have a high and holy mission to perform; go forward successfully, and may heaven prosper your work.

As for you, brother Hunt, we do not know what you are trying to twist yourself into, whether Professor, Author, Critic, or what; but whatever you aim at, in God's name be a *man*, there is nothing higher than that.

We had formed the resolution to say nothing about this subject, and although we have for once departed from it to please the Corporal, we now return to it, and to a work which is too high and pressing to be interrupted for altercation with our neighbors.

ART. II. — *An Address Delivered before the Macomb County Medical Society.* By HENRY TAYLOR, M.D.

GENTLEMEN: — When we first contemplated the organization of this Society, the opinion generally prevailed that the law provided for such organizations. But it would seem that our legislators (and, we are happy to think, for some wise cause) had concluded that medical men could get along without its protection; consequently, with one general sweep — with one final dash, obliterated for all coming time, everything like law-sustained medical societies; having incorporated such a clause in the constitution of our State government.

Well, gentlemen, we will not stop to question the wisdom of our legislators, or to complain of any injustice to ourselves. Like themselves, we also think that we can get along and do without their aid. Like the helpless infant, the time has been when we stood in need of their fostering and maternal care. But now, since we have attained our present mature and more manly growth, we are able to stand alone, to depend upon our own strength, and bid defiance to their want of care and protection.

Hence, gentlemen, the charge can no longer be urged against us, that we are a privileged class of men — that we have rights not common to all men — that we have exclusive privileges which are *anti-democratic,* and inconsistent with a free government.

For more than half a century, have these *sticklers* for *equal rights,*— these advocates for *unbridled* liberty, been making their appeals to community to enkindle a prejudice, and create disapprobation of the medical profession, — accusing them of monopolizing the healing art, however pleasing or profitable they might think to make it to themselves, and thus withhold from them the pleasure of contending, arm to arm, and on equal ground, with death, and of wrestling with the diseases and sufferings of their fellow men. Nor were these looked upon as unjust causes of complaint by the *psudo wise* men of the times — the self-styled statesmen, — the men who always knew that they had claims that they never could impress upon others or make them understand —, that of themselves being wise and useful men. The *patriotism* of these *good men* was touched, their love for *freedom* and *democracy* aroused, and they stood forth as champions of equal rights — pledged, if placed in power, to defend and redress an oppressed and injured people. These pledges were looked upon as the harbingers of better times, and the choice of these men as legislators, had for its tendency to let the " oppressed go free." That all, regardless of qualification or fitness, might share, and share alike with the learned and skillful in the most important and fearful of all responsibilities and trusts confided to man—that of the life and safety of a fellow being.

What a day of jubilee to Quackery was this! when the Homœopathist, Hydropathist, Eclectic, Thomsonian, Uriscopic, and Stick Doctors could raise their heads as high, in keeping with the law, as the regular physician, though all Heaven wept, and *all* — *all* but Satan and themselves, turned from the loathsome sight, pregnant with feelings of *pity* and *disgust!* But, gentlemen, it is our privilege to take a stand more suitable to our own taste — more congenial with the high claims of the medical profession, than that to which our legislature has invited us—that of the society and fellowship of such *creatures*. Who would not " rather be a toad, and live upon the vapors of a dungeon," than in the fellowship of the loathsome quack? But shall I be accused of prejudice? Shall I be considered as acting from selfish motives, or self-interest, in thus denouncing the false pretenders? I ask, what are his claims above the robber or the pirate? The robber asks for your money, or your life. If you will surrender the one, you may keep the other unharmed. True, he has no right to either; but there is some liberality in the demand, compared with that of the quack; for he asks for your money at the expense of your life. Surely, this is the greatest wrong, and betrays the greatest depravity. The robber knows that he has no just claims upon your money. The quack also knows that he is unable to relieve your sufferings, or to arrest your disease, upon which your life depends. The robber knows that he is trifling with your rights. The quack is aware also, that he is trifling with your safety. The former involves your money, the latter your life. We will crowd the comparison no farther, but leave to the wisdom of our legislators, the comparative claims of these august disputants. But how stands the comparison with the pirates? The quack sometimes takes your money and spares your life. Cannot this also be said by the pirate? The quack may sometimes suffer you to pass with both money and life. The pirate may take from the rich and give to the poor. The pirate meets you as a bold and open villain, and while you are possessed of full mental and physical power, invites you to defend yourself. The quack meets you in the mean and cowardly character of an impostor, and when dispossessed of both mental and physical power. The former takes our life and then our money,—the latter our money and then our life. And we will here also leave this comparison, and let an injured God, and an indignant world decide for these inhuman, unfeeling, and villainous schemers. But shall we be condemned for withholding our companionship from them, who will hold so just comparison with those so truly hated and despised of our race? Let truth and reason command, and we pledge to submit and obey.

Did our legislators for a moment think that the blow so violently aimed at our head, might recoil back on their own, or the heads of others? Had they ever read the *thrilling* misfortune that befell the disappointed and unfortunate *Ichabod*, set forth in a beautiful manner by the learned poet?

> " Ichabod he digged a pit,—
> He digged it for another,
> But Ichabod fell into it —
> That pit he digged for 'tother."

I would seriously inquire if this act of the legislature has proved equally harmless to others as it would seem to have done to ourselves. I would ask, have community been benefitted by it? True, they are at liberty to choose to whom they wll commit their sacred trust. But are they safe in making this selection? Are they competent to make a reliable and worthy choice? How is the man who is unskilled and without experience, to decide between the skillful and learned physician, and the vile and ignorant *pretenders*. The learned and skillful man would urge his claims with modesty and reserve. Not so with the vile deceiver. He intends to be benefitted by the deception, and is regardless of its effect on others. How, I would ask, is the suffering invalid to decide under such circumstances? He is altogether unlearned in the art. He is only sure that he must have relief or die. The learned and worthy physician, will only promise the sufferer that he will be faithful and do his best to relieve: he is more noble than to trifle with his credulity. The other, in the true spirit of quackery, promises, unhesitatingly, a prompt and doubtless cure. It requires but little reflection to comprehend that this unfortunate sufferer is in a dilemma, that calls for more wisdom than he can command, to extricate himself from. But in the absence of all evidence, other than the bare statement of these two, we can readily perceive into whose hands the unfortunate patient will fall and equally sure of the hopeless fate that awaits him. I ask if such instances do not urge the want of protection to community? Now, it is obvious that if the learned physician had those evidences that would and did exist under law-sustained medical societies, evidences that he had been examined by a competent board of censors—men competent to judge, and sworn to judge impartially—or if the tendency of the law has not been to destroy all evidences in such instances, it had been in the power of the skillful man to give satisfactory proof of his professional worth, which evidence had turned the scales in the instance before alluded to, and the otherwise duped and deceived sufferer, relieved and saved. The evil here complained of, is the license given to deception. The legalizing of fraud, the multiplying of schemes to rob the ignorant and credulous, and for creating a pestiferous influence, more destructive and deadly than that of the Bohon Upas. Is not community already calling loudly for relief? Has not quackery waded sufficiently deep in the blood of its slain? The regular physician asks for no protection from the laws. He needs none. He could not be benefitted by any protection other than that which he is sure to receive from a grateful and beneficent people.

But community have a right to ask redress for those wrongs—wrongs that could not exist, if none but competent men could, or should be allowed to take upon themselves such important responsibilities — responsibilities upon which chiefly depends and rests the life and safety of her people.

But gentlemen, in these conceded wrongs, can we, as members of this most deserving profession, claim no part? Have we discharged our duties in the community in which we live, and for whom we labor, as truly becomes faithful and trusty men? I fear not. I think not. I fear that a fearful blame would rest on us. The fault is not with the profession, but *us*, as its representatives. Why have we been so negligent as to suffer men to drink so deep of their absurdities, as thus to poison their understandings? Why have we left them so much in the dark? Have we, when opportunity presented, enlightened or instructed as it was competent for us to do? Or have we thrown a deep mystery around the art, the tendency of which, might be to mystify it? Or have we been fearful that we might expose such light as would enable others to relieve the afflicted at our expense? Is our art so frail as this? Are its resources thus limited ? He knows little of the healing art that judges it thus; and he who would enshroud it with mystery and charms, betrays no better knowledge of its greatness. Community ask for light, for truth, and for reason. They are entitled to it; — they ought to have it; — we ought to give it them. Ourselves, as well as they, would be benefitted by their possession of it. It should be as much our pleasure to give, as theirs to receive it. The fact of our withholding from them, this light, should be looked upon as our want of understanding — a want of fitness to take upon ourselves the discharge of its great and important duties.

When it shall become common to make these requirements, and when we shall consent to respond to them, the days of quackery will cease to exist, for light will assume the place of darkness, upon which all their hopes depend. The intelligent physician can give a satisfactory explanation of the laws that govern him in the discharge of his trust. He can impress it upon the understanding of his auditors. He can make known the beautiful and harmonious rules by which he is governed. A knowledge that will impress the mind with pleasant and useful understanding, and enlarge the heart with an idea of the sublime grandeur, of the wisdom and goodness of the beneficient authors of these blessings. But the unlearned and unprincipled deceiver has no plan; — he knows no law; — he has only the ability to deceive and misguide, and being called upon to express himself, must fail for want of understanding. Hence the worth of the enlightened physician would he appreciated, — his ingenuity and industry commended, his zeal and learning rewarded. But, of the quack, his shame and ignorance would be made known, — his foul deception and base heartlessness would be apparent, — his reckless disregard for the life and happiness of his fellow man, would be visible. He would only be known as he is despised.

"And if thou hadst no name to be known by, I would call thee *devil.*"

Nor is this neglect our only fault. Have we not failed to take that decided stand that would tend to show our appreciation of the great worth of our calling. Being in a legal view placed almost on a level with the charlatanist. We have appeared dispirited. We have hesitated to throw our influence together. We have failed to keep up our organizations. We have not, as we ought, kept up the high distinction betwixt the learned physician and ignorant pretender. We have in some instances, mingled with, and counselled them, thus crouching to their level, — forgetful of the fact that the man is known, and estimated by the company he keeps. These, and other faults which might be mentioned, have detracted from the high character we should maintain, and that exalted worth to which the greatness of our profession has entitled us. These acts of ours have thrown a foul stain upon our profession, for which we justly have incurred the contempt of the slow and moving finger of scorn directed at us. What was our duty in the premises after the entire responsibility was thrown upon us? It was that of defending and protecting the character of the profession.

This was now left with us alone. Hence it required a greater zeal. Before it did not require so much from us, for we had assistance from another source. We had had the aid of others to do that which was now left to us alone? Were we now at liberty to slacken in our efforts after this additional burthen had been thrown upon us? Such a course would only be looked upon as cowardly and mean; none but an indolent and stupid spirit would prompt to such resort. No! we should stand up to our profession. We should claim for its dues. We should crowd around its standard, and proclaim to the world its greatness. We should direct its opposers to its lofty and towering heights, and bid defiance to their levelling tendency. We should unfurl its noble and majestic banner to the breeze, on which is inscribed in large and indelible capitals: " *Heaven's greatest and best gifts to afflicted humanity.*"

In conclusion, gentlemen, I am proud to know that a higher and nobler feeling exists in the ranks of our profession, over the entire world. There has been a simultaneous struggle of its advocates, to raise it to that level to which its exalted worth has entitled it. The mighty minds of intelligence have swept off that rubbish under which ignorance and vice had attempted to cover it. It has burst forth like the fires of the great Vesuvius to a more perfect day. I rejoice, gentlemen, to meet you here. I am proud of the honor of being one of your number, engaged in the accomplishment of this great enterprise of medical reform. I most devoutly hope that you may merit the approbation of your brethren for your zeal and ability, and that your last may be your best days in the consciousness of a well-spent life, and that you may long live in the esteem and gratitude of a well-served people!

ART. III.—*Medullary Cancer of the Knee. Amputation—Death— Autopsy—Microscopical Observations—Remarks.* By W. BRODIE, M.D., Detroit.

Mr. —— Scherzel, aged twenty-two years, was admitted into St. Mary's Hospital, September 22nd, 1853, suffering from disease of the right knee. Previous to May, he had always been a healthy man. About that time he was on his passage from Germany to the United States, when he felt a slight pricking pain in the inner condyle of the femur, and passing through the end of the bone, which soon began to enlarge. Upon his arrival in Detroit, being destitute, he was taken to the Wayne County Poor House, and placed under treatment.

His friends not being satisfied at his not regaining his health, brought him to the Hospital in this City, where he was first seen by Dr. Pitcher and myself.

At this time the knee was considerably enlarged, the skin was smoothe and distended, and the joint had the appearance of effusion having taken place.

There was considerable tenderness of the parts, yet the leg could be flexed upon the thigh, partially, when done so by the hand, without producing much pain.

The disease gradually progressed, in contempt of all treatment. Tumors formed in the popliteal space, and upon the condyles of the femur. These were elastic and pressure made upon them produced little, and, at times, no pain.

About the end of October he complained of great pain in his foot, and likewise in the popliteal space. His body had now considerably emaciated. Erysipelas attacked the knee, and extending, involved the leg and foot. On his recovery from this, he was attacked with the prevailing fever, (Typhoid) which continued through November into December, and left him with his lungs weak, and a copious, thick expectoration. About the middle of this month, slight hectic symptoms appeared, which were soon combatted.

His general health seemed now to improve, and being abundantly satisfied that his only hope of recovery was in amputation of the part, it was decided to do so at once, and on the 29th instant, assisted by Dr. Pitcher, who administered the chloroform, Drs. Stebbins, Batwell, Davenport, and Christian, I removed the knee by the circular operation, making my first incision at the union of the middle with the lower third of the femur, in order to be above the contaminated soft parts; but, owing to his great emaciation, the muscles contracted so much that the limb was taken off at the union of the middle with the upper third. The stump was then dressed and the patient put in bed, when he soon recovered his usual spirits. For ten days he improved in his general health, the stump progressed in healing, and at the time of his death was entirely closed.

After the tenth day he had more fever, the expectoration became more copious, his appetite began to fail, and on the 21st day of January, 1854, he died.

No autopsy of the body was made. After the diseased limb was removed, it was thoroughly examined. Upon dissecting off the skin, superficial fascia, and adipose tissue, a most interesting specimen of medullary disease presented itself, involving the condyles of the femur and extending up the shaft of the same, together with the origin of the vasti muscles, insertions of the biceps, fascia, ligaments, adipose tissue, and glands surrounding the joint and occupying the popliteal space.

Upon opening into the joint, the semilunar fibre, cartilages and synovial membranes were found in their usual healthy and moist state, but the anterior and posterior crucical ligaments were undergoing degeneration, even to their origins from the head of the tibia, yet the tibia itself was unaffected.

The ligamentum patellæ was distended, so that the patella was drawn up above the joint, and was involved in the cancerous mass. The patella was not implicated.

The popliteal glands were so enlarged as to make the course of the artery and vein torturous and much diminished in size. One of the glands, the size of a hen's egg, had so pushed itself before the popliteal nerve, as to distend it and carry it backwards, like the string of a viol over its bridge. This no doubt gave rise to the extreme pain complained of in the ancle and foot.

The measurements of the knee, before the integument was removed, and afterwards, have been lost, so that I cannot give them correctly, but the appearance of the knee was that of a man's head.

Through favor of my friend Dr. Andrews, of the medical department of the University, to whom the preparation was sent, as a pathological specimen for the museum, I am indebted for the following microscopical observations:

"Upon examination the cell walls could not be discovered, but the nuclei alone were visible, as in some cases described by Paget. The nuceli were nucleolated, and lay in a granular substance. Very few fibres were to be found.

" The osseous part of the tumor did not present the regular bone structure, but rather a granular mass without definite formation.

"The above appearance plainly indicates, and even demonstrates, the nature of the disease, and renders the case exceedingly interesting."

There are two leading points of interest connected with the case, viz: 1st. The rapid growth of the malignant disease, and its complication with erysipelas and typhoid fever. 2nd. The particular location, unpreceded by the implication of any other part.

As regards the first, the disease appeared in May, by a pricking sensation passing through the condyles of the femur. In December, it had advanced so far that amputation was necessary to save life. The erysipelatous inflammation did its part in depressing the vital energies, and the typhoid fever followed to complete the constitutional disorganization. In my humble opinion, deceased would have recovered from the amputation had not the lungs been so much disorganized and depressed by the fever.

2nd. Sir Benjamin Brodie, in Chap. viii. of his valuable surgical observations on the diseases of the joints, says, "In the cases which have fallen under my observation, carcinoma of the bones has never occurred as a primary disease, but has always been preceded by carcinoma of the breast, or some other glandular organ, but in Case 73 of the same Chapter, is related one in which the same form of disease occurred, without any account of previous malignant degeneration of any one organ or tissue. In this the primary seat of the disease was in the head of the tibia, instead of the condyles of the femur."

In the case of Scherzel, no trace of malignant disease could be found, except in the knee; nor could I learn that it had before existed in any of his family connections; and, what is still more interesting in his case is, that no provocation was given by blows, or otherwise, as a nucleus for its origin. The treatment of the case was such as the varying complications demanded—at all times supportive in its character. However, a detail will add no particular interest to the case itself.

Detroit, Feb. 15th, 1854.

Art. IV.—*To the Editor of the Peninsular Journal of Medicine:*

Sir:—I take the liberty to send you a report of one or two medical cases, which you are at liberty to publish, if you think them worthy of that honor.

CASE FIRST.

Mrs. B., about twenty years of age, a healthy and vigorous woman, for the first time pregnant, began to be afflicted near the close of the eighth month of gestation, with a peculiar numbness and tingling in the middle and ring fingers of each hand. This affection gradually increased in intensity proportionably with the enlargement of the mammæ, until the hands were rendered almost useless. The affected fingers were constantly distended with blood, and the patient complained of a good deal of pain in them. The application of warm water was intolerable, but cold water afforded great relief. After Parturition, the fingers soon got better, but the nails were sore for sometime. As I do not recollect having seen a similar case recorded in any of the books or journals, I was much interested, and took some pains to ascertain the cause of the peculiar symptoms. I soon found that there was an enlargement of some of the axillary glands, which appeared to be affected through sympathy with the mammary glands. These undoubtedly pressed upon the axillary plexus of nerves, thus causing a partial paralysis of the parts supplied by some of its branches. It is singular that the middle and ring fingers of each hand were the only ones affected. What would you infer from this, Mr. Editor? You are better posted in anatomy than I am. Which branch of the plexus was pressed upon?

CASE SECOND.

Same patient, lingering and laborious labor. Cause, rigidity of the os uteri. After the patient had been forty hours in hard labor, and was nearly exhausted by her long continued and intense sufferings, but little progress having been made, I thought I would try the effect of the inhalation of Chloroform. What was my gratification at finding that as soon as the patient was fairly under the influence of the remedy, the os uteri began rapidly to dilate, so that in less than two hours she gave birth to a living female child, weighing seven pounds. This child has spina bifida, and as I have it now under treatment, I may at some future time report upon it. For the present, Adieu. Yours with Respect,

JOHN C. NORTON.

ART. V.—*To the Editor of the Peninsular Journal of Medicine:*

Sir:—If you deem the annexed worthy of a place in your Journal, you are at liberty to insert it.

$$\text{R}\!\!\!/ \quad \begin{array}{lll} \text{Gum Acacia,} & \text{3} & \text{iv} \\ \text{Aqua Pura, (Boiling) f} & \text{3} & \text{ij} \\ \text{Alcohol,} & \text{f 3} & \text{ss} \end{array}$$

Pour the water on the acacia, and agitate frequently, until it is dissolved, then add the alcohol (which is to keep it from souring) and cork tightly.

I find this an invaluable preparation for burns, and excoriated surfaces. When poured (and spread) upon the denuded parts it produces anything but a disagreeable sensation, the water soon evaporates, and leaves a thin transparent artificial epidermis, which posesses a considerable degree of elasticity, and if not exposed to a cold temperature, it will not exfoliate until displaced by the formation of an epidermis beneath. I have used it in a number of cases, also on my own person, and have found it agreeable and effectual.

Lowell, Michigan, January 23.　　　　　　　　Z. E. Bliss.

On the Analyses of Waters. By Prof. S. H. Douglass, of the University of Michigan. A Report to the Board of Water Commissioners of the City of Detroit.

LABORATORY OF THE UNIVERSITY OF MICHIGAN,
February 11th, 1854.

To the Board of Water Commissioners of the City of Detroit.

Gentlemen—On the the tenth day of November last I received from J. Houghton, Esq., Superintendent of your City Water Works, three stoneware jugs, containing water from the following localities, viz.:

No. 1. From the iron pipe at the residence of A. C. McGraw, on Jefferson avenue, between Rivard and Russell streets, collected January 25th, 1854.

No. 2. From the wooden logs at the residence of Dennis Cuyle, corner of Orchard and Fifth streets, Crawford Park, collected October 5th, 1853.

No. 3. From a well at the residence of Amos T. Hall, on Woodward avenue, Park lot 11, collected October 5th, 1853.

These waters were accompanied with a request to have them analyzed, and to report the result to you at my earliest convenience, with such suggestions, founded on the analyses, as I should conceive important to be taken into consideration in the construction of the new Water Works. Having completed the analyses, I herewith submit the result.

Before proceeding to consider the composition of the waters above named, it may not be inappropriate to make a few remarks on the varieties of water in common use for domestic purposes; the impurities of each variety, and the sources of those impurities.

These waters may be considered under three varieties.

First.—Rain water, which includes water derived from rain, dew, hail, snow, or frost. When secured before it has come in contact with the earth, or any substance that can impart impurities to it, this is the purest natural water. It contains only a small quantity of air, carbonic acid, and ammonia. Not holding in solution any of the earthy salts, its tendency to dissolve other material with which it may come in contact is very greatly increased. For this reason, as ordinarily secured, it is far more deleterious than any water in use. Thus falling upon tin roofs, and being conveyed by tin conductors, with lead soldering, to cisterns, a very perceptible quantity of the poisonous compounds of the latter metal, derived from the soldering, are invariably found dissolved in the water. This I have found to be particularly the case with the water collected from roofs that have been painted with white lead. Collected from shingle or gravel roofs, the evil does not exist to the same extent; yet, in being conveyed through tin conductors, with lead soldering, or lead pipe, is clearly perceivable. I do not hesitate to say that rain water, collected in the ordinary mode, used as an habitual drink, must prove highly injurious to health.

Second.—River water. This stands next in purity to rain water. When its source is considered, it must be evident that the water of all rivers must be very far from being pure. The water of all our rivers, lakes, ponds, and oceans, has at one time existed in the air in a state of vapor, from whence it has been precipitated, in a pure state, as rain or snow. This water, coming in contact with the earth's surface, and frequently penetrating its strata, becomes impregnated with the soluble matter of each particular stratum. For instance, in leaching through a limestone or chalk formation, it would become charged with lime; or, in passing over a magnesian limestone, with lime

and magnesia. Thus it will be perceived that this second variety of water must contain variable ingredients ; and that a
knowledge of the composition of the water becomes an index to
the geology of a. district, and a knowledge of the geology an
index to the composition of the water.

Third.—Spring or well water.—Inasmuch as all the water of
springs and wells has come in contact with, and leached through
the earth, and usually very little time has been allowed for the
separation of the clay, sand, &c., held mechanically in suspension, this variety may be considered the most impure water in
use. This is more particularly the case with the water from
wells dug in a clay soil, and in large towns, where surface filth
accumulates in great abundance.

WATER AS A SOLVENT.

In what form of combination are these earthy salts held in
solution ? This is a question of some considerable practical
importance, and one with which all should be familiar. In some
few cases, the water dissolves the substance directly, as silica
(sand) and the sulphate of lime (gypsum) ; while, in other cases,
in order that the water should become a solvent, it must contain an excess of carbonic acid gas, or the salt must be in the
form of a bi-carbonate. Thus pure water will dissolve little or
no carbonate of lime (limestone), but allow the water to take
carbonic acid, and convert the carbonate into a bi-carbonate ;
and it will readily dissolve a hundredth part of the limestone.
It becomes a " hard water." By long exposure of this water
to the air, or by boiling it, the free carbonic acid escapes as a
gas ; consequently, the water loses its power of holding the
lime in solution. It becomes turbid and milky, and the lime is
deposited. Hence, the calcarious deposits in the vicinity of
" hard water " springs, and the calcarious incrustations on the
inside of boilers. This carbonic acid is derived, in part, from
the atmosphere, and in part from the soil. In the decay of
vegetable matter, the carbon of the plant unites with the oxygen
of the air, to form the acid. Hence, we find it very abundant
in open, porous soils, highly charged with decaying organic

matter. Water leached through such soils would acquire carbonic acid, and, coming in contact with limestone, would dissolve it in great quantity. A "hard water" would be formed. Boiling expels the carbonic acid, and the lime is no longer dissolved. The water is made soft. If, however, the water is made "hard" by the presence of the sulphate of lime, the sulphate is not affected by boiling. In this case, the lime may be precipitated by the addition of carbonate of soda or potassa. An insoluble carbonate of lime is formed and precipitated while the sulphuric acid unites with the soda. Hence, the great practical importance of knowing the precise condition of the lime held in solution—that is, whether it is a carbonate or sulphate.

Waters holding in solution the sulphates are liable to a form of spontaneous decomposition, highly deleterious to health, when they come in contact with organic matter, either animal or vegetable. All animal and vegetable matter contains hydrogen. In ordinary decomposition, this gas is liberated; and if, in the nascent state (at the moment of being set free from a previous combination), it comes in contact with the sulphates, it decomposes them, uniting with the sulphur, to form sulphuretted hydrogen, or hydro-sulphuric acid. This is a very noxious gas, and its foul odor is perceived in the exhalations from bilge water, cesspools, drains, &c. Hence the necessity of avoiding contact with organic matter when the water contains the soluble sulphates. It should not be conveyed through wooden logs, or pumped through wooden pumps. The disinfecting property of chloride of lime depends upon its power to decompose and destroy this hydro-sulphuric acid.

THE ANALYSIS.

In conducting any analysis, the first object with the chemist is, to determine what substances are present. This is called the qualitative examination, or analysis. In the case in question, an indefinite quantity was taken, and, having been divided into several parcels, the proper tests were applied for the detection of every substance liable to be present in natural or mineral waters. This qualitative analysis resulted in the detection of the following substances :

	Number One. From Iron Pipe.	Number Two. From Logs.	Number Three. From Well.
Silicic Acid (Flint) -	Present,	Present.	Present.
Oxide of iron, -	'Present.	Present.	Present.
Lime, - \ -	Present.	Present.	Present.
Magnesia, - -	Present.	Present.	Present.
Potassa, -	Present.	Present.	Present.
Soda, -	Present.	Present.	Present.
Chlorine, - -	Present.	Present.	Present.
Sulphuric Acid, -	Present.	Present.	Present.
Phosphoric Acid, -	Present. `	Present.	
Carbonic Acid, -	Present.	Present.	Present.
Allumina, - -	Present.	Present.	
Hydro-Sulphuric Acid,		Present.	Present.

Having thus fixed upon the presence of certain substances, attention was next directed to the determining of the quantity of each of these substances, or the quantitative analysis.

The total quantity of solid matter in a definite quantity of water, after filtration, was determined by evaporating to dryness' 3500 grammes (nearly one gallon) over a water bath. The following table will give the result :

	Number One. Iron Pipe.	Number Two. Logs.	Number Three. Well.
Solid matter in 3500 grms.	·3432	·3893	7·2000

In determining the quantity of the several substances indicated by the qualitative analysis, six parcels of water were carefully weighed out. The object in taking so many parcels was, to avoid the errors that might arise from the accumulation of impurities in the use of chemicals. From number one the chlorine was extracted; from number two the silica, iron, lime, and magnesia; from number three the iron, magnesia, and lime precipitated on boiling, and which are supposed to exist as carbonates, and the same elements held in solution; from number four potassa and soda; from number five sulphuric acid; from number six allumina and phosphoric acid.

In determining the quantity of these substances, it must not be supposed that they were obtained and weighed in the forms above expressed, for this was the case with but a single substance, silica. All the rest were weighed in the form of some one of their combinations, and the quantity of the element sought determined by simple calculation. This process is based on an invariable law in chemical science, that bodies unite in certain fixed and definite proportions. Thus chlorine was weighed as a chloride of silver. Now, one hundred parts of the chloride of silver *invariably* contain 24·72 parts of chlorine, and 75·28 parts of silver. Lime was separated, as a carbonate of lime; magnesia, as a phosphate of magnesia; potassium as a chloride of platina and potassium; sulphuric acid as a sulphate of baryta, &c. In this manner, the chemist attains to a degree of minuteness that would appear, to an unpractised person, wholly incredible. Thus a good balance will turn on the 1-000 part of a grain (equal to three-tenths of an inch of fine hair). One-thousandth part of a grain is a weighable quantity; and yet the one-thousandth part of a grain of chloride of silver contains but the 1-4000th part of a grain of chlorine, a quantity too small to be weighed, but one which may be calculated. It may be proper to state that the balance used was Robinson's, of the best German manufacture. To avoid friction, the pans and beam are suspended on knife edges, and highly polished carnelian.

The following table will exhibit the quantity of each substance in 1,000 grammes of water :

	Number One. Iron Pipe.	Number Two. Logs.	Number Three. Well.
Silica (Flint), -	·00500	·00583	·02370
Oxide of Iron, -	·00500	·01330	·00625
Lime, - -	·03528	·03192	·33590
Magnesium, -		·00045	·08910
Potassium, - -	·00127	·00127	·10460
Sodium, - -	·00245	·00245	·28740
Chlorine, - -	Trace.	Trace.	·74890
Sulphuric Acid, -	·00550	·00680	·21420
Phosphoric " -	·01430	·02385	*
Carbonic " -	·01766	·01060	·17635
Allumina, - -	·01050	·01050	*
Hydro-Sulphuric Acid,		Trace.	Trace.
Oxygen, with K. & Na.	·00111	·00142	·00960
Total, - -	·09807	·10839	1·99600

In determining the manner in which the above substances are combined among themselves to form neutral compounds, the precipitates formed, on boiling, were first considered as carbonates ; and then recourse is had to the law that governs the distribution of acids and bases, *i. e.*, the strongest acids unite with the strongest bases.

The following table will give the result of this calculation for 1,000 grammes, as before :

---

* Not determined.

	Number One Iron Pipe.	Number Two. Logs.	Number Three. Well.
Chloride of Potassium	....	....	·11000
Chloride of Sodium, -	....	....	·72520
Chloride of Magnesium,	....	...	·34760
Sulphate of Potassa, -	·00283	·00283	·10450
Sulphate of Soda, -	·00750	·00750	....
Sulphate of Lime, -	....	·00254	·23260
Phosphate of Lime, -	·03110	·05192	....
Allumina,	·01050	·01050	....
Magnesia, -	....	·00073	....
Silica (Quartz). -	·00500	·00583	·02370
Carbonate of Lime, -	·03300	·00510	·39190
Carbonate of Iron, -	·00814	·02160	·01020
Total, - -	·09807	·10865	1·99570

From the above table, a very marked difference will be perceived in the composition of the water taken from the wells and that from the iron pipe or logs. The large quantity of the chloride of sodium (common salt), chloride of potassium and magnesium found in the former, clearly indicates its surface origin. The two last salts are cathartic in their properties, and the habitual use of water holding them in solution in any considerable quantities must prove injurious to health.

In addition to the above impurities, the wells of Detroit, being dug in a clay soil, and usually in back yards, would be liable to contain organic matter in the process of decomposition. This would be particularly the case during the warm season, when sickness is most likely to prevail. The use of water containing this organic matter would predispose to disease, and materially aid in the spread of epidemics. No doubt a careful examination would show that, during the prevalence of the cholera, that disease was more fatal, and prevailed to a greater extent among those using the water of the wells than among those in the habitual use of river water. My limited acquaintance with the distribution of water in your city, and with the localities where the disease was most prevalent, does not enable me to furnish examples in confirmation of this position. From Dr. Terry I obtain the following case in point:

" During the prevalence of cholera in Detroit, in the summer of 1850, I was called to see the wife of Mr. T. F., whom I found in a state of collapse, from which she did not rally, but died in about twelve hours. My attention had been previously called to the effect of well water in developing cholera; but, in this case, there had been such other apparently exciting causes, that I did not even inquire in regard to the water used by the family. The next day I was called to see the two sons of Mr. F. and found them under the care of two physicians. One was severely sick, and the other in a hopeless state of collapse, from cholera. They had been under treatment some hours when I arrived. The first one recovered, and the second died in a few hours.

" I then, for the first time, learned that two persons in the adjoining house had died of the same disease within two days, and my attention was at once directed to the water used by these families, which proved to be water from a well common to both. Mr. F.'s family consisted of himself, his wife, two boys, and a daughter, the children all under seventeen years of age, the daughter the younger. Mr. F.'s employment was at a place where he had access to, and used the water of the river. All the rest used the well water. To recapitulate, Mrs. F. and the elder boy died; the younger just escaped, and the girl had severe diarrhœa, which would have soon developed cholera, had not immediate precautions been taken. I prohibited the use of the well water, and from that time there were no more cases in the family. On the same street, immediately opposite, there were certainly two deaths (and I think three) from cholera, in a house in which well water was used. It was reported that other instances of the same kind occurred on the street, but for this I cannot vouch.

"ADRIAN R. TERRY, M. D."

I have also been informed by Professor Palmer, of Chicago, that this disease has been observed to be most fatal in that city in those districts where well water was used, although the most high, and apparently the most healthy. The lower districts, containing such quantities of surface water and filth as entirely to preclude the use of well water, were supplied with water from the lake by carts, and were comparatively free from this disease.

Again, the city of Sandusky is situated on a clay soil, underlaid by a limestone, and is supplied with water mostly from wells dug in this tenacious clay. The water must not only be highly charged with lime and other earthy salts, but likewise contain large quantities of decaying organic matter, derived from surface drainage. I am fully of the opinion that the fearful ravages of cholera in that city may be, in a great measure, attributed to the use of impure water.

It is a well established fact, that, in the city of Cincinnati, of all persons who used the water of certain springs during the prevalence of cholera, not one escaped fatal attacks of the disease.

Other examples might be given, drawn both from this country and Europe, illustrating the effect of water on the spread of epidemics, as a predisposing cause; but this is not the place for a lengthy discussion of this subject.

The chemical analysis of the river water leads to the following useful conclusions:

1st. The carbonates are found in very small quantities. As very little precipitate is formed on boiling, the water cannot be improved as to its "hardness," by the application of heat.

2nd. The sulphates and phosphates are the most abundant

salts held in solution. The presence of the former, for reasons already stated, would forbid the use of wood conducting logs. That hydro-sulphuric acid is formed by the spontaneous decomposition of the sulphates, is shown by the presence of this noxious compound in the water taken from the logs.

3rd. The analysis of number one, from the iron pipe, shows it to be water superior to that of most other cities. Thus an examination of the annexed table will show that it contains less solid matter in the gallon than either the Croton or Cincinnati water, but more than the Fairmount or Long Pond water. In estimating the value of your city water, as compared with the water of other cities, due allowance must be made for the fact that the total solid matter is materially increased by the presence of silica, allumina, and iron, elements that can produce little or no injury ; while the chlorides, much the most injurious compounds, are entirely absent. The presence of such large quantities of silica and iron is accounted for by the fact that Lakes Superior and Huron are formed, for the most part, in a basin of ferruginous sandstone and igneous rock. It will also be observed that the carbonate of lime is more abundant in the water collected in February than October. This arises, doubtless, from the change of temperature, the cold water holding much more lime in solution than when warm.

Analyses of Natural Waters: Showing the Quantity of Compound Ingredients in Grains Troy in an American Standard Gallon (58372 Grains) of each of the Specimens.

	Schuylkill River, Fairmount.	Croton River.	Charles River.	Spot Pond.	Long Pond, Boston Water Works.	Mystic Pond.	Ohio R. at Cincinnati.	Detroit River. Iron Pipe, Collected in Feby.	Detroit River. Logs, Collected in Oct.	Detroit Well.
Chloride of Potassium,	·1470	·1670	·1547		·0380	·1590				6·4192
Chloride of Sodium,		·3720	·0420		·0323	27·9110				42·3200
Chloride of Calcium,	·0094				·0308					
Chloride of Magnesium,		·1600		·3969	·0764	·1544	·4773			20·2846
Chloride of Allumina,										
Sulphate of Potash,										
Sulphate of Soda,	·0570	·1530	·3816			1·2190	0125	·1651	·1651	6·0982
Sulphate of Lime,		·2350	·2624	·2276	·1020	·9768	·7738	·4376	·4376	16·4915
Sulphate of Magnesia,						·4478			·1482	
Sulphate of Allumina,									·0426	
Phosphate of Lime,		·8320	·0973	·1081		·2810		1·8148	3·0298	
Phosphate of Allumina,										
Allumina,										
Silicic Acid,	·0600	·0770	Trace.	Trace.	·0800	·5559	·2694	·6127	·6127	
Carbonate of Lime,	1·870	2·1310	·1610	·3722	·0300	·9894	3·2615	·2917	·3402	1·3830
Carbonate of agnesia,	·3510	·6620	·0399	·1420	·2380	1698		1·9257	·2076	22·8698
Carbonate of Manganese,		Trace.			·0630					
Carbonate of Iron,	Trace.						Trace.			
Salts of Soda, with Nitric and Organic Acids,	1·6436	1·8650	·5291		·5295		1·3215	·4750	1·2605	·5952
Total Solid Matter,	4·2600	6·6600	1·6680	1·2468	1·2220	34·7671	6·7361	5·7226	6·3343	116·4615
	Analyzed by Prof. Silliman, Jr.						Analyzed by J. M. Lock.	Analyzed by Prof. Douglass.		

The purity of water is not simply a matter in which is involved health and convenience in domestic economy; for, to the manufacturer, where water is used as a solvent, it is exceedingly important that it should be pure. " Brewers often go to an enormous expense in boring deep wells, in order to obtain a supply of soft water, for extracting all soluble matter from the malt and hops they employ. Dyers also bore wells, in order to obtain a supply of soft water, as certain colors cannot be dyed where water, containing the ordinary impurities, comes in contact with the dye-stuffs. Bleachers, again, require pure water; and many other branches of manufacture might be mentioned where pure water is absolutely indispensable."

You have requested me to direct my particular attention to the propriety of using lead service pipe in the conveyance of river water. I approach this subject with great reluctance, for I am well aware of the important bearing it has upon the health of your city, and equally well aware that, at present, there is no little discrepancy of opinion among scientific men as to the circumstances in which lead pipe may be safely used. This disagreement arises, in part, from the difficulty in determining precisely what water does not corrode lead, and, in part, from the evil effects of the lead on the system, so nearly resembling diseases produced by other morbific agents, as not always to be clearly distinguishable from them. Not having made any experiments myself to determine the action of water on lead, except in the case of rain water, I shall be compelled to rely on the experiments and views of others. I have already deprecated the use of lead pipe for the conveyance of rain water. No one will question the impropriety of thus using it. It is said, however, that most spring and river water contains a sufficient quantity of the neutral salts to form an insoluble lining on the inner surface of the pipe, which most effectually protects it from further decomposition. Thus Dr. Christison states that "water containing 1-000 or 1-1200 part of salts, may be safely conveyed in lead pipes, if the salts are chiefly sulphates and carbonates; and that lead pipes cannot be safely used when it contains 1-4000th part of saline matter, if this consists of muriates."

At the request of the Board of Consulting Physicians of the City of Boston, Prof. E. N. Horsford, of Cambridge, in 1849, examined, with great care, the relations of lead to air and water, and gives the following as his conclusions :

" A coat of greater or less permeability forms in all natural waters to which lead is exposed. The first coat is a simple sub-oxide, absolutely insoluble in water, and solutions of salts generally. This becomes converted in some waters into a higher oxide ; and this higher oxide, uniting with water and carbonic acid, forms a coat soluble in from 7,000 to 10,000 times its weight of pure water. The above oxide unites with sulphuric and other acids, which sometimes enter into the constitution of the last coat; uniting with organic matter and iron rust, it forms another coat, which is in the highest degree protective,"

Dr. Horatio Adams, in a lengthy and very able report, before the American Medical Association, at its annual meeting, in 1852, deprecates the use of lead pipe for the conveyance of water, under any circumstances. Having shown, both by analysis, and its effects on the system, that lead is present in the Cochituate water drawn through lead pipes, also in the Croton water, the New Orleans water, the Cincinnati and Louisville water, he concludes—" That it is never safe to use water drawn through lead pipes, or stored in leaden cisterns, for domestic purposes ; and that any article of food or drink is dangerous to health, which, by any possibility, can be impregnated with saturnine matter."

Gmelin, a distinguished German chemist, does not differ from Christison.

On the whole, as it is, at least, doubtful, whether the solid matter contained in any of the varieties of natural water, will effectually protect lead from dissolving, and especially as the water of Detroit river contains less solid matter than either Christison or Gmelin consider necessary for that purpose, I am inclined to discourage the use of lead service pipe, at least until it can be clearly shown that no evil results therefrom. Block tin service pipe, or lead pipe, lined with tin, would not be liable to the same corrosion. I would, therefore, recommend it as a substitute for the lead pipe.

SELECTIONS.

Norwood, on the Therapeutical Powers of Veratrum Viride.

[Dr. Norwood has placed at our service his pamphlet on Veratrum Viride. As the subject is exciting much attention, we publish the body of it entire, notwithstanding we have given some parts of it before. We hope physicians will test the remedy and report to us their experience with it. It can be had of Higby and Dickinson, Detroit.—Ed.]

Veratrum viride, as a therapeutical agent, had excited comparatively little interest previous to June, 1850; and it was noticed for a time after that date, more on account of the extravagance of the claims set up for it as a remedial agent of superior powers, than because of any belief that it was possessed of peculiar and valuable properties. If we recollect correctly, it was about the year 1835 that Dr. Charles Osgood's interesting article on the powers and properties of veratrum viride made its appearance. The only additional information he conveyed was that it is destitute of cathartic powers, which give it a superiority over the Veratrum Album or European Hellebore, in the treatment of cases where active cathartics are inadmissible. Be this as it may, it is certain, and cannot be successfully controverted, that prior to June, 1850, it was not known positively to possess any superiority over veratrum album; indeed the one was supposed to answer the same purposes as the other.

Why Dr. Osgood ceased to give further notice of its powers we are not prepared to say; whether his silence grew out of a want of confidence in its remedial powers, or from death, we are wholly ignorant. We do not wonder at the violent and drastic effects he witnessed; but we rather wonder, from the large doses given, that he obtained any beneficial effects. Be this as it may, if it possesses the powers and properties we attribute to it, and is adapted to the treatment of the symptoms and diseases indicated by us, the discovery must be eminently valuable. Greatly enlarged experience and observation have strongly confirmed us in the belief of the correctness of what we stated on a former occasion, namely, that when its powers and properties are fully known and understood, it will constitute a new era in the treatment of disease.

In July, 1844, we first used it in the case of Mrs. L. She had been laboring under a severe attack of pneumonia typhoides for several days. Calomel, blisters, Dover's powders, &c., failed to afford relief. This case having annoyed us by its severity and obstinacy, and opium producing unpleasant effects without relief to the pain, we determined to make a trial of the tincture of veratrum viride. We withdrew all other remedies, and put her on tea-spoonful doses of the tincture, to be repeated every three hours.

We gave her a teaspoonful at 11, A. M. About 1, P. M. we were sent for in haste, as the medicine, or something else, was acting drastically. We found the patient vomiting every few minutes: skin cold and covered with perspiration; great paleness, nausea distressing; complained of a sense of sinking and exhaustion. After the vomiting had ceased, the pulse was found not more than 60 per minute, full and distinct.

In a few cases, in which nausea was great and the vomiting frequent, we have found the pulse very slow, small, and almost imperceptible at the wrist; but as soon as the vomiting and consequent exhaustion subside, the pulse will be found slow, full and distinct. The nausea or vomiting, when in excess, can be readily and certainly relieved by one or two full portions of syrup of morphine and tincture of ginger, or laudnum and brandy.

In this case, before administering the tincture of veratrum viride, the skin was hot and dry; pulse 130, small and soft; circumscribed flush on the cheeks; pain severe; breathing hurried and difficult; cough frequent; expectoration scanty. The very striking effects of the medicine, the great reduction in the frequency of the pulse, and the sudden breaking up or arrest of the disease, in this and another case, profoundly enlisted our attention, and led us from that period to observe more particularly its powers.

The second case in which we used the veratrum veride was that of Mrs. M., who was also laboring under a severe attack of pneumonia. Pulse from 130 to 140 beats per minute; pain violent, and extending from the right side, near the spine, to, and under the sternum; tongue red on the edges and tip, and covered in the centre with a thin, dark, dry fur; bright scarlet circumscribed flush, appearing first on one cheek, and then on the other, rarely on both at the same time; the end or tip of the nose and chin frequently red; very pale around the mouth; expectoration scanty; mucus streaked with blood; cough frequent and very harrassing; great increase of pain under the sternum during a paroxism of coughing; decubitus on the back; breathing labored and difficult. Did not see her till the fourth day: she had been bled, and otherwise treated, with little or no relief. Applied a blister, and gave a camphorated powder to allay the cough and violent pain, and to excite diaphoresis. At the expiration of three hours, to commence with the tincture of veratrum viride.

The first portion excited intense nausea, violent emesis, great paleness, coolness and a sense of sinking or exhaustion. The patient and friends becoming alarmed, another physician who lived much nearer than myself, was sent for in great haste, but when he arrived the nausea and emesis had ceased; the patient was comfortable, pain and febrile symptoms subdued, pulse 65, full and distinct. The doctor was surprised to find the condition of the patient so different from the representation given by the messenger. The disease was really broken up and a crisis and resolution brought about. Our friend, the doctor, ordered a little paragoric and quinine, in which we fully concurred on our arrival, as there was entire relief of all active febrile and inflammatory symptoms.

Deeply impressed with the peculiar effects of verat. viride, we determined to make farther and careful trial of it in pneumonitis. The third case in which we administered it was that of Mr. T., who was taken sick when on a visit to his friend in this section of the country. We ordered the tincture given every three hours, beginning with eight drops, to be increased one drop at each dose until nausea, vomiting or some other visible effect was produced. On the dose reaching twelve drops it induced vomiting with but little nausea. The pulse was reduced from 135 to 78 beats per minute; the surface, from being hot and dry, became cool; and the severe pain was now but slightly felt on taking a deep inspiration. The interval between the doses was extended from three to five hours; but as twelve drops induced too frequent vomiting, the quantity was reduced to seven drops and continued three days without any return of the symptoms, when the case was dismissed and the patient was soon able to return home. This case was one full of interest on account of the success and promptness with which the violent symptoms were removed and the disease cured.

We might report any number of cases, but as many of them have already been given by others, we will confine ourselves to such facts only as may tend to illustrate particular points. We continued our experimental trials with various doses from three to twelve drops, increasing or diminishing them according to circumstances, until we acquired a perfect knowledge of its effects, and could graduate them at will.

We ascertained that in cases which had run on for sometime, or in which emetics and cathartics had been freely used, a very small quantity was necessary. Where tartar emetic has been given, it is almost sure to act harshly and drastically. Where tartar emetic had been taken, we would therefore always give a full portion of syrup of morphine, at least one hour before entering on the use of the veratrum viride, and in such cases would not commence with more than six drops for a male adult. Free venesection increases very materially its activity, especially its unfavorable or drastic effects. No one should think of following a large bleeding with the veratrum viride, unless with the greatest caution. The depressing influence of the loss of blood upon the brain and nervous system generally, cannot fail to render the use of so potent a sedative as veratrum viride exceedingly hazardous. The administration under such circumstances, of an agent capable of reducing the pulse from 130 or 140 down to 75, 70, or even 50 beats in the course of a few hours, cannot be too carefully watched.

But, to proceed: We soon discovered, to our surprise, that in almost every instance, so soon as nausea or vomiting was excited the pulse became slow, full and distinct, the skin cool and often soft and moist, and in some cases bathed in a most profuse prespiration, with entire relief of pain in a number of cases, and materially mitigated in others. The cases in which there was no abatement of pain were very few. The mouth and tongue grew moist, breathing and expectoration more free and easy, and by continuing the remedy, in doses short of the nauseating point, from one to three days longer, there would be no return of the symptoms in a large majority of the cases in which the disease was subjected to early treatment. In a small number of cases, if not continued longer, the symptoms would return on a suspension of the remedy. In very few cases we have had to continue the tincture from five to twelve days. These cases are exceedingly rare, and were often treated with other remedies, or suffered to run some time without any treatment. We had, by a continued series of experiments and observations, arrived at the fact that, in nearly every case, we could reduce the pulse to any point we wished; that by putting the patient under its influence, we could predict with certainty that the pulse would range between 56 and 85 beats per minute.

In 1846 we were called to see Mr. E., in consultation with Dr. J. A. Stewart. Mr. E. had been laboring under a severe attack of pneumonia for several days. The remedies prescribed were entirely approved of and continued for a time, but failed to relieve. The threatening aspect of the case was such, that it was thought prudent to inform his parents, at a distance, of his perilous condition. At this critical juncture, we observed to Dr. S., that we had been using an article in a number of cases of pneumonia, with a success and peculiarity of effect we had never been able to obtain from any other remedy, and proposed to use it in the present case. We immediately put Mr. E. on the use of the veratrum viride, to be given every three hours—the quantity to be increased one drop at each dose until nausea or vomiting occurred. At 8 o'clock A. M., commenced with seven drops. The third portion excited severe nausea and free vomiting, with great paleness, coolness, and moisture of the surface. During the occurrence of these interesting and striking effects, we were notified that Mr. E. was vomiting freely, was much worse and was thought to be dying. We found, however, that what had caused so much alarm to the patient and his friends, was to us a source of gratification; for, after the effort at vomiting was over, and nausea relieved, the pulse was reduced to 63 beats and the pain relieved.

In this case, a pulse of from 120 to 130 beats, was reduced in twelve hours, to 63, and all the febrile and inflammatory symptoms were relieved. This was to us an occasion of thrilling and exciting interest. Dr. S. was the first physician to whom we had stated our belief in its powers, and he now stood before us witnessing the most commanding demonstration of the powers of the agent over a disease of acknowledged fatality, and under the most unpromising circumstances. Who would charge us with wanton enthusiasm? or who would fail to be enthusiastic on such an occasion? The portion was reduced to one-half, and continued several days without any return of the symptoms, and the patient rapidly convalesced.

We were at one time impressed with the belief that nausea or vomiting, one or both, was essential to the control of the heart. Called in February, 1847, to see a son of Mrs. T., laboring under a violent attack of pneumonia; we put him on the use of veratrum viride every three hours. Although 12 years of age, his general slender health and deformed chest, having been severely afflicted with asthma, induced us to commence with a very small dose, that we might avoid any drastic effect of the remedy. The first portion given was two drops, to be increased one drop every portion until the slightest nausea was experienced, then to lessen or discontinue the remedy, as the case might require. On taking the third or fourth portion, Mrs. T. discovered that he was getting very pale, and the skin was cool and moist, and the pain scarcely felt only on taking a full inspiration. The slowness of the pulse, and the palor and coolness of the surface alarmed her, and she sent for us. We found him pale, cool, moist, and with a pulse beating 35, full and distinct. When put on the tincture, in the morning, his pulse was 120 to 125, skin hot and dry, frequent and labored breathing, pain severe, great thirst. In the short space of twelve or fifteen hours the symptoms were subdued, and by continuing the tincture in doses of from two to three and four drops, there was no renewal of the symptoms.

Since the above, we have been able, in a number of cases, to succeed in reducing the action of the heart and arteries, without exciting the least nausea or vomiting, by commencing with a very small dose.

In 1850, we determined to announce to the world the fact, that *the great disideratum had been discovered: an agent by which we could emphatically say to the heart and arteries, thus fast shalt thou beat, and no faster.* Aware of the fate of many remedial agents urged upon the attention of the profession, and which have proved valueless, we withheld our notice until we had, by the utmost care and observation, acquired the conviction of its being as much a specific in pneumonia typhodes, as quinine is in intermittent fevers. We leave it to an enlightened profession to judge whether or not the agent has failed to answer or equal the representations made.

We now began to reflect upon the fact, that in a very large majority, if not in every disease of violence, a frequent pulse is manifest, and that we judge in a great measure, of their intensity, by its frequency and the condition of the vascular system. We asked ourselves the question, if veratrum viride will control arterial excitement, break up and arrest pneumonia typhodes, why should it not succeed in arresting other fevers and inflammations? Believing, as we did, that the altered and vitiated condition of the secretions were the consequence of increased and perverted circulation, and that the degree of their morbid condition might be measured by that of the vascular system, we concluded that the veratrum viride would cure other febrile and inflammatory affections by its specific action on the heart. We were therefore led to test the veratrum viride in a number of diseases.

In nearly all, if not in every acute disease, especially of a febrile and inflammatory character, we find the frequency of the pulse and the derangement of the vascular system in proportion to the force and severity of the case. There is scarcely an exception to the rule. Why this is so we do not know. The fact cannot be denied; and in order to restore health, we must, of necessity, control the circulation, directly or indirectly. Now, veratrum viride will almost invariably effect this, whatever may have been the disturbing cause. The how and the why, we do not understand. We look upon the universality of its application, to be exactly defined by the universality of the occurrence of increased cardiac action. In testing its powers, we did not confine our experiments to febrile and inflammatory diseases of an idiopathic character, but extended them to traumatic lesions in which fever and inflammation had supervened, and our labors were crowned with a success that we little dreamed of realizing. Its power of controlling arterial action, in febrile and inflammatory diseases, and in traumatic lesions, we consider established beyond a doubt.

It stands unrivalled in palpitations of the heart, for promptness and certainty of relief. It is a specific in the painful affection of the testicle consequent upon metastasis in mumps. We have not failed, in a single case, to obtain relief from the pain and fever in twelve hours, and prevented a return of the symptoms, by perfect rest and a continuance of the tincture for three or four days. How far it will succeed in orchitis, from other causes, we are not prepared to say. It affords us no ordinary pleasure to record its value in the treatment of the inflamed mamma of lying-in females. If taken in time, in these cases, it may be relied on to control the fever, pain and inflammation of the gland, so as to prevent suppuration in almost every instance. It is valuable in inflammation of the brain. In hooping-cough, accompanied with high febrile excitement, it has no equal. In convulsions generally, it is highly valuable. In asthma and rheumatism its effects are peculiarly striking, especially in the acute forms. In chronic rheumatism we have not used it. In puerperal fever our experience is limited, but the few cases in which it was used stamps it a reliable agent in that disease. We have found it of great value in the treatment of typhoid dysentery, and would feel unable to combat that disease without it or some other remedy of equal power. Its effects on the system are in perfect antagonism to those of scarlet fever. Combined with the diuretic treatment, we do not believe it can be equalled by any other plan of treatment that has ever been adopted in scarlet fever.

When we reflect upon the powers of veratrum viride to allay pain, irritability and irritation, and more especially irritative mobility, in connection with its influence over the heart's action and deranged secretions, it is truly difficult properly to appreciate its value.

We must confess, that notwithstanding the time and space already occupied, that we have scarcely entered the threshold, much less exhausted the subject. It would take a volume to unfold the powers and effects of veratrum viride, and the almost innumerable cases to which it is peculiarly applicable. The powers and properties of veratrum viride, when fully known and understood, will open new fields for thought and investigation, and give greater scope for practical research in all that relates to the pathology and treatment of disease, than any agent that has ever enlisted the attention of the medical world; and we are persuaded that it will completely change many of the existing views of pathology, and simplify the treatment of disease to an extent unparalleled in the history of medicine.

We now enter on the most important and interesting part of our subject, viz—its value in the treatment and cure of Typhoid Fever—a disease whose fatality renders big with interest any thing proposed for its cure. The treatment of typhoid fever is a matter in which every individual is deeply interested. Might we not ask with emphasis, what country, what community, has not felt and heard of the destructive mortality following in its wake? and has not the cry been echoed back by every tongue and breeze—a remedy to stay the fell destroyer's progress! When we have presented as much of facts and evidence as we deem sufficient on the occasion, you will be able to judge, and others can determine, whether a cure has been discovered and the destroyer stayed or merely checked; when the value of veratrum viride in pneumonia typhoides and other malignant and fatal diseases, is embraced in the subject, it becomes doubly interesting and important. In 1850 we first entered on a trial of the tincture of veratrum viride in the treatment of typhoid fever. It was due to our patients and to justice that we should proceed with caution. We accordingly, at first, gave it in mild and moderately severe cases, avoiding its use at first in all cases of unusual severity and malignancy. We first used it in the case of a negro boy of Mrs. W., which was uncomplicated and yielded readily. When called, on the third day of the disease, the bowels had been moved sufficiently by a cathartic of calomel, followed by repeated portions of camphorated Dovers powder, without abatement of the symptoms. The skin was hot and dry, great thirst, severe pain in the forehead; the eyes dull, heavy and ecchymosed; tongue covered in the centre with a dark thin fur, tip and edges very red and dry; pulse 127, small, soft and with a quickness in the stroke, that indicated greater frequency than really existed. The patient was ordered a six drop dose, to be increased till nausea or vomiting occurred. By mistake, the dose was not increased. After continuing the treatment twelve hours, there being no abatement in the symptoms, we were notified of the fact and wrote to increase until an impression was made, and that we would see the patient in twelve hours. During the absence of the messenger, Mrs. W. discovered that the dose was to be increased, and did so, and when this reached eight drops there was free vomiting, with a subsidence of all febrile symptoms, the severe pain in the head excepted. At the expiration of twelve hours, we found the boy with a skin cool and moist, thirst materially abated, and the pulse reduced to fifty-six beats. A blister was applied to relieve the unmitigated pain in the head, and the veratrum viride was continued four days without any return of the symptoms.

Other mild cases were treated with the same rapidly favorable and successful results. We were thus emboldened and warranted in extending it to the treatment of cases much more severe and malignant, as were those of Mr. R., the son of Mr. W., the two at Dr. Q.'s, and that of Dr. T.'s—all of which, except the first, were published at length in the January number of the Augusta Medical Journal in 1851.

While on a visit to Georgia, in July, 1851, we were asked by Dr. M. to look at a negro woman of Mr. T.'s. She had been sick a number of days, with no abatement of the symptoms. Pulse 116, skin hot and dry, tongue red and dry, great thirst, more or less delirium, and a peculiar nervous motion, or more properly, a tremor and inability to hold the head still or to take a drink of any thing out of a tumbler with her own hand. The owner was exceedingly uneasy about the condition of his negro, as a great many had fallen victims to that disease. We might have noticed the gurgling noise, sickness at the stomach, and spinal tenderness, which had resisted the use of blisters to the stomach and spine, as well as cupping of the same, together with an alterative treatment of calomel. On being asked our opinion, we observed to Dr. M., we thought the fever could be cooled and the pulse reduced. By request, we remained five hours, put her on the use of the tincture of veratrum viride —gave her seven drops at 12, eight at 2 P. M., and nine at 4 P. M. In half an hour after the third portion nausea and vomiting were excited moderately. The pulse was reduced to 80 beats per minute, the skin became cool and moist, and the nervous tremor or motion very much relieved. The Doctor observed, that the pulse was reduced as low as he wished it; the dose was consequently reduced to four drops, to be given every three hours. A son of Mr. T. was also sick of typhoid fever. His case was mild, the pulse at the highest numbering but a very few beats over one hundred. When the effects on the negro woman were known, he was quite anxious to take it also. Accordingly, he was ordered it every three hours, beginning with seven drops; to be increased one drop. The third dose excited severe nausea and free emesis, producing cool and moist skin, and reducing the pulse to 58 beats per minute. The portion was then reduced to four drops, at intervals of three hours. The next morning, at 9 o'clock, found the negro's pulse 80; delirium entirely gone, and full relief of all nervous tremor; skin cool and moist; tongue moist, and little or no thirst. The son's pulse was from 58 to 60, other symptoms in unison.

The above was an occasion of interest and solicitude to us, for the time, and our feelings can be much better imagined than expressed. Dr. M. dismissed the cases within thirty hours after we first saw them, the medicine to be kept up for a few days, and he to be notified in case of change for the worse. Dr. W. saw them, and Dr. S., then a student, was also present. Dr. W. has since used the veratrum viride extensively, and with great success. This circumstance led to its introduction into that region, Coweta, Troup and Heard, as Dr. M. practiced in the three counties. The letters of Dr. M., Dr. Ridley, and Dr. Renwick, are testimonials of their opinions of its value and beneficial effects in the treatment of typhoid fever, &c.

We were called with Dr. P., to see a negro girl of Judge B.'s, on whom he was attending. The girl was severely sick with typhoid fever, which had been unusually fatal in that region. The pulse was from 120 to 130, when at the highest; tongue dry, and red on edge and tip, dark brown or black in the centre; great tenderness of the abdomen; gurgling or rumbling and tympanitic abdomen; decubitus on the back; feet drawn up; knees separated; muttering and delirious while inclining to sleep, especially during the night; tendency to diarrhœa; tip of the nose peculiarly sharp or pointed—had been treated with calomel, turpentine, and camphorated Dover's Powder. It was on the eighth day we saw her, and, with desire of Dr. P., commenced giving the tincture every three hours. The patient being ten or eleven years of age, we commenced with two drops, and increased each dose one drop. In thirty hours the pulse was reduced from 110 to 90 beats per minute, surface became cool, and mouth and tongue moist. In fifty hours the pulse was reduced to 70, at which time she was nauseated and vomited—it was kept at between 75 and 85, till she was fully convalescent, and did not exceed that point, unless suspended, or given at too great intervals.

This was a case of no ordinary interest, as in that immediate section many had denied the efficacy and the powers of the veratrum viride, but had witnessed the mortality of the disease under every other mode of treatment. This closes the history of three cases we assisted in treating in Georgia. We will again turn to our own, and an adjoining county, and give the cases of most interest.

On the 14th July, 1852, we saw, in consultation with Dr. C., Mr. C. It was the sixth day of his relapse. Pulse 120, small, soft and weak; gurgling on pressure, and tenderness in the right iliac region; bowels flatulent and slightly tympanitic; burning in the palm of the right hand; edges and tip of tongue dry and red—slight white fur on the tongue, which we attributed to calomel; preternatural wakefulness. Had been treated with alterative doses of calomel and Dover's powder—had taken an emetic. Gums slightly distended from calomel, fœtid or mercurial breath, and a number of small ulcers on the cheeks and tongue; skin dry; bowels inclining to diarrhœa, but readily controlled. By consent, was put on the tincture of veratrum viride every three hours, to be increased slowly, and to avoid emesis, as he was opposed to taking it till it produced this effect. This is a great error; for those who take it till free emesis is excited, and the liver properly aroused, convalesce much faster. Commenced with three drops, and increased one drop every portion given, till six were taken, and slight nausea produced. It was then reduced to three drops or more, according to effect. On reaching six drops, the pulse was reduced to 80, and kept from 80 to 85. By continuing this treatment for a number of days, the pulse was reduced as low as 70 in the morning, with the skin rather cooler than ordinary, and towards sunset it would get up to 80 or 85, and the skin would be rather warm, and accompanied with more or less restlessness till midnight, and then pass off. It was suggested to try a few portions of quinine. The morning on which he took the quinine, the pulse was 70, skin cool, mouth and tongue moist. A portion of quinine was given at 9 and 11. Before 1, his pulse was 130 to 135, and skin hot and dry, and a general aggravation of all the febrile symptoms. The veratrum viride was resumed in full portions for a few doses, which soon subdued the excitement, and was continued. Convalescence was slow but perfect. It is an error, not to reduce the pulse as low as sixty in many cases. There is as much febrile excitement in some, with a pulse of 80, as there is in others with a pulse of 90 or 100; consequently, when this is the case, the convalescence will be extremely slow. In such cases, the veratrum viride should be given till free emesis is excited, and the pulse should be kept at 60 or under.

On the 19th of July, 1852, we were called into an adjoining district, to see a negro woman of Mr. G.'s, in consultation with Drs. T. and McD.

We saw her at 8 A. M., on the 20th, the 12th day of the disease. She had been treated with all the remedies usually resorted to, without relief. She was slightly mercurialized; supposed to be three months advanced in pregnancy; pulse 130, extremely quick and weak, so much so that it was difficult to count; tongue dry and red on the tip and edges, with a thick dark fur in the centre. The papillæ that were not covered with fur, were elevated, enlarged and flattened at the top; thirst extreme; great heat in the region of the stomach, and complaining of internal heat and burning; extremities cold, with general coldness of the surface, except over the region of the stomach; answered questions in a quick and hurried manner — would invariably change some part of the body before giving an answer. Discharges from the bowels dark and muddy, mixed with slime; more or less tenderness and gurgling on pressure in the right iliac region; tendency to diarrhœa slight. On the ninth day from the attack, there was a sudden and decided change for the worse, and brandy and quinine were freely given to sustain the action of the heart and arteries, and the surface was thoroughly rubbed to keep up external warmth.

We have given such a description of the treatment and of the patient, at the time of our first visit, as will be fully endorsed by the physicians in attendance. Two cases had just terminated fatally in the same family, and two others in a family not more than six hundred yards distant. We could not complain of the reputation that had preceded us; but the standing of the medicine was any thing but favorable in that region of the country. The previous and threatening mortality, the severity of the case, the new remedy, the unfavorable prognosis of the physicians in attendance, naturally excited the deepest interest, and curiosity was wrought up to the highest point as to what course would be pursued. By consent, every remedy was discontinued, both internal and external, and the tincture of veratrum viride ordered every three hours, to be increased *pro re nata*, which we superintended in person from 9 A. M., till 5 P. M. Three drops were given at 9, which nauseated and vomited pretty freely before 12. The first matter thrown up was a large quantity of mucus and slime, followed by a quantity of dark, green bile, or bitterish fluid, on the ejection of which she expressed considerable relief from the unusual burning or heat in the region of the stomach. Four drops were given at 12, which excited free emesis in from thirty to fifty minutes, bringing up an abundance of thick yellow bile. After this paroxism of vomiting had subsided, the extremities and surface generally became warm, or, in other words, there was a general diffusion and equal distribution of heat. She expressed perfect relief from internal heat or burning, followed by a general feeling of agreeable coolness; but three drops were given at three o'clock, which excited slight nausea, and perhaps a slight but single paroxism of vomiting. What we had achieved when we left (at 5 P. M.) was the relief from unusual heat in the stomach, severe thirst, general restlessness, an equal diffusion of heat and greater fulness and distinctness of the pulse. Instructions were left to continue the veratrum viride in three or four drop doses, as she might be able to bear it, avoiding too much nausea and vomiting, if possible.

After leaving, we sent a message back to give twenty or thirty drops of laudnum, one hour before the next portion, to prevent nausea or vomiting, if possible.

That night, as a matter of course, was passed by us with more or less anxiety and interest. On reaching the patient the next morning, the viride was exciting very little nausea, the pulse was reduced to 120, more full and distinct, and all the other symptoms were slightly improved. We were not satisfied with the small quantity of the veratrum viride we were using; we therefore ordered an enema of four ounces of cold water and six drops of the tincture of veratrum viride every six hours, and the three drop doses, every three hours, to be continued, thus making, in all, forty-eight drops in the twenty-four hours. The enemata were ordered to be given between the portions by mouth. The nausea and vomiting were kept up for a time after each enema, but not to an extent that required them to be suspended, and which subsided after a few repetitions of the enema.

The morning following, which was the fourteenth day of the disease, the pulse was down to 100, and with a like improvement in all the symptoms. The morning following, the pulse was reduced to 85, and all the other symptoms were greatly mitigated, so much so that we were not to see her for the next forty-eight hours. On Sunday morning, at 9 A. M.. (the seventeenth day of the disease,) we were at our post, with our pleasing anticipations disappointed, blasted, and for the time, scattered to the winds,—but to fight the battle at far greater hazard. Found her flooding; pains severe and frequent. Requested Dr. T. to examine the condition of the uterus; found the os tincæ soft and dilated, so that he could discover a substance or body presenting; gave her a portion of ergot; the fetus was thrown off within half an hour, and flooding ceased. By this time the pulse had reached 135 beats per minute, was peculiarly quick and feeble; number of respirations 63 per minute; skin hot and dry, the heat of that peculiar acrid kind called "calor mordax;" thirst greatly aggravated. The veratrum viride was increased to five drops every three hours; spirits of turpentine to be given every six hours, in fifteen drop doses, in a little warm sweet milk to cover the taste, which excels any vehicle we ever tried. The enema of cold water to be continued every six hours, and the viride increased to eight drops. When we left, at four in the afternoon, there was slight moisture of the surface; the pulse was 130, more full and distinct; breathings a little less frequent and hurried. On the day following it was reduced to 98 beats per minute; on the following day it was reduced as low as 85, with a like improvement of all the symptoms. The remedies were continued, and she rapidly and perfectly convalesced. It did appear that Providence brought us safely through the most critical of all the cases we have met. It also appeared, that so soon as the fœtus was thrown off, she was much less susceptible to the impression of the veratrum viride.

There are many points of interest in the above case, which are well worthy of particular notice. In the first place, it had been treated by two skillful physicians, with all the ordinary remedies. On the ninth day, the stage of collapse or exhaustion set in so rapidly and to such an extent, as to render brandy, quinine rubefacient and frictions necessary, to keep up the actions of the heart and arteries as well as the external warmth. After the free use of the above, from Saturday till Tuesday, we find there was no relief, but rather a continuance and aggravation of the symptoms. On Tuesday there was a withdrawal of all the remedial agents in use — was put on a few drops of the tincture of veratrum viride, at no time for the first 24 hours exceeding four drops. This was attended with relief from internal heat and burning, a general distribution of heat on the surface, and the pulse rendered slower, fuller, and more distinct, &c. The only change made which seemed to add to the good effects, were enemata of cold water, containing six drops of the tincture of veratrum viride. In the mean time she aborts with a renewal and aggravation of all the symptoms; to meet which there is added to the treatment 15 drops of spirits turpentine; the dose of veratrum viride increased, by mouth, to five drops, and by enemata to 8 drops. Again, the lessened susceptibility after the abortion, whereas, under ordinary circumstances, bleeding increases this susceptibility; true, the loss of blood was comparatively small, yet taking into account the length of time she had been sick, it might be said to have been relatively large. These are facts and circumstances for reflection and investigation.

We will add, for the sake of brevity, that all the cases were treated previous to January, 1852, except a very few. Since the first of June, 1852, we have been called to see seven cases of typhoid fever, in consultation, all of which were cured. We had noted down eleven consecutive cases of this fever, eight of which we saw in consultation, one had been seen by another physician, and two had been seen by no other physician. We notice those on account of their great severity, and more especially from the fact of a large majority of them being patients under treatment by other physicians. We are in possession of a large number of cases of typhoid and other diseases, which have been treated with unvarying success with the veratrum viride. Dr. B. treated 23 cases, without the loss of a single one — all in the same family.

The properties and powers of veratrum viride are the following: 1st, acrid—This property is very limited and confined to the fauces. 2. It is adanaigc, deobstruent or alterative: this property it possesses in a marked and very high degree; not equaled by calomel or iodine in this particular, which well adapts it to the relief and cure of many diseases hitherto beyond the reach of any remedy. Of this class of diseases, those which we think will be much benefitted by it, are, cancer and consumption. 3d. It is actively and decidedly expectorant, so much so that we rarely add any other article. 4th. It is one of the most certain diaphoretics belonging to the materia medica: it often excites great coolness or coldness of the surface; in some cases the skin is rendered merely soft and moist; in other instances, the perspiration is free, and at other times it is most abundant; but notwithstanding its profuseness, it does not reduce or exhaust the system, as many diaphoretics do when in excess, and therefore need not excite alarm nor be suspended on that account. 5th. It is nervine, not narcotic, under any circumstances, as since our first article, we have taken it more than twenty times to test its varied powers, and we have taken it in all quantities, from the production of free emesis down to the minimum dose. This property renders it of great value in the treatment of painful diseases and such as are accompanied with convulsions, morbid irritability and irritative mobility. For example—pneumonia, rheumatism, puerperal fever, convulsions generally, and palpation of the heart, &c. It is one of the most certain and efficient emetics known, and is peculiarly adapted to meet that indication in hooping cough, asthma, croup, scarlet fever, and in all cases where there is much febrile and inflammatory action. It often excites severe nausea and frequent vomiting, which, taken in connection with great paleness, often alarms the patient and by-standers; but these effects, when in excess, are readily relieved by one or two full portions of morphine and tincture of ginger, or of laudanum and brandy. One grand and leading feature is, that the exhaustion which follows it, is not excessive and permanent, but confined merely to the effort. Again, the matter, first ejected, is a large quantity of thick, slimy mucus, and soon after, the liver is called on to pour forth its own fluid in abundance. 7th. The seventh property is its most valuable and interesting, and for which it stands unparalleled and unequalled as a therapeutic agent. So much has already been written on what we call the sedative — arterial sedative —properties of the agent, or the power it possesses of controlling and regulating arterial action, that we shall not again run over the amount of evidence on this part of the subject. By virtue of this and other powers, the treatment of disease has been much simplified, and when the effects, recorded in the case of Mr. G.'s negro woman, shall have been fully considered, we may bid adieu to much of the supposed necessity for stimulants in the treatment of atonic or asthenic cases. We challenge the medical world to produce its equal, as therapeutic agent, for certainty of effect, for extent of effect, or for peculiarity of effect, and the ease and safety with which it may be administered to small and great. In small portions, we have found nothing to equal it in exciting and promoting appetite.

The usual interval with us is three hours between the portions. In ordinary cases of pneumonia, we usually continue it three days after the symptoms have subsided. In typhoid fever, and many other diseases, it requires to be continued much longer. For the satisfaction and information of the profession, we would state that it may be continued indefinitely, or any length of time, in moderate doses, or short of nausea, without the least inconvenience. The only objection that could be urged, is the increase of appetite, or desire for food. It is not cathartic—it is like all other remedial agents, subject to the same rules and regulations, making it out of the question for a person to lay down any but general directions for regulating the dose. In a male, twenty-five drops is the largest quantity we have known to be required to excite emesis, and 16 drops in the female when given in the manner and at the intervals we have directed. There need be no danger apprehended of its exciting inflammation of the stomach—we have given special attention to that particular. It is peculiar and at the same time interesting in its effects. The fact of its acting as a sedative on almost every other portion of the system, diminishing the vascular and muscular action and motion of every other part, and increasing that of the stomach. We have seen it produce emesis in very susceptible persons, and the contractions of the stomach were so rapid as to be almost continuous and uninterrupted; but a strong alcoholic tincture of ginger and morphine would afford more prompt and immediate relief than any other articles that we have ever used. We have never seen a case that failed to be relieved by the above remedies in thirty minutes. The great advantage of the remedy is that it does not exhaust longer than the effort to vomit is continued. A great many remedies leave the patient in an exhausted and enfeebled condition, aside from the effort or immediate action—not so with the veratrum viride. Again, tartar emetic should never be given with it, in any form or manner. The only cases in which we have seen the tincture of veratrum viride purge, were when given in combination with tartar emetic, or with Coke's hive syrup. In most of these cases it excited a violent cholera-morbus. We would not think of giving the tincture of veratrum viride where tartar emetic had been used, without preceding it with a full dose of morphine or laudanum at least one hour. We have known many fall out with the veratrum viride when it was not at fault. Again, venesection when a large quantity of blood is drawn, increases materially its effects, whereas opium and morphine lessen or diminish them. If a patient had been bled freely, preceded or followed by a liberal use of tartar emetic, and then followed up with full portions of the tincture of veratrum viride, we should anticipate and prepare for drastic, if not hazardous effects.

We feel fully assured, that we can confidently offer to the world the desideratum so long sought and wished for, namely, an agent that will certainly and undoubtedly control and subdue morbid aterial excitement, the great frequency of the contractions of the heart and arteries, so especially belonging to all acute diseases, and the removal of which has been as difficult as its presence was universal in all severely acute diseases. Dr. Bass, writing us on the subject, observes, "It seems to act directly upon the heart and arteries, as manifested by a diminution of the force and frequency of the pulse; it relieves irritation, congestion and inflammation — establishes the equilibrium of the circulation — excites free diaphoresis and expectoration, which well adapts it for the treatment of pneumonitis, pneumonia typhodes and asthma — in which diseases I have used it effectually, or in other words, with unparalleled success." Dr. I. Branch, in writing us on the same, states, "I will simply say, I regard it as one of the most important articles of the materia medica. You never made a more just and appropriate remark, than you did when you said, it would say to 'the pulse thus fast shalt thou beat and no faster.' I have used it in many cases of the severest sort of typhoid fever, with the happiest effect; it will cool the surface, reduce the *frequency* of the pulse, while at the same time it does not diminish its volume or strength. Indeed, I have sometimes thought that the volume and strength of the pulse was increased, in atonic cases, under the use of this article. The following will serve as an illustration of its use and effects: When called to a case of typhoid fever — with a hot surface, frequent pulse, great restlessness, in a word, with all the symptoms of such a case — if the patient be an adult, I commence with giving him eight drops of the article every two hours, and increase the dose a drop or two at every succeeding dose, until slight nausea is produced, never fearing but that when this effect is produced I shall have a cool surface, an infrequent pulse, and an absence of all febrile excitement. I then continue more or less of the article, until the case is broken up." Dr. J. A. Stewart, in a letter on the same subject, writes thus: I do not believe any remedy or combination of remedies possesses the same powers in pneumonia or pleuritis as yours — it not only lessens the frequency of the pulse, bnt exerts a curative influence on the disease, and with regard to its lessening the frequency of the pulse, I unhesitatingly say, without fear of successful controversy, that it will control the pulse in *any* and *every* case where it is morbidly excited. I regard your "remedy" as peculiarly adapted to the treatment of pneumonia typhodes, pertussis, typhus fever with increased action of the heart and arteries. Mr. Rodgers, in whose family you practice, was attacked with typhoid pneumonia about the time you left home. And Drs. Agnew and Traynham attended him, and when all hope his recovery was lost, his family recollected that some of them had been rescued from an untimely grave by your remedy — urged the physicians to give the "drops." Neither of the physicians having the medicine, they determined to send to me for it; and, with only ℥ ij of the tincture, both of the physicians assured me they had saved Mr. Rodgers, and would not take less than five dollars for the remnant of the two drachms."

We challenge the world to discredit the above. We pledge ourselves, and stand ready to demonstrate the powers and effects claimed. We have staked our reputation for veracity and medical skill on the above, and we are perfectly willing to abide the verdict of a liberal and enlightened profession and an intelligent community. Truth is omnipotent. The above was not got up in a day, or a corner, but is the result of years of laborious investigation, and of time and money spent to prove and test the certainty and correctness of our experience, and the conclusions reached, the world can either receive it or reject it.

We will, for the benefit of many who have written us, state the diseases in which we have used it with success, and leave the matter with the profession for further experiment and application from analogy. We do not hazard any thing of opinion or reputation, when we assert that it is a speeific in pneumonia, in the qualified terms we have stated; we say the same of convulsions accompanied with high febrile excitement, also of palpitation of the heart. In typhoid fever it has more than answered our moist sanguine anticipations; we assert the same of puerperal fever, rheumatism and asthma. In the spring of 1851, we were called in consultation with Dr. Stewart, to Dr. G.'s child, who was well nigh run down with hooping cough, fever and diarrhœa. We advised the tincture of veratrum viride, which acted like a charm; since which time, Dr. S. has written us a letter highly extolling it as unparallelled in the treatment of hooping cough. We have seen no case of metastasis to the testicle in mumps, that was not relieved of pain and fever in twelve hours. It may be styled *the remedy* in croup, when there is great vascular derangement. We have used it with great success in inflammation of the brain, also in typhoid dysentery. It is a valuable emmenagogue. In the inflamed breast, we give it with a confidence bordering on a certainty of success. In epilectic convulsions we have confidence of obtaining great relief from it. We look with confidence to being able to cure consnmption, by a timely and judicious use of it. We trust that even cancer will be robbed of its terrors. We are anxious to test its powers in yellow fever and in phlegmasia dolens, &c.

In conclusion, we will state to the profession at large, that we have endeavored to give a faithful and unexaggerated account of a portion of the cases in which we have used it, with a statement of its powers and properties. We know that we have like passions with other men, and that we are liable to be mistaken, that we are liable to be carried beyond the bounds of truth and soberness, as well as others, in our great desire to advance and consummate as far as we may, the honor and perfection of our science. But we feel confident, that when all is cool and calm — when every property and power is put to the test of fair and proper trial —that every effect and power claimed by us as belonging to and possessed by veratrum viride, will be emphatically confirmed and established by the profession. We have not made any effort to distinguish between its primary or direct and its secondary or indirect effects. If we have succeeded in getting the profession awakened to its properties and enlisted in the investigation of its application and adaptation to the treatment of disease, we congratulate ourselves that we have achieved much with our feeble efforts, and that ere long we shall see embodied, by much abler pens, all the inestimable and unparalleled powers belonging to vetatrum viride.

Extract from "Doctors' Commons." An Address. By S. W. BUTLER, M.D., President of Burlington Co. Medical Society, Vermont.

Gentlemen, you may think it bold and presumptious, that one of my age and standing in the profession, should use the language I do here. But, I announced it as my intention at the start, to seek some guiding star, some way-marks, by which to thread my path through the mazes that lead to the goal of professional ambition, and, if in my field of vision, there are unsightly crags and projections that will aid me, I presume I may use, while I endeavor to avoid them.

It is because I regard these flaws as unmitigated evils, because I earnestly deplore them, and because I think that every influence should be brought to bear, that may tend to draw more closely the cords that bind us together as men, and as *practitioners of medicine*, the "noblest of all professions, but meanest of all trades," that I venture to bring forward, for your consideration, the following plans. Should they at first view, seem utopian, and impracticable, I pray my professional brethren not to

˙udge and condemn them too hastily. Albeit they are the outburst of
the youthful and ardent temperament of one who hopes and believes,
that he is sincerely desirous of advancing the best interests of his chosen
profession, they are nevertheless, the result of a good deal of study and
observation, as well as of much intercourse with his professional brethren.
I believe the plans to be perfectly feasible, and that they will bear investigation.

The policy which I advocate, is founded on the principle of *association*,
and whatever, if any claim, it may have to originality, can be so, in only
part of its details. For, in our State Society founded eighty-eight years
ago, in our county Societies, in our National medical organization, as
well in all such associations, at home, and abroad, the principle is recognised, and by its very existence, triumphantly vindicated, for, had it not
been found to work well, it would long ago have come to nought. It
has come to be a general rule as well in the eyes of the discriminating
public, as in our own, that he, and he only, is the respectable physician,
who not only acknowledges fealty to some form of professional association, but who takes an *active* interest in the proceedings of such organizations. The man who holds the license of a Medical Society, merely
for the purpose of placing himself under the ægis of legal protection, is
a "marked man," even in the eye of the public.

I have reason to know that plain farmers' wives, read with interest, the
meager reports, of our too often meager proceedings, which are published
in the newspapers, and they know who of the physicians in their neighborhood are present at those meetings, and what part they take in them.*

The city or village newspaper, which in an "item" chronicles the fact
that any number of physicians, either in a simply social, or in a more
public capacity, met as physicians, and had "a good time," in so doing,
spreads abroad the intelligence who constitutes the *profession* of the
place or neighborhood.

The day has long gone by, when a man could attain eminence in any
profession, or command the respect of any community, without hard
study, and close application, and he who by his attainments is entitled to
respect, is as irresistably drawn into association with men of kindred
tastes, as are particles of matter by the law of attraction.

The apparent exceptions to this rule, are like malignant growths in
the human organism, whither the disorganized cells convey and deposit,
their morbid material, gathered alike from the fountain head of human
intelligence, and from "those members of the body which we think to
be less honorable." And, if one of these exceptions should claim precedence on the score of a more liberal pecuniary support, it is, as if a
cancerous breast should exult over its healthy fellow, or a morbidly enlarged organ over one free from disease — for money thus acquired, is
unhealthy materia., and will as surely eat into the vitals, "as doth a
canker."

---

* I would here respectfully suggest the propriety of having the proceedings
of our society published by the Secretary in *extenso*, or, so far as may be
proper for the public eye, in the newspapers of the day. I believe good would
result from it.

Notwithstanding these facts, it is well known that there are some physicians who are backward about connecting themselves with our societies, and many others, who, too often honor our appointments in the breach rather than in the observance. I would, by increasing the inducements to association, bring these men into the societies, and thus enlarge the sphere of our influence, and, at the same time, make more apparent the difference between us, and the horde of pretenders, who like jackalls beset our paths. I would have some bond of union, other than the mere abstract principle of association — some *nucleus*, around which we may cluster in a sort of "social crystalization." It is extremely difficult to form an attachment to an abstract principle, " Where the *treasure* is there will the heart be also."

In making an application of the foregoing suggestions, we will briefly consider them in reference to —

1. Our State Medical Society.
2. Our County Medical Societies, and
3. Our City or Village Associations.

First, then — I advocate the formation by our State Medical Society, of a Library, Pathological Museum, and Cabinet of Natural History. The Medical Society of Virginia, at its annual meeting in April last, laid the foundation for such a collection, and appointed a curator.

" Many hands make light work," and the principle once established, and the labor heartily engaged in by the members of our society, I believe that such a collection could be made at a very trifling expense, and that it would steadily grow, and be of permanent value to the profession, and to the State. Books and specimens in Pathology and Natural History would flow in, and the hills and valleys of Sussex would vie with the plains of old Cumberland and Cape May, and our large towns and cities would compete with both in adding to the common stock. Every contributor to such a collection, would have a *personal* and an abiding interest in it, and our Annual meetings would be vested with a new interest. Indeed, once a year, would be found too seldom for these reunions of the profession of the state. These collections too, particularly those in the pathological and natural history departments, would inevitably call forth communications and essays which would give to the transactions of the Medical Society of New Jersey, an interest which would attract the attention of neighboring states, and indeed of the profession everywhere. These essays might always be written in a form suitable for binding, and thus be preserved in the archives of the society.

The establishment of such a collection was a favorite project of the late Dr. James Paul, of Trenton, and had the proposition to that effect, which was brought before the Society at its Annual Meeting in 1852, been favorably received, I have reason to know that this valuable library would now have been the property of the State Society.*

For the accommodation of such Library and Museum, I would ask, *and expect*, that the legislature of the State would appropriate to the use of

---

* I am happy to say that most of this Library is now in possession of physicians in this county.

the Society such room or rooms in the State Capitol as might be needed, and where all the business meetings of the Society could be held. The Society is a State institution, having a general, and not a local interest, and one which it is to the interest of the government to foster and protect, and which *it will do* if we are true to ourselves, — and if we evince a disposition to engage heartily in such a work, I have no fear but the appropriation would be promptly and heartily made. Legislation has reference to the future, as well as to the present well-being of man, and I ask in all candor, if such action as that proposed on the part of our State Medical Society and Legislature, is not fraught with benefit to the profession, and through them to the whole people of New Jersey.

But, it is objected that such a collection at the State Capitol would be of little or no value to the profession in remote sections of the State. I answer, that legislation has reference to the greatest good to the greatest number, and, with the present and prospective facilities of travel, together with the necessarily frequent communication with the State Capitol, the large majority of the physicians of the state would have comparatively ready access to the collection. Besides, the advantage to the profession at large, which would result from the *attractive force,* so to speak, of such a library and museum, would far counterbalance all such objections. These objections are not of sufficient force to prevent our National and State Legislatures from collecting, at their respective seats of government, extensive libraries for the use of legislators; and no one questions that, notwithstanding the outlay from the public funds necessary to establish and keep up these libraries, the money is well expended, and that they will be of lasting advantage to the public. These libraries are often consulted by public men during the recess between the sittings of the legislatures. What valid reason is there why physicians should not have equal facilities for consulting an extensive library of medical authors?

In reply to the objections that the extensive medical libraries of the cities of New York and Philadelphia would render the proposed collection unnecessary, I would simply say, that it would be as reasonable for our legislature to rely on the extensive public libraries of those cities as for us to do so; and, besides, we would not, and *could* not feel that freedom in resorting to, and using those libraries, that we would in resorting to one of our own. To my mind, the argument, in any view, is clearly in favor of such a collection as the one proposed.

Second.—I advocate the formation, by our county medical societies, of similar libraries and museums, on a scale, of course, proportionate to the extent of the sources from whence they are to be drawn. Interchanges of duplicate copies of books, or specimens in pathology or natural history, might often be made with the state or other county societies. For the county libraries and museums, I would ask, and expect accommodations in one of the public buildings in the county, for the same reason that I would ask such accommodations in the state capitol. Here, the county meetings, which ought to occur as often as once in three months, should be held. The several advantages to be derived from such collections, enumerated under the first head, are as applicable to this, and need not be repeated.

Third, and lastly.—I would carry the same principle as far as practicable, into our cities, towns, and villages. Wherever there are two or three physicians, I would have them hold a room in common, in a public part of the town, easy of access, and known as "*the doctor's room.*" Here let each physician deposit, for the time being, such books from his own library, and such specimens from his cabinet as he can spare, each marked with his own name, and the whole properly secured in glass cases; each physician being provided with keys to open them. Then, at suitable hours each day, let this room be thrown open to the public. Let there be here skeletons of the human frame, wired and natural, for the inspection of the curious non-professional inquirer. Let the room be attractive in size and furniture, and be a common resort at all hours for the profession of the place, where they may meet, as they have opportunity, for social converse, and where they may hold frequent stated meetings of a professional character, and where, in the larger towns and cities, there may be, on proper days, certain hours in which the physicians, in rotation, could meet, and prescribe for the poor. I need do no more than mention the advantage of such an arrangement to the medical student. The physicians might agree to subscribe for different medical periodicals, and thus have the advantage of receiving medical intelligence from various sections of the country, and from abroad. The profession and the public, too, would thus often enjoy the advantage of reference to valuable collections in mineralogy, botany, conchology, etc. etc., and the body of physicians in the place would, necessarily, command more entirely the respect and confidence of the public. The trifling expense of furnishing such a room is not to be thought of, in view of the great advantage that would result.

Such frequent intercourse among physicians as the proper carrying out of these plans would require, would make them too well acquainted with each other to render it possible, except in very rare cases, that any serious misunderstanding should arise between them, and the medical profession would present the grand spectacle of the devotees of a benevolent and useful science laboring *unitedly* and earnestly to promote the welfare of mankind. Then would this temple of science present to the popular view one massive structure, whose integral parts are fused into a whole, against whose broad and deep foundations the surges of popular superstition and error dash in vain, and whose fair and faultless proportions, as they loom up against the gathering clouds, bid defiance to storms and tempests.

EDITORIAL AND MISCELLANEOUS.

Meeting of the State Medical Society.

The second annual meeting of this Society will be held at the Medical College, Ann Arbor, on Thursday, the 30th of March. This will be on the same day with the Medical Commencement. After the conferring of the degrees, and the delivery of the address to the graduates, the Medical Society will be called to order, and adjourned to meet after dinner In the afternoon the Society will listen to an address from the President, George Landon, M.D., of Monroe; and the subsequent sessions will be occupied in listening to the reports of committees, and the reading of papers, and in miscellaneous busi—

ness. Persons having papers to read are requested to call on the Secretary as early as possible, in order that the arrangements for reading them may be properly made. All physicians of this or adjoining states, on becoming members, are entitled to present papers. Members preparing papers, but not able to be present, can forward them to the Secretary, who will place them among the transactions, and read them before the Society. All regular physicians of this and adjoining states and Canada may become members on receiving an election, and paying one dollar initiation fee. It is believed that the time has now come for the profession to take its defence into its own hands, and that its dignity and future prosperity depend on the energy with which it maintains its organization. This meeting will be one of unusual interest and importance, and a full attendance is desired from every part of the state. The county medical societies, and other local medical organizations, are entitled, by the constitution, to send delegates. It is hoped that all such organizations will not fail to have their representatives present on the occasion.   \   E. ANDREWS, M D.,

Ann Arbor, Feb 19, 1854.   Secretary.

Medical Commencement and Junior Exhibition.

The close of the Medical Session, the conferring of degrees, the meeting of the State Medical Society, and the Junior Exhibition of the Literary Department all occur in the same week. As this is a state institution, medical men of every section have an interest in it, and are by the Faculty cordially invited to be present at the examination, and other exercises, which will take place. The following programme will give an outline of the proceedings :

TUESDAY, MARCH 28.

Forenoon.—Examination of canditates for the degree of M.D. upon their final theses. *Afternoon*—The same. *Evening*—Address before the Serapion.

WEDNESDAY.

Forenoon.—Examinations on theses continued. *Afternoon.*—The same. *Evening.*—Junior exhibition of Literary Department.

THURSDAY.

Forenoon.—Medical commencement, conferring degrees; address to the graduates; calling of State Medical Society to order. *Afternoon*—Meeting of State Society; address by the President. *Evening.*—Meeting of State Society; reports of committees and reading of papers.

FRIDAY.

Forenoon.—Closing session of the State Society; adjournment.

Works Received.

We acknowledge the receipt from Blanchard and Lee, publishers, Philadelphia, of *Buckley on Bronchitis and Pneumonia,* and *Carpenter on Alcoholic Liquors;* also, new editions of *Fowne's Chemistry for Students, Bennett on the Uterus,* and *Laurence on the Eye :* all of which came too late to be carefully examined for this number; but we shall acquaint our book-loving readers with them in our next.

Reply to the Attacks of Dr. Charles Coldwell.

This is a small pamphlet, in very spicy style. Respecting the merits of the quarrel which gave it birth, we know nothing, and desire to know nothing. By Lunsford P. Yandell.

Western Medico-Chirurgical Journal.

This journal contains the novel feature of a popular department. It seems to be conducted in a sound orthodox style.

J. F. Sandford, M.D., Editor, Keokuk, Iowa.

Medical News and Library.

Published by Blanchard and Lea, and sent gratuitously to all subscribers of the *American Journal of the Medical Sciences* who pay in advance.

Disease of the Uterine System as a cause of Physical Degeneracy.

A contemptible pamphlet, whose object we shall not further by publishing its author's name. It gives no scientific information, but is designed solely to catch patients for the author.

THE

PENINSULAR

JOURNAL OF MEDICINE

AND THE COLLATERAL SCIENCES.

| VOL. I. | APRIL, 1854. | NO. X. |

ORIGINAL COMMUNICATIONS.

ART. I.—*Observations on the Cause, Nature, and Treatment of Epidemic Cholera.* By A. B. PALMER, M.D., Prof. of Anatomy in the University of Michigan.

(CONTINUED FROM PAGE 252.)

2. Of the Nature of Cholera, the limits of these observations will allow but a brief consideration.

The external features or symptoms of the disease are too familiar to require particular description, and only sufficient reference will be made to them to render the remarks upon treatment intelligible.

The disease is usually divided into *four* stages. These stages, as is the case with the more or less arbitrary division into stages of most other diseases, often run into each other, and are not always well defined; neither do they all exist in every instance, but in their general outlines may commonly be observed.

First. *The Premonitory* Stage, marked by general lassitude, dull pain above the eyes, sometimes constrictions in the calves of the legs, disturbed digestion, abdominal uneasiness, slightly coated tongue and diarrhœa. This stage is not always observed, and when it is, is liable to vary much in the number, severity, and duration of the symptoms; but it usually may be traced continuing from one to several days before the full developement of the disease, or the arrival of the

Second Stage, which is marked by active vomiting and purging of a fluid soon becoming of a rice-water appearance, great thirst, coldness of the surface, severe spasmodic pain caused by cramps, particularly in the abdomen and extremities.

In the commencement of this stage the pulse is sometimes a little excited and not unfrequently quite firm, but it soon becomes more and more feeble as the impression of the poison is more profound, and as the exhausting discharges continue. Towards the latter part of this stage, the surface becomes much shrunken and more or less blue. When the disease is severe this stage only lasts a few hours—in less violent cases, a day or more—when, if re-action and improvement do not occur, it passes into the

Third, or Stage of Collapse, marked by loss of circulation, laboured respiration; the skin being shriveled, livid, and bathed with cold perspiration. The discharges sometimes continue in this stage, though less profusely; at other times they are suspended either from exhaustion of the fluids of the system, or from a suspension of nearly all vital action. The pain and cramps sometimes continue in this stage, while in other cases they cease; the patient becoming more quiet and comatose. During some part of the second stage a ringing in the ears usually occurs, and the voice becomes husky and peculiar. These symptoms usually continue throughout the disease, the huskiness of the voice increasing in the third stage until the patient is only able to articulate in a whisper. Those who survive the active onset of a severe attack, especially if the disease pas . . . . are liable to the

Fourth Stage, or . . . . .ve .ever, generally accompanied by protracted local congest. . . . . . .w forms of inflammation of the brain and spinal marrow, or of the .bdominal viscera.

Occasionally cases of . holera Morbus, or what is called English Cholera occur, and also serous vomiting and purging during the progress of miasmatic fevers, which in their external symptoms are almost the same as genuine epidemic or Asiastic Cholera; yet differing, as I apprehend, in the essential cause, and certainly as it regards fatality—the former class of cases being generally (always, so far as my experience extends) amenable to treatment, even if the treatment be not commenced until an advanced stage, while the large mortality of the latter when the same apparent advanced condition is permitted to occur, is too well known. Dissimilar causes not unfrequently produce similar, though perhaps not in every respect identical effects, and these cases of sporadic and accidental cholera are presumed not to be produced by the specific poison which gives the epidemic variety its virulence.

If we are unable to ascertain the precise nature of the Cholera poison, we are quite as much in the dark as to the particular manner in which it produces its effects. Among the various speculations on this subject the Zymotic theory seems at present to be in the ascendent.

This theory, as its name implies, supposes that the blood, and perhaps other fluids of the system, are acted upon by the poison in the manner of a *ferment,* and that the poisoned or fermented blood and other fluids being applied to the nerves and other parts, produce the phenomena of the disease.

Whether this fermentation takes place, or whether the poison remains distinct, either preserving its original quantity or multiplying itself in the system, attaching itself to, and impressing the solids—however these things may be, it appears that early in the train of morbid effects a strong impression is made upon the nerves of organic life, modifying, diminishing, and in severe cases, rapidly overpowering their vitalizing influence. That portion of the brain and nervous system which is engaged in thought and sensibility, is left comparatively undisturbed— while all the functions depending upon the organic nerves, such as nutrition, secretion, exudation, circulation and respiration; and their consequences, as animal heat, &c. — are either enfeebled, suspended, or greatly modified.

Nutrition is entirely suspended — Glandular Secretions, particularly of the liver and kidneys, are either suspended or greatly diminished. The circulation of the blood is much retarded, apparently, to a great extent at least, by spasm of the smaller vessels; the vital fluid retiring to and congesting the internal organs. Respiration is diminished and labored; the blood, consequently, is not well oxygenated, and animal heat is reduced.

Usually at the same time, and in some instances preceding most other symptoms, there is a high degree of irritation of the mucous membrane of the stomach and bowels; and this whole membrane, as well usually as the cutaneous surface, transudes a copious serous fluid, consisting of the thinner parts of the blood, and containing a large portion of its salts. The blood thus becoming deprived of its more fluid portions, of its salts, and above all, of its oxygen, and being moreover loaded with urea and bile from the suppression of the secretions of the liver and kidneys, becomes unfit for the uses of the system;—and when the disease in a grave form arrives at this stage, uninfluenced by treatment, collapse and death are the almost inevitable consequences. When from the less severe form of the disease or great powers of endurance, a patient survives these conditions, the train of morbid actions has been of such a character as to cause more or less inflammation in most cases. The stomach and bowels, the lungs, the membranes of the brain, and spinal marrow, are the most frequent seats of the inflammation.

Without entering minutely into the morbid anatomy of Cholera, it may be stated that the only morbid appearances approaching to uniformity found in the bodies of those dying in the collapsed, or asphyxied state, is that of congestion.

Most of the vital organs are found in a congested condition. The membranes of the brain, particularly of its base and of the spinal marrow —the whole system of nerves, particularly the organic—the stomach and bowels, with much uniformity, and often the kidneys, liver, &c. The lungs are the most frequent exceptions to this general congested state; these organs being often found emptied of blood and collapsed. This bloodless condition of the lungs is produced by obstruction of the right ventricle of the heart, this side of the heart being often found filled with black and sometimes fibrinous clots,—while the left side is usually empty. In consequence of this condition of the heart the blood is kept from going to the lungs, but is not prevented from returning.

3. Treatment of cholera.

The prophylactic management of this disease, so apt to be fatal when it has made an attack, and usually so easily prevented, is of the first importance; and of course consists in the avoidance of its causes.

These have already been referred to and need not to be repeated in detail, though one or two particulars may be worthy of a more special notice.

The views taken of the mode of propagation of the cholera poison, and the local character in many instances of the predisposing causes which give that poison its potency, and particularly my own observation while acting as the medical adviser of the Board of Health of Chicago, have impressed me with the great importance of giving special attention to the localities where the disease makes its appearance, and to the groups of persons among whom it selects its victims.

If in such localities, many are crowded together under unfavorable hygenic conditions, every such condition should if possible be instantly removed, and a dispersion of the persons should take place; due regard being had to the safety of others among whom they may be sent. If those having been particularly exposed to the poison are well washed in person and changed in apparel, and are placed in cleanly and well ventilated apartments, none will be likely to suffer from them, even should the persons thus having been exposed and removed, themselves experience an attack. The propriety of such procedures and their influence in arresting the progress of the disease and saving life cannot be questioned, or too strongly insisted upon by those who have charge of the public health.

In a preceding part of these observations, the use of alcoholic drinks was simply mentioned, on the authority of Dr. Carpenter, as a predisposing cause of cholera; but as there is a popular opinion somewhat prevalent, that these drinks act as preventives to the disease, the question may, with propriety, be referred to in this connection. From all just principles of medical reasoning, we should conclude that the use of an article which impedes the proper normal transformation of elements and tissues, and obstructs the elimination of decomposing and effete matters from the system, which retards respiration and the combustion of carbon in the lungs, rendering the blood dark and carbonaceous, (as shown by the experiments of Prout and others,) and which also quite often severely irritates the stomach and bowels; could not be a preventive of such a disease as cholera, but on the contrary, would be a predisposing cause of a disease, which, though it be produced by a peculiar poison, yet seems to require a degree of impurity in the system to give that poison activity and effect, and in which the train of morbid actions in its course, developes conditions similar to those which that article is known to produce, and all experience upon the subject confirms these conclusions of reason, and shows that spirit drinkers are more liable to attacks, and that the disease is more fatal with them than with those who abstain. Most certainly my own observations sustain this view.

It may be alleged that the exciting and stimulating effects of these drinks in moderate quantities, may enable the system more effectually to resist a morbid influence; and this might be true if the only effect of alcohol was stimulating; and further, if that stimulation could constantly be kept up at a uniform and proper point; but alcohol has other effects than stimulation, and as we have seen, of a deleterious character, and that stimulation cannot be kept uniform. By the fixed laws of the vital economy, all unnatural excitement is followed by a corresponding degree of depression, and the whole vital condition and movements of the spirit consumer are ever fluctuating and unsteady. If, then, the excitement would resist the morbid influence, the subsequent depression would favor the production of its effects. Both reason and experience show that the belief in the preventive virtues of alcohol in this disease, is fallacious, and affords an example of those popular delusions which our enlightened profession should labor to destroy.

There are no known specifics for destroying the cholera poison or preventing its effects, and all medication should be avoided, unless symptoms occur. The system should be kept in as uniform and healthy a condit. ion as possible, and the mind calm and confiding, yet active and cheer- ful.

In approaching the subject of the curative treatment of cholera, we come upon a variety of procedures and a mass of remedies advised by respectable authority, which are truly embarassing to the inexperienced practitioner, desirous of making a judicious choice. Indeed, the plans of treatment which have been employed, are almost as numerous as the combinations of which remedies are susceptible. This fact, taken in connection with the nearly uniform results of the different modes of treatment, as shown by statistics upon a large scale, (from forty-five to fifty-five per cent. of mortality being the general fact) would seem at first view, to show that there is little power, or at least choice, in remedies. Still, there is doubtless a choice of remedies, and treatment has unques- tionably a great influence over many cases of the disease. Indeed, there are few diseases more susceptible of being influenced in their results by treatment, than this. Very few, where the services of a prompt and skillful physician can be made more valuable than in this.

It would seem strange that a disease so uniform in its cause, and iden- tical in its essential nature, and withal, so much influenced by remedies, should remain such a length of time under investigation, without a course of treatment being found, upon the adoption of which, the pro- fession generally would agree. But, though the disease is thus essen- tially uniform and identical, there are numerous varieties as to several particulars, and more than this, contradictory elements and conflicting indications in each case, — and the arrival at fixed truth, when the prob- lems are complicated and dependent for their solution upon numerous observations made by many persons, is necessarily a slow process. We must be content to labor and to wait, and should regard as valuable every contribution to the result, however small. In the mean time, while authority is undecided and contradictory, every practitioner, in determining for himself, is necessarily thrown off the ground of general experience upon that of principle, and his own observation.

In this spirit I shall proceed in attempting to give a description of the treatment of this disease, which my experience and reflection have led me to regard as the best of which I have any knowledge. I feel, how- ever, a great difficulty in giving a clear and intelligible discription of this treatment. Indeed, in the details of proper management, so much de- pends upon the peculiarities the particular case presents, the different degrees of rapidity with which it passes through the different stages, the constitutional and special condition of the patient in various respects, the different manner in which remedies are borne, the special impression made by them, &c.—so much of the appearances of the patient can be learned only by experience; and in the doses and timing of medicines, so much must be left to the judgment, that a full and correct representation of the treatment cannot be made. As the best means, however, of approximating to such a representation, I shall first express some general views of indications and the means of fulfilling them, based upon pathological and therapeutical principles, and afterwards attempt a more minute and specific account of the manner in which I would apply these principles — of the special mode of procedure in the treatment of cases.

In the absence of a fixed and positive pathology, at least such a pathology as reveals clearly the nature and succession of the essential morbid actions, and points unerringly to the proper remedies, and in the absence also of ascertained specifics, the attention of the practitioner should rest upon such morbid conditions as he believes to exist, and his efforts should be directed to the correction or removal of such conditions; and if no means of acting upon the primary or essential diseased state are within his knowledge or reach, he must content himself with doing what he can for the correction and removal of the obvious disturbances of the functions, and thus by putting the system as nearly as possible in its normal condition, prepare it to endure the shock of the morbid cause, and assist it as the sailor would a disabled ship, to weather the storm.

It has already been intimated that the cause of cholera makes an early and decided impression upon the ganglionic system of nerves, those nerves presiding over the respiratory, circulatory, secretory and assimilative functions; and that as a consequence these functions are, each in its peculiar mode, but all more or less, seriously disturbed. The stomach and bowels are generally the seat of such serious irritation, and the source of such peculiar and profuse discharges as to be regarded by most of those who have written upon the subject, as points of a primary and principal morbid impression. But, whether this be the case, or whether these symptoms are the result of impressions upon the nerves of organic life, the symptoms themselves are of the gravest importance, and in a large majority of instances, require first, and most imperatively, the attention of the physician; for, if this irritation be not allayed, and these discharges be not controlled, medicines are not retained in the system, and the patient is soon exhausted and carried beyond the reach even of hope.

It must, however, be borne in mind that this irritation and these dis-

charges are 1.   ..e sole causes of the depression and collapse; in fact,
that in some c: the most rapidly fatal cases, no evacuations occur; and
that diminished circulation, diminished respiration, diminished animal
heat, and diminished glandular secretions are much more constant symptoms than profuse evacuations; and, therefore, that in the treatment, other
conditions than the vomiting and purging are entitled to constant attention.   In this view of the subject, the following leading indications are
presented:

1st. To arouse and maintain the sensibility and proper action of the
organic nervous system; and

2nd. To excite and correct the action of those organs whose natural
functions have been suspended or perverted, whether from a direct impression upon them, or by the failure of that nervous influence upon which their
integrity depends; and in a more particular manner when the gastro-intes-
tinal irritation and exhausting discharges are present, the indication is to
allay that irritation and arrest the discharges.

Now, by what means shall the first indication be fulfilled?   Unfortunately we are yet but little acquainted with any direct beneficial influence of remedies over the organic nervous system.   When this system
is debilitated and deranged in chronic diseases, hygenic regulations are
more efficient than any known specific medicines.   But here the most
prompt action is required.   There is in cholera so much prostration, such
an appearance and real danger of rapid sinking and fatal exhaustion, so
much spasm and pain, and such profuse discharges, that stimulants and
anodynes are resorted to almost instinctively, and alcohol and opium are
given, often with far too much freedom and too little discrimination.

There can be little doubt that opium, alcoholic mixtures, chloroform,
&c., particularly when given in free doses, tend to depress rather than
exalt the energy of the nervous system of organic life.   Though this
may not be the effect of these articles uniformly and in all doses, it certainly is often, and generally, when administered in large quantities.   If
alcohol in certain quantities and under certain circumstances does temporarily excite these nerves, still by depriving the blood of its oxygen,
diminishing the natural effects of respiration and retarding other vital
changes, its secondary effects become often powerfully depressing.   The
same is true of opium and other narcotics in a greater or less degree.
These facts should not be lost sight of for a moment, and while these
articles may be useful, and opium particularly, even in pretty free doses,
quite essential for fulfilling these indications, regard should always be paid
to their depressing effects upon the vital powers.   No language can be
too strong in condemning their use in large quantities, in the advanced

stages of the disease. Both principles and experiences go against the practice, and facts under my own observation have convinced me that many lives have been sacrificed by it. Alcohol is very seldom useful in cholera under any circumstances. It not only fails to meet the indication of sustaining the vital powers, but it also usually fails to exert a beneficial influence over the vomiting and purging; in fact, it increases the irritation of the mucous membrane, and disposes it as well as the brain and other parts of the system to inflammation and its consequences, in case the patient survives the earlier stages of the disease.

Opium in proper doses and combinations in the earlier stages of cholera, before the vital powers are much exhausted, and while irritation of the stomach and bowels is the most prominent symptom, is *the great* remedy in the disease; or at least one of the prominent and essential items of a correct treatment. It is by far the most potent remedy we possess for allaying that irritation, arresting the flow of fluids to the mucous surface and controlling the debilitating discharges; and when from its use these effects are produced, the system generally by proper other aids, is enabled to rally and struggle successfully against the morbid influences. But when the powers of life are low, when the blood is deficient in oxygen, loaded and black with carbon; the free administration of an article which in full doses produces even in healthy persons similar effects, can but be productive of severe and fatal results. I dwell upon this point because of its exceeding importance, and will recur to it again when describing the particular mode of managing cases.

In selecting stiumlants then, to arouse the nervous energy, we should prefer those which will not diminish the oxygen of the blood, as some of the most constant and dangerous symptoms are produced by such diminution. Opium, alcohol, chloroform, and ether, as already stated, have. to a greater or less extent, that effect.

With reference to this indication, we shall experience better results from such articles as coffee, quinine, mustard, ammonia, capsicum, camphor, cassia, valerian, and oil of turpentine.

An emetic dose of salt and mustard is strongly recommended by some, and may have a good effect in arousing these organic nerves and changing the train of morbid actions; but this, if resorted to at all, should only be considered as preliminary to other treatment, and the period of quiet succeeding its immediate operation must not be neglected for the introduction of other remedies.

But there is another system of means for answering this indication of arousing the nervous energy, which is worthy of attention. We know that when the functions of the organic nerves are overcome and suspended by a poisonous dose of prussic acid, opium, alcohol, or chloroform, the most effectual means of rallying it into action are, sudden dashings of cold water upon the surface, cold affusions continued for a short time, and repeated, and the abundant inhalation of fresh air, improved by the addition of the vapor of ammonia or oxygen gas.

We might infer that this same system of means would be useful in cholera, and in many cases it has been so found. When these cold applications are used, during their intermissions, reaction should be encouraged by frictions, warm flannels and sinapisms.

I have used these cold affusions only in a few cases, and most of those were in a condition not favorable for the success of any treatment; but I have generally been able to procure a degree of re-action, and the result of the experiments made, impressed me favorably with the remedy. I regard it worthy of further trial.

To fulfil the second general indication, viz.: That of exciting the dormant, and correcting the morbid action of the different distinct organs, such as the liver, stomach, kidneys, &c., thus endeavoring to restore, as far as possible, their different functions to their normal condition, a variety of means must be used.

To correct the exhalent and other functions of the stomach and bowels, to allay the irritation and arrest the profuse discharges, opium, in my opinion, as anticipated by preceding remarks, is the chief remedy. In order that it be retained and have a speedy effect, abstinence from drinks in considerable quantities must be enjoined, and the medicine given in minute division, triturated with some other substance; and its effects may be aided by counter-irritation over the epigastrum and indeed the whole abdomen, and sometimes by various astringents. The acetate of lead, is, upon the whole, the most useful of the astringents; but it affects the purging more than the vomiting, and controls this symptom much more manifestly when given by enema, after an impression has been made upon the stomach with opium. When thus used in a moderate quantity of fluid, and combined with a quantity of laudanum, varying with the condition of the patient and the amount of opium previously taken, the effect is often most happy.

To excite the liver to its natural secretion, thereby relieving the blood of much of its effeté matter, and usually changing the whole character of the disease, calomel should be given in repeated doses. The use of this article I consider of exceeding importance. My observations upon it have been careful and abundant, and I think I cannot be mistaken. The discharges may often be checked without its use, and temporary improvement produced; but unless the secretion of the liver be excited, (and calomel when properly given and retained tends powerfully, and far more than any other article, to excite that secretion,) the cholera discharges will generally again return, and severe consequences follow. The indication for calomel exists in the early stages of the disease and continues present until the symptoms are controled, the action of the liver restored, or until a sufficient quantity is given to produce all the beneficial effects of which the medicine is capable.

I am by no means insensible to the injurious effects, both proximate and remote, which the free, or even moderate use of mercury, under many circumstances, produces. I do not belong to that class of practitioners ever seeing some " liver complaint," or " bilious obstruction," and hurling heroic doses of calomel, or everlasting " blue pills" at these, so often, immaginary difficulties. But mercury is a medicine of power, and has its uses; and cholera is one of the diseases where its remedial virtues are greatest. In this disease it seldom produces salivation or other remote injurious consequences, and even if it did much more frequently, considering the extreme danger of the patient and the good effects it produces, we should be justified in its use.

To excite the action of the kidneys, diuretics may be given whenever the stomach will retain them, and when they will not interfere with other more necessary remedies, or produce any other unpleasant effects. Oil of turpentine and spts. nit. dulc. are among the best articles of. this class.

To counteract the derranged state of the sanguinous circulation, which is always great in the full-formed stage, amounting to a degree of obstruction in the capillaries and a very general internal congestion of organs, various means have been suggested and practised. Any course which will contribute to the first indication—that of arousing the organic nervous energy—will do much to acomplish this; but there are other means acting more directly in effecting this object, among which is blood-letting.

This may seem a desperate remedy, and certainly should be used with the greatest discrimination and caution. There is however much testimony in its favor entitled to the highest respect, and my own experience enables me to express the opinion with confidence, that there is a class of cases occurring in the robust and vigorous, marked by a degree of hardness of pulse, by a violence of pain and cramps, without very free discharges, where, at the proper time—the early stage of congestion —duly aided by other means, and these, perhaps, stimulants, it will operate most beneficially. McIntosh has long since shown, and his observations have been abundantly confirmed, that bleeding in the congestion or cold stage of intermitting fever affords the greatest temporary relief, and would be generally indicated in the cold stage of the ague, were it not for the more remote consequences—the continued debility and impoverishment of the blood which would follow.

I have resorted to bleeding in cholera only in a small proportion of cases, as the large majority of those I have treated in the disease have been foreign emigrants, debilitated from recent sea voyages, or others whose vital powers were low; but whenever I have practised it under the circumstances described, I have been pleased with the result. The cramps, pains, blueness, and oppression of breathing have been relieved, and all the symptoms taken a milder form.

Another means for the relief of this congestion in cholera, less hazardous in its effects, is the use of dry cupping. The cups should be applied along the spine and over the abdomen. A large cup or common tumbler suddenly applied on the stomach will often produce a marked effect in allaying the nausea and vomiting and enable the stomach to retain medicines until they can make an impression.

Nearly akin to this and to blood-letting, combining in some degree the advantages of both, and avoiding some of the disadvantages of the latter, is the ligation of the extremities, near the trunk, thereby detaining for a time a portion of the blood in the vessels of the limbs, and when the necessity for its detention has passed by, allowing it to return into the general circulation.

Whether the blood may not be deteriorated by this detention, so as to be in danger of producing unpleasant effects, has often suggested itself to me, but I have not been able to discover evidence that this is the case, and if it be not, this plan must possess some advantages over blood-letting. I have practised it frequently and with satisfactory results. Besides the general effects, it often relieves in a marked degree the cramps in the limbs thus treated.

Sinapisms, frictions, external warmth, and other modes of cutaneous irritation, directly conduce to the relief of congestion, and sometimes act beneficially in arousing nervous energy.

I have a strong impression, hardly amounting however to a definite and positive opinion, that the good effects of pretty free doses of quinine in many cases of cholera, depend upon its removing internal congestion, and equalizing—freeing, as it were—the restrained circulation. That it has an immediate effect in relieving the symptoms of congestive, miasmatic fevers, somewhat aside perhaps from its anti-periodic influence, is quite certain—and the analogy between the cold or congestive stage of a miasmatic fever, and the algide stage of cholera is quite apparent.

At all events, whatever the mode of its action,— whether by sustaining the nervous energies, relieving the system of capillary and visceral

·congestion, or, in some mysterious way, by neutralizing the effects of the cholera poison, as it seems to neutralize the poison of periodic fevers, it has a beneficial effect in the disease, and in most cases, after the stomach is somewhat quieted by opium, and an anodyne influence is produced, the chances of recovery are enhanced by the administration, in divided doses, of a scruple or more of quinine.

To correct that condition of the blood which arises from deficient respiration, and from a loss of its watery and albuminous portions, and its salts in the discharges; free, full inspirations of the freshest air must be encouraged, and a solution of common salt and bi-carbonate of soda may be given, when the stomach will, without inconvenience, retain it; and chicken broth or beef tea, well salted, must not be omitted.

Saline solutions have not only been given by the mouth, to correct these conditions of the blood, but they have likewise been injected into the veins, and in this, the object aimed at is commendable; but the operation of injecting the veins is a delicate and dangerous one, even under the most favorable circumstances of superior apparatus and skillful hands, and cannot be adopted with benefit in general practice.

We have now passed over the leading indications in the treatment of cholera, and have referred in general terms to the principal means by which those indications are to be fulfilled, and it now remains to attempt a more particular account of the details of procedure — of the particular stages and conditions indicating particular remedies and combinations, and the dose and timing of each article or compound applicable to the various conditions which occur. In doing this, it will be necessary to refer again to the different remedial agents just considered, and something like repetition cannot be avoided; but it is better that many things be repeated, rather than to fail in giving a distinct idea of the treatment to be pursued. It is not easy to combine in the same train of remarks, the pathological and therapeutical principles involved, and the minute details of procedure.

In an active and severe case of cholera, the disease passes through so many stages in so short a time, and these stages are so variable in their duration, and each requires such modifications of treatment, the patient, in order to be skillfully managed, must be visited very frequently,— the amount of medicines taken and retained, and every symptom and condition must be particularly enquired into, and if the memory be at all treacherous, should be carefully noted down. The nurses must be faithful and sensible, and must have the most definite and explicit instructions in every particular. The physician must be cool and collected, and must have every faculty of his mind fully awake

and concentrated upon the work. He who cannot come up to these requirements, who has not the health, or the vigor, or the courage,—who
has not indomitable perserverance and sleepless vigilence, and who,
moreover, has not some definite ideas of the proper treatment, and some
confidence in remedies, will consult his own peace of mind and the interests of community, by avoiding, as some do, the treatment of all
cases of this disease.

When, during the prevalence of epidemic cholera, a patient is affected
with the premonitory symtoms of the disease, and especially if diarrhœa
be present, he should immediately be sent to bed in a comfortable and
well-ventilated room, with warm cover, adapted, however, to the temperature. The state of the skin should be enquired into, and if not in perfect condition, as regards cleanliness, a warm bath, or sponging with
warm soap and water or saleratus water should be used. An anodyne,
consisting of from one to three grains of *opium* with the same amount of
camphor, well triturated with sugar, (or its equivalent in laudanum),
should be immediately given, and if the discharges are inclined to be
watery, colorless, and destitute of bile, four to six grains of calomel or its
equivalent of blue pill, must be added. This dose must be repeated in
from an hour and a half to three or four hours, if the discharges are not
completely arrested, and the sensations of abdominal uneasiness removed.
After twelve or fifteen grains of calomel are given, unless the symptoms
assume considerable severity, this article may be omitted, but the anodyne must be continued until a decided narcotic influence is produced,
or until all symptoms of the diarrhœa are removed. Should the diarrhœa not yield readily, acetate of lead or tannin should be added to the
opium in from two to four grain doses, or what is still more effectual,
enemas of ten grains of the lead with a teaspoonful of laudanum in three
or four ounces of some simple fluid, plain water answering every purpose,
at a temperature a little above that of the room, must be given and repeated once an hour, or oftener if not long retained, and if the discharges
are not arrested. In many cases, a few grains of quinine (two or three)
given at first with each dose of the opium will cause the latter article to
be borne better, and the combined effect will be an improvement upon
that which will be produced without the quinine. I have often prescribed pills, containing sulp. morphine one-fourth of a grain, and sulph.
quinine two grains, one to be taken and repeated once in from 1 to 4 hours
as may be required; and these doses in a majority of cases, will be quite
sufficient to arrest all the symptoms. Mercury, however, should not be
omitted where any considerable severity of symptoms exist, and where
the cholera tendency is manifest in the colorless condition of the dis-

charges; for, though without the mercury, the symptoms may be arrested, they are much more liable, after a few hours to return; when this article is not used. Where mercurials however are used with the opium, such returns of the symptoms are exceedingly rare. When by these means the discharges are completely arrested, the next day a mild laxative of syrrup of rhei., or equal parts of the syrrup and tinct. of rhei., or castor oil, with a few drops of oil of turpentine and tinct. opium, may be given with advantage. A simple anodyne should follow its operation if there be pain or a tendency to a continuance of the catharsis. At the commencement of the treatment, or any time during its course, a sinapism to the abdomen may be useful. The blandest diet should be insisted upon, and the patient kept quiet until restored. These means are almost as certain to arrest the disease, if resorted to and persevered in, during the *first stage*, as quinine is to arrest an ordinary attack of intermitting fever.

When the cholera is prevailing, physicians should strongly advise those who depend upon them for medical advice, to keep about them medicines adapted to the disease, and should give them instructions respecting their applications, in case of emergency; but still to send for advice as soon as possible after symptoms appear. Many lives may in this manner be saved.

But the premonitory stage is sometimes absent, or so slight as not to receive attention, and is frequently so neglected, or so short in duration, as not to become the subject of treatment, and the case passes into the second stage—the full development of the active disease occurs before aid is sought. In the early part of this stage, before the deep blueness occurs, and while considerable warmth is present, especially if the disease seems to be of a forcible character, with some pain and spasms, the treatment may commence by a moderate bleeding, or safer, by ligation of the extremities, detaining in that manner, a portion of the blood from the circulation. Several cups may be applied over the stomach and abdomen; all drinks, in larger quantities than just sufficient to wet the passages, must be instantly and peremptorily prohibited, and, whether the preceding means be used or not, the following powder administered in a teaspoonfull of water:

> ℞ Opii., grs. ij.
> Gum Camphor, grs. jss.
> Submuriate Hydrg., grs. vij.
> White Sugar, grs. xv.
> M. Triturate very thoroughly.

The minute division of the medicines by trituration, I regard as very important. All the ingredients, when thus treated, will diffuse themselves readily, and will be extensively and speedily applied to, and will readily act upon, the stomach,— while, if the opium and other articles be given in pill or coarser powder, they will be much more liable to be rejected before they have time to act, or if retained, their effects will be more slow and cumulative, and that of the opium may be too profound at a later period, when a powerful narcotism would be liable to be fatal. If the treatment be commenced at a *very* early period in the second stage, and the circulation and respiration is still comparatively good, a quarter of a grain of morphine may be added to the first dose of the above powder. If there be evidence of matters upon the stomach not rejected, or if there be much cramp and retching, without the power of free emesis, an emetic dose of salt and mustard, or of sulph. of zinc, may precede the administration of the powder, and in that case, the temporary calm after the vomiting must be seized upon to give the powder. When the vomiting is spontaneous, the calm succeeding it is the most favorable moment for administering a dose. When the dry cups come off they must either be re-applied, or the regions of the stomach and bowels covered with a strong sinapism. Sinapisms may also be applied to the extremities. If the first powder be rejected before it has had time to make an impression or be absorbed, another should be immediately given, omitting the morphine, however, in the second dose, if the first was retained as long as ten or fifteen minutes, or if there is evidence of any portion of it having been retained; and after the second dose, it is not usually safe to add morphine to the two grains of opium, however frequent the vomiting may be. These powders may then be continued, sometimes varying the proportions by increasing the calomel and diminishing the opium, repeated once in from one to three hours, according to the severity of the symptoms, *until either the discharges are arrested, a visible degree of anodyne influence is produced, or the blue stage occurs.* After one or two doses of the powder are given, and the vomiting is somewhat abated; and especially if the treatment had commenced at a later period of the disease, three or four grain doses of quinine should be administered once in two or three hours until a scruple or half a drachm has been given. Should the discharges be arrested or very matetrially abated, as they usually are after a short time under this treatment, the stomach will be in a condition to retain other articles, and other indications besides that of arresting the discharges can be attended to. Should a considerable degree of narcotism be present, a strong infusion of coffee must be given liberally, and continued until the symptom is no longer sufficient to excite uneasiness. Should there be much depression, carbonate of ammonia may be added to the quinine or given by itself, and should the surface be dark, with considerable depression of the vital powers, common salt and flour of mustard, in doses of from ten to fifteen grains each may be given once in from one to two hours. At the same time, a few spoonfuls of chicken broth, or beef tea with rice water, well salted, may be given quite frequently, say every half hour. In the meantime, some twenty to thirty or more grains of calomel has probably been given in the powders, and if so, no more will usually be required; but if rice water discharges still occasionally continue, five or six grain doses of calomel may be continued without the opium, or with a quantity of it so small as not to be incompatible with the safety of the patient. The extent to which opium may be safely carried, cannot be defined, and must be carefully judged of in each case by all the lights which close observation and experience can afford. If the treatment be commenced later in the disease than we have been supposing, opium must be used more sparingly, and as the point at which treatment has been commenced, advances towards or into the blue and collapsed stages, less and less must be used, until none can, with safety or a prospect of success, be given.

Acetate of lead, in from two to four grain doses, may sometimes be given alternatively with the opium powders, especially if the purging be out of proportion to the vomiting. But the stomach has certain capacities for the enduring of medicines, beyond which, it cannot be plied with impunity. We cannot pour promiscuously into that organ when irritated as in this disease, every article for which there seems to be an indication; and according to my observation, when acetate of lead, by the stomach, has been added to the treatment just described, the effect has not usually been as satisfactory as without it. In the condition however, above referred to, when the purging is more severe than the vomiting, and continues after a partial calm has been effected by anodynes,— or in the latter and lower stages of the disease, when this exhausting discharge continues, the effect of *enemas* of the lead, given as directed when describing the treatment of the premonitory stage, with such quantities of laudanum as may be borne, can scarcely be too highly praised. Tannin may be used as a substitute for the lead,— is often quite as effectual, and not unfrequently is borne better by the stomach when used in that way. I have not unfrequently combined tannin with quinine, where the latter article was indicated, and purging was present, without producing unpleasant effects upon the stomach, and with a manifest impression upon the purging.

The above course of treatment, when commenced *before the blue stage has thoroughly set in*, will, according to my observations, in a very large proportion of cases, I should say, in fair constitutions, in nine cases out of ten, succeed in arresting the disease and procuring a favorable reaction. The after treatment should be simple. If the bowels are not open after twenty-four or thirty-six hours from the period of reaction, a gentle laxative of castor oil, with the addition of small quantities of oil of turpentine and laudanum, or an aperient of some of the preparations of rhubarb, in divided doses, may be given. If the stomach seems loaded, as it not unfrequently is at this period, with bile, a gentle emetic of salt and mustard will sometimes procure great relief. If the urinary secretion is not soon restored, or indeed in anticipation that it may not be, when the stomach and bowels become quieted, spts. nit. dule., may be given in half tea-spoonful doses in water, frequently repeated. Bland nourishment and drinks may be allowed and the patient kept quiet. Sometimes gentle tonics may be useful. In some rare instances, after not very severe cases of cholera, but rather more frequently after the graver cases, the kidneys fail to perform their functions entirely, and the patient dies comatose from the poison of urea in the blood, notwithstanding stimulating diuretics and electricity may be used to prevent the result.

Where mercurials have been pretty freely used, and alcoholic stimulation has been avoided, it is seldom that severe congestions and inflammations of the brain and other organs occur, after attacks which have not passed into the collapsed stage. Whenever these cases do occur however, treatment must be conducted on general principles, bearing in mind that though there be inflammation, it occurs in a system much debilitated by a severe disease. If the brain and spinal marrow, and their envelopes, be the seat of the disease, blisters, mild mercurials, and iodide of potash, would be indicated. If the stomach and bowels be the seat of the inflammation, blisters, a few minute mercurial doses, with small doses of morphine, followed perhaps by a mild laxative of castor oil, and this succeeded by the following mixture will be well:—

> ℞ Oil of Turpentine.
>   Tinct. of Opium, aa f ℨ i j ss.
>   Gum Arabic.
>   Sugar,   aa. ℥ ss.
>   Camphor Water,   f ℥ ij.
> M. for an emulsion. A teaspoonful
>   once in 3 or 4 hours.

These secondary symptoms are varied and sometimes protracted, requiring a variety of management, often embracing ultimately a general tonic course.

But cases of cholera are frequently not seen until they are far advanced into the cold and blue stage, or have actually passed into the collapsed condition.

While the pulse remains at the wrist, there is sufficient hope to demand strenuous efforts, and even after it has disappeared patients occasionally recover. The practitioner of close observation, of acute discernment, and of much experience in cholera, will be able almost at a glance to determine the probable fate of his patient, for there is a discernable point beyond which if he pass, all the chances are against his recovery.

If bordering upon the full collapsed or asphyxied state, opium, as has already been stated and repeated, must not be given, or only in very small quantities. If the purging still continue, an enema of a solution of acetate of lead, (15 or 20 grains,) with perhaps a half teaspoonful of laudanum may be used, and repeated, with or without the laudanum, as circumstances may require. The cold affusion, or the rubbing in ice, may here be tried, followed by warm frictions, sinapisms, and warm blankets. The fullest inspirations of the freshest air must be insisted upon, and warm coffee, quinine, and carbonate of ammonia, two or three grains each of the last two, once an hour or two, alternated with doses of from ten to fifteen grains each of salt and mustard, may be given, not omitting the frequent administration of chicken or beef tea, well salted. Dry cupping along the spine may be added to the treatment with advantage. Besides these means, six or eight grains of calomel should be given once in an hour or two, until some twenty or more grains are used; not with reference so much to any immediate effect, as to act after several hours upon the bilious secretion, should the vital powers be kept up for that length of time; for, without that action upon the liver, the cholera discharges are liable to continue or return.

Of the treatment of the fully collapsed state I have nothing to say. I have seen a few such cases recover—that is, cases where the pulse could not be felt at the wrist, and where the loss of voice, the blue and shrunken condition of the surface, the extreme sunken and lustreless eye, and the slow, laborious breathing, corresponded with that condition of the arterial circulation; but these are exceptions so rare, that the influence of treatment is not ascertained.

In describing the treatment of the active or vomiting stage of cholera, it was mentioned that drinks should be avoided excepting in teaspoonful doses, or quantities just sufficient to moisten the mouth and throat, and the subject is again introduced here in order to make it more prominent.

This I regard as an essential item of treatment in most cases. The objection to the drinking is, that while fluids in considerable quantities are taken into the stomach, vomiting will continue, and medicines will not be retained. A teaspoonful of ice water, or a very small piece of ice may be taken frequently, and will answer all the purposes of quenching thirst of a larger quantity. So important do I consider this point, that I would not take the responsibility of a case — would abandon a patient whose friends would not enforce the restriction, where vomiting or the danger of vomiting existed.

Time is so essential in the treatment of cholera, that it is very important that every practitioner have about his person several articles of medicine, particularly if the powders of opium, camphor, calomel and sugar, which I have recommended, be used, they should be very carefully prepared, of good materials, thoroughly triturated, and put up in packets, accurately weighed. In a large practice much time and many lives may be saved by such precaution.

The views of cholera expressed in the preceding pages are the result of no small amount of observation and experience, and are presented to the profession with a good degree of confidence in their general correctness; and though possessing no distinct features strikingly novel, they are nevertheless brought forward with the hope that they may contribute in some small degree to the establishment of more definite and rational principles in regard to this still obscure and mysterious affection. The treatment recommended has been tested in a large number of cases, and the results have been such as to establish my confidence in the power of remedies over the disease.

It is to be regretted however that, as yet, no means have been discovered of answering an indication which is above, and would supersede all those we must now labor to fulfil, viz.: that of directly neutralizing the cholera poison; and although all alleged specifics have failed to establish their claims as such, although the late Ozone, and charcoal and sulpher bubble burst, leaving but a feeble trace behind, yet we may hope, that in the advancement of science the hidden nature of the cholera germ will be discovered, and a remedy found which will directly destroy its effects. He who shall be so fortunate as to make this discovery, must ever be regarded as among the great benefactors of mankind—will indeed occupy a high niche in the temple of fame, and in celebrations of the triumphs of our art, his name will be pronounced in the same sentence with that of Harvey—and Hunter—and Jenner.

ART. II.—*Inguinal Hernia and imperfect descent of the Testicle of the right side, Orchitis.* By E. K. Phillips, M. D.

Having noticed a case of strangulated inguinal hernia, reported in the July number of the Peninsular Journal, (which I have just received, having to wait for the reprint of that number,) by Wm. Brodie, M. D., and presuming the Doctor to have forgotten some of the particulars of the case, I am led to make the following report:

October 29th I was called to see David G., aged forty years, a farmer, had resided in Michigan one year on a new farm.

On my arrival, I was informed he had been troubled with a hernia since a boy, that it had been strangulated once or twice, and been treated by his old family physician in the State of New York; he thought it then strangulated, and sent for me.

Upon examination, I found to all appearance an omental hernia of the right side, which was by little force applied in the course of the inguinal canal placed within the internal ring, which being done, the fingers of the left hand were placed over the internal ring to retain all there, while a compress was being prepared, but upon a slight movement of the fingers, nearly all of the mass was observed to slip back to its former situation with considerable force, causing some pain, though the tumor was somewhat lessened in size.

There being no symptoms of strangulation, such as vomiting, or obstruction to a free passage of the bowels, I directed fomentations of warm water, rest in a recumbent position with knees raised, gave an anodyne, and left him with positive instructions to send for me if any unpleasant symptoms should occur.

Heard no more of the case until in the night of 2d November, I was roused and informed that Doctor Brodie, of Detroit, was on his way to see Mr. G., and requested me to meet him there as soon as possible. Accordingly, on my arrival, I informed the Doctor of all I knew about the case, having seen it but once.

Upon a second examination, the tumor was found to have slightly enlarged since my former visit.

Doctor B., after endeavoring to return the mass through the internal ring by the taxis, for a reasonable time declared the necessity of an operation; while the subsequent dressings were being prepared, the patient suspecting that in all probability he would be minus one testicle, informed us that the one on that side would be in great danger. Whereupon another examination was instituted, and the fact ascertained that the scrotum contained but one testicle. The knife was not used.

The patient afterwards gave as a reason for not speaking about the situation of the testicle till that late period; "that he supposed that in all cases of hernia the testicle of the affected side occupied that locality.

November 3d, swelling materially increased. The treatment consisted in the use of leeches and occasionally a saline cathartic during the sthenic form of the orchitis, after which tincture iodine was made use of which reduced the size of the organ.

Adhesion having taken place, held the testicle nearly over the internal ring, and prevented the application of a truss till I made one expressly for him, having a concavity nicely fitting and gently pressing upon the convexity of the testicle, which was applied, and I have had no farther trouble with that hernia.

Rochester, Michigan, December 4th, 1853.

Art. III.—*To the Editor of the Peninsular Journal of Medicine:*

[We do not endorse all the sentiments of this correspondent, nevertheless we admire his stormy eloquence, and give it place, because its peculiar style may be useful to the reader though he may not be prepared to adopt all the thoughts.—Ed.]

St. Louis, Mo.

Sir:—John Randolph, of Roanoke, said in a letter to a friend, "make to yourself an idol, and, in spite of the *decalogue*, worship it." Every young man in commencing life should have, like Moses, a promised land where, though finally he may not repose his bones, he may, at least, approximate, and die *in sight* of the treasures beyond. He should fix upon some star of hope which shall tell him, as of old, where his first-born honors lie, and what his last reward shall be. He should say, "I will be this, or shall attain that," and should mark out his course in strict conformity with his ambitious resolution. Then let him strike for the goal, bend with matchless energy and perseverance every obstacle to his purpose, and ride joyous on the gale, though he sweeps over heaven and rushes through hell. I would like to have him, as he begins his youthful career, draw a skeleton of his future course, and say, "here is my starting point — this is the way in which I go — and yonder is my destiny; now I am almost a worthless cypher — then I shall have striven to be a jewel of precious value." Oh, how far above the present strata

of men would the succeeding generation be, did we all cast our early aspirations in such a mould as this! But what avails it me to take the point and compass, and draw my tortuous figure? It will do me no good, for I am like a bird that is shorn of its wings, which cannot fly.

* * * * *

Quackery. Let me urge upon you a different acceptation of that term, and consider briefly the truthful import of that word. In what consists a quack? In my opinion, it is very much distorted by medical men, and is made to include under its withering ban many an aspirant for immortality, who holds no part nor parcel with the branded class. It is generally thought if a man is enrolled under the banner of M. D., that he is descended from the gods, and superior to all crime. There is a charm in those words which render its bearer invulnerable. But, as I view it, his high title should be of no avail, farther than as presumptive evidence. If I saw him outstep the demarcation of integrity, saw him careless in his studies or heedless in his observations, I would not shield him from the merited opprobrium, though he showed his descent from ·the first institution of the land. But I would delight to recognize that one who, whether or no upheld by the parchment of the schools, is zealously working for the glory of his profession and the salvation of man.

Nor is the quack an empiric, as he is often too worthily and too honorably styled; for an empiric is one who has experience for his guide.

The essence of quackery is deceit, humbug, and scientific ignorance. There is a species of quackery indulged in by most, but which is nevertheless not the more praiseworthy — the hieroglyphic character of our prescriptions, to conceal some objected medicant, and a very common propensity of not telling *all* the truth. This I have participated in on suitable occasions, with the idea that it was harmless in its nature and pregnant with good, but notwithstanding, is it right? From the above, I may be thought to withhold my support from the dignity of our profession, and to favor the progress of the charlatan, but let my thoughts, my words, and *deeds* assure you of an opposite conclusion. There is perhaps no person in the world who sets a higher value on the position, the qualifications, and attainments that should characterize physicians than myself, and never shall my voice or act lower the standard of our colors. The preliminary education requisite, previous to attending medical schools is too limited, and as a consequence, hundreds of young men are yearly thrown out upon society with diploma in hand, wholly unqualified for their expected duties. The most of them occupy an indifferent sphere through life, and die forgotten and unknown; whereas

had th.. .:ade themselves familiar with the various departments of literature ...d science, and cultivated strict habits of thought, they might
have reached an honored eminence, and departed this life with the
regrets of the world.   At all events, whether or not they were recognized
by fame, they would practise with a skill of which they are now entirely
ignorant, and send many less patients to the kingdom of God.

Some months ago, a young man who had attended one course of lectures, proposed to study medicine with me.   I inquired into his past life
and literary progress, and found him like many others, woefully deficient
therein.   I told him he should base his medical superstructure on a
thorough classical, historical, and logical foundation, that he might have
so much the more an accomplished mind; he should dive deep into
mathematics, for the bedside of the sick often demanded the solution of
some of the most intricate known problems for the relief of discomfort
and the preservation of life; metaphysics and philosophy should receive
his careful attention, and be his constant companions, for deep thought
and continued study should pre-eminently distinguish the physician.
A fearful responsibility rests upon us when attending the afflicted, that
we add not to their sufferings nor shorten their days.   When he heard
these things, "he went away sorrowful;" like the young man who
came to Jesus and said, "good master, what shall I do to have eternal
life ? "

When I compare the quantum of talent engaged in medicine, with
that of the law, I am not flattered.   It shall be my effort to swell the
list of scientific pursuers, and to ennoble that calling which has, and still
will grace with immortal triumphs the lives and names of its most ardent
disciples.   Beneath the streaming folds of our professional banner, there
let me daily bow and humbly worship.   Oh, would that I could penetrate the very center of the comprehensiveness and profundity, of the
source of truth, clothe myself in its gorgeous habiliments, and be presented to the world a glorious embodiment and unqualified perfection of
knowledge!   Futile wish, but I would like to be a god.   G.

SELECTIONS.

Foreign Correspondence of the Nashville Journal of Medicine and Surgery.

Action of the Academy of Sciences of Paris, in regard to experiments with the Per-Chloride of Iron in Aneurisms. By W. F. WEST-MORELAND, M. D., of Georgia.

PARIS, RUE DE BUCI, Dec. 20, 1853.

The treatment of Aneurisms, by coagulating the blood contained in the aneurismal tumor, has, for a great while, been attempted, but without any veritable success, until a few years past. This subject has for some time occupied many surgeons, and recently numerouse xperiments have been instituted in search of agents the most proper to determine this happy result. Thus, we have had proposed, and rejected within that time, numerous methods, as Acupuncture, Electro-puncture, &c., &c. But my object in this communication is not so much to discuss the merits, or demerits of either of these procedures, as to bring before the profession all the facts known in regard to the new method, which, for the past six or eight months, has created much attention in France. I allude to the method known as that of Pravaz, which consists in the injection of the per-chloride of iron in the aneurismal sac, coagulating the blood, and thus obliterating the artery.

It was the 10th of January, of the present year, that this new method was made public, by a letter of M. Lallemand to the Academy of Sciences. In this letter he gave the experiments made by himself and M. Pravaz upon animals, some of which are the following: In an experiment upon the carotid of a sheep, the injection of four drops of the concentrated solution of the per-chloride of iron, transformed into a solid clot all the blood contained in an inch and a half of this artery. Eight drops of the same liquid coagulated the blood contained in three inches of the carotid of a horse. The sheep was killed, though months after the operation, and the post mortem showed the artery entirely obliterated for three inches in extent, and the clot almost entirely absorbed. No other lesions were found. The experiment upon the horse was equally successful. After numerous trials, M. Pravaz estimated that two drops was sufficient to coagulate one teaspoonful of blood. He insisted that there should be no more injected than sufficed for the coagulation of the blood to be acted on; that an excess would produce symptoms of intoxication, dissolution of the clot, with violent inflammation of the sac, or parts operated on. The instrument used in these operations was a very small trocar, made for the purpose, with a small syringe attached, the piston being depressed by a screw; each half turn of the screw ejecting one drop of the liquid. The only precaution insisted upon in performing the operation was, to use compression above and below the point selected for the operation during, and four or five minutes after, the injection.

These experiments were soon after repeated at Alfort, by M. M. Giraldes and Debout, but, as will be seen, not with the same success. They intercepted between two compresses the blood contained in three inches of the carotid of an ass, in which they injected six drops of the per-chloride. Seeing no effect, in a few minutes they injected eleven more, making in all seventeen drops. This produced complete coagulation, with extreme hardening of the artery. The injection of fifteen drops of the same liquid into the blood contained in the same extent of the carotid of a horse, produced a similar result. Other experiments were made, with like results. In most of the cases, the artery became extremely hard; and in one case, thin and distended, in a manner to offer, forty-eight hours after the operation, an extreme dilatation. These operations were not without danger to the general health, as two of these animals, detained after the operations, were found to have fever, with other general symptoms. In one of them, killed thirty days after the injection, pus was found in the artery. Pravaz was greatly concerned at these results, which put in peril his discovery. He attributed the bad results of the experiments at Alfort to the large doses employed, and insisted strenuously upon the employment of just enough of the liquid to coagulate the blood to be acted on. After making other experiments, he adds, that " we cannot notably pass this limit without symptoms of intoxication, dissolution of the clot, and inflammation, with consecutive ulceration." He advised, for an aneurism the size of a hazlenut, the injection of three or four drops of the liquid; and in a few minutes, if the pulsations continued, to repeat the injection.

We now-come to speak of its application to the treatment of aneurisms in the human subject. The first case, although attempted without any rule, and the manner of operating being very imperfect, yet we have an admirable cure. This operation was performed the fourth of February, by M. Raoult Deslongchamps, for an aneurism of the sub-orbital artery, the size of a pigeon's egg. He punctured the tumor obliquely with a very small bistoury; a small quantity of blood was discharged, but without jet. He introduced in the incision a small glass syringe, and made the injection of the per-chloride of iron, without calculating the amount injected; the syringe being removed, some drops of blood were discharged; the pulsations of the tumor continued. The next day he injected ten or twelve drops of the liquid, but having no way of measuring it, he was not certain as to the amount. The syringe was introduced through the incision made the day before. This time the pulsations ceased, and the tumor gradually disappeared, without any unfavorable symptoms. It is necessary to add, that the diagnosis in regard to this tumor was contested by some surgeons, they thinking it an erectile, rather than a true aneurismal tumor. This appears probable, from the announcement of M. Raoult Deslongchamps, a few months ago, that there had appeared another tumor in the same place, which he hesitated not to call an erectile; but adds, that he is still of the opinion that the first was aneurismal.

The next operation was performed by M. Niepce, in March, and reported to the Academy of Sciences the 25th of April, by M. Lallamand. I will give his analysis of it. This was an aneurism of the poplitial artery. Five minutes after the injection of the per-chloride of iron, the tumor became very hard; the pulsations had entirely ceased. The syringe was removed without the loss of a drop of blood. The next day, and the days following, violent inflammation manifested itself in the parts operated on. The eleventh day, fluctuation was observed at the internal side of the tumor; a slight puncture gave issue to a small quantity of purulent matter. After this, all inflammatory symptoms disappeared; and the twentieth day after the injection, there was nothing remaining but a small hard tumor, the size of a hazlenut.

The 9th of May, M. Lallemand reported another case, operated on by M. Terres, of Alias, followed by success; but unhappily, as in the last case, the report is too concise. This was a varicose aneurism at the bend of the elbow. The clot was promptly hardened under the influence of the injection; the pulsations ceased in the tumor, and in a few minutes also in the radial and ulnar arteries. Inflammation of the sac ensued, and a slight puncture a few days after, gave issue to a small quantity of purulent matter. An eschar was detached from the walls of the sac without any hemorrhage. After this, cicatrization made rapid progress, and in a short time the patient was cured. Thus, in the two last cases, and this time for true aneurism, the injections appeared to have been followed by radical cures. But M. Lallemand, far from feeling himself flattered by such success, looked upon it in rather a different light. He alleged, that in the operations of M. M. Niepce and Terres, there was three times as much of the per-chloride injected as was necessary to produce the proper coagulation, as stated by M. Pravaz.

The next case reported, was by M. Malgaigne. The injection was not made by himself; but from the unfavorable result, the patient was induced to enter his wards a few days after. This was a mason, 25 years old, with an aneurism at the bend of the elbow, the size of a hazlenut, the result probably of a wound of the artery in venesection. Five drops of a solution of equal portions of water, and the per-chloride of iron was injected without any result. In a few minutes five drops more were introduced. Immediately after the last injection, there was violent pain of the whole arm, and in a few minutes the arteries in the fore-arm ceased pulsating; the hand became cold and bluish. The next day there was gangrene of the thumb. In this situation the patient entered the wards of M. Malgaigne. Forty-eight hours after the operation, the fore-arm was entirely mortified. M. Malgaigne, still hoping to save the life of the patient, proposed amputation, which was rejected; but the eleventh day after the injections were made, he submitted to the operation, without any good result. The greater portion of the fore-arm had sloughed before amputation was performed. Death occurred in a few days.

The first case operated on at Paris was by M. Velpeau, on the 25th

of May, M. M. Roux, Malgaigne, and several other surgeons of distinction
being present. This was an aneurism at the bend of the elbow, of considerable size. He injected eight drops of the solution prepared by M.
Dubuisson, of Lyons, without any apparent hardening of the tumor.
Compression being removed, the pulsations re-appeared in the tumor,
and in the arteries of the fore-arm. No accident occurred. Twenty-one
days after the first injection, M. Velpeau made another of ten drops.
Coagulation complete was not obtained, yet the tumor appeared to
increase in size. Inflammation of the sac ensued, and seven days after
the last injection, it was thought prudent to ligate the artery. A few
days after the ligation of the artery, the tumor bursted, discharging a
small quantity of purulent matter. The patient recovered.

A short time after the above case of M. Velpeau, M. Lenoir operated
for a poplitial aneurism, the size of a hen's egg. He injected at first
seven drops of the liquid, without any success, the pulsations continuing
as before. No accident occurring, twelve days after he injected sixteen
drops of the same solution, and again without apparent alteration in the
tumor. Attributing this want of success to the bad quality of the agent
employed, he furnished himself with a solution prepared by M. Dubuisson, of which he injected at first six drops; seeing no result, in a few
minutes he injected six more drops. The pulsations still continued both
in the tumor and arteries. During five days the patient felt no pain or
uneasiness, either in the leg or poplietal space; but on the sixth day,
there appeared suddenly a dull pain in this region, followed by chill,
fever, &c. The next day there was decided inflammation around the
tumor; and notwithstanding anti-flogistic treatment, the most absolute,
the patient died ten days after the last operation. The autopsy showed
effusion of blood in the poplietal region; the femoral vein was filled with
sanies, the color of the lees of wine; the sac contained a clot adhering to
its walls, more consistent in the centre than at the circumference.

The 26th of July, M. Soule, of Bordeaux, operated for an aneurism of
the femoral artery, three inches in diameter. He injected six drops of
the per-chloride, but thinks there was but four that entered the sac, as he
found some in the trocar after its removal. The tumor immediately
became hard. To favor success as much as possible, compression was
maintained fifteen minutes after the operation; but when it was suspended, pulsation immediately re-appeared in the tumor. No accident
occurred. The 1st of August, five days after the first injection, he made
another of seven drops of the same solution. Violent pain was instantly
produced in the region of the aneurism; the sac became inflamed, and
increased in size. There was partial coagulation. Inflammation increased,
and on the 7th of September, M. Soule, fearing hemorrhage from ulceration of the sac, ligated the artery. The patient recovered. We have no
account whether the sac was ruptured or not. The solution employed
in this case was not prepared by M. Dubuisson.

A few days after this last operation, M. Soule tried this method on a
small aneurismal tumor of the posterior tibial artery, near the internal
maleolus, the result of a wound of the artery. The external wound was
closed only by a clot, consequently there was frequent hemorrhages.

He injected several drops of the solution, and introduced some lint wetted with this liquid, retaining this by a bandage slightly compressible. Three days after, seeing no effect from the per-chloride, he excised the tumor; but being unable to seize the artery to ligate it, he used compression from the bottom of the wound, by means of the charpie, wetted with the liquor of Pagliari. This treatment was successful.

A case of the same kind was treated by M. Alquie, of Montpelier. The cubital artery having been wounded one month after there was a tumor the size of a pigeon's egg, with pulsations, &c. He made an injection of six drops of a solution of equal quantity of water, with the per-chloride of iron. At first there was no change in the tumor; but night coming on, violent pain commenced in the region of the aneurism. The next evening there were chills, with tumefaction of the fingers, &c. The fourth day after the operation, the hand and fore-arm were extremely red; the pulsation in the tumor was very distinct, and threatened a rupture of the sac. The humeral artery was ligated, and nine days after, hemorrhage from the wound made it necessary to ligate the ulnar artery with a collateral branch of considerable size. The patient recovered. Not being able to obtain the reports of the three following cases, I give the result as presented to the Academy of Sciences a few days ago, by M. Malgaigne. One was an aneurism of the carotid artery, operated on by M. Dufour. The injection was followed by violent inflammation of the parts; the tumor became gangrenous, and in a short time ruptured, giving rise to fatal hemorrhage. A short time after, M. Jobert made the injection for an aneurism of the femoral artery. Violent inflammation, gangrene of the whole limb, and death was the result. M. Berrier, of Lyons, made three injections of twenty-five drops each, into an aneurism of considerable size, of the brachial artery. Fifteen days elapsed between each injection. No unpleasant symptoms followed either operation; nor was there any apparent change in the tumor.

The last case operated on in Paris was by M. Malgaigne, and reported a week or two past. This was an aneurism of the brachial artery, and was two inches in diameter. He injected six drops of the liquid, without any apparent hardening of the tumor. Compression was used during several minutes, above and below the aneurism; but when removed, pulsations immediately re-appeared, both in 't and the arteries below. No accident occurred for four days; but on the fifth the tumor increased in size, and became the seat of some pain. Two days after the first unpleasant symptoms, the pain became excruciating; this increased with the tumefaction of the tumor. Eleven days after the injection, M. Malgaigne ligated the artery. A few days after this, a slight puncture of the tumor gave issue to a large quantity of thick black blood. In a few days the incision in the tumor was enlarged, and there was extracted a clot of considerable size. After this, all unpleasant symptoms subsided, and in a short time the patient was cured.

I notice in the journals of last week a case reported by M. Valette, of Lyons. The injection was made for an aneurism of small size, of the brachial artery. Twenty drops of the per-chloride was injected; the tumor immediately became hard; pulsations ceased; no inflammatory symptoms occurred; and the tumor gradually disappeared, leaving un-controverted evidence of a radical cure.

Such, then, is the statistics of results of this new method: Fourteen operations, four deaths, four cures, one without any apparent effect, and five failures, with accidents which made it necessary to ligate the artery. Much has been said in regard to these experiments. Each case has been analyzed, and the manner of operating condemned or approved, agreeably to the opinions entertained by writers, of the peculiar action of this remarkable substance. For the past six weeks, the subject has occupied particularly the Academy of Sciences; and in some of its sittings, the discussion has been exciting. At the last meeting of this body, the subject was called without any one responding, all seeming to feel the inutility of such a discussion, and the impossibility of arriving at any definite conclusions in regard to its action, except by experimentation. It is apparent to all that the surgical applications of this substance thus far has failed to give satisfactory data. The experiments have been made under circumstances so diverse, and by experimenters differing so much in opinions, that it is impossible to draw any conclusions in regard to its action, farther than that it does coagulate the blood.

It is necessary to add that the per-chloride has been extensively applied for the treatment of varicose veins. Its injection into these veins appears to be less perilous, and have been followed by better results than those made for aneurisms. It has also been employed in capillary hemorrhages with considerable success.

From the American Medical Monthly.

Chloroform in Delirium Tremens. Report of ten cases. By W. M. CHAMBERLAIN, M.D., Astoria, L. I.

Few men who have not "written a book" upon the subject, are satisfied with the pathology of the nervous system. In reviewing the literature of Delirium Tremens, we are obliged to conclude that terminology, has been indefinite, diagnosis inexact, pathology inadequate, and the net result confusion and uncertainty.

Eberle and Coates tell us that, whatever the disease may be, insomnia is its index; that stimulus is unnecessary; that opium is the *remedium magnum;* and sleep, *coute qui coute,* by its power, the indication. In a neighboring hospital, Dr. Gerhardt taught that nervous depression is the key to all the phenomena; and support, by stimulation and nutriment, the one thing needful. Dr. Klapp and others support a different theory, if we rightly interpret a practice which admits of giving 30 grains of tart. ant. et potass. in the course of a few hours. Consistently they add, free " venesection is a useful adjunct."

Again, we are told that the disease is simply poisoning by alcohol. Elimination by the skin and kidneys is the cure. The physician prescribes a bucket of cold water and a tin cup; nature supplies the appetite; all indications are thus easily answered, and recovery is almost certain.

Another says that the disease is self-limited, and "let it alone" is the corollary.

One finds phrenitis or meningitis pretty uniform, and "exhibits" a coronet of leeches, the ice cap, cold affusion, and blisters. Another sees the exciting cause in depraved secretions, retained bile and urea; and calomel, with diuretics, is his sheet-anchor.

One insists that recumbency is indispensable, and compares the value of bed-straps and straight-jackets; a second orders the largest liberty of speech and motion; and a third, alive to the necessity of relieving the brain by the muscular system, visits his patients with a rope's end. Spearmint-tea is remembered as a specific by other practitioners. Assafœtida, valerian, camphor, ether, and chloroform, have their devoted partisans, who sought nothing further from the pharmacopœia. The results of the same methods in different hands have been distractingly various. An eminent man, in charge of one of the largest and best lunatic asylums in the country, tells us that, under the "let-alone" plan, he has lost but one patient in seventeen years, and that one moribund at admission; while one of our city institutions, retaining splendid medical skill, in its annual report for 1852, admits 27 deaths from delirium tremens. Another hospital, in a distant city, reports, for 1853, 162 cases of delirium tremens, and 88 of debauch, admitted; and in this number 52 deaths from delirium tremens. If all certificates of death from "apoplexy," "epilepsy," "congestion of the brain," &c., by which credit and the feelings of friends are wont to be shielded, could be carefully analyzed, unexpected statistics would appear.

What is to be said of such diversity? It cannot be supposed of many of the modes of treatment above enumerated, that they were inapt to the particular cases upon whose favorable issue their credit stands; or that, in those cases, the particular medication was a matter of no importance. We may not so stultify our teachers. It must be concluded that different authors, giving their own experience in different forms of disease in the drunkard, have claimed a generic name for widely differing conditions. The fatuous insanity of intoxication, the sthenic delirium-e-potu, the spasm and epileptiform convulsion, which mark the toxic effect of alcohol on the surface of the brain; the true delirium tremens, with prostration and anæmia of the cerebral mass; the slow paralysis of intellection and motion deepening into coma, which attends retention of bile and urea; the pain and peculiar delirium of cerebritis; and the persistent vigil of mania, have been confounded, perhaps not in the mind of the physician, but certainly in the definitions of the author. They do, indeed, so alternate and complicate each other, as to tax to the utmost the most acute observation, and the best-instructed judgment. Though we may well doubt whether the elements of present science have been sufficiently appreciated, yet the hope of a complete rationale and therapeutics of logical induction must be deferred to another age. Suggestions to be elaborated and facts to be compared, are present desiderata.

With this feeling, we are disposed to offer some cases, observed and imperfectly recorded, without any view to such a report. They are extracted
from our " Case Book," not as a challenge to criticism, or a buttress to
any theory, but in the hope that they may illustrate the use and power
of the great narcotic, opium, and the greater sedative, chloroform. In
some of them these agents were employed almost without stint or limit,
and the effect, in suspended and restored animation particularly, we
have not seen elsewhere so fully detailed. They occurred in the Penitentiary Hospital on Blackwell's Island, under the direction of Dr. Wm.
Kelly, late resident physician, in whose fate, cast away upon the Atlan-
tic, while we now write, the many who have loved and honored him
feel a deep and painful interest.

A few belong to the period since Dr. K.'s resignation, during which
the writer held the medical charge of the island. Most of them were
observed and treated by himself personally,—a few by associates in
duty there.

During the year 1853, 960 persons, in the various stages of debauch,
were sent to the hospital by the police courts of the city. Almost uniformly such belong to the lowest class in society—prostitutes, thieves,
" fighting-men," and broken-down vagabonds, who revolve in fixed orbit
through their dens of vice and the charitable institutions of the city.
Excess, privation, exposure, and chronic disease, are the staple facts of
their lives.

They arrive at the hopital generally on the second, often on the third
day after they have been arrested, or picked up by the police. Meantime, they have been confined in the station-houses and in the "Tombs,"
in cells often dark, cold, wet, and comfortless; cut off from all stimulus;
unable to take, and sometimes to find food; oppressed with their de-
gradation, a prey to " horrors," and the scarcely less horrid vision of
months imprisonment. It is not strange, then, that a large number of
aggravated cases of delirium tremens occurs among them. Of the 960
mentioned above, but 200 are counted on the books of the hospital as
delirium tremens. It was intended to exclude from this list every equiv-
ocal case; and of the remaining 760, credited with debauch simply,
it is believed many might, with much propriety, have been counted as
subjects of the graver malady.

It may not be amiss to introduce the elements of an average case of
debauch, in this connection. They are somewhat as follows:

A. B. presents herself at 5, P.M. She is pale, weak, and tremulous;
has been drinking constantly and largely for a week. Since her arrest,
36 hours have elapsed. She has had no sleep, and has been unable to take
food. Her pulse indicates irritation and asthenia. The skin is cool,
the tongue moist and pale. Last night she suffered frightful hallucina-
tions. She craves liquor, dreads the coming night, and fears she shall
die. From the warm bath she is removed to a warm bed. Three pints
of warm infusion of hops are given her. This acts gently but effectually
in three ways: first, as an emetic; second, as a diaphoretic; third, as a
hypnotic. When her stomach is quiet, after the vomiting, two or three
compound cathartic pills are given her. An hour or two after, she is

offered some bread and tea, or some beef-tea; and still later, is required to drink a full draught of ale, containing a drachm of laudanum. Early in the night, she sinks into comfortable sleep, which continues till late in the morning. The bowels move, the nervous disturbance is abated, the appetite returns. She has a pint of ale with her food during the day, sleeps well again, and is discharged on the morrow, to recoved, her perfect strength and health gradually. The case thus managed is a slight affair; neglected, it would probably have been delirium tremens. Those hereafter cited are delirium tremens, except the second of extreme severity; and must not be considered, in any sense, *average*. The appeal to chloroform was held to be dangerous, and never accepted save as the "*ultima ratio medendi.*"

On admission, patients receive a warm bath, a bed, and light food, if they desire it, from the attendants, before the evening visit of the physician, at 7, P.M. The "punch" mentioned in the reports, except where otherwise specified, consists of a pint of milk, two ounces of brandy, and q. s. of sugar. The chloroform employed was that manufactured by Powers and Weightman, Philadelphia. These items premised, we submit the cases for what they may be worth.

The first is Delirium Trmens; cure, relapse, and final recovery, without the aid of chloroform.

CASE I.—Oct. 31st, 1853, 7 P.M.

Physique.—T. S.; 35; white; Irish; butcher; height, 5 ft. 6; weight, 140 lbs.; skin, hair, and eyes, dark; features course; frame, athletic; temperament, bilious-lymphatic; general condition pretty good.

Symptoms.—Slight gastric irritation, headache, anorexia, quick pulse, dry and warm skin, constipation, slight delirium and tremor.

Treatment.—Emesis, by inf. hum. lup. hot; slight catharsis, by Haust. nigra. Laudanum, gtt. 120, to be repeated according to indications. Ale, Oj., containing tr. hum. lup. f. ℥ii., to be given in four draughts, at intervals of an hour.

Nov. 1. Took 360 gtt. tr. opii. Fell asleep at 12½, and remained so until 5, A.M. Febrile disturbance controlled. Is now, 8 A.M., awake but quiet. ℞ Tr. opii, gtt. 120. Ale and tr. hum. lup. as before. 8, P. M. Went to sleep at 9½ A. M.; continued so for three hours; is now calm and rational. ℞ Ale, Oj.

Nov. 2. Slept all night; seems about well.

Nov. 8, 7, P.M. After one week of apparent health, under the strict discipline of the hospital, and without stimulus, except as by medical order, ale, Oj., daily, he became, this morning, uneasy and wild. Delirium incoherent, busy, and apprehensive. ℞ Tr. opii, gtt. 60. Punch, Oj., containing Sp. Vin. Gall., f. ℥ii.

Nov. 9. Did not sleep last night. Is now in much the same mental condition. Constitutional disturbance slight. ℞ Tr. opii, gtt. 60. Punch, Oj. (s. v. g. f. ℥ii.) To have as much punch as he can drink through the day, and sulph. morphiæ, gr. ss. hourly. 5, P.M. No improvement; very delirious; screams and prays incessantly. Increased the stimulus, giving him whiskey (which he prefers) *ad libitum.* 9, P.M. More quiet; pupils contracted; pulse 80; strong; evidently under the effect of opium and morphine. Respirations seven per minute. Slight spasms of the extremities. To be carefully watched.

Nov. 10. Slept all night; is now, 9, A.M., sleeping. To have ale, Oj., on waking.

Nov. 11. As above.

Nov. 12. Seems well again.

Nov. 14. Discharged, cured.

In the following case, chloroform was employed. After due preparation, treatment was commenced with narcotics and stimulants. Diligent use for 30 hours showed the insufficiency of these agents. A single administration of chloroform "jugulated" the disease. This case is introduced as the type of a large class.

Case II.—Aug. 10, 1853, 7, P.M.

Physique.—I. P.; 28; white; Irish; butcher; height, 5 ft. 10;. weight, 145 lbs.; temperament, bilious-nervous; condition, good.

A habitual drunkard for many years. Has been drinking brandy freely, and working in ice-houses. Presents the ordinary characters of delirium tremens. Is perfectly wild and unmanageable.

Treatment.—After freeing the stomach and bowels, ordered tr. opii, f. $\bar{3}$i. every hour, for five hours, unless he should sleep; and a small quantity of stimulus.

Aug. 11, A.M. Treatment continued; no sleep or improvement. 10, P.M. No improvement. Chloroform administered with ease, and happy effect.

Aug. 12. Slept nine hours.

Aug. 20. Is well.

The third case was more aggravated than either of the preceding. True delirium tremens, partially subdued during the first night of observation, progressive in intensity during the following 36 hours, under the ordinary treatment; becoming critical on the third night; resisting the repeated use of chloroform; persistent, under the full effect of opium, on the fourth day and evening; and finally subdued by the anæsthetic on the fourth night.

Case III.—Dec. 23, 1853, 7, P.M.

Physique.—S. B.; aged 32; white; English; height, 5 ft. 8; weight, 165 lbs.; book-keeper; dark hair and eyes; regular features; rather full habit; bilious-lymphatic temperament, with tokens of the scrofulous diathesis. A man of habitually intemperate habits, for the past three months in a constant debauch.

Symptoms.—Little or no excitement; skin and bowels inactive; prostration well marked; tremor of limbs and tongue so great, that he cannot stand, lift a glass to his lips, or articulate his words. Motions not unlike those of chorea.

Treatment.—Emesis, with inf. hum. lup. ℞ ol. ric. f. ℥i. tr. opii, gtt. 100. Punch through the night.

Dec. 24. 9, A.M, Slept two hours; is quiet, but wandering. Tr. opii, gtt. 120. Punch and ale. 7, P.M. Condition and treatment the same.

Dec. 25, 9, A.M. Did not sleep at all. Is more delirious. Continued stimulus. ℞ Tr. opii, gt. 40, every hour for five hours. 10, P.M. Very delirious; skin blanched; perspires abundantly. Chloroform by inhalation. Anæsthesia continues but fifteen minutes. Repeated four times in two hours, without permanent effect. Condition as before inhalation, or somewhat worse. Ordered him to be freely fed with strong milk punch,, and to take gr. opii, gtt. 50.

Dec. 26, 9, A.M. Did not sleep at all. Continue opium, gtt. 20,. hourly, and stimulus. 10, P.M. Sleepless and furious; pupils a point. Chloroform by inhalation, to the approach of stertor. Spasm and laryngismus during its exhibition. Effect transient. Repeated: effect permanent.

Dec. 27. Slept 7 hours. Is calm and rational, still under the effect of opium.

Dec. 28. Delirium tremens no longer. Under treatment for constitutional syphilis.

The fourth case is more violent than the preceding, but otherwise a parallel (except in the *internal* use of Chloroform), until the night of the 25th of January. At that date, after anæsthasia had been vainly invoked, the prognosis became unfavorable. Renewed inhalation was followed by unforeseen asphyxia; but it would appear that, even at that alarming moment, the disease was conquered, and the final convalescence initiated and secured.

Case IV.—January 23rd, 1853, 7, P.M.

Pysique.—H. J.; aged 38; white; Scotch; architect; height, 5 ft. 11; weight, 170 lbs.; robust; well developed; of good constitution; health uniform, except when disturbed by excess.

Present condition.—"Has been on a long spree;" very much excited, talkative; facetious; eye wild; limbs tremulous; tongue ditto, and pale; skin warm, rather dry; pulse 80, full; conversation coherent. "Has had no sleep for three nights."

Treatment.—Full emesis, by warm infusion of hops, followed by tr. opii, gtt, 75, when the stomach became quiescent. 10, P.M. Condition the some; effect of opium not perceptible; same dose repeated. 12,P.M. Pupil free; general condition the same.

Jan. 24th, 9, A.M. Slept but little; appears much as last night; bowels not open. ℞ Comp. cath. pil. iii., and an enema of warm water at 3, P.M.; milk punch, Oj. Appetite good. 7, P.M. Bowels freely moved during the day; is now quite calm, rational, quiet, and disposed to sleep; skin normal. No further treatment.

Jan. 25th, 5, A.M. Called to patient, who is confused, wild, noisy;

insists upon getting up. 7, A.M. Condition the same. Desiring to try sedation' by chloroform, ordered ℞ chloroform ℥ i, mucil. acaciæ, f. ℥ viii, sumat, f. ℥ i, sing horis. 4, P.M. Has taken f. ℥ vi, as above, with happy effect; is much more quiet; has been gently restrained in bed, and fed *ad libitum*. 7, P.M. Delirium increasing (often observed at the approach of night); is very restless and noisy; disturbs the house, and requires forcible restraint. Applied the bed-straps, and administered chloroform by inhalation to the approach of stertor, twice, without permanent good effect. Left him at 8, P.M., with a rapid and feeble pulse; prostration and excitement great; having ordered tr. opii, gtt. 60, milk punch, Oj, containing s. v. g. f. ℥ iv, to be given as rapidly as possible. 12, P.M. Condition the same; repeated above. 3, A.M. Do. do.

Jan. 26th, 9, A.M. No improvement perceptible; pupil quite fine; pulse rapid and feeble; excitement great and constant; continued the punch, without the opium. 4, P.M. Has remained screaming, struggling, and convulsed during the day; surface bathed in cold perspiration; pulse exceedingly rapid and feeble; muscular activity still great; face wears an aspect almost cadaveric; has been forced to take two pints of punch, containing 8 oz. of brandy, during the day. There seems no prospect of this spasmodic activity ceasing, except with the total loss of power. Administered chloroform by inhalation; spasm and laryngismus very great; anæsthesia brief, and followed by no good effect. Repeated. Respiration suddenly *suspended* at the instant when it was becoming stertorous. Having no aid at hand, the pulse was not questioned. Performed artificial respiration by elevating and depressing the ribs. Function rallied in a few moments, becoming gradually stronger and more easy.. Left the patient at 7½, entirely quiet, and inclined to sleep. Before inhaling the chloroform, he took tr. opii. gtt. 75. 10, P.M. Quite quiet: has had an hour's sound sleep. 12, P.M. Has slept an hour and a half. Ordered punch freely, and tr. opii, gtt. 75, if he should become wakeful.

Jan. 27th, 9, A.M. Quiet and dozing; has slept four hours; taken a pint of punch and six ounces of brandy since last note; continued treatment.

Jan. 28th. Sleeps continuously; is otherwise well.

Feb. 2d. Discharged from treatment, cured.

Case five was in itself less severe, but tells a very similar story for chloroform.

CASE V.—Dec. 13th, 1852, 7, P.M.

Physique.—H. L.; aged 60; white; Irish; height, 6 ft.; weight, 170 lbs.; dark hair and eyes; fair skin; well developed; of strong constitution; bilious-sanguine temperament; health generally good. "Has had yellow fever and phagedenic chancres, but no other sickness which confined him to bed."

Present condition.—Drunk. ℞ pulv. ipecac. Ði, to be followed by a full draught of inf. hum. lup.; tr. opii, gtt. 70; ale, O ss.

Dec. 14th, A.M. Did not sleep last night; is up, and walks about the ward; eats well; bowels regular; appears strange, but hardly delirious. 6, P.M. As above. ℞ punch, Oj, s. v. g. f. ℥ v.; tr. opii, gtt. 150. 12, P.M. In raving delirium; chloroform by inhalation; anæsthesia and sleep followed.

Dec. 15th, 10, A.M. Slept three-fourths of an hour after the chloroform, and no more during the night. Repeated stimulants and narcotics of last night. 10, P.M. In the same condition of furious delirium; chloroform by inhalation; spasm and laryngismus during its exhibition; slept an hour and three-quarters after. 12, P.M. Re-administered chloroform; at the point of stertor patient *ceased to breathe; pulse at wrist imperceptible;* cold affusion restored him, and he immediately dropped asleep.

Dec. 16th. Slept all night, and continues asleep; is well and rational.

March 2d. Died of pneumonia.

In the following case, after an hour and three quarters of futile anæsthesia, to the point of stertor, having in view the issue of the preceding cases, we determined to proceed to the *verge* of asphyxia. This *occurred* suddenly, and by it the disease was as suddenly vanquished. Artificial respiration completely restored life and all its organic functions. The patient slept, and, after eight hours of sleep, rose again to the level of consciousness and reason, perfectly well.

Case VI.—Feb. 9th, 1853, 7, P.M.

Physique.—C. C., aged 36; white; native of Maine; height, 5 ft. 7 in.; weight, 170 lbs.; laborer; eyes black; hair do, thick and coarse; well developed; athletic; bilious-sanguine temperament. A drunkard for several years, and for six months past almost constantly intoxicated. Drinks brandy.

Present condition.—Bewildered, not delirious: tremor of tongue and limbs excessive; skin florid, hot; pulse 100, soft. From ancle to middle third of the thigh, on right side, red, swollen, and hot. ℞ cold water dressing. "Has not vomited since last drink." 7½, P.M. ℞ inf. hum. lup. Oiij; prompt emesis follows; vomiting persistent. 11½, P.M. Haust. nigra, f ℥ ii; tr. opii, gtt. 75.

Feb. 10th, 1, A.M. Still continues to vomit at intervals; tr, opii, gtt. 75. 2½, A.M. Tr. opii, gtt. 60. 4½, A.M. Do. 6½, A.M. Do. 7, A.M. Fell into uneasy sleep, with intervals of waking and delirium; pupil contracted, iris active. 11, A.M. Tr. opii, gtt. 60. 3, P.M. Do. 8, P.M. Has slept quietly for two hours; no stimulus has been given; patient has taken a little food; bowels freely open. 10, P.M. Quiet, with intervals of sleep.

Feb. 11th. Has slept most of the night; inflammation of the skin and cellular tissue of the leg subsiding; is quiet, but not much disposed to sleep. Tr. opii, gtt. 60. 10, P.M. Has remained in the same condition all day; is still quiet and rational; tremor of limbs passed away. ℞ Tr. opii, gtt. 60.

Feb. 12th, 9, A.M. Seems about well. 12, M. Wild and wandering. 8, P.M. More delirious than at any previous note. Tr. opii, gtt. 125. 9½, P.M. Delirium furious; entire surface bathed in cold perspiration. ℞ brandy freely; tr. opii, gtt. 75; patient has taken more than an ounce. 10, P.M. Ordered chloroform, ℥i; inf. lini. f.℥ viii; sumat, f ℥i sing. horis; brandy continued freely.

Feb. 13th, 6, A.M. More quiet; has not slept; is weaker. ℞ 30 drops of laudanum and an ounce of brandy every hour, the brandy in egg nogg. 10, A.M. More calm; continued treatment. 3, P.M. Still wandering and watchful; has taken a half pint of brandy and 250 drops of laudanum since morning. ℞ sulph. morphiæ, gr. i. 8, P.M. No better; pulse weak and rapid; surface clammy and pale. Chloroform by inhalation to stertor; no permanent sleep or anæsthesia. Patient was kept under its influence for an hour and forty-five minutes, without benefit, when it was determined to push its effects. After a few seconds of stertor, *respiration was instantly suspended;* pulse 0; artificial respiration for a few moments is followed by quiet and continuous sleep.

Feb. 14th. Slept uninterruptedly all night.

Feb. 15th. Sleeps almost continuously; functions all regular.

Feb. 17th. Discharged from treatment, cured.

Case seven is double. The first attack was managed with comparative ease by chloroform, and its subsidence was marked by some of the symptoms of cerebral inflammation. The second is remarkable. Opium, for a time, secured quiet, but could not, even in extreme quantity, procure sleep. The phenomena of anæsthesia were unusual. Asphyxia, in the other cases, was a sudden invasion; in this it advanced, by slow progression, for several minutes after the inhalation was supended. We watched it until it was consummated in death. Re-animation was more difficult than before, and the disease was not cured. The conflict of narcosis and delirium tremens, during the following night, was extremely interesting. After what was thought to be a cure, on October 30th, the disease was re-instated, and as to its subsequent character we are much in doubt. It was treated as delirium tremens with cerebral inflammation.

CASE VII.—June 28th, 1853.

G. S., aged 35; white; native of Long Island; height, 5 ft. 10; weight, 160 lbs. A sinewy, athletic frame, bilious nervous temperament; for fourteen years in the naval service; of intemperate habits, indulging periodically in a "spree" once in 3 or 4 months. Has been drinking very freely for four weeks. Is rational, but much excited. Tremor of limbs excessive; pulse full; face wears a dark, venous flush.

June 29th. Came in late last night; received no treatment except a small dose of laudanum. This morning free emesis and catharsis. Excitement great; delirium furious. Ordered tr. opii, gtt. 60; whiskey, f. ℥iv; milk punch, Oj. 9, P.M. Is worse; perfectly uncontrollable. ℞ sulph. morph., gr. i. 11, P.M. Chloroform by inhalation, preceded by a draught of brandy, f. ℥ii. Complete anæsthesia secured.

June 30th. Slept half an hour under chloroform, and remained quiet and dozing all night; this morning fell into a sound sleep. 6, P.M. Slept until 5, P.M. Ordered punch freely, sulph. morphia, gr. i.

July 1st. Slept all night; is rational, and apparently well.

July 3d. Complains of slight pain and dizziness in head; has no other trace of his late illness. Ordered C. Cups, ℥iv, to temples.

July 6th. Discharged, cured.

Oct. 20th. Re-admitted. Has been drinking freely for a fortnight. Appears much as at previous entry. Functions, except the nervous, not much disturbed. Pulse full, 100. Ordered emesis, with hop-tea, but failed to secure it. It was not thought worth while, at that hour, to make another attempt with a different agent. ℞ Tr. opii, gtt. 120. Repeated at 9, P.M., and at 11, with sp. vin. gall f. ℥iv.

Oct. 27th, 9, A.M. Slept very little; is quiet, but busy and wakeful. Determined to procure sleep by opium and stimulus, if possible. 11, P.M. Took 120 gtt. tr. opii, at 9, A.M. Repeated at 11, 6, 7, and 9, P.M. Ale and punch freely through the day and evening; condition as in the morning. A little while since became suddenly alarmed; started up and passed rapidly along the scale of excitement and delirium until he became perfectly incontrollable. Pupils fine. Chloroform, by inhalation. Violent spasm, with opisthotonos and epileptiform convulsions during exhibition; the body remaining rigid for a moment or two; consciousness and motion returned together, and immediately. Chloroform again. Spasm less; laryngismus so great that its adminstration was suspended. Respiration very slow and labored; *becomes more and more difficult; finally ceases altogether.* Artificial respiration by pressure upon the thorax attempted unsuccessfully for nearly two minutes. Insufflation, followed with pressure, was maintained for some minutes, when the natural breathing was resumed, and continued at seven respirations per minute, stertorous. Slept 20 minutes. When he woke s. v. g. f. ℥ iv. was given, and chloroform again administered; little or no spasm of any sort followed. Slept a few moments. Woke and talked incoherently for a short time, then gradually settled into a profound but uneasy slumber. Respirations 5 per m. Pulse feeble, 130. 1, A.M. As bad as ever. Raves and throws himself about the bed incessantly. Is evidently narcotized, though sleepless; for, in the moments of fitful sleep and exhaustion, which alternate with his paroxysms, he drew but 4, 3, and, in one case, 2 inspirations in a minute. During the paroxysm respiration was very rapid; this condition continued until 3 A.M., when he became more quiet. Slept in longer intervals. Was very narrowly watched until 6, A.M., when I left him overcome with sleep. Pupils still contracted.

Oct. 28th. Sleeps, but is restless. Takes stimulants freely. 6, P.M. Has slept all day. Pupils normal. Pulse 110. Volume and force normal. Is quiet and almost rational. ℞ Tr. opii. gtt. 60. s. v. g., f. ℥ iv.

Oct. 29th, A.M. Slept all night. Continued treatment. P.M. Slept until noon, when he dressed himself, went to the carpenter's shop and worked the remainder of the day; apparently as well as usual. Returns this e\ - - ;, complaining of pain in the head and dizziness. No physical s:., .. in this connection perceptible. Ord. C. Cups to temples, ℥ iv.; tr. opii. gtt. 60. Repeat at 8 P.M. In the course of the night became incoherent and delirious again. It was thought to be a relapse of Delirium Tremens, occasioned by his exposure and fatigue during the previous afternoon. The strictly cerebral symptoms did not engage attention particularly at the time.

Oct. 30th, 9, A.M. Complains of the pain in the head, which was not sufficiently considered, and has not slept at all during the night. Ordered him punch and laudanum. 10, A.M., becoming more violent. Increased the stimulus. 11, A.M., do. do. 12 M., as above. At this stage, pupils being slightly contracted, no marked heat of the head, or febrile disturbance, *suspecting, only*, that cerebral inflammation might have supervened, ordered emp. vesicans, 5 by 4, to nape of the neck; sinapisms to feet and legs; hyd. chlor. mit. 1 gr. hourly; all restraint to be removed, the patient being watched to prevent injury to himself or others. Tr. opii. gtt. 100. Calls for liquor, and will not be pacified without a drink. 6, P.M., bowels have moved and blister has drawn; patient still very much excited and voluble. The delirium is active and busy, but seems less intense. 10 P.M., more quiet, and seems inclined to sleep.

Oct. 31st. Slept 2½ hours during the night. Delirium persists, but in a milder form. Has taken upwards of 16 grs. hyd. chlor. mit., in varying quantities. From this date the delirium seemed to wear off, not in such manner, however, that the effect could be assigned to any medication employed. Hygienic conditions were enforced, and opium, with brandy, continued.

Nov. 2d. Slept all night.

Nov. 5th. Discharged, well.

The successful issue of the following case is clearly due to chloroform. Life was saved at its extreme hour.

CASE VIII.—April 26th, 1853.

F. E. æt. 49; white; stage-driver; native of Mass.; height, 5 ft. 5 in.; weight, 150. Nervous-sanguine temperament. Habitually temperate. Has led a life of hardship and exposure, but has usually been well. This is his "first attack of horrors." "Has been drunk for a week." *Present condition.*—Has acute bronchitis of no great severity. Bears the marks of constitutional depression, with great nervous excitement. Bowels constipated; stomach irritable, vomiting every thing taken. Pulse very feeble; tongue moist, red, and tremulous. Is very delirious, but good natured—the passion of fear predominating.

Treatment.—The notes do not mention in what way the bowels were moved—probably by enema. The patient was fed with ice and brandy in small quantities, and tr. opii. gt. 120, at 9 P.M.

April 27th, 9 A.M. Slept none at all. The brandy and ice have nearly controlled the vomiting, which now occurs at infrequent intervals. Pulse 70, feeble. Tongue heavily furred and dry. Pupils natural. Con.

tinued treatment, ordered punch, Oj. and tr. opii. gtt. 60, to be repeated at 12 M. 4, P.M., still raves, and struggles with his attendant. Continued punch freely. ℞ Tr. opii, gtt. 60. Repeat hourly until nine o'clock. 10, P.M., has taken tr. opii, gt. 360. Find him standing in his bed, trembling with apprehension at the slightest noise. Pupils very fine. Ord. punch, *ad libitum*, to be soothed, not restrained.

April 28th, A. M. Has not slept. Remained quiet through the night. Calls for whiskey. Is tractable, though wild. Ord. whiskey, f. ℥ ii. tr. opii, gtt. 60, hourly, until noon, and punch freely. 9, P.M., is worse. Delirium is now violent. Pulse feeble, uncertain, about 70. Respiration 28; irregular. Ordered s. v. g, f. ℥ iv., tr. opii, gtt. 120, to be repeated at 10. 11 P.M., no amendment. Chloroform, by inhalation. Anæsthesia transcient. Repeated at frequent intervals for two hours. Left him quiet and inclined to sleep.

April 29th, 8 A.M. Slept two hours. Is now quiet, but very weak; raves incessantly, and says he shall surely die if he cannot have whiskey. Ord. whiskey, f. ℥ iv. Pulse 90, feeble. 10 A.M., has been diligently plied with whiskey and punch. No amendment visible. Chloroform again. Produces spasm, but no sleep. Continued the inhalation one hour. 5 P.M. Appearance unfavorable. Face haggard; eyes protruding; chin tremulous; tongue flabby, pale, and moist. Pulse extremely feeble. Gave him ale in full draught, with tr. lupulin, f. ℥ iii., and tr. opii, gt. 120. Ord. emp. vesic. 3 by 3, to nape. 7 P.M., no change for the better. Ord. punch, Oj., and whiskey, f. ℥ iv. 8 P.M., tr. opii, gtt. 120. In restless and desperate delirium. 9, P.M., ditto, Tried to quiet him by soothing talk, with partial success.

April 30th, 8 a.m. Slept a few minutes at a time, in all about one hour, last night. Pulse very feeble; tongue dry. Delirium presists. Ord. stimulants, *ad libitum*. 12 M. An hour since, watching his opportunity, escaped from the ward; was brought back with difficulty. 9 p.m. continued treatment. Patient no better: to be carefully watched and to take tr. opii, gtt. 120, through the night.

May 1st, 9 A.M. Evidently sinking. Pulse very feeble; tongue less dry. Delirium constant; is very difficult to manage. Continued stimulus. 12 M. ordered tr. opii, gtt. 120. Pupil normal. To have egg-nog instead of punch; as much as he can be made to take. Pulse can scarcely be felt at wrist. 4 p.m., no improvement. 6 p.m., face livid, pulse at wrist 0. Heart's action extremely feeble—70. Can, with difficulty, move in bed: says he must die. Calls for liquor, and takes sp. vin. gall. f. ℥ iv. at once. 8 p.m., pupil contracted: has taken no opium since noon. Chloroform by inhalation. The heart extremely feeble; *its action becomes less—less—wavers. Chloroform continued. Respiration 4—8. per minute. Limbs spasmodically convulsed at intervals. Heart's action stronger; pulse returns—fuller — respiration more steady. Patient sleeps—semicomatose.* In five minutes wakes again. Chloroform again administered, for ten minutes, at the end of which comes quiet and profound sleep. Limbs perfectly relaxed. 12, midnight, still asleep.

May 2nd. Is better. Has slept all the time since last note; now is wakened only to take food and brandy.

May 4th. Has slept constantly—as above.

May 9th. Is well.

In case nine, we have again chloroform, attended with both asphyxia and syncope. From both the patient was restored. So far as we can trace the influence of the anæsthetic, it seems to have been favorable. The death which followed was clearly by exhaustion.

Case IX.—September 24th, 1853, 7 P.M.

Physique.—A. H., white, Irish, aged 36; height, 5 feet 2 inches; weight, 110. Has a dark skin, hair, and eyes; bilious temperament; good constitution. Health has been uniform, except when disturbed by periodical excess in drinking during the last eight years. Comes in after eight days of continued debauch during which she says she has eaten scarcely anything and has had no sleep for 72 hours. *Condition.* —Tremulous and excited, delirious, but can understand and answer questions. Remains muttering to herself incoherently: tongue coated; pulse and skin about normal. Ordered punch, Oj. and brandy, f. ℥ iv., tr. opii, gtt. 60, to be followed by 30 more in two hours.

September 25th. Slept none last night. Condition as above. Nervous disturbance is the only prominent feature of her case. ℞ Tr. opii, gtt. 60, to be followed by 30, hourly. Punch and brandy as last night. 8 p.m., called to patient by the report "that she has had a fit." She permits no one to approach her, is pale, feeble, and very wild. From the account of attendants, has evidently suffered elipeptiform convulsions. She is resolved to make her escape from the ward. Ordered restraint— tr. opii, gtt. 60, brandy ad libitum. 10 p.m., no improvement. Gave her tr. opii, gtt. 50, two ounces of brandy, and proceeded to administer chloroform to deep anæsthesia, resuming the administration whenever she seemed about to pass from under its effects. This was continued for half an hour. During the progress of anæsthesia, subsultus came on, deepening in intensity, until it amounted to general spasm of the muscles. This ceased, when the effect of chloroform was completely secured, and in the reverse order attended the progress of re-animation. Did not think it best to repeat the inhalation. Ordered attention and urgent support, with punch, &c.

September 26th. No sleep last night, was more quiet, and seemed occasionally to doze. Pulse 120—feeble. Ordered chloroform internally by the following formula: ℞ Tr. opii, f. ℥ i. camphor, f. ℥ i., chloroform, ℥ ii. tr. hum. lup. f. ℥ iii., to take a tablespoonful every 2nd hour. Stimulants continued. 10 p.m., patient remaining in the same condition, it was determined to try inhalation again. After giving a drachm of laudanum, it was commenced. At first it produced spasm similar to, but more violent than on the previous night. It was suspended at complete anæsthesia, and the patient seemed to pass into sound sleep. Woke in ten minutes. Inhalation resumed, with the same symptoms. After a few inspirations *the subsultus and respiration ceased simultaneously and instantly.* The head was thrown back over the pillow, the eyes open and fixed, the face pale and cadavaric. *No pulse, no sound at the heart.* Cold affusion failed to recusitate, mechanical motion of thorax and trachea also. Insufflation by the mouth was promptly resorted to, and maintained for ten minutes, when the natural function and consciousness were completely restored. She was watched, in the hope that at the gate of death the vicious circle of her dreams might have been broken, but we were soon convinced that the delirium was as high as ever. Ordered brandy, ad libitum, and tr. opii, f. ʒ ss.

September 27th. Patient is bright this morning, says she is well, her appetite is good. Has not slept, though quiet. A pleasanter delirium than yesterday; seems occupied with her household affairs. Ord. tr. opii, gtt, 50, once in two hours, and as much punch as she can be made to drink. In the course of the morning she rose and walked in the ward. 9 p. m. Fiercely delirious again, requires restraint with straps. Continued treatment.

September 28th, 5 a.m. Conscious and rational—dying. 5h. 10m. died. *Autopsy* shows nothing of importance, a normal brain, neither anæmec nor congested, a little serum under the arachnoid and in the ventricles, hardly more than usual in death from any cause.

Case ten is one of sedation by the internal use of chloroform.

CASE X.—January 13th, 1853, 7 p.m.

Physique. J. M., 39, white, Irish. Height, 6 feet 3 inches, weight, 166 ℔s., shoemaker. A man of immense proportions and strength; an animal, passionate nature, bilious sanguine temperament, and uniform health (except when disturbed by drunkenness), in all climates and circumstances. A soldier in the British and American armies, and a bully of the town. Has been twice treated for delirium tremens in this Hospital. Present condition good. Functions, except the nervous, all regular. Says he has " been drinking day and night for three weeks, all the time." Is sane, but much alarmed and shaking badly. Ordered emesis, with inf. hops; ale, Oj.; tr opii, gtt. 150.

January 14th. Slept most of the night. Skin warm and dry; pulse a little accelerated; face flushed. Ordered pulv. ip. co. ʒ i; 10 grains every two hours. Ale, Oj. 7 p.m. Skin soft, moist, pulse has lost its excitement; is somwhat delirious; pupil free. ℞ Tr. opii, gtt. 100; punch, Oj.; ale, Oj. 10 p.m. Is furious, attempting all manner of violence. Confined him in bed and continued treatment, tr. opii, gtt. 20, hourly.

January 15th. Has not slept during the night. Is still furious. Pupil small; administered chloroform by inhalation, three times, without permanent advantage; anæsthesia very transient. ℞ chloroform ʒ i., in mucil. acaciæ, f. ʒ viii. ʒ i, hourly. Under this medication patient became calm, and remained half asleep during the day. Toward night delirium returned. Ord. continued support and stimulus and tr. opii, gtt. 30, every second hour.

January 16th. No sleep as yet. Resumed chloroform internally, as yesterday. After the third dose, the patient fell into a doze. Ordered tr. opii, f. Ʒ i.

January 17th. Slept most of the night. Is conscious, rational, and doing well. January 20th. Quite well.

The foregoing pages contain all which we have seen of asphyxia and syncope, after chloroform. Will they not justify the assertion that death from these causes should seldom occur? Other cases might be presented illustrating varieties and complications in the disease; others still, detailing idiosyncrasies in the patient; but with these our present purpose ends.

In producing artificial respiration we have not found it necessary to lift the epiglottis and draw forward the tongue, according to the proceeding of M. Ricord. Neither have the galvanic battery and the use of diffusible stimulants been imperatively required.

Finally, if any should expect the suggestion of a scheme for managing the various forms of disease comprehensively classed " Mania a potu," we would answer, the subject is large and difficult. Science does not yet fully illuminate it. In the field of Nervous Pathology, speculation has projected theories, observation has gathered facts. Each has done good service. The science of the physician equips and instructs the doctor, the art of the doctor endorses and seals the physician. The mind which commissions all its faculties and reviews all their work, will not rest in any system of rules, which must be in a great measure empirical.

The management of these cases should be, *par excellence*, independent. "See with your own eyes, and judge with your own judgment," is the maxim of a much-respected teacher. With present light upon this point, we shall resort to chloroform only when other medication fails, and *then* we shall not hesitate to seek any measure of its full effect which the occasion may indicate.

EDITORIAL AND MISCELLANEOUS.

Organization of the North-Eastern District Medical Society of Mich.

In accordance with a call previously made, a meeting was held at Romeo on the 8th of March, for the purpose of organizing a consolidated or district medical society. The meeting was organized by electing Dr. Philo Tillson, of Romeo, Chairman, and Dr. Jared Kibbee. of Mt Clemens, Secretary.

On motion of Dr. H. Taylor, it was voted that this society be called the *North-Eastern District Medical Society of Michigan.*

It was also

Resolved, That the district embraced in the bounds of this organization shall be the counties of Oakland, Macomb, Lapeer, St. Clair and Sanilac.

Resolved, That the members of the Macomb County Society, and of the Lapeer County Society, in good standing, be considered members of this Society.

Both of which resolutions were adopted

It was moved and carried that this Society adopt the form of the constitution and by-laws of the State Medical Society, as its own constitution and by-laws. so far as their provisions are applicable to a local organization, provided, that at the next meeting of this Society, said form may be modified at the pleasure of the Society.

It was moved and carried that this society adopt the code of ethics recommended by the National Medical Association.

It was also moved and adopted that a committee of two be appointed by the Chair to revise the form of the constitution and by-laws adopted by the State Medical Socicty, so as to adapt them to the wants of this body, and present them at the next meeting for approval. The Chair appointed Drs. Andrews, and Leete, of Romeo, as the Committee.

On motion, the Society proceeded to an informal ballot for officers. After the ballot, on motion of Dr. Taylor, Sen., of Mt Clemens, Dr. Philo Tillson, of Romeo, was declared unanimously elected President of the Society.

Dr. F. K. Bailey, of Almont, was declared unanimously elected Vice President; Dr W Brownell, of Utica, Secretary; and Dr. S L. Andrews, of Romeo, Treasurer of the Society.

It was moved and carried that the President be requested to deliver an address on some medical subject before the Society, at its next meeting. Also moved and adopted that when this body adjourns, it will adjourn to meet at Romeo, on the second Wednesday in June

On call, the following gentlemen addressed the meeting with a series of remarks which were received with enthusiastic cheering; viz, Drs. E. Andrews, of Ann Arbor; Tillson, of Romeo; Mignault, of Mt. Clemens; Bailey, of Almont; H. Taylor, Sen., of Mt. Clemens, and Brownell, of Utica.

The Society then appointed Dr. H. Taylor, Sen., Dr. A. E. Leete, and Dr. P. Tillson, delegates to the meeting of the National Medical Association, to be held at St. Louis, in May next.

The Society then, without adjourning, took a short recess re-assembled in the dining-hall of the American hotel, where they partook of an entertainment together, and by free and convivial conversation, kept up the enthusiasm of the occasion. After recess, a business session was again held, and the following resolutions were offered and unanimously carried.

Resolved, That we regard our Peninsular Medical Journal as a work deserving our highest commendation, and we pledge ourselves to support it by contributions and subscriptions, and most cheerfully recommend it to the profession at large.

Resolved, That whereas the Medical Department of the University of Michigan stands pre-eminently high in the esteem and confidence of the National Medical Association, and whereas this result is chiefly attributable to the zeal, erudition and industry of the members, of its Faculty — therefore,

Resolved, That we tender them the thanks of this Society.

Resolved, That we regard the report of Dr. Z. Pitcher on medical education, read before the National Medical Association in May last, as having contributed largely to this honorable position; and that his untiring zeal, and earnest and successful devotion to the honor and advancement of our profession in various other respects, justly entitle him to the warmest thanks and most cordial congratulation of this Society, and of the profession throughout our country.

The meeting then adjourned.   JARED KIBBEE, M. D.,
                                                Secretary.

Detroit Medical Society.

At the regular semi-monthly meeting of the Detroit Medical Society, held on Thursday evening, December 29th, 1853, the following resolutions were adopted:

Resolved, That among the objects of pride and the sources of hope to the medical profession in this State, the College of Medicine in the University of Michigan has stood conspicuous, if not pre-eminent.

Its past success, and so its present prosperity have given, and do give, assurances that the hope thus inspired would ripen into fruition. That a wise, faithful, and protracted system of instruction, as contemplated in its incipient organization, would send forth from that point, as the mental luminary of the medical commonwealth, a healthful and healing influence, which would reach and bless through illuminated media, the remotest and humblest citizen of the State

This faith in our public teachers of medicine,—this confidence in the plan on which that part of the University was organized, remained firm and unshaken until a lecture or "Medical Platform," by J. Adams Allen, M.D., was brought to the notice of this Society by one of its members, (Dr. Robinson) in an article read by appointment, as one of the exercises in the regular course of its proceedings.

Believing that the opinions embodied in the aforesaid lecture, which seems only to have been sanctioned by the authority of a single name, if suffered to go abroad as the sentiments of the College Faculty, will seriously impair the confidence of the Medical Profession in the orthodoxy of its Professors, we therefore further

Resolved—That the Faculty of Medicine in the University of Michigan be requested to state whether, and to what extent, *as a body,* they entertain, approve, or sanction the expression and dissemination of the dogmas, or doctrines, paradoxes, or opinions contained in said Lecture.

Resolved—That the proceedings be sent to the Editor of the PENINSULAR JOURNAL for publication, on being verified by the signature of the President and Secretary of this Society.

MORSE STEWART, *President.*

Detroit, Dec. 29th, 1853. EDWARD BATWELL, *Secretary.*

The foregoing resolutions were adopted by the following vote of the members present :

In favor of the resolutions—Drs. Brodie, Klein, Christian, Kieffer, Spence, Inglis, Batwell, and Stewart.

Against their adoption—Drs Gunn, Brown, Davenport, Robinson, Johnson.

The State Medical Society.

This body held its Second Annual Meeting at Ann Arbor, March 30th. The meeting was well attended and enthusiastically conducted. The publication of its proceedings will commence in our next.

Medical Commencement.

The Annual Commencement of the Medical College of the University of Michigan was held on the 30th instant, a full account of which will be given in our next.

Annual Convention of the Serapion.

SERAPION HALL, March 28th, 1854.

DR. ANDREWS, SIR :

The Second Annual Convention of the Serapion was held at two o'clock. second Vice President, E. F. Dorland, in the Chair. The minutes of the last Annual Convention were read. The following members of privilege of the Serapion, were admitted to the degrees of Fellows of the Serapion :

Messrs E. F Dorland, E. Winchester, O. Peak, W. J. Moody, E. Storck, D. Hall, E. C. Taylor, W A. Peck

George R. Bates was elected Corresponding Secretary for the ensuing year. Messrs Hall, Taylor and Storck, were appointed to select subjects and nominate committees to report at the next Annual Convention.

Messrs Darland, Peck, and Fanner, were appointed upon the first Committee:—Subject, Efficiency of the Medical Science in the Cure of Disease during the last century, compared with its previous success.

Messrs Lockwood, Winchester, and Aborn, were appointed on the second Committee : — Subject, The Natural Sciences,—their claims, relative and abstract, on the medical man.

Messrs Andrews, Hall, and Fisher were appointed on the third Committee:— Subject, Specifics—their limitation and real value. After a few appropriate remarks, in the Committee of the whole, on the state of the Society, and the profession generally, the Convention adjourned to meet in the evening at seven o'clock, to listen to an address from Mr. Peck.

ORRIN ABORN, Secretary.

Announcement of Another Session at Geneva Medical College.

This institution, which it was feared would never re-assemble, announces that it will be re-opened on the 4th of October, 1854, and continue sixteen weeks.

NOTICES OF WORKS RECEIVED.

Carpenter on Alcoholic Liquors.

A valuable little work, already favorably known to the public. It is the successful competitor for the prize of one hundred guineas offered for the best essay on the use and abuse of alcoholic liquors. The author, Dr. Carpenter, is the well known English Physiologist of that name, whose fame rests, not so much on original discoveries of his own, as on his clear and agreeable manner of combining the results obtained by others into sensible, practical, useful text-books for the world. The work is provided with a preface from the pen of the well known Dr. Condie of Philadelphia, author of a work on the diseases of children. This work is remarkable as a specimen of that happy style which deals in facts and principles which interest a professional man, and is couched in language which is perfectly comprehensible to a layman. We are particularly pleased with the correctness of the physiological reasoning on the use of alcohol as a stimulus, preparatory or subsequently to any unusual exertion, either mental or physical. Two errors are committed by men here, sometimes, we are ashamed to say even by professional men. One is the *habit* of stimulating the recuperative power after all unusual exertions. Now, the power of self-recovery in cases of fatigue, ought, in a sound man, to respond spontaneously, in proportion to the necessity of the occasion; and any one who has watched his own system, when going through a series of severe exertions, must have observed how rapidly the recuperative power increases under the demand of frequent effort, but if, instead of habituating the system to react against exhaustion by its own spontaneous force, a man accustoms himself to arouse the reaction by stimuli, he impairs the natural connection between the demand for vital force and the power of supply. He has taken out one of the wheels of his physiological machinery, and put a bottle in its place. The same remark may be made respecting the habit of using stimuli to prepare one for every unusual exertion. In a perfect physical and mental man all the voluntary powers, both of mind and body, ought to respond to the mandates of the will, with an energy commensurate to the emergency that demands them; but he, who, instead of training his powers thus to awaken at the trumpet of will, accustoms them to be aroused only by a dram, puts a disturbing force between himself and his own faculties,—he is no longer his own master.

Another still more disastrous error is by the combined power of will and alcohol, to force the system into efforts beyond its natural power of endurance—a transgression which, if frequently repeated, ultimately recoils terribly on the offender. Nevertheless, Dr. Carpenter justly observes that this physiological sin may sometimes be morally justifiable, in certain extreme emergencies, as in efforts to avert shipwreck or other impending destruction. The present danger may be so great that every possible means of arousing and sustaining *present* effort must be brought to bear, and the certainty of injury, and the risk of ultimate death from the succeeding exhaustion must be braved. To those who differ from these sentiments of Dr. Carpenter's little book, we accord all charity, but, for our part, except in such emergencies as Dr. C. specifies, we have always held the use of alcohol, as a strengthener before unusual efforts, or as a cordial after them, to be exceedingly un-scientific, and to the young, whose organic habits are forming, disastrous.

Published by Blanchard and Lea, Philadelphia.

Buckler on Fibro-bronchitis and Rheumatic Pneumonia. Published by Blanchard and Lea, Philadelphia.

This work was originally presented to the Committee on Voluntary Communications for the American Medical Association in 1853, and was by that, committee rejected. It now appears as a neat volume of a hundred and fifty pages. The peculiar doctrine advocated by this work is that certain forms of pneumonia, which are found are, pathologically speaking, rheumatic inflammations of the white fibrous framework of the bronchi. This suggestion is certainly an interesting one, and deserves from the profession a fuller investigation. The book is a modest one It first simply explains without argument, the doctrine of the author; the bulk of the work is occupied with detailing twenty-seven cases illustrating his position, and closes with an analysis of the cases, and remarks upon the treatment. The style of argumentation is not strong, but the body of facts presented is on that account more available and valuable. The observation and permanent record of these facts we consider to be the chief value of the book, for it is by the accumulation and careful collation of cases alone, that the existence or frequency of rheumatic inflammation of the bronchi can be clearly determined. So brief an essay as the one before us, of course cannot settle the doubts of the profession, nor establish the positions of the writer immoveably, but it may elicit examination and leave its facts in the track of useful investigation. We are glad to see the work, for we think the white fibrous tissues in the lungs and bronchi are not exempt from liability to rheumatic irritation, and we desire that investigation may settle to what extent this may proceed, and of what importance it may be either alone, or as complicating other diseases, or producing simple inflammations.

In conducting this investigation, great care, however, is necessary, on account of the great number of circumstances whose changes and combinations like the permutations of arithmetic are almost endless. Hence, it does not follow from a few cases in which cessation of rheumatism in a limb is followed by bronchitis, that necessarily a true rheumatic metastasis has taken place, for besides the numerous chances of accidental coincidence, it may happen that the derivative effect of the bronchial affection has relieved the articular rheumatism, or vice versa an attack of articular rheumatism may on a similar principle during its continuance keep in check an impending attack of bronchitis or pneumonia, which latter diseases, may develop themselves in full force as soon as the rheumatic attack subsides. This is a specimen of the difficulties which will surround the examination, nevertheless they may be overcome, and we are glad to see a beginning made.

Fowne's Chemistry for Students.

This is, we should think, a very excellent small text-book for students. It is illustrated by over one hundred and eighty wood cuts. It devotes a large space to organic chemistry, that mountain of facts, which modern science has thrown into the pathway of chemical students.

Published by Blanchard and Lea, Philadelphia.

Bennet on the Uterus. Fourth American Edition.

This is from the third and revised London Edition. Concerning this extensively known work it is superfluous to speak. The present edition contains several improvements over those which were taken from the first two English editions. The work itself, is established as a part of medical literature, and no physician's library is complete without it.

Published by Blanchard and Lea, Philadelphia.

Medical News and Library.

Published by Blanchard and Lea, for one dollar a year, and furnished gratuitously to all subscribers of the *American Journal of the Medical Sciences*.

History of the Epidemic Yellow Fever at New Orleans.

By E. D. Fenner, M. D., President of the Louisiana State Medical Society, etc., etc. This is a history of the late epidemic, at New Orleans, and contains considerable information of value. The author persists, that even in the late epidemic, quinine properly used was valuable, but not so efficacious as in previous years. The number of cases was about 27,143, of which about 29 per cent. died, constituting about 8 per cent of the entire population of the city.

THE

PENINSULAR

JOURNAL OF MEDICINE

AND THE COLLATERAL SCIENCES.

| VOL. I. | MAY, 1854. | NO. XI. |

Transactions of the Peninsular State Medical Society. Instituted, 1853. *Second Annual Meeting.*

MORNING SESSION.

The Society met at the Medical College University of Michigan, Ann Arbor, at 12 M., March 30, 1854. The President and Vice-President being absent, the meeting was called to order by the Secretary, and on motion, Henry Taylor, M.D., of Mt. Clemens, was elected President, *pro tem.*

It was moved and carried that the regular order of business be suspended to attend to the admission of delegates and new members.

The following delegates were then found present:

Drs. S. L. Andrews, of Romeo, H. Taylor, of Mt. Clemens, and Wm. Brownell, of Utica; all from the North Eastern District Medical Society.

Also Drs. E. Dorland, and W. A. Peck, representatives of the Serapion Society of the University of Michigan.

The following gentlemen were then proposed and elected Fellows of the Society.

Dr. P. Klein,	of	Detroit.
" A. Murray,	"	Niles.
" J. D. Alexander,	"	Wayne.
Prof. A. B. Palmer,	"	Chicago, Ill.
Dr. C. M. Stockwell,	"	Port Huron.
" S. L. Andrews,	"	Romeo.
" D. Winchester,	"	Canada West.

* " E. Thornton,   "
* " G. W. Topping,   "
* " S. S. Cutter,   "
  " H. C. Fairbank,   "   Grand Blanc.
  " E. P. Christian,   "   Detroit.
* " J. W. Phelps,   "

The following gentlemen were then recognized as members, having become so since the last meeting.

Dr. J. P. Foster,   of   Unadilla.
 " P. Tillson,   "   Romeo.
 " J. C. Gorton,   "   Detroit.
 " D. F. Mitchell,   "   East Saginaw.
 " W. W. Collins,   "   Waterloo.
 " G. H. Chase,   "   Ann Arbor.

It was moved and carried that there be a committee of three appointed by the Chair to nominate officers for the ensuing year. The Chair appointed Drs. W. Brodie, E. Andrews, and W. Brownell, as that committee.

An invitation was then presented to the Society by Prof. Douglass, for the members to attend an entertainment to be given in the evening by some of the Professors. It was moved and carried that the invitation be accepted.

The society then adjourned until 2 P. M.

AFTERNOON SESSION.

At 2 P. M., the Society re-assembled. Dr. H. Taylor, in the Chair. The Secretary called the roll, and the following members were found present.

FELLOWS.

Dr. S. L. Andrews,
 " J. Andrews.
 " E. Andrews,
 " C. F. Ashley,
 " J. D. Alexander,
 " W. Brodie,
 " W. Brownell,
 " J. H. Beech,
 " E. Batwell,
 " G. H. Chase,
 " W. W. Collins,
 " S. S. Cutter,
 " S. H. Douglass,
 " S. Denton,
 " H. C. Fairbank,
 " J. P. Foster,
 " J. C Gorton.

Dr. —— Holley,
 " D. F. Mitchell,
 " A. Murray,
 " A. B. Palmer,
 " J. W. Phelps,
 " A. C. Roberts,
 " H. B. Shank,
 " A. Sager,
 " Stebbins,
 " C. M. Stockwell,
 " M. K. Taylor,
 " E. Thornton,
 " G. W. Topping,
 " H. Taylor,
 " Wm. Upjohn,
 " D. Winchester.

* Residence not stated.—They are requested to forward them to the Secretary.

Dr. H. Taylor,
" S. L. Andrews, ⎫ From the N. E. Dist. Med. Society.
" W. Brownell. ⎭

Dr. E. Dorland, ⎫ From the Serapion.
" W. Peck. ⎭

The minutes of the last meeting were then read and approved. The committee for nominating officers for the ensuing year, then reported the following nominations:

For President,   Dr. H. Taylor,   of Mt. Clemens.
" Vice-President,   " A. Murray,   " Niles.
" Secretary,   " E. Andrews,   " Ann Arbor.
" Treasurer,   " S. H. Douglass,   "   "

The Society proceeded to ballot for these officers, when a majority being for them, it was moved and carried that they be declared unanimously elected.

The next business in order being the reports of Standing Committees, the committee appointed to establish and report a system of observations on the Meteorology of Michigan, presented the following:

Report of the Committee on Meteorology. By M. K. TAYLOR, M. D., Chairman.

To the President of the Peninsular Medical Association:

The Committee to whom was referred the subject of Meteorology, and the establishment of a system of observations throughout the State of Michigan, and to report the same at the present Session, submit the following:

Owing to the limited number of persons engaged in this State in connection with the Society, in making observations on the Meteorological phenomena, few generalizations can be made at the present time, or more be done than to present the facts as they have transpired, in as condensed a form as possible, and leave to future observers the pursuit of this interesting branch of natural science in its relations to medicine and general sanitary measures.

Immediately after the appointment of your committee at the last session, efforts were made to enlist a sufficient number of persons in the more important localities of the State, in these investigations; but few, however, expressed a willingness to do so.

The subject matter, therefore, of this report is mainly derived from the observations of Dr. M. Stewart, of Detroit, furnished by Dr. L. Davenport; those of Dr. J. C. Norton, recently of Rockford, Ill.; the report of Mr. Blodgett, of the Smithsonian Institute at Washington, "On the climatic conditions of the summer of 1853," and the observations of the Chairman of your committee.

With a view of facilitating our operations, a letter was addressed to Prof. Henry, of the Smithsonian Institution, proposing to purchase blank charts as there prepared, for our use; but he, in return, declining to make a sale, offered to furnish the requisite quantity free of charge or postage, when sent direct from that Institution, the only remuneration asked being copies of our proceedings in detail or otherwise, as might best suit the convenience of those engaged.

This arrangement still remains, and is the best that can be effected under existing circumstances; but could we have a system of our own, independent of any other, much labor in copying might be dispensed with. As the matter now stands, triplicates of each monthly return have to be made out, one being for the Smithsonian Institution, one for the observer's own use, and the other for the benefit of the Society. This, however, is quite overbalanced, with those having sufficient leisure, by the advantages arising from a connection with that central Institution.

The period of observation at Brooklyn extends from August 15th, 1852, to the present time; that furnished from the Detroit observations from July 1st, 1853, to November 1st, and that at Rockford from Nov. 1st, 1852, to January 31st, 1853. These are, of course, all too limited in extent to afford any reliable basis of comparison, except, perhaps, in the amount of aqueous precipitation.

The mean temperature at Brooklyn for the period referred to, is 44.01 deg., with an extreme range of 108 deg.; being from 98 deg. on the 21st of June last, to 10 deg. below zero on the 23d of January, this year. The difference between the temperatures at Detroit and Brooklyn is not sufficiently marked to be worthy of comparison at the present time, but with reference to Rockford, it is different, and is herewith presented.

Station.	Month.	deg.	Month.	deg.	Month.	deg	Mean.	Entire Range.
Brooklyn, - - -	Nov. 1852	39	Dec. 1852	31	Jan'y 1854	29	30 00	59 degrees.
Rockford. - - -	" "	32	" "	26	" "	30	27.33	57 "

With regard to the extreme temperature of the past summer, a few facts furnished by Mr. Blodgett are worthy of notice. According to his report, it appears that the attainment of highest temperature occurred in those States south-westward of Tennessee on the 19th June, with a maximum of 79 deg.; reached Ohio and this State on the 21st and 22d, with the maxima of 95 and 97.; and New York and Savannah on the 23d, with the maxima of 92 and 93 deg,;

On the 29th and 30th of the same month, another extraordinary wave of heat, so to speak, passed over the central portions of the United States. In the latitude of Washington, the thermometer rose to 99 deg. and a fraction, while in this State the maximum of heat was on the 28th, or one day previous, when the thermometer rose to 91 deg. ·

With one or two exceptions during the past season, this excess of temperature has been very regular in its recurrence one or two days earlier in the western than in the eastern States.

The next instance of excessive heat occurred in August on the 10th, when the thermometer rose to 94 deg. at Brooklyn, and 96 deg. at Detroit. The highest point at Montreal occurred a day later, and at Philadelphia two days subsequent. From a further examination, it appears to have passed over the continent in a south-westerly direction, reaching Camden, South Carolina, on the 15th, where the temperature was at 92 deg., and Austin, Texas, on the 17th, with a maximum of 99 deg.

The extreme ranges for 1853 have been such as to attract the attention of nearly all observers, both in regard to temperature and humidity, by which an unusual number of facts have been elicited in relation to the prevalence of epidemics and the public health generally, during these extremes.

In a letter recently received from Mr. Blodgett, Superintendent of the Smithsonian Meteorological observations, he states that the line of excessive mortality, temperature and humidity, can be readily traced in the United States wherever they have existed in the past season.

In our own State, and the north-west generally, the humidity has been low when compared with other sections. At Brooklyn, the only point in this State where the humidity has been observed and reported, the mean of saturation has been 73 per cent. at 2 P.M. It was lowest in the month of April, the mean for which is 63 per cent, and highest in November, when it attained 85 per cent.

The mean degree of saturation does not seem to sustain any definite relation to the amount of aqueous precipitation in this climate; for in the month of April we had 5.03 inches of rain,—in May, with a mean of 65 per cent. of saturation, 7.00 inches of water, and in November, but 5.43 inches. It would seem to be influenced to some extent, however, by the degree of cloudiness, for in April the number of days during which no clouds were visible at the regular hour of notation was five, and the completely cloudy days numbered but three, but in November there were no entirely clear days, and seven completely cloudy. The mean per cent. of humidity for the months of July, August and September, was 71' 77 and 79 per cent. respectively. These are the months which are regarded usually as being the most unhealthy, but this, as a general thing, has not obtained the past season in this State.

The amount of aqueous precipitation for the past year, including rain and snow melted is 37.14 inches. Seventeen and forty-six hundredths of this quantity fell in the months of April, May and November, thus allowing but 19.68 inches to be distributed through the other nine months of the year.

There seems to have been, during the time referred to, a remarkable difference in the amount of water precipitated on the eastern boundary of the State, and in the interior. Thus, at Detroit, the sum for the months of June, July, August, September and October, is 13.55 inches, and at Brooklyn, 11.89, showing a difference of 1.66. This difference has been pretty constant in each month, as will appear from the table herewith presented. Whether this shall be constant and for each year, remains to be seen.

1853.	June.	July.	August.	Sept.	Oct.	Total.
Detroit, - - - - - -	2.56	2.23	3.59	2.58	2.59	13.55
Ann Arbor, - - - - -	0.71	1 10	3.96		-	
Brooklyn, - - - - -	1.50	1.71	3.95	3 23	1.50	11.89
Battle Creek. - - - -	1 00	1 56	1 00			

The difference between Detroit and Battle Creek is still greater for the summer months, being 2.22 inches.

The amount of snow for the same year, and in fact for the past two years has been moderate, as will be seen by reference to the appended tables.

From the observations made at the regular hours of 7 A. M., 2 P. M., and 9 P. M., upon the winds, it appears that 69 per cent. are westerly — the south-west currents greatly predominating.

A table showing the number of observations in each month, and the prevailing currents is appended to this report.

The connection which the atmospherical currents seem to sustain to the greatest degree of cold is this: The wind, succeeding some storm, during which it has been more or less variable, settles in the north-west where it remains until the temperature has been materially lowered, thence gradually changing to the westward, settles in the south-west, at which time the climax of cold is experienced. If the wind remain in this quarter for any length of time, however, the temperature readily becomes modified.

May we not suppose in this instance that the excessive temperature is in a measure due to the north-westerly winds, having passed over the, interior of the continent farther to the southward, and thence being returned to us by the prevailing south-west current, over an already frozen surface?

The total number of days during 1853, in which the cloudiness has been complete is 62, and the number of entirely clear days, or those on which no clouds were visible at the hour of observation is 49.

It is not, however, from minor matters pertaining to our observations, like the latter for instance, that the greatest practical benefits to medical science are to be derived, though each may have its appropriate influence in the final summing up. But to the temperature and degree of saturation, together with local or general causes operating directly through these, must we look for an explanation of the excessive mortality of the country at one time, and the general healthy condition at another. The facts elicited by the Hygrometrical observations for the past season throughout the Union and adjacent territories, seem to point in a very marked manner to these conditions in confirmation of this statement.

Throughout the Gulf coast, where the pestilential diseases have been raging to the greatest extent, the humidity has been at a high per cent. The same was the case in New York during the time that so many were stricken down so suddenly with that cerebral congestion.

It cannot be the high temperature alone that effects such remarkable changes on the constitution, for in those locations where the temperature has been equally high and the per cent. of humidity low, no unusual mortality has been witnessed. This may be better understood, perhaps, by a glance at the peculiar circumstances as they exist at such times.

If the temperature stand at 90 deg., and the point to which a thermometer will be lowered by the process of evaporation stand at 70, the degree of saturation is but 33 per cent., and as a matter of course, evaporation is very rapid. This process thus operating from the surfaces of the body, gives us the benefit of a temperature of 70 deg. only, but if the thermometer stand at 90 deg., and there be but 3 deg. difference between it and the temperature of evaporation, the saturation is 88 per cent. with a corresponding arrest of the transpiration of the fluids from the surfaces of the body and consequent retention in the system of their morbid constituents.

In our own State where the humidity has been low, as indeed has been the case in the entire north-west, as a whole, the public health has been remarkably good — unprecedented, perhaps, in the same locations since the settlement of the country, and hardly equalled by any other section of the United States of the same extent and number of inhabitants, either at the present or any former period.

An unusual opportunity will be presented the coming two years for a systematic investigation of this subject in this Peninsula. By an act of the Legislature at its last session, provision was made for the enumeration of the inhabitants, and with that the ratio of mortality. This taken in connection with a well arranged system of observations must develope many interesting facts which cannot be derived from any other source. It is to be hoped that so rare an opportunity for scientific research will not go unimproved by the profession of this State, and those who seem to be best qualified to prosecute them, and to whom the greatest benefits will be likely to accrue, will enter into the subject with that zeal apparently demanded by the circumstances.

Nor is it to be supposed that these investigations are without their daily reward. Quite the contrary is the case.

With these careful observations of the dew-point or lowest degree of evaporation may we determine the approach of storms almost with the same certainty as with the Barometer. There is, however, this difference in the use of the respective instruments: The Barometer shows the perturbations of the atmosphere preceding and attendant upon storms, and the wet bulb that condition of the air most favorable to their developement and precipitation of rain under slight disturbing causes, which the Prince and Power of the elements in these latitudes seldom fails to have at hand.

Thus, if the dew-point is observed to be rising rapidly so as much to exceed the mean for the particular month at the hour of observation, or if there be not more than five degrees difference between it and the standard thermometer when the latter is ranging at 70 and upward, rain may be confidently expected. It may not fall at the particular point of observation, but will be sufficiently near to be recognized readily, and materially affect the readings of the instrument. Such has been the case at least during the past two years in the central portions of this State. Very probably in those localities near large bodies of water, some modification may be necessary in the general statement.

With a view of furthering these investigations in our State, if the Society shall deem them of sufficient importance to merit such, a table has been prepared from the Tables of Elastic Force of Aqueous Vapor, by Reynault, and the Psychometrical Tables of Prof. Guyot, on the Centigrade scale, for the determinations of the per cent. humidity from observations with the Fahrenheit Thermometer, at a glance. It is not considered a part of the report, but is offered with it if desired. Other tables showing the peculiar features of the climate of Michigan for the past year are also herewith presented. M. K. TAYLOR,

Chairman.

Year and Month	Mean deg. for the Month	Highest deg.	Date	Lowest deg.	Date	Mean deg, Humidity for the Month at 2 P.M.	Lowest per ct. in the Month	Date	Prevailing wind	Entire Amount of aqueous precipitation, including snow melted.	Amount of snow in inches and hundredths	Number of days on which snow or rain fell.	Greatest amount of snow on the ground at one time.	Number of entirely clear days.	Number of entirely cloudy days.
1852—September,	60.60	89	1st	32	29th	0.49	0.32	3d	S.W.	3.29*		11		3	1
October,	53.01	79	1st	36	31st	0.54	0.24	10th	S.W.	3.57		6		7	4
December,	30.80	54	6th	6	14th				S.W.	3.87	5.00	11	4.50	2	12
1853—January,	28.95	48	8th	—5	26th		0.30		S.W.	1.24	6.25	3	6.00	10	12
February,	29.18	49	1st	5	6th	0.63	0.36	4th	S.W.	2.59	13.75	11	6.50	5	9
March,	35.75	58	20th	5	14th	0.65	0.44	26th	W.	1.60	5.00	12	2.00	5	7
April,	44.99	73	27th	31	10th	0.67	0.51	14th	N.E.	5.03		17		6	3
May,	56.98	84	28th	41	12th	0.71	0.57	30th	W.	7.00		14		4	5
June,	67.66	98	21st	58	25th	0.77	0.72	28th	W.	1.50		8		4	0
July,	64	86	15th	51	16th	0.79	0.51	28th	W.	1.71		10		5	0
August,	71.70	94	10th	48	25th	0.72	0.54	15th	S.W.	3.95		11		1	0
September,	62.78	86	5th	33	29th	0.85	0.44	30th	S.W.	3.24		8		7	3
October,	45.60	70	16th	26	24	0.81			W.	1.50		5		0	4
November,	40.09	59	20th	21	25th	0.73		22d	S.W.	5.43	0.75	13	0.75	2	7
December,	27.74	53	11th	2	24th				W.	1.17	15.00	10	4.00		10
Yearly Mean,	48.84					0.73									
1854—January,	19.68	41	20th	—10	23d	0.80	0.65	30th	S.W.	2.78	2.00	14	0.50	2	5
February,	26.79	49	12th	—8	4th	0.74	0.50	20th	W.	1.57	5.50	8	2.25	4	8

Table of winds, showing the number of observations of the wind from the respective points named below in each month, from August, 1852, to February, 1854, at Brooklyn, Mich.

Months.	South.	South West.	West	North West.	North.	North East.	East.	South East.	Calms.	Total No. observations.
1852—August, - - - -	9	30	8	19	4	2	4	12	28	86
September, - - - -	9	30	8	19	4	2	4	12	28	86
October, - - - -	20	30	26	11	4	7	0	2	13	133
November, - - - -		56	19	4	2	9	0	16	12	122
December, - - - -	4	40	30	14	1	0	0	1	18	123
1853—January, - - - -	5	31	23	17	7	1	0	6	12	105
February, - - - -	8	16	29	12	4	6	0	8	8	88
March, - - - -	8	8	13	11	9	5	14	6	15	87
April, - - - -	5	8	26	9	6	6	0	9	18	88
May, - - - -	11	9	20	0	2	3	6	8	18	93
June, - - - -	3	25	20	0	0	0	1	8	27	84
July, - - - -	4	13	13	5	4	1	4	8	30	89
August, - - - -	2	15	6	10	1½	1	2	11	42	90
September, - - - -	5	28	9	13	1	1	1	3	29	89
October, - - - -	2	17	24	11	2	1	1	2	27	87
November, - - - -	7	28	10	10	1	4	1	11	15	87
December, - - - -	4	15	23	11	5	3	1	6	16	84
1854—January, - - - -	3	28	16	6	0	1	3	4	16	67
February, - - - -	10	9	16	8	1	5	0	15	6	73
	119	428	326	190	52	66	42	138	353	1714

It was moved and carried that the report be accepted, and the thanks of the Society be tendered to the committee for the able manner in which it had discharged its duties.

The President having announced that the subject of the Report was before the Society for discussion, Dr. Andrews inquired what relation was found to exist between humidity and the prevalence of epidemics. Dr. Taylor replied that a very close connection could be traced between the lines of excessive humidity and the track of certain epidemic diseases over the country.

Prof. Palmer remarked that this was a most important subject, and a very valuable report, and it was to be hoped that when the Society came to make up its committees for the ensuing year, it would reappoint this one, and endeavor to devise means of connecting its observations with observations on the prevalence of diseases of various kinds; in short, to establish such a corps of investigators as should be able ultimately to put us in possession of the complete relations of climate to pathology.

The Report of the Committee on Epidemics being then called for, Dr. M. A. Patterson, of Tecumseh, Chairman, read the following

Report of the Committee on Epidemics.   By M. A. PATTERSON, M. D., Chairman.

The Committee on Epidemics respectfully report, that during the past year the State has been remarkably free from epidemics, and the information on this subject in possession of the undersigned is so meagre, as scarcely to entitle the committee to report.   To present the few, and not very important facts collected during the year by the committee, would be but a waste of time, and until some system is adopted to unite the medical practitioners of our State in an effort to consolidate their individual observations and experience, we can have no well grounded expectation of obtaining a satisfactory history of the epidemics of Michigan.   We are, therefore, of opinion, that the design of the Society in creating one committee, will be best promoted at this time, by suggesting a plan to obtain the requisite details hereafter; and, with this view, we respectfully recommend the adoption of the following resolution.

Resolved, That the Society shall be a "Committee of the Whole" on Epidemics, and each member is hereby required to keep a record of such epidemics as may prevail under his immediate observation, carefully noting their special peculiarities and treatment, and annually transmit an abstract of his observations to the President of the Medical Faculty of the University of Michigan, in season for said Faculty to condense the information thus obtained, giving each practitioner credit for details furnished, and to present the same, in the form of a Report to the Society, at each annual meeting, and that to ensure the response of the profession, the Faculty be requested to send a circular to various parts of the State, asking information on epidemic and endemic diseases, and the success of the treatments instituted.

Resolved, That a Committee be appointed to wait upon the members of the Medical Faculty of the University, and report whether said Faculty will perform the duty requested of them by the above resolution.

M. A. PATTERSON,
Chairman Committee on Epidemics.

P. S.—The Committee request to be discharged from the further consideration of the subject.

On motion, the report was accepted, and the committee discharged. The question was then put on the passage of the resolutions, and they were passed unanimously. The President appointed Dr. Ashley, of Ypsilanti, as the committee to confer with the Faculty. After a brief interval the committee reported that having consulted with as many of the professors as were present, they were found ready to undertake the duty contemplated in the resolutions.

Prof. Palmer then offered the following:

Resolved, That this Society request the Faculty to forward to the Committee on Epidemics of the National Medical Association, the information obtained as contemplated in the preceding resolutions.

The Committee on the Geographical Distribution of Diseases, being called for, reported verbally that owing to the neglect of the profession to respond to the circulars and letters sent out, it had been impossible to collect sufficient materials for a report.

The report was accepted and the committee continued.

The reading of voluntary papers being next in order, the following paper was read.

Hints on the Diagnosis and Treatment of Diseases of the Vesciculœ Seminales. By J. H. BEECH, M.D., of Coldwater.

Mr. President and Gentlemen:

In calling your attention for a few moments to diseases of the "vesciculæ seminales," we cannot expect to reward your patience by remarkable developments or astute reasoning; but as special pathology has become the absorbing topic of this era, we humbly submit a few facts and thoughts for your consideration and enlargement. We are not aware that the symptomatology of these reservoirs has ever been segregated, although their autopsic phenomena have been described by various observers.

The "seminal vesicles," being situated in regard to the male organs of generation in the same relation as the billiary vesicle to the liver and digestive system, can but exercise similar functions, and like it, liable to affections which are secondary to those of organs with whose "*orgasms*" they sympathize, and whose secretions they receive. Being also lined by mucous membrane, they participate in those constitutional affections, producing congestions of mucous surfaces.

That these organs are seldom diseased *per se,* is undoubtedly true; but that they may be thus circumstanced, we as certainly believe.

They are largely supplied by nature with circulating media, and nervous energy, and we opine, exert more influence when diseased, upon the human organism, than has generally been accorded to them.

Their arterial system, derived from the hypogastric, hæmorrhoidea media, pudica, (both before and after passing around the sacro-sciatic ligament,) the ischiatica and obturatoria, furnishes a supply of arterial blood from so many sources that deficiency is not likely to occur.

While the vesicles receive filaments from the ischiatic and obturator nerves, which we may suppose sufficient to control nutrition and general sensation, they participate in the special sensations of the penis, by branches from the internal pudic nerve.

Furthermore, the communications with the great ganglionic system are not less free than of other organs, on whose diseases much study has been bestowed. The character of the symptoms is such that unmixed cases of vescicular seminal disease do not often present themselves to the medical profession, as pathogena of other organs, not more important in health, or annoying in disease. Those whose idiosyncrasies or circumstances, render them obnoxious to affections of these organs, reluctantly disclose their ailments; often, perhaps, being hindered by well-founded suspicions that some private fault of former times may have provoked the attack. There are some individuals who exhibit perpetual zeal in the care of their generative functions. If all parts are not in perfect order, *they* speedily lay the matter before their medical adviser, in all its details and minutiæ; but this is not the class among whom we shall find primary disease of the "vesiculæ seminales," but among persons of sedentary habits, living virtuously, but with free diet, etc., who are not naturally disposed to bestow excess of "honor on their uncomely parts," and disinclined to expose their private ills. We believe, also, that the use of tobacco promotes in an eminent degree, a tendency to disease of the seminal vesicles. The symptoms which we believe belong to the subject of this paper, are a sense of heaviness and congestion of the lower part of the body, lancinating pain situated on either side, high above the "tuber ischŭ," which is supposed by the patient to be fatigue from much sitting. The pain is sometimes referred to the hips, or, said to be darting through the pelvis diagonally.

There is frequent desire to evacuate the bladder *without* "ardor urinæ" or the tardiness of flow incidental to inflamed or enlarged prostate; and excessive uneasiness when hardened fæces distend the rectum. Involuntary seminal emissions first call the attention of the victim, to the fact that the discomfort which has attended him is more than the legitimate result of fatigue.

Sometimes erections are frequent and annoying, accompanied more by an itching or sense of titillation referred to the rectum or perinæum, (or perhaps a burning sensation,) than by sexual desire. If there be seminal emissions, whether attended by normal or abnormal conditions, the sensations of heat or smarting pain may be extremely severe for several minutes.

The quantity of fluid emitted is small and changed in consistence, according to the variety and stage of the disease. Here, we presume, (for we have not been favored with the proof,) the microscope would afford efficient aid in diagnosis. If digital examination *"per ani"* be made, the prostate is found somewhat tender, perhaps, but the seminal sacs can be reached by pressing higher and on either side, and are still more sensitive. If the bladder be partly distended, the vescicles can be reached more readily, but the contents of the urinary bladder must not be allowed to give us false impressions when the vescicles are enlarged. There is not necessarily tenderness of the testicle and spermatic cord; no hæmorrhoidal congestion, or soreness of the urethra. If purulent, or other matter distend the organs, the pain extends higher and towards the "crista ilium," or renal regions, to which the patient may refer the difficulty; but disorder of the kidneys is not otherwise apparent. Exploration "per urethræ" does not reach the exact seat of pain, unless inflammation extends to the orifices of the ejaculatory ducts; it then produces the same smarting or burning sensation mentioned as succeeding seminal emissions.

The victim of vescicular disease is restive, impatient and sometimes suffers extreme mental depression or delirium. The physician seeing so much of nervous disorder, and so few signs of disease appreciable to his usual modes of inquiry, after the "res contra-naturam," gets neuralgia strongly depicted and is supported by the habits and temperament of his patient. Walking, although not immediately productive of distress, except in acute inflammation, generally is followed by an increase of all the symptoms, and fatigue evidently aggravates the tendency to priapism, or involuntary emissions. The diseases of these parts may extend to the testicle, along the "vas deferens," and can be traced by the tenderness along the cord and epidydimis, but in this case, the pain from the passage of semen commences with the orgasm; whereas, if confined to the "vescicles" and their ducts, the pain is not felt until late in the copulative act, or after the ejaculation.

Is this smarting or burning produced by closing together of the mucous surfaces of the emptied organs, and thereby of evidence an inflammation of the membrane? The particular form of disease must often be diagnosed by general symptoms, to wit: tuberculous or schirrous cachexy might guide our judgment. Confirmed consumptives often exhibit excessive sexual propensities, and may not the irritation of tuberculous deposites in these and other organs of the generative system produce the desire, which, compared with the wasted vigor of the body, is most assuredly morbid! Gouty diathesis would lead us to suspect earthy concretions, and in gouty persons an "ardor venereus" is often observed similar, and perhaps allied in cause to that before mentioned. Rigors and hectic phenomena give intimation of purulent accumulation, and adynamia of gangrenous destruction.

Of treatment, we can say but little, without doing violence to our good opinion of the therapeutic skill of the members of this association. With the appropriate remedies, constitutional, local and revulsive, for the pecific form of disease existing in such case, the "anaphrodisiac" should e combined. The success of distinguished and ingenious gentlemen in :theterism of the fallopian tubes, gives us reason to hope that topical atment may yet reach the "vesciculæ seminales."

It was moved and carried that a copy be requested for publication.

The following paper was then read.

General Blood-letting or Fashion in Medicine. By WM. BRODIE, M. D.

Amongst the numerous therapeutical agents which are employed by physicians in the treatment of disease is venesection, and if I may use the expression, the most abused and most neglected of the entire materia medica.

The time has not far past when blood-letting was resorted to in the treatment of nearly every case of disease, and without doubt, for want of due discrimination, resulted in great injury to the patient, if not causing death.

The tendency of the human mind is to launch into extremes, and it is only necessary to decry a well-known and valuable property, when it is laid aside and condemned to lasting obscurity. The antithesis is equally true, and hence obscurity becomes pregnant with some implied virtue which is emblazoned forth as the desideratum of all perfection.

This state of things holds equally good (and I say it with sorrow) in the profession of medicine, as with the multitude, be they learned or ignorant.

The nature of our institutions is progressive and popular, and hence arises a tendency to discard old things that are well-known, and launch into a sea of experiment. Consequently, views and opinions become facts, before experience can concede them worthy of any notice.

When confined within proper limits, this progressive and emulative spirit is commendable, but when employed in search of novelty, should be equally condemned.

The science of medicine is progressive not only in its therapeutical, but in all its varying branches, and no one is worthy of greater honor and commendation than he who by patient and persevering investigation can render to his professional brethren a more certain method of saving the lives and health of his fellow man.

Upon this point I can quote no higher authority than Sir Benj. Brodie, who says, " I am not one of those who would be trying indiscriminately all the new remedies which in these days are being constantly brought before the public; nor can I think well of this modern fashion of resorting on all occasions to novel methods of treatment.

" I see many practitioners who would always rather give a new medicine than an old one, but I advise you if you wish to succeed in your profession and be useful to the public, to pursue a different course. Make yourselves master of the old remedies, learn how to handle them, and what good they will do, and as a general thing, have recourse to them in the first instance.

" If the old remedies fail, and you are at a stand stilll, then, and not till then, have recourse to the new ones.

" If you always begin with new remedies, you throw away all the valuable results not only of your own experience, but of the experience of those who have gone before you. You have to begin as it were *de novo*, and the first consequence of this will be that you will not cure your patients, and the second that you will have none to cure. When old remedies fail I say that it is not only not unreasonable, but proper that you should ascertain what can be done by new ones; but it is very unwise to employ the latter, when there are sufficient reasons to believe that those already in use will answer the intended purpose. I should be very sorry to see the march of science impeded by an unjust apprehension of experiments and innovations; but surely there is a broad enough line between a discrete and prudent use of new remedies, and that indiscrete and hasty use of them which we find to prevail in the practice of the medical profession at present."—*Clinical Lectures, page* 305.

It often happens that the use of a remedy is pushed too far, and applied too indiscriminately, hence in many cases it fails to produce the desired result, and we become dissatisfied. Consequently it is thrown aside as worthy of no purpose.

A result of this kind has fallen upon venesection, and hence it has passed to a great extent into oblivion. Without doubt the changes in the diatheses of disease have in a great measure warranted this, but not in my opinion to the extent it has been carried, and were this remedy resorted to in the commencement of disease, we should cut short much that is now prolonged and tedious.

The principal indications for the use of this agent are those of a congestive and inflammatory character, whether local or general, and although these conditions may be brought to a favorable termination without its aid, yet were it resorted to in their first stages, a lingering, complicated result might be abbreviated.

The late Dr. Gallup, of Woodstock, Vermont, maintained even to his death that the first remedy for Tubercular Pthisis was blood-letting, and although in many cases he carried it too far, (or rather the disease had advanced beyond the proper time for its use) yet without doubt many are now living to thank him for its timely application.

A resort to the lancet, was almost a hobby with this celebrated physician, and its use was followed with general success.

In his time, and in the section of country in which he practised, diseases may have been more of an inflammatory nature than at the present day, and yet, I think much was owing to his nice discrimination.

W. Cumming, Esq., M. R. C. S., writing in the *London Lancet,* of November, 1853, on the subject of general blood-letting, after discoursing upon the too general freedom in which it had been used, says "the increased knowledge of diseases, showing that many are not inflammatory but dependant on want of blood and strength, the recognized power of calomel and antimony to control inflammation with other cases, have removed this error in practice, but seem likely to carry us to an absurdity in the opposite extreme. Unfortunately it is too true that even well educated members of our profession are too apt to misuse or neglect a good remedy from the powerful influence of mere fashion. At the pres-

ent time there seems to be a prevailing prejudice against general blood-
letting amongst practitioners of medicine, forsooth, because there are
epidemics which are characterized by marked debility, and because many
slight inflammations will get well without it, (and indeed without any
treatment at all) they relinquish a most valuable means of controlling
diseases, one which used within proper limits, with care and discretion,
may prove of the highest service."

[J. T. Mitchell, F. R. C. S., in the January number of the *Lancet* for
1854, writing in reference to the paper of Mr. Cumming, remarks " that
Mr. Cumming is evidently a careful observer, a judicious reasoner, and
a cautious practitioner. He clearly perceives the error into which too
many of the modern school have fallen, in totally rejecting what is by
far the most important and valuable remedy in the hands of the physician,
when wisely adopted in the acute and sthenic diseases, regulating quantity
and frequency by the urgency of symptoms and state of the patient. True
it is that much can be done by antimony, calomel and opium, but these
all act far better in highly acute cases after an early well-adjusted bleeding, than when bleeding had been omitted. Moreover, I am well
persuaded that in modern times many a case of inflammatory disease
has been lost by the omission of this highly essential remedy on the first
appearance of the acute symptoms, and by trusting alone to large doses
of antimony, &c., the list of cases of permanent, lingering, distressing
chronic disease, has been extensively increased.

"I am convinced that this remedy is decried to a most injurious extent,
and therefore, I gladly add the result of a long experience to that of Mr.
Cumming.

"Large and repeated bleedings have no doubt killed many a patient, or
have left many a sufferer in an anæmic and pitiable condition, but observing the 'just medium' with this remedy is a very different thing."

The above quotations from such authorities shew that English physicians are no more exempt from the popular feeling in regard to this
remedy than ourselves.

We have been guided altogether too much by the opinion that for
venesection to be beneficial we must have fever, or in other words an excited circulation, a full, hard, or bounding pulse, but such is not the case.
We are often consulted on cases in which the patient complains of simple
pain, severe in character, and involving some of the many visceral organs,
but unaccompanied by any febrile action: to abstract a portion of blood
in such is to entirely remove the pain and relieve the patient. How is
this? Pain is most frequently the precursor of inflammation, the first
speaking symptom of congestion. To bleed is to relieve the hyperæmia

and establish reäction, thereby enabling the oppressed organ to reëstablish its normal function.

Several cases have occurred under my personal observation, in which the above views have been fully corroborated.

Rev. Mr. ——, a young Catholic clergyman, was received into St. Mary's Hospital, complaining of severe pain in the apex of the right lung, accompanied with a small hacking cough. The pain, however, was the chief complaint. A physical examination of the lungs, detected the primary symptoms of tubercle. General bleeding was resorted to twice, and each time the relief was marked and positive. Tonics were then administered with nutritious diet, when he soon left as far as could be observed a healthy man.

Mr. ——, a Norwegian, was admitted into the same place under similar circumstances, with the exception that the disease was farther advanced and accompanied with a bronchitis of some weeks standing. He was placed under the same plan of treatment, excepting that cups were employed instead of the lancet. He was discharged apparently recovered. I have seen him since, and he has had no return of his previous difficulty.

A short time since, I was consulted by one of the members of this society, who complained of a general aristriction of the system. His pulse was slow and labored, and his sensations were that some inflammatory action was impending, (he being liable to such.) I advised him. to be bled, to which he readily assented. After removing about 12 oz. of blood, he felt quite relieved, and has been perfectly well since, as far as that condition was concerned.

Now, had the above cases occurred in private practice, the good people would have raised their hands in condemnation of such treatment, and be sustained by men calling themselves doctors of medicine.

I would not say but that they would have been remedied by other means, but the plan adopted was much more brief and safe. The physician must always bear in mind that not only has he the disease itself to consider, but the results of that disease upon the patient's after existence. It is not enough to say we have cured the disease, but that we have so cured it as to free them from after consequences; and in my opinion, many die from consumption from neglect of sufficient depletion in inflammatory diseases of the thorax and lungs.

It should be our highest endeavor to treat disease upon sound pathological deductions, to discard all fashion in our remedial agents, to make good use of all well-known and tried remedies first, to discard novelty, and act independently; then, instead of physicians bowing to the popular will, community will look up to the physician and render that respect due to his talents and profession.

It was moved and carried that a copy of this paper be requested for publication.

Prof. Palmer remarked that the sentiments of this paper deserved serious consideration, and in many parts of the country such a prejudice had grown up against blood-letting, as to deter many practitioners from it, even when it was most urgently required, by the fear of losing popu_larity. Practitioners ought to maintain their integrity and independence, and in cases where the lancet was required for the patient's recovery, to insist that he submit to it, or else leave him.

Prof. Denton remarked that in this region he had not found so strong a prejudice; that he used the lancet freely whenever it was required, and seldom met any serious opposition to it. He highly approved of the sentiments of the previous speaker in respect to insisting on the giving up of foolish prejudices on the part of the patient and his friends, where if e and health were at stake.

The following paper was then read by title.

Historical Notice of the Territorial and State Medical Societies of Michigan. By Z. Pitcher, M.D.

The following sketch of the origin, duration and dissolution by legislative decree, of the former Territorial and more recent State Medical Society may furnish some information of transient interest to the younger members of the profession, and will afford us an occasion of making some remarks upon the comparative value and relative utility of incorporated societies and voluntary medical associations, when regarded as means of professional improvement.

The first act, in relation to the medical profession, passed by legislative authority in Michigan, which was then vested in the Governor and Judges of the Territory, was dated the 14th of June, 1819, and signed by Lewis Cass, Governor, and A. B. Woodward and John Griffin, Judges of the Territorial Courts, and was entitled "An Act to incorporate Medical Societies, for the purpose of regulating the practice of Physic and Surgery in the Territory of Michigan." The act itself was preceded by the following preamble, notable for its true presentment of the objects or purposes for which such societies should be established, especially now that the law makes no distinction between the mountebank and the medical philosopher. It was brief, but to the point; and reads thus: "Whereas, well regulated Medical Societies have been found to contribute to the advancement and diffusion of true science, and particularly of the healing art, therefore, Be it enacted," &c.

This law, besides authorizing the organization of a Territorial Society and of societies in the different counties thereof, exempted the members of each from serving as jurors and from doing military duty in time of peace. It granted authority to the Censors to examine students and to issue diplomas under the hand of the President and seal of the society, and to the societies power to hold real and personal estate, to make by-laws and regulations relative to the affairs, concerns, and property of said societies, relative to the admission and expulsion of members, relative to donations or contributions, as they or a majority of the members at their annual meeting shall think fit and proper: Provided that they be not contrary to the laws of this Territory or of the United States. They were empowered also to raise funds for the purchase of a Medical Library, for apparatus, and for the encouragement of useful discoveries in Chemistry and Botany.

Fines and pecuniary penalties were authorized to be imposed upon persons engaging in the practice of medicine in violation of the sections of this law, prescribing the qualifications pre-requisite to their receiving a diploma or license from the Territorial or County Medical Society.

Some years later, but before the State had thrown off its Territorial exuviæ, a more stringent act was passed, designed to prevent the intrusion of unqualifed persons into the ranks of the profession. It never fully met the expectations of its friends.

After Michigan became a State and was admitted into the Union, a code of laws was prepared by the late Wm. A. Fletcher for the consideration of the legislature. This code, as modified by the legislature and finally adopted, retained essentially the provisions of the Territorial Law in relation to medical societies, except an abatement in the rigor of the penalties to be imposed upon illegal practitioners of medicine.

At the same session of the legislature, a law was enacted, whereby that violation of sepulchre essential to the study of anatomy, was made a penitentiary offence, which might be expiated by a year's residence in the penitentiary, or by the payment of a fine of two thousand dollars. By the present laws of the state, the midnight assassin and the inquiring medical student are liable to become inhabitants of the same cell, in the Michigan State Prison.

That part of the Fletcher code which related to medicine, continued to be law, till 1844, but proved to be of such trifling validity that the members of the State Medical Society, on consultation with Dr. M. A. Patterson, then a member of the state legislature, and with Dr. Kibbee, his senatorial colleague, addressed a memorial to the legislature requesting the passage of an act, repealing so much of the revised statutes as related to the practice of medicine. The physicians of the State were made, in a particular sense of the word, a law-less set of fellows, by this act, till a new version of the statutes took place, under the supervision of the Hon. Sanford M. Green, now one of the judges of the Supreme Court, on the cold-water side of the liquor law. At this time, the former State Medical Society was reinstated, or set up anew, the former law, in most particulars, re-enacted, and some additional force, as will appear from the following extract to one or two of its sections, designed to restrain the illegal exercise of the functions of a physician. A step was also taken at this time towards legalizing the study of Anatomy.—*See Chap. 36, Title 8, Rev. Statutes.*

" SEC. 33. Whenever the medical department of the university of Michigan shall be organized, said department shall be entitled to the exclusive privilege conferred upon the medical society of the state by the preceding section.

" SEC. 36. Every person who shall falsely represent himself to be a duly licensed physician or surgeon, and shall procure himself to be employed as such, shall be deemed guilty of a misdemeanor, and on conviction thereof shall be punished by imprisonment in the county jail not exceeding one year, or by a fine not exceeding one thousand dollars, or both in the discretion of the court.

" SEC. 37. If any person professing or holding himself out to be a physician or surgeon, shall be guilty of any neglect or mal-practice, an action on the case may be maintained against such person so professing, and the rules of the common law applicable to such actions against licensed physicians and surgeons, shall be applicable to such actions on the case; and such mal-practice or neglect may be given in evidence in bar of an action for services rendered by such persons so professing."

These provisions of law were so far rendered nugatory by a decision of one of the judges of the Supreme Court, who held that any man who styled himself a doctor was a doctor in the eye of the law, and legally entitled to the professional honorarium, that the members of the medical profession made no resistance to their total and final repeal, when the legislature was moved thereto by infinitesimal potentialities, which took place in 1852.

The transactions which have taken place in the medical organizations provided for in the laws above referred to, have never tended in any considerable degree to advance or diffuse true science. This, however, has been rather the fault of the laws themselves, and of the times in

which they were enacted, than of the men who were appointed to execute their provisions.

In the exercise of authority derived from the Governor and Judges,
the physicians of the territory met at the City of Detroit, on the 10th day
of August, 1819, and formed the Medical Society of the Territory of
Michigan, and elected the following named persons as the officers
thereof:

President,	William Brown,
Vice-President,	Stephen C. Henry,
Secretary,	John L. Whiting,
Treasurer,	Randall S. Rice.

At the first Annual Meeting, held January, 1820, a Board of Censors
was elected, consisting of,

E. Hurd, | S. C. Henry, | R. S. Rice.

A code of by-laws was also adopted at this meeting, one of which so
clearly foreshadows the opinions now more explicitly enunciated on the
subject of preparatory education for medical students, that I am tempted
to copy it for present use.

"9. The President, Senior Censor, and Secretary, shall form a board
to examine students in the preparatory branches of education, and give
a certificate previous to their entrance on the study of medicine. They
shall keep minutes of their proceedings, and lay them before the society
semi-annually. If a student has had a collegiate or academic education,
his moral character only shall be a subject of inquiry. This certificate
shall permit him to study with any member of this society."

When a student became a candidate, or rather an applicant for a diploma, the mode of his examination and the subjects he was to be questioned upon were fully set forth in the code of by-laws.

Owing either to the features of the times or the characteristics of the
individuals then most active as members of the society, special provisions
were made in the by-laws of the society, for the discipline of sinning or
refractory members.

The following list of names taken from records includes all who ever
held the office of President:

William Brown,	from August 10, 1819, to January 10, 1826.
William Thompson,	"	Jan.	10, 1826, "	"	9, 1827.
Stephen C. Henry,	"	Jan.	9, 1827, "	Feb.	5, 1833.
John L. Whiting,	"	Feb.	5, 1833, "	Jan.	8, 1836.
Marshall Chapin,	"	Jan.	8, 1836, "	Jan.	10, 1837.
D. O. Hoyt,	"	"	10, 1837, "	"	9, 1838.
Zina Pitcher,	"	"	9, 1838, "		1851.

Except the time the society was in a state of asphyxia, from the repeal of the Fletcher to the adoption of the Green code.

During the time of my connection with the State Medical Society, and I presume at all others, efforts have been made semi-annually, to infuse a working spirit into its members. Notices were uniformly published in the newspapers of the city, some twenty days in advance of the time and place of the annual and semi-annual meetings. Yet a bare quorum for the transaction of business could be got together, and not always that.

This nerveless condition of the old society may be thus explained. The organic law stood in the way of the vitalizing process. Only two permanent members could be elected annually. The design of the statute appeared to be, to make the working men out of the delegates from the country societies. Many of the counties had no organization and others were so remote that the delegates could not, without great sacrifice, attend the sessions of the State Society. Unavoidably, it remained a mere local affair, and was wasting of atrophy at the time it received the *coup de grace* from state legislature.

The history of this society furnishes one evidence of a general truth, which is, that the legislation of a government deriving its powers from the consent of the governed, in order to have any binding validity, must be an exposition of the popular sentiment, however erroneous that sentiment may be.

Legislative efforts to establish conformity in matters of religion, now of more than doubtful utility, may, in former times, when the power was less directly derived from the people, have produced beneficial results, may have developed a higher order of talent in those who ministered in holy things, and possibly have produced more striking examplars of christian learning and piety in the body of worshipers. So perhaps in medicine. But in the existing state of things, when power inheres in the masses, it is futile to expect an organic expression of sentiment antagonistic to their own. The populace, on the subject of medicine, are ignorant, and will not sanction legislation which does not address itself to that ignorance. The medical profession, then, in order to secure that position in the estimation of this public to which it is entitled, must set itself to work to supply an obvious want in the public mind, by disseminating that kind and degree of knowledge which will enable them to appreciate the cardinal truths in physics, the normal laws of health, and the abnormal deviations, with the therapeutic rules for their restoration. In this way only can we prevent their being made the victims of quackery, or secure legal sanctions for its repression.

If men, in their preference for the sympathetic treatment of wounds, &c., choose, as many did in the time of some of the later crusades, to cure a wound by the application of an ungent to the lance, by which it was inflicted, or please to believe in the efficacy of Perkins' metalic tractors, or that "a small dose of *Gold* taken internally, produces excessive scruples of conscience," (Jahr's Manual) there seems to be no way of preventing their perpetrating such absurdities and entertaining follies, except by educating them so that they shall be able to discriminate between truth and error, or their analogies, the conscientious physician and the designing knave. When, by whom, and how this is to be done, are questions which interest the community more than they do us. I submit, however, to the members of the Society, whether the initiative should not be taken by the medical profession, who are most perfectly aware of the existence and of the evils of quackery, and of the nature and modus operandi of the remedies to be used for its suppression.

My reflections, during the preparation of this sketch, have led me to contemplate the causes which bring about changes in the phases of moral, social, and political life; all of which are expressed in the idea of advancement, which I find to be natural acts, educed from the nature of man, who labors in obedience to rules laid down by the Author of his being. The remarkably aphoristic saying of Wordsworth, that "the boy is father of the man," as the type of a general truth has a manifold application. The completion of one period in the life of the individual, is succeeded by new wants, and new powers of ministering to their gratification. The manifestation of the same law in communities or nations, constitutes social progress, and in the geological and animal world, has been termed development.

On examining into the legislation, on the subject of medicine in Michigan, and the action of the medical societies under the various laws of the Territory and the State, you may see a want of adaptation between the laws and the persons or bodies on whom they were designed to operate, showing the existence of an instructive transition movement in the medical mind, urged by the wants of the times.

The analogies between the natural and moral world, every where hold good. What at one time constitutes the primitive rocks of the globe, at another furnishes the elements or materials of newer and more horizontal strata; in the meanwhile, uplifts, dislocations and distortions of strata take place, symbolical of the struggles by which old thoughts, old forms of speech, and old modes of civilization, become moulded into new shapes, and a prime new relation. As the debris of antecedent things, become the soil and furnish the aliment of those which spring of the dust of antiquity.

There must have been within certain periods of man's history, not only a propriety, but necessity for an alliance between the religious organizations of a people and their form of government, or that union would never have been permitted to take place. And without the fostering care of the State, medicine may never have reached its present position in the learned professions. But in the process of time, it came to be a question whether the strength, pertaining to the organizations created by law, did not tend to abate from the vigor of the individuals who entered into their composition. Jealousy at length on the part of those excluded from these affiliations, but who were aspiring without adequate preparation to become the high-priests of medicine, began to weaken the respect of the public for the bodies, because the individuals composing them, did not always show themselves to be men. Super-added to this feeling, the apprehension of a monopoly came in, which led the people in the blind exercise of an attribute of sovereignty, to tear away the pillars of the æsculapian temple, and leave the individual members of the profession to stand or fall, as they might or might not, have strength to do.

Hence arose the necessity of more perfect individual culture, and the importance of voluntary associations as a means to that end.

Let us then put on the strength of a full-grown individuality, taking care that in our love for liberty we shun licentiousness, so that each part and member being perfectly developed, we may reconstruct a living temple, comely as the stars and enduring as the eternal hills.

DETROIT, April 30, 1854.

It was moved and carried that a copy of this paper be requested for publication.

The following paper was next read.

Psora, Malaria, or Michigan Itch. By WM. BRODIE, M. D.

The study of cutaneous diseases has ever been fraught with much difficulty, constituting as they do a distinct class by themselves, and embracing so many peculiarities, it is no wonder that writers upon the subject should differ so widely in their opinions; and although every author on the subject has endeavored to include all varieties peculiar to the cutaneous surface, still it is no matter of surprise that some may have been omitted.

The subject of this paper is one that we find no description of in treatises of skin disease; at the same time, it is one of common occurrence in this section of our country.

It is common as I am informed in the State of Ohio, as well as in Michigan, and its leading features consist in the excessive pruritus which it occasions.

Upon examination of a patient suffering from this disease, we find as a general thing his appearance is languid, and it may be emaciated; his spirits depressed, and his circulation weak and low; to sum the whole, he would be judged as laboring under some one of the various forms of malarious fever.

The secreting system is deranged, and the assimilating organs are weakened and debilitated. In some cases the appetite is poor, in others voracious. In others, the disease will show itself in an otherwise healthy person, but this is rare.

The local symptoms of the disease reside in the skin, the color of which is a dirty white, almost a bronze. Upon examination of the surface of the body, we find it covered with small black specks, which specks are small points of blood which have exuded from the abrasion of the summit of a small papulæ, which papulæ is generally the color of the cuticle, and slightly raised upon it in some cases a slightly reddened base is found.

This eruption is generally dispersed about equally over the body, excepting those parts which are constantly exposed to the atmosphere, or covered with the hair, as the head.

A favorite location of the disease is upon the abdomen and anterior of the thorax, where the eruption is more free.

The great peculiarity of this eruption is the excessive pruritus which attends it. This condition is augmented by heat, and is more troublesome at night than in the day, doubtless owing to the warmth of the bed; yet, it persists during the whole time, and patients describe the sensation produced by rubbing it, as of a pleasing character.

The diagnosis of this disease is only to be confounded with Prurigo, Lichen, and Eczema, but mostly with Prurigo. This is described by Cazenave and Wilson, as a disease non-contagious, whereas Michigan Itch seems to possess this property, although I do not feel positive that it is so. Papula are not a necessary feature of Prurigo, whereas, they are of Michigan Itch. In Lichen the pimples are solid and prominent, also discolored, and the itching is of a tingling character.

From Eczema in the papula being solid, whereas Eczema, it being a vesicular eruption, the vesicles when being broken produce a thick scab, and have a great tendency of coalescing. If vesicles occur in the former, they stand prominent, and after bursting dry up.

From Scabie, in not having the undermined ragged state of the derma, and the presence of the acarus scabiei.

The causes of this disease arises mostly in the systems of those afflicted, and its predilections are not with any particular age or sex. In those seen by myself, they have been mostly males. It occurs mostly in the fall, winter and spring months, but less in the latter, than the two former. In summer I have not seen it, yet I am informed it does occur.

Prurigo, on the contrary, is mostly seen in the spring and summer months.

Want of cleanliness, doubtless has much to do in keeping up the irritation, still I do not think it originates it in any way.

What I consider as directly producing it, is malaria. The influence of this poison upon the economy is of such a debilitating nature that it renders the entire secerning and secretory systems unhealthy, consequently the whole organization is impoverished, the skin necessarily becomes dry and hard, the dermal terminations of the nerves become irritated, and hence arises the constant itching which irritates and destroy the patient's comfort, the exposed part of the skin being excepted. Why I have considered malaria as the chief cause of this disease, is derived from the history of the patients. I have not yet seen a case but that has been preceded by intermittent fever in some of its varying forms. Moreover, it is decidedly a disease of the west, especially in Ohio and Michigan, where intermittents are rife; and for the same reason I should expect to meet with it in Indiana, Illinois, &c.

In Ohio, I am informed, it is known as the Ohio Scratches, and was common more than 25 years ago.

The Prognosis is favorable, it being amenable to treatment, and not destructive of life.

In the treatment of this disease the first indications are to relieve the pruritus, and second, to raise the standard of health.

The first can be brought about by the administration of diaphoretics, sponging the surface with alkaline washes, and painting the surface with the tincture of iodine.

The second, by a judicious use of tonics, as the sulphate of quinine, the chalybeates, and the vegetable bitters, together with good diet, bathing and cleanliness.

A common remedy used by the inhabitants to appease the pruritus, is the juice of the Lactuca elongata, seu Wild Lettuce or Trumpet Milk-weed, this is rubbed over the parts, and is said to stop it at once, for a time.

It was moved and carried that a copy of it be requested for publication.

The following paper was then read.

An Account of a Double Monster Resembling the Siamese Twins.
By E. ANDREWS, M. D.

The singular monstrosity now before us, was presented to the Museum of the Medical College, by Dr. H. Taylor, of Mt. Clemens. You perl

·ceive that the two infants are joined by a connection extending from the lower third of the sternum to the umbilicus, being that sort of monstrosity called anterior duplicity. The junction is almost exactly in front of each fœtus, placing them face to face; still, the connection extends a little farther on one side of the mesial line than on the other; hence, these subjects by a slight effort can be placed side by side like the Siamese Twins, which celebrated pair are united by a connection exactly similar in form and position to this. Unlike them, however, both these specimens are females.

As soon as the specimen was received, I made a partial dissection to ascertain the form and peculiarities of the internal organs. On cutting through the skin, the abdominal muscles were found deflected from their course, so as to wind around the connecting band to gain their usual insertions. The two sterna were attached firmly to each other at the junction of the middle with the lower third. The arrangement here was singular. Instead of the conjoined sternum extending downward between the two chests, it bifurcated, and the two branches extended to the right and left in the form of a firm cartilaginous arch. To the circumference of this arch the costal cartilages of the lower ribs were articulated. From the inferior surface depended a thin membrane separating the cavities of the two chests. The thorax contained two pairs of lungs perfectly unconnected with each other, and two hearts, each perfect and distinct, and each having the proper position in relation to its own body.

There were also two pericardial sacs, whose cavities had no communication with each other. The two sacs lay in contact, and the double serous membrane formed by the adhesion of one to the other, was the membrane above referred to, as depending from the arch of the sternum and separating the cavities of the two chests. On cutting into the abdomen, two peritonœal sacs were also found, which being in contact in front, formed a thin serous partition between the two abdominal cavities, exactly like that between the two chests. Unlike that, however, this partition was perforated, there being a large foramen of an inch in diameter at the lower part, through which the two cavities were continuous. No viscus, however, passed through this opening, and neither the stomach nor intestines had any communication with each other. The only common viscus was the liver. This organ extended across from one body to the other, without even a constriction to mark its double origin. The peritonœal septum extended over it in the form of a falciform ligament, connecting it to the diaphragm. There were two gall bladders, and two umbilical veins. The cord was single and contained five vessels, of which I am led to conclude from the records of other cases, as well as from their own appearance, that three of them must have been arteries, and two of them veins. The fear of injuring the external appearance of the specimen, deterred me from tracing them up with the scalpel. This case, so far as we can judge, is almost similar to that of the Siamese Twins. The mode of junction in that celebrated pair is the same externally, and when either of them coughed, the connecting band is said to have dis- dlstended in its whole length, showing a peritonœal cavity through it. If the liver extended through, and the pericardiar were in contact as in the case before us, an attempt to separate them by surgical means, as has been proposed, could have but the faintest possible chance of terminating otherwise than fatally.

Another case resembling this, is described by Cruveilheir, and is figured in the plate which I here exhibit. In his case the union of the viscera was quite intimate. There was but one heart and one pericardi- um. The heart had four auricles and two ventricles, and sent off two aortæ. The liver he describes as resembling two livers adhering together by the border. The stomachs and duodenums were separate, but termi- nated in a common jejunum The lower part of the small intestine, however, divided again, and terminated in two colons.

It may be proper here, also, to recall to mind the famous Ritta Christina. This was a female infant, the lower half of which was single, while from the single waist sprung two perfect chests, with the corres- ponding arms, necks and heads. At the time it was presented for bap- tism, a grave theological question arose as to whether this was one child or two. As it had two heads, it was decided to be theologically two babies, and one was baptized under the name of Ritta, and the other, of Christina. The monster lived eight months.

While upon the subject of monstrosity, it may not be amiss to men- tion one which recently appeared before the medical class, and which has already been described in several medical journals. A case precisely similar is also figured in the Cyclopedia of Anatomy and Physiology. It was an instance of arrested development of the anterior part of the pelvis and its viscera. This part of the body seemed not to advance beyond that fœtal state in which the visceral cavities are open in front. The pubic bones did not reach each other, but seemed to have a loose liga- mentous connection; the penis was exceedingly short, and was open from the urethra upwards throughout its whole length, showing a mere groove. At the upper part of this groove the openings of the seminal ducts could be perceived. The anterior wall of the bladder was entirely wanting, and the posterior wall red and irritated by contact with the air, bulged for- ward in the form of a tumor. The surface constantly secreted mucus, and on the lower part the orifices of the uretus were plainly to be seen with the urine dripping from them. This was a case of montrosity by arrested development. It comes under the same class as the cases of non-formation of the front wall of the chest, leaving the heart exposed, or absence of the anterior wall of the abdomen, causing all its viscera to appear externally. An interesting case of this exposure of abdominal viscera in which the intestines and liver were entirely uncovered, was shown me formerly by Dr. Taylor, the same gentleman who presented this specimen before us.

It was moved and carried that a copy be requested for publication.

Dr. H. Taylor being called upon, gave the following history of the case.

"Being called to attend in the case which resulted in the delivery of the specimens now before the Society, I found it an example of tedious labor, the patient having at first endeavored to do without a physician, but at length finding that no progress was made, had sent for me. I waited for a considerable time, as the symptoms were not urgent, to see if patience and the natural efforts would not suffice, but no progress whatever resulting, I made an examination and discovered two heads presenting together at the superior strait, whose combined diameters, lying as they did in one plane, were too great to allow either of them to engage. Greatly relieved at this discovery, I supposed I had found the whole source of difficulty, and that by changing the position enough to allow one head to present at a time, everything would go on prosperously. I accordingly made efforts to accomplish this object, but greatly to my chagrin there was some invisible obstacle. As soon as I pushed back one of the heads, the other retreated with it, and then both would come down again as before. After being foiled thus a long time, I at length began to push my hand farther, and having with some difficulty reached the shoulders, I there discovered again, as I supposed, the cause of trouble. The arms of the infants were folded around each others necks, they lying face to face. I carefully disentangled them, and then again endeavored to make one slide past the other. But to my astonishment the same trouble occurred; when one was thrust back, the other retired with it, and when they came down to the strait, both came obstinately together. Meanwhile the pains increased in frequency and force, and as I could reach nothing which threw any light on the matter, I at length flexed one head until it lay in the hollow of the neck of the other. In this position the combined diameters being reduced, they became engaged in the strait, and notwithstanding my shame at having two infants born together under my charge, they were delivered both at once. The cause of the trouble was then apparent, as you see in these specimens. The placenta was large and oblong, and the cord was single. The cord was pulsating, but they never breathed. After these were disposed of, a third infant was found in the uterus, which was soon born and lived several hours."

In the discussion which followed, the Society requested Dr. Stockwell, of Port Huron, to describe a case of monstrosity which had occurred under his observation. Dr. Stockwell rose, and remarked:

"The case alluded to, occurred near Port Huron. I was not present at the birth, but sometime afterwards was called by the father to prescribe for a sore on the infant's back. On examination, I found it obviously a case of *spina bifida*, with also a tumor on the back of the head, which was soft, and apparently communicated with the brain. The child was exceedingly low and feeble. I devised means of protecting the raw surface of the fissure in the spine from the friction of the clothes, and with directions how to treat it in other respects; informed the parents that there was but little hope of its ever recovering so as to be free from disease. I did not see it again for some time, when being sent for, I found it better in almost every respect. The *spina bifida* was cicatrizing in a healthy manner, but the tumor on the head was increased. In the process of time the cleft in the spine was entirely closed up, but the tumor of the head still enlarging and seeming to have fluid at its apex, I explored it with the lancet. A quantity of serum escaped from the puncture, which, being evacuated, showed within the cavity a smaller tumor having convolutions like the surface of the brain; in short, appearing like a cerebral hernia protruding through the canal which occupied the pedicle of the tumor. From this time it went on increasing rapidly, occasioning great uneasiness and irritability which threatened to wear out the patient. After long delay and careful counsel it was decided to risk the removal of the tumor. This was done, first by cutting through the scalp around the pedicle which exposed a prolongation of the dura mater. This was divided, and the whole removed. On examination, the neck of the tumor was found to contain a pedicle of brain substance, showing that a cerebral hernia had been removed. The wound healed up, and the patient is now well both of the tumor and of the *spina bifida*."

It was moved and carried that the order of business be suspended to hear the report of the committee appointed to ascertain if the faculty of the University would act as committee on epidemics. The committee reported affirmatively.

Dr. Brodie offered the following resolution, which was adopted.

Resolved, That a Committee of three be appointed to revise the Constitution of this Society, and draw up by-laws for the government of the same; said committee to report at the next annual meeting.

Dr. Pitcher then offered the following resolution, which was unanimously adopted.

Resolved, That this Society request of President Tappan, a copy of his able and valuable address to the graduates of the Medical College, for publication.

(TO BE CONTINUED.)

SELECTIONS.

From the Report on the Health and Mortality of Memphis for 1853.

[The statistics and considerations here presented, ought to be considered carefully by all physicians who are in the habit of indiscriminately advising phthisical patients to "go south for their health."—ED.]

	DEATHS FROM PHTHISIS TO TOTAL MORTALITY.	DEATHS FROM ALL PULM. DIS. TO TOTAL MORTALITY.
Philadelphia	14.84 per ct.	28.57 per cent.
New York	17.50 " "	28.08 " "
Havana	19.50 " "	25.07 " "
Boston	15.13 " "	23.97 " "
Baltimore	18.20 " "	23.33 " "
Charleston	18.27 "	22.73 " "
Mexico City	2.45 "	16.76 " "
Norfolk	11.01 "	12.78 " "
New Orleans	9.37 " "	13.87 " "

Again, in volume V. of the Transactions of the American Medical Association, page 579, the same distinguished writer invites attention to certain tabular statements, which exhibit some most unexpected and remarkable results, and says: "One of the most signal is the great prevalence of phthisis in the island of Cuba; that beautiful island, to which so many of our countrymen are conveyed—to die. This is not only the case with the city of Havana, where it constitutes *more than one-fourth of the entire mortality,* but in many of the rural districts, the *average* of the four I have given, being upwards of twelve per cent. I bear witness from personal knowledge, that this is of the native population, originating there, and influenced greatly, as it is everywhere else, by moral and hygienic conditions; and I do not speak with more emphasis than truth, when I say that, to send a patient to Cuba with *phthisis,* after a certain stage is set in, is but to send him to his grave." So, too, the "Statistical Reports on the Sickness, Mortality, &c., in the Troops in the United Kingdom, the Mediterranean and British America, &c., &c.," supply us with very similar facts. It was found that a body of selected soldiers, subject to no severe duty, and exposed to no hardships, lose, annually, a larger proportion of their number in the Mediterranean, by consumption, than in the United Kingdom. This inference, however adverse to generally received opinions, is strikingly corroborated by the prevalence of consumption, and other pulmonary affections, among the residents of Malta. It was also ascertained that of the diseases and deaths among the British troops in the West Indies, that at least twice as many cases of consumption originated in that climate, as in Great Britain. Sir James Clark asserts that phthisis is more prevalent among the troops in the British West India Islands, than at home; that whilst one and a half per cent. of those serving in these colonies, were attacked annually with consumption, only one and a half per cent. of the dragoon guards, serving in England, suffered. The evidence of Sir William Burnet, and other medical officers of the royal navy, tend to the same result. In both the windward and leeward islands, twelve per one thousand annually suffered; in Barbadoes as much as fifteen; whereas, in Nova Scotia, New Brunswick, and Canada, not more than seven per one thousand annually die of consumption. In an exceedingly interesting paper, on the effects of Climate on Disease, by William F. Carrington, M. D., United States Navy, in which these facts are stated, the writer remarks, that so far from the natives of these islands being exempt from the disease, on the contrary, its great prevalence among them has been long a matter of notoriety, and he further says, "In all tropical countries, both east and west, great heat appears to have a powerful effect in producing tuberculus disease."

In his report, Dr. Sutton says, "It will be remembered by many members of the American Medical Association, that the late Professor Drake, in offering a paper on 'The Connection between Climate and Pulmonary Consumption,' remarked that, 'the facts obtained by extensive inquiries and observations, had led to results very different from what he had anticipated.'" In conversation with Doctor Grant, as to the results thus obtained by Professor Drake, Doctor Grant kindly offered to write out the substance of the remarks made to him by Professor Drake on the subject. The following is Doctor Grant's letter:

MEMPHIS, January 17, 1854.

DEAR SIR,—The substance of the remarks made to me, by the late Professor Drake, of Cincinnati, on the relation of *climate and phthisis pulmonalis*, was, that his conversations with medical men, and his own observations, had led him to conclude that this disease was much more prevalent in the *southern* portions of the Mississippi valley than was generally believed—that the results of his investigations, in this particular, were not in accordance with his pre-conceived opinions, or with the opinions inculcated by most medical writers on this subject—that *tuberculosis* of the *lungs* was infinitely more prevalent in the *temperate* latitudes of this great valley, than he had found it to be in the rigorous climate of *Canada*.

It may not be amiss to state, that Doctor Drake made these remarks to me on his return from the last southern tour made by him, for the purpose of collecting the material for his "great work."

Respectfully,   GEORGE R. GRANT.

DR. QUINTARD.

It is much to be regretted that the paper by Doctor Drake, was with-held by him from publication. His powers of observation, and analysis, together with his acquaintance with the topography of every section of our country, would have placed in the hands of the profession, a most valuable guide on this subject. We cannot conclude our remarks on the subject of phthisis pulmonalis, without a reference to the researches of Doctor Forry.

"It is seen," says Doctor Forry, "that, with the exception of catarrh, and influenza, the annual ratio of pulmonary diseases is lower in the northern than in the southern regions of the United States. It is in the middle districts of the United States, however, that pneumonia, pleuritis, and phthisis pulmonalis, are most prevalent, the peninsula of Florida having a lower average than any other. It is found, too, that the same law obtains in regard to the mortality arising from this class of diseases, the deaths per 1,000 of mean strength being as under:

PHTHISIS PULMONALIS.		PNEUMONIA, PLEURITIS, & CATARRH.	
Northern Regions	2.1	Northern Regions	0.5
Southern "	4.4	Southern "	1.8

The high mortality of the southern regions is caused by the middle division of the United States, the average on our southern coast being comparatively low. Taking the statistics of the posts in east Florida, and those on the lower Mississippi, the ratio of phthisis pulmonalis is found to be only one and seven-tenths, and that of the remaining lesions of this class, to be no more than seven-tenths per one thousand of mean strength.

It is also ascertained that these diseases are of a more fatal tendency in the southern, than in the northern regions. In the latter, the ratio of mortality from phthisis pulmonalis is thirty-two, and in the former, forty-two per hundred cases; and as regards pleuritis and pneumonia, the difference is much greater, the average mortality in the northern being nine, and in the southern, twenty-six per one thousand cases.

These statistics show, that as regards pleuritis and phthisis pulmonalis, the ratio of cases and deaths is greater in our middle regions, including the south-western stations, than at either extreme. In endeavoring to account for this result, much may, perhaps, be due to the circumstance that the subjects are generally from the northern states, or from Europe. It may be safely asserted, as has been already remarked, that the majority of cases of consumption at our southern posts, supervene upon febrile diseases, more especially in constitutions broken down by intemperance, bearing the same relation to fevers as those other sequelæ—dropsy, jaundice, and the various chronic lesions of the viscera. On the lower Mississippi—a class of posts which present the highest mortality—the average of phthisis pulmonalis is low, owing very probably to the circumstance that fevers are of the most fatal tendency, terminating either in speedy death, or rapid recovery. At the south-western stations, and those along our middle coast, the malarial poison acts more slowly, thus developing by a gradual deterioration of the constitution, a tubercular form of consumption, general opinion to the contrary, notwithstanding. It follows then, that a continuous residence in the south, so far from being beneficial in this disease, will often hasten its fatal issue.

From the Eleventh Annual Report of the Superintendent of the New York State Lunatic Asylum, for the year ending November 30, 1853.

To the Managers of the Asylum:

GENTLEMEN—In accordance with the regulations of the Institution, the following report is respectfully submitted.

	Males.	Females.	Total.
Number of patients at the commencement of the year, ...	215	210	425
Admitted during the year, ...	251	173	424
Whole number treated, ...	466	383	849
Discharged, ...	227	176	403
Remaining November 30th, 1853, . .	239	207	446
Average number resident during the year, . .			423
Discharged, recovered, ...	95	74	169
much improved, . . .	11	10	21
improved, ...	26	19	45
unimproved, ...	76	53	129
Died, ...	19	20	39
	227	176	403

Statistics of the Asylum, from its opening, January 16th, 1843, to December 1st, 1853.

Total number of admissions, ...		3,923
" " discharges, ...		3,477
" " discharged recovered, ...		1,625
" much improved, . . .		55
" improved, ...		598
" unimproved, ...		753
" " died, ...		446

Ages of those admitted, and of those discharged recovered, during the year ending November 30th, 1853.

AGE	Admitted.			Discharged recovered.		
	Males.	Females.	Total.	Males.	Females.	Total.
From 10 to 20, - - -	23	12	35	13	6	19
" 20 to 30, - - -	80	48	128	23	25	48
" 30 to 40, - - -	59	51	110	18	24	42
" 40 to 50, - - -	44	39	83	20	10	30
" 50 to 60, - - -	28	15	43	16	5	21
" 60 to 70, - - -	10	6	16	2	3	5
" 70 to 80, - - -	7	2	9	3	1	4
Total, - - - - -	251	173	424	95	74	169

PROBABLE CAUSE OF DERANGEMENT.

	Males.	Females.	Total.
Intemperance and vice,	61	3	64
Masturbation,	56	1	57
Spiritual rappings,	10	4	14
Puerperal,	..	15	15
Domestic trouble,	5	25	30
Change of life,	..	11	11
Dyspepsia and constipation,	13	55	18
Defective training,	2	2	4
Grief,	6	11	16
Malaria,	3	3	6
Phthisis,	6	3	9
Hereditary predisposition,	4	..	4
Fatigue and anxiety,	..	10	10
Predisposition from previous attack,	9	8	17
Epilepsy,	6	..	6
Business perplexities,	12	..	12
Menstrual irregularities,		17	17
Injuries of head,	5	1	6
Old age,	3	1	4
Religious excitement,	3	2	5
Want and destitution,	3	5	8
Want of occupation,	1	..	1
Seduction,	..	3	3
Disappointment in love,	2	4	6
Excessive venery,	4	..	4
Miscarriages,	..	3	3
Chorea,	1	..	1
Fright,	1	..	1

PROBABLE CAUSE OF DERANGEMENT.—(Continued.)

	Males.	Females.	Totals.
Disappointed expectations,	1	..	1
Loss of sleep,	6	5	11
Measles,	..	1	1
Erysipelas,	.	2	2
Coup de soliel,	1	..	1
Disease of heart,	..	1	1
Disease of ear,	1	..	1
Tumor in brain,	..	1	1
Remorse,	1	1	2
Child bearing,	..	2	2
Pleuritis,	1	..	1
Pneumonia,	1	..	1
Congestion of lungs,	1	..	1
Intemperance of father,	2	..	2
Neuralgia,	..	1	1
Loss of property,	1	..	1
Novel reading,	..	2	2
Deafness,	..	1	1
Hysteria,	..	3	3
Scrofula,	1	..	1
Pregnancy,	..	5	5
Chronic diarrhœa,	1	..	1
Acute rheumatism,	..	1	1
Excessive depletion,	..	1	1
Congenital imbecility,	1	..	1
Unascertained,	16	9	25
Total,	251	173	424

Duration of insanity, previous to admission, of the one hundred and sixty-nine cases discharged recovered.

	WELL.		USUAL HEALTH.		
	Male.	Female.	Male.	Female.	Total.
Under 1 week,	12	6	..	..	18
" 1 month,	15	6	..	..	21
" 2 months,	10	9	..	..	19
3 "	5	10	2	..	17
4 "	4	1	..	..	5
5	2	2	..	..	4
6	4	5	1	..	10
7	..	2	..	..	2

From the Boston Medical and Surgical Journal.

Glucosis—its Treatment. By Geo. J. Ziegler, M.D.

A recent number of the Journal contains a description of a case of diabetes, and some interesting remarks on it and its treatment, and more especially with the sesqui-carb. of ammonia.

The view of the pathology of this peculiar affection, which limits the primary derangement to the stomach, is one, however, which does not seem to be strictly in accordance with the more recent investigations on the subject, as it is now well known that this organ is not the only one concerned in the healthy evolution of saccharine matter, but that the liver is also actively engaged in the elaboration of the same material. When, however, it is generated in undue quantities, from the excessive or morbid action of the two organs thus principally concerned in its healthy production, it does not necessarily follow that they are primarily affected, but it may be, rather, that they are thus forced into an undue and more exclusive physiological effort, in consequence of an antecedent deficiency in, or a previous deranged condition of the blood, which furnishes these, as well as the other organs, with the materials and elements for their nutrient and functional operations, and this supply being probably in such cases disproportionate, exclusive and exalted action results. Hence, seemingly, it is to this fluid that attention should be specially and primarily directed for the discovery of the fundamental aberration. When, however this saccharine substance is thus produced in abnormal quantities, its elimination from the economy, by those great emunctories, the kidneys, is a purely conservative process; and, further, this latter is now known to be frequently occurring, even under ordinary circumstances, if there should happen to be a disproportionate relation between the normal production of this material and the aeration of the blood, either directly or indirectly, from deficient innervation, or otherwise, as it then appears in the renal fluid and is thus expelled, while frequently when in excessive quantities other secretions as well as the general system are more or less charged with it.

The proximate state or glucosic diathesis being thus, it is believed, general, instead of local, it appears to be entitled to a more comprehensive and expressive designation, and therefore, in accordance with such views and medical nomenclature, and to indicate more definitely its nature and extensive relations, I have in a former paper, denominated it, as above, *glucosis*, from glucus, sweet, glucose or grape sugar being the product; the gastric, hepatic, renal and other concomitant affections but subsequent and secondary or tertian states or *effects*.

It is not, however, the design in this article to specially discuss the pathology of this peculiar affection, except so far as it seems necessary for present purposes; but rather, to more particularly invite attention to that all-important subject, its treatment, which must necessarily, however, be based on correct principles only deducible from just views of the former. Therefore, as connected with this, and to more clearly expose those which seem to be of fundamental importance, some of such will be briefly noticed. In the first place, then, respecting the nature of this aberration, which is now pretty generally considered to be of a more purely chemical character, and the result of an undue exaltation of a special chemico-vital process; and, hence, secondly, its treatment has mostly been based on chemical principles. These views have been sustained by therapeutic experience, as it has been found that usually the most efficient agents for its prevention and modification, are those which possess the common property of azotization, or in containing more or less nitrogen. Still, the fact respecting the compound and complex nature of the agents thus employed, and the difficulty and even improbability of their decomposition, or sufficiently so to yield their nitrogen, has been too completely overlooked, and therefore hygienically they could be useful only in preventing further saccharine production, though as asserted not even so positively, whilst therapeutically they were still less, and more indirectly efficient.

Again, in consequence of such views, the treatment has too frequently been thus chemically limited, to the too great exclusion of the more positively vital. In the case reported however, the relative importance of these principles was generally recognized, as will be seen by the two indications given, viz: one for hygienic, the other for therapeutic measures, the latter of a two-fold character, and which, though in the main unobjectionable, still it is belived, might be usefully extended. This is presented by Dr. Jewett as follows: "The next indication appears to be to introduce into the stomach a highly-*azotized substance*, and at the same time a *diffusable stimulant*, to exalt, if possible, that organ." He then adds, "both of which ends appear likely to be attained by *ammonia*." In accordance with these indications the sesqui-carb. of ammonia was administered, but without the desired effect, notwithstanding its peculiar constitution, the powerful chemical properties ascribed to it, and the fact that it has been thus employed with asserted success.

The apparent discrepancy between the remedial influence of this agent at one time, and its failure at another, may, however, it is believed, be explicable on general principles, connected with its constitution, chemical affinities and medicinal properties, and their relation to the nature of the affection and material under consideration, as it undoubtedly is very valuable in numerous instances, but of which in this particular one, except under certain circumstances, and then only indirectly and to a limited extent, there is very great doubt. This will be more clear from a slight examination of the principles upon which the remedial influence of this agent depends. These are two-fold, viz: first through its constituent elements, or chemically; and second, by virtue of its stimulant property, or, for brevity and contradistinction, vitally. The abeyance of the former and activity only of the latter property of this agent, in the glucosic affection particularly, though sufficiently apparent from the constitution and relations of the ammonia and sugar, may be still more clearly exhibited by a very general retrospect thereof. This will show that the former already possesses an abundance, and its due proportion of one of these elements, viz: hydrogen, the affinity for which must be active to prevent the formation or cause the decomposition of the latter, which it is well known

is a compound of carbon, hydrogen and oxygen, in nearly equal proportions. The constituent elements of the ammonia, however, are less, both
in their number and proportions, consisting of two only, nitrogen and
hydrogen; thus (NH_3); but if the elements of the acid to form its salt
above mentioned, be added, they will be greater in the former respect;
thus the carbon and oxygen of the carbonic acid, (CO_2) neces ary to the
constitution of the carbonate of ammonia. These are, of course, merely
general remarks, designed rather to exhibit the *elements* than their equivalent proportions, the latter not being esteemed strictly essential to the
argument. The nitrogen, therefore, in the ammonia, having its full supply of the element hydrogen, and *vice versa*, and the affinities of the
carbon and oxygen in the carbonic acid being also satiated, and the two
thus aggregately combined in the salt, their several and mutual affinities
are necessarily in these respects entirely neutralized; consequently there
could be little or no affinitive action between these elements in the ammonia and those in the sugar. This slight consideration of chemical
principles, therefore, exhibits the fact, that this salt of ammonia, or itself
alone, cannot be very useful chemically as a remedial agent for preventing
the formation, or decomposing this saccharine substance after it is
formed; and, hence, a very important therapeutical indication is thus
entirely unfilled and lost.

In those cases, however, in which the state of the system, giving rise
to the excessive evolution of saccharine matter, is dependent on local or
general debility, the more purely stimulant or vital properties of ammonia, properly aided, may in some instances be sufficiently powerful to
improve the systemic energies and correct the more immediate deranged
condition. The want of success, therefore, with this agent, does not
seem to have been in consequence of the incorrect interpretation of the
indications, but because it is incompetent to fulfill them.

The principles thus cursorily noticed not only exhibit some of the deficiencies in the present plan of treatment of this glucosic condition, but
inductively point towards those principles which seemingly promise to
lead with great certainty to such correct conclusions as to more positively
indicate the true and only reliable hygienic and therapeutic means.

In the first place then, the derangement to be prevented or eradicated,
is one in which a substance of a definite chemical nature is elaborated,
composed, as before stated, of the elements carbon, hydrogen and oxygen.
This saccharine material is now known, however, to be a true physiological product, and only connected with a morbid condition when produced in excessive or deficient quantity, or not normally disintegrated.
For this latter process, it requires certain other chemical elements, or, as
mostly believed, only an additional quantity of one of its own elements
from the atmosphere, viz., oxygen. It is therefore reasonable to infer
that, in a state of derangement with the excessive production or non-
destruction of this material, this physiological process is modified or accelerated in consequence of a deficiency of one or both of these elements, an excess of the saccharine, or that the morbid influence is sufficiently great to overpower and destroy the usual chemico-vital affinities.
Two indications, independent of the hygienic, are therefore presented,

viz., first, to supply a due proportion of the chemical element or elements required, and, second, to exalt and regulate the vital energies sufficiently to induce the healthy organic metamorphic processes of formation and decomposition. To determine what the former are, it is only requisite to refer to such as are active in the normal destruction of this saccharine matter. It is now almost universally considered that aeration of the blood is effected by its oxidation: or in other words, that the oxygen of the atmospheric air, directly or indirectly, unites with, causes modifications of, and disintegrates the various materials contained in that fluid; and that the other principal atmospheric element, oxygen, is mostly passive, or a mere diluent of the former. When, however, this exalted glucosic condition supervenes, and the saccharine matter is evolved in undue quantities, the principle, on the other hand, is almost as generally recognized that it is in consequence of the deficiency of this agent, nitrogen; hence the treatment has been directed to its introduction, and experience has amply testified to its propriety and necessity. Now, as I have heretofore stated, I believe that in the physiological as well as in the therapeutical, which must necessarily be based on the former processes, both of these elements are more or less essential. Hence, therapeutically, the correct principle seems to be, to introduce into the economy a substance composed of such elements, oxygen and nitrogen, and which by readily undergoing decomposition will supply them in a *nascent* state, thus exciting the more active play of the mutual affinities between them and the constituent elements of the sugar to prevent its formation or cause its decomposition, and the subsequent production of those substances so essential to the healthy condition and functions of the combined organs and parts of the body. Some of these affinitive re-actions and relations may be thus cursorliy noticed. The elements oxygen and nitrogen, (NO) and those of sugar $(C.H.O)$; the hydrogen and nitrogen for ammonia (NH_3), carbon and nitrogen for cyanogen (C_2H), and oxygen superadded for cyanic acid (C_yO), the two aggregately, cyanate of ammonia, which with the addition of HO is considered to be isomeric with urea. Besides these, the other associations of carbon and oxygen, and hydrogen and oxygen, for carbonic acid (CO_2) and water (HO), may be mentioned. It will thus be seen that the agent ammonia, which for curative purposes is introduced in its compound state into the system, may be actually generated therein from its elements, principally derived from the material thereof, and all its primary as well as secondary advantages thus more directly obtained.

Independent, however, of these chemical relations, the other highly-important indication still, to a certain extent, exists, viz: to prevent and rectify that diathesis or proximate state, giving rise to the excessive production of saccharine matter. This can be more immediately fulfilled by those hygienic and thrapeutic measures which tend to exalt and regulate the vital processes, among the latter of which are, as is justly observed, the diffusible stimulants. The fulfillment of these compound chemical and vital indications seems, therefore, to require a great diversity of agents; yet, following out the course naturally indicated with regard to the deficiencies, physiological processes and aberrations, it is evident that it requires but a simple and more purely chemical agent composed of the definite elements specified, though possessing superior and unique general physiological properties. Now, fortunately, there is a known agent thus constituted and endowed. This obviously is the protoxide of nitrogen, or nitrous oxide (NO), the particular constitution, properties and general applications of which, have been, for present purposes, sufficiently enlarged upon in my former papers; and I am induced to refer to it again in the present relation, only from a sense of duty and a strong conviction of its usefulness in this glucosic state, believing that it not only answers, but will fulfill, all the indications therein required. Still, though I have thus hastily glanced at some of the reasons for this opinion, I do not wish it understood that it now depends exclusively upon mere inference or speculation, as the constitution and general stimulant property of this agent is well known, and I have proved to my satisfaction, and so stated in published articles, so that others might have the benefit of, and test the correctness of such observations, that it does undergo decomposition in the blood, removes sugar therefrom, forms urea, which is deficient in this affection, regulates the renal as well as general secretion, modifies the action of the liver and alimentary canal, corrects organic aberration, and speedily restores the general hæmatosic and vital equilibrium. Therefore, though I have never had an opportunity of treating the exalted glucosic state, known by the indefinite term "diabetes," as it is somewhat rare, I have treated successfully, with the agent recommended, those minor conditions attended with the moderate saccharine contamination of the renal fluid.

It is also probable, from the consideration of the physiological disintegration of this saccharine material, that oxygen, superadded to, and inhaled with the atmospheric air, might exercise a favorably-modifying influence over its production and the general affection. Either of these agents, by surcharging liquids with them, may also be introduced into the circulation through the stomach or other parts of the alimentary canal.

In conclusion, and in relation to such therapeutic investigations, it will be proper to state that, when all other means fail, except occasional and accidental ones, in preventing or correcting this or any other biological aberration, it is believed to be not only justifiable, but the duty of medical men to resort to a judicious system of experimentation, to endeavor to discover thereby, some more certain and reliable hygienic and therapeutic means. And first, this should be done with those substances to which induction points, which reason selects, and of which judgment approves; particularly if, within themselves, they are exceedingly powerful, yet are capable of being so carefully employed as to avoid all danger of further deranging the organism, and thus of more speedily accelerating the dissolutive processes.

Philadelphia, March 6th, 1854.

Correspondence of the Boston Med. Journal.

Alcohol in Medical Practice.

MESSRS. EDITORS,—In the Journal of February 8th, I notice some remarks by Dr. Gilman, of South Deerfield, on "Alcoholic Liquors in the Practice of Medicine," which, by your leave, I wish to examine. He says "there is no subject upon which the whole community, including the medical faculty, so much need light, as they do on the proper medicinal use of alcohol." I agree that *more light* is much needed on every subject connected with the science of medicine; but I think as much probably exists in regard to the use of alcohol, as is known in regard to many other equally useful and remedial agents. As an agent of value, it has been recommended and extolled by many to whom medical science owes much. He proposes three questions for discussion, two of which I will notice.

1. "Are alcoholic liquors indispensably necessary in the practice of medicine?" I think they are. Alcohol is a diffusible stimulus. It increases the force and activity of the nervous system, when depressed by various *depressing* poisons; and, so far as my experience goes, strengthened by the recorded testimony of many able observers, it does this more efficiently than any other known remedy. The bite of the rattlesnake, so deadly and rapid in its effects if not quickly counteracted, so far as I can learn, is not so amenable to any other treatment as the "alcoholic;" and is enough, I think, if there were no other instances, to establish the fact, that alcoholic liquors are "indispensably necessary in the practice of medicine." But there are other instances where they are necessary. Who has not seen their good effects in cases of fever accompanied with great prostration of the nervous forces? In *delirium tremens*—not *delirium ebriosorum*—they are at times surely indispensable. Solly, in his work on the Brain, page 280, says, "The plan of treatment which I have found on the whole most successful in *true* delirium tremens, is to give the stimulus which the patient prefers from being most accustomed to: this is usually porter and gin in the hospitals; brandy or wine, or both together, in private practice. And revolting as it is to our feelings as moral beings to pour in the very poisons which, by their *habitual* use, have reduced the man to the level of the brute, still as medical men it is our *duty* to *preserve* life by those means which we *know* are capable of doing so." The italics are my own. It is not "indispensably necessary" for me to instance other cases (for it would occupy too much space), in which alcoholic liquors have been used with profit by almost every member of the profession.

2. "If they are necessary, to what extent?" I am unable to say to what extent. As well might we ask to what extent we should use opium, calomel or any other remedy, or to what extent bleed. We should use them *all* whenever necessary, and at no other time, and to the extent the necessities as each case require, and no further; we should be ruled by judgment, and not by *prejudice*. Dr. Gilman declares he has not used alcoholic liquors in his practice for "five years past." Possibly in a practice of even *five* years they might not be required; but if they should, they ought by all means to be used, and not discarded because when used as a *beverage* they *invariably* do harm. If this is the reason why some do not not use alcoholic liquors in their practice, I must say that it is contrary to that wise discriminative policy, that should ever characterize the physician.

In the above remarks, I do not wish to be understood as advocating the use of alcoholic liquors as a beverage; for when thus used they truly "out-venom all the worms of Nile," and every good citizen should feel in duty bound to use every effort, consistent with reason and common sense, to prevent their baneful effects. But while we do this, as medical men, we ought by all means to use everything known to be of value.

Carthage, Ill., March 19, 1854.   ' GEO. W. HALL.

From the Boston Medical Journal.

Raising Leeches in France.

[The Paris correspondent of the *New York Daily Times* furnishes the following interesting information respecting a successful mode of propagating and raising the leech in France :]

The raising and propagation of leeches has for many years been a necessity in France, for the supply furnished by her marshes gave out thirty years ago. Out of her abundance she used to export; and now she is forced to make up her deficiency from abroad. Other countries have in their turn been exhausted — Italy, Germany, and Spain; and of late, certain districts of Asia have been laid under contribution. Still, all over the world, the yield has been seriously diminished, and prices have risen to such a point that the poor cannot pay them; and the hospitals even are alarmed. The Academy of Medicine has voted prizes to persons who would discover methods of propagation; and lately a sum was placed in the hands of the Prefect of the Seine, to make experiments with a model leechery in the suburbs, A. M. Borne has just sent to the Academy an account of his establishment at Rambouillet, where he seems to have met with extraordinary success in encouraging the reproduction of his "pupils," as he calls them. They are fed three times a year; they bury themselves in the earth late in the autumn, and pass the winter in a state of torpor. They mate early in the spring — on St. Valentine's day probably — and lay their cocoons in May, to hatch in September. The young ones are fed upon the "less substantial blood of calves." The are extremely voracious, and in two years weigh ten times their primitive volume. M. Borne has built conveniences for the reception of the cocoons, and for their artificial incubation. By care and tenderness he has succeeded thus far in preventing any epidemic or sudden mortality in his reservoirs. The leech is very apt to be carried off by sudden disorders, and history mentions the loss of a colony of 18,000 in one winter; of the destruction of 60,000 by a hard frost, and of the consumption of 200,000 in Soloque, by a flock of wild geese. M. Borne has taken extraordinary precautions against any invasions of the sort. In the middle of his ponds is a light-house or look-out, where a man is constantly stationed, armed with guns and other means of defence; the edges of the ponds are guarded in such a way as to keep out all aquatic enemies, such as water-rats, moles, and frogs; traps are set for the trochètes, glossiphonies, hydrophiles, and dytisques, which nourish a traditional animosity toward all leeches. Marauders and poachers are also keenly watched. In short, M. Borne hopes soon to be in a position to furnish France a supply sufficient to render any further importation useless; and later he expects even to be able to export for his own account.

EDITORIAL AND MISCELLANEOUS.

Irregularity of the Mails.

We often receive information that subscribers fail to receive all their numbers. We assure them that they are faithfully mailed, and were it not from our knowledge of the similar experience of other periodicals, we should be astonished at the carelessness, which in the post-office department, sends amiss so many printed documents. We shall do everything in *our* power to have the journals go safely, but the imperfections of the P. O. Department are beyond our reach. If subscribers who fail to receive all their numbers will notify us, we will make good their deficiency.

Death of Dr. Briggs.

We regret to learn of the death of Dr. J. Briggs, of Schoolcraft. Although we had but little personal acquaintance with him, yet by reputation we understand him to have been an ornament to the profession, one whose loss is deeply felt in the western part of the State, and whose social as well as scientific excellence was of priceless value to community.

Annual Report of the Managers of the N. Y. State Lunatic Asylum.

We have received this pamphlet and have selected some tabular statistics from it, which will be of value to those who are interested in studying the nature of insanity.

New Orleans Medical and Surgical Journal.

The death of the former editor has caused this journal to pass into the editorial care of Dr. Bennet Dowler. Mrs. Hester, the widow of the late editor, is proprietress. We trust that the gallant men of the South will give that journal a good support.

Address to the Graduates of the Kentucky School of Medicine. By R. J. BRECKINBRIDGE, Professor of Materia Medica, and Clinical Medicine.

This document is full of enthusiasm for medical science, as Kentucky documents always are. It makes an important distinction which ought to be more thought of among those who clamor about what they call the uncertainty of medicine. The distinction is this: The *nature of the effects* of medicines, as a general rule, are certain, but the question whether those effects will prove superior or inferior to the opposing effects of the disease, is to be decided anew in every new case; it is a question of relative power. The situation of the physician is like that of a soldier. The action of his weapons is known, and sure, but whether that action will be sufficient in a given case to beat the enemy, depends upon the enemy's relative force and strength of position. This is an important thought for those who talk and think vaguely on medical un-certainty. The only fault of the address is that it puts it forth too modestly, and claims too little for the real strength of its position.

Health and Mortality of Memphis.

A pamphlet by CHARLES T. QUINTARD, A. M., M. D., Professor of Physio-logy and Pathological Anatomy in the Memphis Medical College.

This report contains some useful hints and statistics. The population of the city is about 15,000, and the mortality for the year only about two per cent. There was scarcely any yellow fever. Some important statistics and remarks respecting the prevalence of consumption in warm climates, may be found in our selections.

Peninsular State Medical Society.

At the meeting held at Ann Arbor, the following resolution was passed.

Resolved, That an assessment of one dollar be made upon each member of this Society, to defray the expenses involved in its operations.

Members who were not present at the meeting, are requested to send their assessment to the Treasurer, Prof. S. H. Douglass, Ann Arbor, by mail.

E. ANDREWS, M. D., Secretary.   H. TAYLOR, M. D., President.

Lawrence on the Eye.

This is a new edition, edited by Isaac Hays, M.D. It contains many im-provements and additions over former issues, and at the same time an unnecessary increase of bulk has been avoided, by leaving out such general details respecting inflammation, etc., as are to be found in all our common text-books on surgery: Among the improvements are new methods of illuminating and examining the retina of the living eye, so as to diagnose its pathological conditions. The whole work contains nine hundred and fifty pages. It is already widely known from former editions, and is obtained by all who pretend to keep anywhere near up to the times in the complex surgery of the eye.

Published by Blanchard and Lea.

Prof. Dunglison's Charge to the Graduates of Jefferson Medical College, Philadelphia.

This address is marked by a high, liberal tone, and a beautiful and spirited style.

THE

PENINSULAR

JOURNAL OF MEDICINE

AND THE COLLATERAL SCIENCES.

VOL. I.	JUNE, 1854.	NO. XII.

ORIGINAL COMMUNICATIONS.

ART. 1.—*Proceedings of the Peninsular State Medical Society,*
Continued from page 513.

Dr. Shank, of Lansing, gave an instructive case in which he had
performed the operation of *Paracentesis thoracis*, and with entire success, notwithstanding the constitution of the patient was exhausted to
such a degree as to promise but little for any kind of treatment.

Prof. Denton remarked, that he was much pleased to find that the
operation which Dr. Shank had performed was coming more extensively
into use. He believed that there were many cases like that related by
Dr. S. in which life might just as well be saved as not, but in which
the patients were suffered to die on account of the groundless fear which
surgeons had of the operation. In cases where the effusion was purulent, he thought the evil of allowing air to enter the cavity was greatly
exaggerated. Such effusions frequently ulcerated into the bronchial
tubes, and were discharged by expectoration, a mode which necessarily
admitted air to the pleural sack, and yet these cases frequently did well.

He deemed the operation to be one which ought to be more frequently resorted to.

Dr. J. Andrews, of Paw Paw, gave an account of a case of a large opening into the cavity of the chest caused by a gunshot wound, where there was a great destruction of the anterior wall. The patient survived, and after the immense suppuration necessarily consequent on the nature of such a blowing to pieces of the tissues, the wound healed. It opened several times afterwards, but finally closed permanently up, and the patient is now well.

Dr. E. Andrews then offered the following paper, which was read by its title, and a copy requested for the use of the Society:

Vital Capacity. By E. ANDREWS, M.D.

The following statistics respecting the amount of air inspired and expired in forced respiration, are offered to the Society, not from any supposition that they will lead to valuable results in the direction claimed by those who proposed this means of diagnosis; but because statistical observations of this and other kinds are always worth preserving in a permanent form, often being valuable as material for reasoning in quite different and unexpected channels.

It is well known that Mr. Hutchinson, of England, in a memoir before the Statistical Society of London, presented an account of an extensive series of experiments to show, that in health, there is a certain law regulating the amount of air which a person can draw into and expel from his lungs in forced respiration. It has also been claimed that a remarkable diminution of this vital capacity, as it is called, unless it can be accounted for by obvious causes, is a very early and alarming sign of approaching phthisis.

He stated that the variation of vital capacity was not in the ratio of the bulk nor weight, but of the height, about eight cubic inches being added to the capacity for every additional inch in height of the person between five and six feet. It is claimed that this law of increase is so regular that from the individual's height, it is possible to tell what his vital capacity ought to be; and that it is cause to suspect consumption if one falls short of the regular proportion, without some obvious cause of the deficiency.

I took with the spirometer the vital capacity of one hundred and nineteen persons, noting the age and height of each. They were nearly all males. Hutchinson's observations were made upon 1923 males. I have thrown my observations into a tabular form and added the column of Hutchinson's observations by way of comparison.

Height.				Vital capacity as observed by me.	By Hutchinson.
ft.	in.	ft.	in.	Cubic in.	Cubic in.
5	0	to 5	1		
5	1	" 5	2	143	174
5	2	" 5	3		177
5	3	" 5	4	165	189
5	4	" 5	5	183	195
5	5	" 5	6	209	201
5	6	" 5	7	234	214
5	7	" 5	8	227	220
5	8	" 5	9	237	228
5	9	" 5	10	240	237
5	10	" 5	11	244	246
5	11	" 6		264	247
6	0	" 6	1	286	259
6	1	" 6	2	316	

From this table, it may be seen, that the increase of vital capacity is much greater with the increase of height, according to my observations, than according to Hutchinson's, his increase being 8 cubic inches for every additional inch in height, and mine 13 cubic inches. The short persons upon whom I experimented, fell below the standard, which he establishes as the average for their height, and the tall ones went beyond it; while the average for persons between five and six feet in height, corresponds with his exactly.

The grand average of all the heights observed, compared with a corresponding average of all the 119 vital capacities correspond nearly with the capacity given for that height in his table. The average height of all the 119 persons tested by me, was 5 feet 8 inches; the average vital capacity was 240 cubic inches, while the capacity for that height in Hutchinson's tables, is 234 cubic inches; a difference of only six cubic inches. On the whole, taking a large number of persons together, I think their vital capacities will give averages remarkably corresponding with his tables; but if separate individuals be taken, a terrible discrepancy is found. Thus of the persons whom I observed between 5 ft. 4 in. and 5 ft. 5 in. in height, the greatest capacity was 250 cubic inches, and the least was 160, a difference of 90 cubic inches — yet the less capacious subject is in perfect health to this day. Of those between 5 ft. 5 in. and 5 ft. 6 in. the greatest capacity was 250 cubic inches, and the least 180, being a difference of seventy. Between 5 ft. 6 in. and 5 ft. 7 in. the greatest capacity was 290 cubic inches, and the least one which was healthy, was 225 cubic inches, a difference of 65 cubic inches. Between 5 ft. 7 in. and 5 ft. 8 in. the greatest was 262 cubic inches, and the least 131, a variation of 131 cubic inches. In the next inch the greatest capacity was 300 cubic inches, and the smallest healthy one was 180, a difference of 120 cubic inches. Between 5 ft. 9 in. and 5 ft. 10 in. the individual variation reached 110 cubic inches. In the succeeding inch, the greatest capacity reached the enormous measure of 350 cubic inches, and the smallest was only 170. Both persons were in perfect health apparently, and yet there was a difference of 180 cubic inches in their capacity. Other departures from the standard were numerous. One person six feet two inches in height, blew 340 cubic inches, and one person only six feet, expelled at one expiration, 360 cubic inches.

From these data, I am inclined to adopt the opinion of others who maintain that this instrument cannot be relied on for diagnosis except where the previous vital capacity of the individual is known, so as to decide whether there is really a diminution going on. At the same time it must be confessed that diseases of the lungs exert a remarkable influence on the capacity. But few such fell in my way in circumstances to be conveniently experimented upon. One person having the asthma, could reach only 150 cubic inches, although he was five and a half feet high, and consequently should have expired 234 cubic inches. Another person who had some symptoms of consumption, blew but 180 cubic inches, although he was five feet eight inches in height. It is proper to state, however, that although nearly a year and a half has since elapsed, the unfavorable symptoms have not at all increased. Another man of the same height, and having also symptoms of consumption, blew but 178 inches, whereas from his stature, he ought if he were sound, to have expired about 236 inches. Only three females were in the list, all of them vigorous and free from any consumptive appearance. The most note-worthy circumstance respecting them, was their small vital capacity, compared with males of the same height, a fact referred to in the books. The average height of these females was 5 ft. 4 inches, and their average capacity 144 cubic inches, whereas the average capacity of males of the same height is 193, a difference of 49 cubic inches.

Dr. Brodie presented a bill of $7,40, for printing circulars and for postage in calling the meetings of the Society. Dr. Brodie offered the following resolution which was adopted:

Resolved, That the account be paid by the Treasurer, and that the balance of the funds in the hands of the Treasurer, be paid over to the Proprietor of the Peninsular Journal of Medicine; also, that the proceedings of the Society be published in that Journal, and that the Editor be the Committee of Publication.

Dr. Brodie then offered the following Resolutions, which were unanimously adopted:

Whereas, Various malignant attacks from different directions, have been made upon the Medical Department of our State University, and as we believe, with the view and for the purpose of lowering its standing and detracting from its just merit,

Therefore, *Resolved,* That we disclaim all fellowship for such motive, and that that Institution is conducted on a principle and with a zeal and ability highly gratifying to this Society.

Resolved, That we regard the Organ of this Society, the Peninsular Medical Journal, as quite indispensable to the necessities of the Profession of this State; that we are fully satisfied with its management, and that we *will* sustain it at all hazards.

On motion, Dr. E. Hall, of Mt. Clemens, was unanimously elected an honorary member of the Society.

It was moved and carried that Dr. M. K. Taylor, of Brooklyn, be continued as the Committee on Meteorology with power to choose colleagues.

It was moved and carried, that Dr. Murray, of Niles, be a Committee to report on the powers and uses of Veratrum Viride.

The following gentlemen were chosen Delegates to the meeting of the National Medical Association at St. Louis:

> Prof. A. B. Palmer, of Chicago.
> Dr. J. Beech, of Coldwater.
> Dr. E. Batwell, of Detroit.
> Dr. W. Brodie,   "
> Dr. C. M. Stockwell, of Port Huron.
> Dr. E. Andrews, of Ann Arbor.

It was moved and carried that Delegates be empowered to choose substitutes in case of being prevented from going in person.

The following members were chosen Censors for the ensuing year:

> Dr. J. Beech, of Coldwater.
> Dr. J. Andrews, of Paw Paw.
> Dr. W. Brownell, of Utica.

It was moved and carried that a vote of thanks be tendered to the officers for their services.

On motion, the Society adjourned to meet at the time of Medical Commencement, in March 1855.

APPENDIX.

Corresponednce between Chancellor Tuppan and the Peninsular State Medical Society.

ANN ARBOR, MICH., March 30, 1854.

DEAR SIR: The members of the State Medical Society have listened with great satisfaction to your Address to the graduates of the Medical Department of the University, and in accordance with a vote of the Society, we would respectfully solicit a copy for publication with its transactions. \

H. TAYLOR, M. D., President.

E. ANDREWS, M. D. Secretary.

To HENRY P. TAPPAN, D. D., President of the University of Michigan.

———

UNIVERSITY OF MICHIGAN,
April 31, 1854.

Gentlemen,—I cannot well refuse the request of the State Medical Society, presented by them through you, that a copy of my Address to the Graduating Class of the College of Medicine and Surgery, be furnished for publication. The fact that a body so respectable and so fully qualified to judge of the propriety of publishing the Address, makes this request, relieves me as an unprofessional man, from the hesitation I might otherwise very naturally feel.

I am very Respectfully,

Yours, &c.,   HENRY P. TAPPAN.

To Dr. H. TAYLOR, President, and E. ANDREWS, Secretary of the State Medical Society.

———

Address to the Graduates of the Medical Department of the University of Michigan, at the Annual Commencement in March 1854. By HENRY P. TAPPAN, President of the University.

The learned professions have their origin in the wants of mankind. Our natural rights — the rights of life, liberty, property, opinion, conscience, character, and the pursuit of happiness. Were there no organized society and government, each individual would maintain them for himself as he best could; but under organized society and government, each individual commits them to the protection of the common law. Hence, the principle of government and legislation, based upon the more general principle of ethics, and the determination of questions of individual and corporate rights amid the complications and collisions of society, require the exclusive attention and devotion of a competent body of men. Thus arises the legal profession.

But man is a being placed not merely under human government, and holding merely earthly relations; in his conscience, he recognizes a Divine government likewise, and, by his religious belief, he is connected with immortal interests and destinies. Hence, the inculcation of religious truths, exhortations to religious duties, and the conduct of an appropriate religious worship, require another body of men who should give their exclusive attention and devotion to these momentous offices. And thus, again, arises the Clerical profession.

Once more. Man is a being whose corporeal organization, intimately connected as it is both with his physical well-being and enjoyment, and his intellectual and spiritual life, is liable to various derangements which tend to impair his activities, to destroy his bodily and mental sanity, and to produce premature death. Hence, the adequate knowledge of his physical structure in all its relations, of the adverse influences which may assail it, of the laws of health, and of remedial appliances, require, also, the exclusive attention and devotion of still another body of men. And thus arises the Medical profession. These three professions having once come into being, can never become extinct, and must ever accompany the history of humanity.

These professions are called the "learned professions," for the very obvious reason, that many other professions, although either directly or indirectly, demanding the aid of learning, may, nevertheless, be prosecuted according to certain rules of art provided by the learning of others; while these, in their very nature, presume no mean acquaintance with science and literature, and an ability to conduct original investigations.

Were it within the scope of the present occasion, it would be easy to illustrate this distinction in reference to all the learned professions. It is given to us now to speak only of the Medical profession.

Since I do not belong to this profession myself, it can hardly be expected that I should treat of it so appositely as one of its erudite and experienced members.

The observations, however, upon which I shall venture, will lie in a region not wholly foreign to me; and if I, at all, trespass into other regions, it will be under those general points of view which are supposed. to belong to all men of science, whatever be the particular determination of their pursuits. Besides, the learned professions have so many interests and subjects in common, that they may be said to constitute one great fraternity, and to hold the privilege, if not bound to exercise the the duty of watching over, aiding, and inspiring each other. Philosophy, ethics, literature, scientific investigations and philanthropy, belong to them all; and he is the greatest in his particular profession, who is the most distinguished in these.

Permit me, then, to attempt to point out in what respects the Medical is a learned profession, and thence to sketch the proper discipline of the student of Medicine.   \

A Physician, in the strictest sense of the word, should be an educated man; and an educated man cannot entirely neglect any branch of human knowledge. But there are, of course, particular branches of knowledge especially required for particular professions and pursuits Those which belong to the profession of Medicine, are found in the three great divisions of Philosophy, Experimental Science, and Ethics; to which must be added those literary accomplishments common to all educated men.

Aristotle has remarked, that "the Philosopher should end with Medicine, and the Physician begin with philosophy," thus making Medicine the complement of philosophy, and philosophy the propædentic. of Medicine.

The truth of this remark is evident whether we consider the field of enquiry belonging to Medicine as a science, or the objects which it contemplates as an art. As a science, it would be complete if making no attempts to cure disease. Now, in a science, purely, we cannot but perceive its close connection with the most instructive questions in philosophy; and hence, as a science, it would take a high place among the sciences, if it never gave birth to any corresponding art. What is its province as a science? The answer is given in one word,—man. Man is its province — man in his physical constitution, from his first generation to his grave; man in his spiritual constitution; man in the union of the physical and the spiritual, with their reciprocal influences; man in all his relations to the outer world, as a part of nature, and the creation of society; man with ideas and sensibilities which connect him with a future state,—it is man, taken under all these points of view, as an organism which requires certain physical appliances, certain occupations, certain modes of life for his proper development and well-being; and who, under all these points of view, may meet with hostile elements and present the phenomena of disease and pain; that abnormal condition in which the ends of his existence appear more or less frustrated, and by which existence itself, is prematurely terminated.

The mere physiologist investigates the laws of the corporeal structure of man; the mere psychologist, the laws of his being; the mere moralist, the laws of deity; while the physician investigates all these in reference to two special ends;—that he may ascertain the general laws which govern his proper growth, and his proper exercise and enjoyment of all the functions of life; and the sources and forms of all those maladies which may hinder his growth and impair or destroy the functions of life. So far, we say, the Physician pursues a special science, which would be complete in its aims, even if no art of healing ever came into being. The Physician, is, therefore led, necessarily, by his science, into all the subtle questions of biology, metaphysics, psychology, anthopology, and of social, moral, and religious influences. An individual may, indeed, discard all these questions, and take up Medicine as an art prepared to his hand by ignorant empirics, or by the scientific investigations of others; but then he becomes a mere medical mechanic, and cannot in truth be a Physician. The proper study of the science can no more be separated from these regions of thought and enquiry, that it can cease to be occupied with man.

What I have here stated is fully borne out by the whole history of medical science. Galen, with whom medical science properly commences — for Hippocrates can hardly be said to have created a science — formed a theory out of certain biological and cosmological principles—principles more or less metaphysical in their character. His whole system was founded upon a certain theory of the vital functions. He divides them into three classes, the essential, the animal, and the natural; the first having their seat in the heart, the second in the brain, and the third in the liver. Then he introduced the *pneuma*, a most subtle portion of the air as the medium through which the vital forces act. But in addition to this, he introduced the old doctrine of the four elements, fire, air, earth, and water, the hot, cold, dry, and moist, to explain the constitution of animal bodies; the various combination of these elements forming the blood or material, and the semen or formative principle. In the first, the watery and earthy elements predominate; in the second, the fiery and æriform. In the combination of the two for the production of animal bodies, the moist element obtains the predominance. In infancy, there is the greatest predominance in the moist element, but with the advance of years, the dry is supplied more and more, and the flexibility of childhood merges into the rigidity of old age. Eating

and drinking keep up the supply of the moist and the dry; respiration
and the pulsations of the heart, the supply of the cold and hot. These
elements by the organs of the animal economy, are separated into the
finer portions which are assimilated, and into the under which are
ejected. Health consists in the admixture of these elements in proper
proportions, and in the normal condition of the organs which assimilate
them. The predominance of the moist element in the animal economy
is shown in the existence of specific humors or watery portions. The
condition of these humors thus come to afford the signs of disease and
to explain its character. The predisposing cause of all disease Galen
represented as a putrefaction of the humors; the putrefaction of the
mucus producing the quotidian fever; that of the yellow bile, the
tertian; and that of the black bile, the quartan. Inflammation arises
from the passage of the blood into those parts which in their normal
condition do not contain it. When accompanied by the *pneuma* it becomes
a spiritous inflammation in distinction from the other forms caused by the
admixture of the bile on the mucus. The humoral pathology, and the
doctrine of animal spirits during fifteen centuries, reigned supreme in
medical science, and even now may be detected in medical theories.
The individuals who may claim to be the founders of modern medical
science, are Stahl, Hoffman, Boerhaave, Haller, and Cullen. They were
not only men of great and varied learning; but they were all distinguished for philosophical genius. Boerhaave followed the old humoral
pathology most directly. Hoffman entirely departed from it; but Hoffman, Stahl and Cullen, are distinguished for the use they made of the
vital principle. Hoffman maintained that the phenomena of living
bodies cannot be explained by the laws of inanimate matter, but depend
upon the constant action of the vital principles, which he regarded as
emanating from the Deity. Both Van Helmont and Des Cartes, had
taught the influence of immaterial principles upon inert matter. Stahl
concentrated all in the *anima*. This at first generates the body, and
this governs its nutrition and protects it against decay. The anima he
seems to have identified with the soul, assigning it two functions, that
of acting with the mind in the production of the phenomena of consciousness, and that of producing all the phenomena of animal life.
His pathology was founded upon his doctrine of the *anima*. All disturbances of its normal action tended to disease; and the symptoms of
disease were signs of the struggle of the *anima* to regain its tone.
Cullen's system, like Stahl's, was founded upon Hoffman's.

Haller's doctrine of irritability and sensibility has its starting point
in Galen's *pneuma*, and Hoffman's vital principle; for as Galen attributed

the pulsation of the blood to the action of the pneuma upon the heart and arterial system, and the impression of rational objects upon the sensorium to the action of the pneuma upon the brain; and as Hoffman held that the vital principle was accumulated in the brain, and thence conveyed life and energy through the nerves to every part of the body; so Haller assigned the brain and nerves as the seat of sensibility, and the muscular fibre as the seat of irritability. All these theories when nicely analyzed, will give us the common idea, of an immaterial vital force.

We have referred to a few of the most celebrated names in medical science to illustrate what indeed the whole history of medical science can be adduced to illustrate, that philosophical genius and philosophical speculation have not only not been separated from it, but have been engaged in founding and building it up.

The peculiar power of philosophical genius and the peculiar nature of philosophical speculation, are shown in the development of metaphysical ideas relating both to the being of man and the constitution of nature. It is by these ideas that we gain true methods of investigation and observation, the laws of reasoning, and those prophetic conceptions which direct our experiments, and enable us to arrange facts in reference to a definite end. These guiding conceptions may be dim and lead to crude theories, and yet, without them, no predetermined advance can be made in science; but investigation is mere groping in the dark, and discovery an accident. Stahl, who conceived of the anima in physiology, likewise conceived of phlogiston in chemistry; and although phlogiston is now set aside, no one can deny that in the dawn of modern chemistry it answered a most important purpose in systematizing experiment and investigation.

It may safely be affirmed, that without philosophic discipline, no one can be prepared to read intelligently, the history of medical science, or to conduct original investigations. A great genius may overleap the necessity of such a discipline; or rather, by a peculiar energy and clearness of mind, he may make it for himself in his own independent thinking; but such cases form exceptions, and afford no rule to men in general.

When we come to consider the nature of the studies belonging to the Physician, there is one particular, at least, which must forever connect these studies with philosophy, and that is, the reciprocal action of the conditions of the living organism, and the states of the mind which dwells within it. Disease is both corporeal and mental, and the two forms tend to produce each other. Anthropology, or that branch of philosophy which relates to the mutual influences of body and mind and, of course, to the influences of external circumstances through the body upon the mind, and the influence of the mind through the body in modifying these circumstances, must belong, peculiarly, to the Physician. Without a profound knowledge of anthropology, it is hard to conceive how the most formidable forms of disease can be understood as a matter of science, or treated as a matter of the healing art. ·

It is evident, too, that the physical conditions under which man is placed must seem to modify many questions of the deepest interest in ethics, jurisprudence, and religion. Physical predispositions to sin and crime, must be taken into consideration to account for their commission, and to measure their turpitude; and even religious affections, and cases of conscience are not to be viewed independently of natural constitution and morbid physical influences. The investigations of the Physician, therefore, have most important bearings upon the moral and spiritual well-being of individuals and of society. Perhaps in no region of human knowledge is a keen philosophical insight more imperatively demanded in connection with the widest and most accurate observation. In Natural Theology, again, where from the ranks of design in the constitution of the universe, we collect evidence for the beings and attributes of an intelligent creator, the enquiries of the Physician find a necessary and appropriate place. No part of nature exhibit these marks of design with so much clearness and beauty as organic bodies, and of organic bodies the human is the noblest. It is by the study of organisms in general, that the Physician gains clearly the great idea of life and the knowledge of determinate laws of organization; but it is in comparative anatomy, in particular, that the harmony of plan, the unity of design, come forth conspicuously in a gradation of subjects which culminate at last in man. Indeed, not only the living organisms come under his view, but the rock embedded fossil, also, which show, in the untold ages of the past, " the foot-prints of the Creator."

A theory of development applicable to the whole universe, and of which the gradation of animal organism is taken to be an exponent, has been made well nigh a popular speculation by the interesting and clever work of an anonymous author, entitled, " Vestiges of Creation." According to this theory, all the forms of matter, and all the phenomena of action whether physical or mental, are but the developments of certain primordial laws. Creation is identified in its elements and laws. All that exists, exists in different stages of growth; and the different degrees of perfection in both inorganic and organic forms, arise only from the different degrees in which the primordial laws are developed.

The organic grows out of the inorganic, the animal organism out of the vegetable, the higher order of animals out of the lower; and man becomes the culmination of the whole not by separate and peculiar laws, but as the higher development of the same laws. The phenomena of the galvanic battery in the laboratory; the phenomena of animal instinct and sagacity, and the phenomena of the human mind, differ not in kind, but in degree; the brain is only a more perfect galvanic battery; and thought, imagination, sensibility, and volition, are only more subtle, complicated, and beautiful electrical phenomena.

This theory, so philosophical in its pretensions, and so clearly at war with morals and revealed religion, can be met only by more acute investigations and a higher philosophy. It is in vain to ridicule it, to laugh at it; it must be met and fairly overthrown. It is here that we feel, peculiarly, the force of the remark of Aristotle, already referred to, that "the philosopher must end with medicine, (or the studies of the Physician,) and the Physician must begin with philosophy." The united studies of the philosopher and Physician alone can meet the theory of development.

In meeting this theory our first aim must be to reduce it within proper limits, by shewing that the organic cannot be developed from the inorganic, and that life is a distinct and peculiar law; that the animal cannot be developed from the vegetable organism, and that each has its distinct determinative law; that one species cannot be developed from another species, and that each one is limited in generative power to its own sphere: that man, beyond all, is incapable of derivation from a lower order; and, finally, that the phenomena of mind bear no affinity to the phenomena produced by any known physical force.

In the second place, we must enter into the human consciousness as both a distinct and a legitimate field of observation. The veritableness of external phenomena, must depend upon the veritableness of the phenamena of consciousness, since all that we know, we know through consciousness. Again, the laws which govern all our investigations are laws of the thinking power, and hence the criterion of all just conclusions must be sought for within the mind itself. Even he who broaches the theory of development, does so by a certain exercise of the thinking powers; and whether he do so by a legitimate exercise of this power must be decided by an appeal to the inherent laws of thought. If he assume that the very conception of the theory is but a necessary result of the law of development itself, then there remains no possible distinction between truth and error. All who think, therefore, under an admission of the distinction between truth and error, must be remanded back to the power of thought as primordial to all knowledge, and to the laws of thought as alone sufficient to give the criteria of truth. If the brain be a galvanic battery giving out all mental phenomena as mere electrical phenomena, then it is hard to conceive how any law can be violated, how any standard of judgment can be required or be possible, or how these questions and difficulties — these agitations and conflicts of thought of which we are conscious, can arise.

The " Vestiges of Creation," is a bold system of materialism. This and all kindred systems, lie within the appropriate field of study of the philosophical Physician. Organic subjects, are peculiarly his subjects of investigation. He is forever conversant with the laws of life, the forms, distinctive qualities, and proper distribution of its products. And as man, the noblest organism is to him the prime object of interest and attention, and to comprehend whom the study of all other organisms is subsidiary, so in the proper study of man he is compelled to become the psychologist also, and to ascend to the fountain head of all philosophy. If he study organization, watching the signs of the disorganizing power of disease and life on the very border of the shades of death, so also, he studies the physical as it conditionates the spiritual, and the mortal as it fades into the immortal. He takes a position, at the same time the most solemn and the most sublime that can be occupied by the philosopher and the man of science.

Thus far we have considered the philosophical bearings of the studies of a Physician taken as a mere devotee of science. When we proceed next to consider him as a man devoted to an art, the art of healing, his fellowship with philosophy is no less apparent. Therapeutics consists of three parts, the theory of disease, the mode of treating disease, and the agents to be employed. But all these must be determined by the physiological doctrines adopted. Thus, Galen's theory of the predominance of the moist in the human constitution, led to his humoral pathology; his humoral pathology led to his treatment by bleeding and purgatives; and the mode of treatment, of course, led to the agents to be employed.

The fundamental principle of Hoffmann's system, is an immaterial vital power. As this was accumulated in the brain, conveyed along the nerves, and distributed into all the fibres; so, with him, the fibres, in opposition to the humoral pathology, became the seat of disease, and disease itself a disturbance of the tone of action. Thus he described disease as either *spasm* or excess of tone, or *atony* or relaxation of tone. Hence his medicinal appliances were either " anti-spasmodica," or " tonics."

The fundamental principle of Stahl's theory was the same with Hoffmann's, but he made a somewhat different use of it. His *anima* or vital power maintained the composition of the body and repairs its waste, by tonic movements in the soft tissues, producing alternate tension and relaxation, and thus directs the movements of the fluids. With Galen he held to the expulsion of morbific matter. Symptoms of disease are signs of the efforts of the anima to resist putrefaction, and to expel morbific matter. Death ensues when the tonic power relating to this matter is too weak to effect its expulsion. Plethora is the most common source of disease. Hence, his treatment corresponded very much with Galen's, and consisted of bleeding and evacuant medicines. But then, his treatment was milder, since he aimed merely to assist the spontaneous efforts of the anima.

The author of the "Vestiges of Creation," who represented the human constitution as "merely a complicated but regular process in electro-chemistry," very consistently describes disease as a derangement of the electro-chemical forces by various external agencies. The treatment on this theory would be to restore the equilibrium of forces, and the remedial agents, I suppose, would be applied externally, and not internally.

It appears, then, that the philosophical ideas which go to shape a system of physiology, and pathology lead to a corresponding medical art. Indeed, if it were not so, the art would be wholly empirical in its character.

There are, in general, two forms of empiricism. The one discarding physiology and pathology, altogether, laboring in the dark to collect remedies for diseases described according to their symptoms. In these cases the remedies are collected like charms and omens upon a few observed coincidences, without any principle by which to establish a real *nexus* between the remedy and the cure. This is the empiricism of ignorance, of mystery, and of superstition.

The other takes up a physiological and pathological theory, but it takes it up without investigation or philosophical insight upon authority, or by plausible conjecture, or by a mere fiction of the imagination confounding shreds of old pathologies to form a mongrel system. The same facility which, at random, constructs systems, lays down rules of art, and discovers potent remedies. It is universally true, that just where sound learning and philosophical acumen are most required, there the sciolist and empirical adventurer are most eager to rush, for the very reason that they find a region most convenient for their displays and undertakings. Despised by the few who are alone competent to judge, they may be popular with the many, because this region being remote from common observation and judgment, affords a hiding place for their shallow pretensions. A man may talk absurdities about the surface of the moon with greater impunity than about the surface of the earth. It is very much on the same principle that empirics in medicine get along and win confidence. There is so much, too, that is really occult in the laws of life, in the nature of disease, and in the *modus operandi* of remedies, that mankind are prone to consider mystery as the appropriate garb of the Physician. The rude Indian who identifies the conjurer with the medicine man, and he who purchases Hygeine pills and confides in their virtue the more readily, because their composition is concealed from him, exhibits the same weakness of human nature.

True philosophy alone, can explode empiricism, by reducing medicine, if not to an absolute science, at least, to a safe and consistent theory; where the Physician interprets and arranges facts by principles, proposes to himself a definite end, and can give a reason for his treatment of disease which will justify him as acting wisely under difficult circumstances, although acting without positive certainty. The Physician who has received a philosophical training, will disenchant the minds of men, wherever he goes, from the sorceries of empiricism, by exhibiting in his practice no mysterious and vain pretensions, and proving to the common eye, that while the highest science is alone adequate to treat disease at all, even the highest science can work no wonders, and can afford relief only by obeying the indications of nature. The empiric succeeds, because he boldly claims the absolute power of curing disease. But who is he who makes this claim? Is he a man of scientific culture? Has he devoted himself to wide and nice observation? Does he reveal the composition of his drugs and explain and prove their potency? No. He merely affirms and parades in the newspapers, fictitious or purchased certificates. And what is he beside the man of philosophic education, of scientific acquirement, of systematic observation, and ripened experience? Is the one pretentious and confident just in proportion to his ignorance; and the other modest and cautious, just in proportion to his accomplishments? Let the contrast be made as strong as possible, and the common sense of mankind will mark the difference and yield their confidence where alone it is justly deserved. A defective education in the accredited doctors of medicine, will do more to multiply empiricism than any other cause. The empiric, under the mystery which he professes, shields his ignorance; while the regular Physician, deprived of this resource by his very position, exposes his incompetency to general observation.

Let the maxim of another then be accepted, that "the Physician must begin with philosophy, as the philosopher must end with medicine," that in fact the Physician and the philosopher are one. There is no field of investigation more rich and curious; there is none which opens more profound questions than that which belongs to the Physician; and we may add, too, that there is none in which a higher order of genius has been exerted, and more illustrious names appear, and where more interesting and splendid results have been attained.

If philosophy belongs to the Physician, the science of observation and experiment belong to him no less. This, indeed, is implied in all that we have said. Philosophy governs all observation and experiment, and, at the same time, proves its own true value in this way. The one is the thought which suggests, the principles which arrange, the light which guides; the others collect the facts, supply the conditions, furnish the materials, reveal the occasions, and provide the field of scientific construction. Science is the joint product of philosophy, and observation and experiment. Physiology and pathology are constructed in this way. Anatomy and Zoology, Botany, Mineralogy, Geology and Chemistry, are perhaps more strictly the sciences of observation and experiment. Sciences so vast and rich, all lie naturally within the range of the Physician, while some of them are in no sense optional to him, but positively indispensible. The Physician is a naturalist, a philosopher, a student of facts and of principles, of nature, and of mind.

As a student of mind, we have seen how extensively psycology and anthropology enter into his pursuits. Nor can ethics be omitted here as furnishing a necessary part of his qualifications. This may be considered under two points of view. First, as comprising the principles which should govern him in discharging the duties of his profession. Secondly, as affording him light in the treatment of certain forms of disease. The oath which Hippocrates enacted from his disciples, contains the chief part of what may be called professional ethics. It in part runs thus: "I will honor as my father the master who shall teach me the art of healing, and convince him of my gratitude by endeavoring to minister to all his necessities. I shall act in a similar manner to all my brethren who are bound by a similar engagement. I shall prescribe to my patients such a course of regimen as I may consider best suited to their condition, according to the best of my judgment and capacity, seeking to preserve them from any thing that might prove injurious. No inducement shall ever lead me to administer poison; nor shall I ever give a criminal advice, or contribute to an abortion. My sole end shall be to relieve and cure my patients; to render myself worthy of their confidence, and not to expose myself even to the suspicion of having abused this influence, more especially when a woman is in the case. I shall seek to maintain religiously both the integrity of my conduct and the honor of my art. To whatever dwelling I may be called, I shall endeavor to cross its threshold with the sole view of succoring the sick, abstaining from all injurious views and corruption, especially from any immodest action. If, during my attendance, or even after a recovery, I happen to become acquainted with any circumstances of the patient's life which should not be revealed, I shall consider this knowledge a profound secret, and observe on the subject a religious silence. May I, as a rigid observer of this my oath, reap the fruit of my labors, enjoy a happy life, and obtain general esteem. Should I become a perjurer, may the reverse be my lot."

The cardinal virtues of gratitude, reciprocity, fidelity, purity and honor, are here taught. A heathen has conceived of them after a manner which a Christian might imitate.

The profession of the Physician is, also, one of the highest benevolence. He is the friend and confidant of families. He holds his walk amid disease, poverty, pain and death. He often enjoys the inexpressible satisfaction of affording relief , bringing back the sick from the borders of the grave, wiping away the tears of the despairing, and giving the oil of joy for mourning, and the garments of praise for the spirit of heaviness. Often, too, he can only weep with those who weep. The finest sympathies of our nature, and the holiest offices of religion, belong to him. In the Campo Santo, at Pisa, there is a beautiful monument erected to a Physician, the work of the celebrated Thorwalden, It is wrought in marble, *in relievo*, and represents an old blind man attended by his wife and dog. A young man of great beauty and a most benevolent expression, with the staff of a traveller in his hand. under the guardianship and direction of an angel, approaches him. The old man raises his head, the wife stands up in eagerness, and even the dog seems conscious of a Heavenly visitation. The meaning is obvious. The good Physician walks through the earth under the direction of Heavenly mercy, to relieve the sufferings of mankind. Is it not a high and holy destiny to lead such a life, and to deserve such a monument!

The manner in which the principles of Ethics — and under this I would comprise the principles of religion also — can be applied to relieve insanity, is plain to those who have had to deal with such cases. Insanity, among other causes, arises from keen disappointment, from vice, and from religious depression or excitement. The medicine here to be employed is not physical, but mental and spiritual. I suppose none will deny, that an acquaintance with man's moral and religious nature, with the principles of morals and religion, and a personal experience of moral elevation and purity, and of religious hopes and enjoyments, must prove invaluable qualifications in him who would administer to a mind diseased. The treatment pursued by such an one, will not be formal and mechanical; nor will it be less philosophical, because, inspired by a sympathy with the wants and fears of all that is spiritual and immortal in the nature of man.

When we have combined in the idea of the Physician, philosophy, science, skill, and virtue, we cannot but imply other accomplishments which wait on these, and which appear in literary culture and refined breeding. The first, which embraces an acquaintance with literature and the power of literary production, naturally complete the idea of an educated man; and the last is essential to the professional man as a man of society. It will be found, I think, upon consulting the history of medical science, that the most distinguished names upon its pages, and those who have contributed most to the advancement of science, were men of thorough classical education, and not unacquainted with the social usages of the world; and who, therefore, had the power of elegantly expounding their doctrines in books and in discourse, and of recommending their profession and extending its influence by the charm of cultivated manners. A high state of civilization in a community in general as well as a high state of education in individuals in particular, must spontaneously give their outward expression in the mutual respects and courtesies of society.

The influence of professional men, and of Physicians, surely, no less than the members of the other profession, upon the culture of society, must be paramount. On the one hand they possess the power of moulding society in the superior endowments with which they are presumed to be furnished; and, on the other, their avocations bring them into constant intercourse with all varieties of men in the most confidential and important relations.

We have thus vindicated the application of the title "learned," to the medical profession, by laying open the scope of medical study. If any should be inclined to the opinion that such a scope of study would require too much of the candidates of the profession, in general, and is possible only to the few, we would reply by asking whether it is not justified by the nature of the profession itself, and by the whole history of its development. An individual may choose to know little or much of any science or art; but the limits of the science or art cannot be determined by his acquirements, but by what it contemplates. An Empiric would make the same objection, and hasten to compound his mysterious drugs. One thoroughly trained Physician occupies a wide sphere, and may bestow unnumbered benefits upon mankind; while an indefinite multiplication of Empirics would never create medical skill. Human life is everywhere of too much value to be trifled with, and the cure of disease is everywhere attended with the same difficulties. If we set up a standard of acquirement, we must be careful to make it a true standard; otherwise, we shall only ensure the reign of mediocrity. A legitimate advance, to any extent, in any science or art, can be made only in view of its true principles and real demands.

It is true, indeed, that skillful Physicians are made with fewer acquirements and accomplishments than have been indicated above, by concentrating attention upon what is more immediately connected with medical practice, and by cautiously and wisely collecting knowledge from experience; and many may be compelled, by unavoidable necessity, to take this course. But skillful Physicians, however made, will be the very men to exalt the requirements of their profession; to regret the circumstances which may have limited their own education, and to recommend to all candidates to make the utmost efforts to become fully embued with the spirit of their pursuits, to reach the highest attainments, and to copy the example of those great men, the memory of whose lives, whenever mediocrity or empiricism prevails, revives to recall the honors of their profession, and to rebuke those who have loaded it with reproach.

The preparations which have been made for medical education in the most enlightened nations, accord with the view we have taken. We refer to the very nations which have produced the great lights of medical science; the men whose books are every where studied, and the principles they contain every where appealed to as fundamental.

We have not space to give an account of these great schools of medicine in detail; and, perhaps, they are too well known to render it necessary. I will only mention that in the schools of medicine and pharmacy in Paris, twenty-five Professors deliver lectures, besides seven who lecture in the Museum of Natural History, in the "Jardin des plantes;" and that in Berlin, thirty-seven professors and teachers deliver lectures in medicine, in addition to those who lecture upon the Natural Sciences in general. It must be recollected, too, that the students who attend these lectures, have received a full preparatory classical and scientific education.

In our own country, the preparations for the higher forms of education, (among which, of course, we rank the professional,) it must be confessed, have not yet reached the completeness of the institutions of Europe. We have, indeed, produced men of the highest distinction in all the professions; but these have, in some instances, gone abroad to complete their education, or if remaining at home, have been compelled to overcome many difficulties which, with more perfect institutions, they would not have encountered.

There is a certain order of mind that cannot be prevented by the most untoward circumstances, from reaching a destiny for which they seem preordained. But one of the greatest benefits of a thorough system of education is that it tends to equalize the condition of men, and to prepare for usefulness, and often to lead to eminence, those who are less distinguished for natural endowments. Men of genius are rare; and we cannot look to them to supply the wants of society in all its varied offices. But there are multitudes whom education can prepare for every useful and honorable station.

The medical profession in our country, has suffered peculiarly from two causes. The one is, that it alone of the learned professions, has been thrown without the protection of law. The clerical profession is held by the ecclesiastical laws of the different denominations which prescribe the course of discipline necessary for admission to the clerical office. The legal profession has its necessary qualifications prescribed by statute. But there is no law of any kind which prevents an incompetent person from practising medicine. Not only may every man be his own doctor, which is, perhaps, a natural right; but every man may also be every other man's doctor.

The other cause lies in the manner in which medical schools are very often constituted and conducted. A number of Physicians, combining for the purpose, procure a charter for lecturing in medicine, and conferring the degree of Doctor of Medicine. Dependent as they are upon the fees of tuition and graduation, and with full power to regulate the course of instruction, they are under the temptation while they possess every facility for multiplying Doctors in the most summary way. The influence of competition upon these institutions is very great; but it is apt to take a wrong direction. Young men are ever too eager to rush into professional life without seriously measuring its duties and responsibilities. They will, consequently, be too readily inclined to seek those institutions which open to them the nearest way to professional degree. Do not such institutions degenerate into mere shops for the sale of academical degrees? And what is the influence of their example but to lower the dignity of the profession, by showing to the world how little preparation is requisite for attaining its highest title? Is it not simony in medicine? The empiric may now stand forth unblushingly, beside the Doctor of Medicine, and tell him that his diploma is only an acknowledgment for so much money received by a corporation of impostors who would palm him upon the world under a name which he does not deserve; while he, nature's doctor of medicine, trusts to an inborn sagacity and skill, and a knowledge which his own independent investigations and experience have given him.

Now let it be understood at once that the University of Michigan, in its Medical School, will not become one of these shops — will not be guilty of this simony; will not lay itself open to this reproach of the empiric. It seeks to make Doctors of Medicine who deserve the name. The condition of so many of the Schools of Medicine in our country has so much lowered the general tone of medical education, that it will require many efforts and much perseverance to elevate it to its true standard. But this Medical School may justly claim to have made a decided and honorable advance both in the requirements for admission, and in the length and fullness of the discipline prescribed for the attainment of a degree.

This School, endowed with the rest of the University by the bounty of the General Government, and fostered by the State, is exempt from all pecuniary temptation to lower its standard. It therefore does not sell its degrees; it labors only to qualify its pupils to receive them. Tuition and the degree, are here indeed given freely, without money and without price; but they are given not for the purpose of cheapening medical education, and thus entering into a successful competition with other Schools by giving away that worthless thing which they sell, and thus acquiring the vain honor of sending forth a large number of graduates. This would be a shameful desecration of our endowment. Tuition and the degree are without price for the purpose of enabling students to employ their means in prolonging their course of study, and securing a more solid and ample preparation for an important and difficult profession, instead of wasting them in the purchase of an empty title.

The Literary and Scientific Department of this University, is closely connected with the interests of the Medical School, and with the interests of any other professional school which may hereafter be established. We hope the time is not distant when that department will furnish many pupils to this; and that young men aiming at the medical profession, will be induced to pursue a preparatory course there, before entering upon the course here. We hope, for the honor of the medical profession, and for the good of humanity, to see the sentiment prevail, that the physician and philosopher are one; and that a profession so useful and necessary, so lofty and honorable, and adorned with so many great names in the whole history of philosophy and science, will redeem itself from the cupidity of the sciolist, and the taunts of the empiric, and reclaim its ancient glories.

Gentlemen of the Graduating Class! The University of Michigan in expressing to you, through me, its sentiments, its aims, and its hopes, does so in the confidence that it is addressing those who have ears to hear, and honorable and manly hearts to yield a cordial response. The very fact that you have remained here to complete your course, and to earn your title to a medical degree, we take as a proof, that you value and approve the discipline we inculcate. May you ever worthily represent this discipline, aid us in maintaining it, and adorn the profession you have chosen.

You now go forth to try your strength in the active duties of life. No longer under the direction of your Professors, you will henceforth be compelled to study and observe for yourselves. Recollect that the practice of your profession is not a mere mechanical art, but a constant study, a developing philosophy, a ripening discipline. The science of medicine has been created amid these very scenes to which you are about to be introduced. While, therefore, you apply the principles you have been taught, you will enjoy the opportunities of testing them, of enlarging your knowledge by fresh experiments and observations, and of advancing yourselves more and more in all those sciences which are naturally connected with your pursuits. It would seem, therefore, to be no difficult matter for you to keep alive the " esprit de corps" of science and philosophy.

Mingling, too, with society under the most interesting and responsible relations, you will find that all the fine sentiments of human nature, all the principles of honor, truth, integrity and religion, will be put in requisition; and that nothing will be unworthy of your attention that can seem to render you attractive to your fellow men, to secure their confidence, and lead them to regard you as friends, gentlemen, companions, wise counsellors, and exemplars of virtue, as well as skillful Physicians. Your profession opens to you the doors of human dwellings, and the hearts of their inmates. Humanity claims you in its deepest anxieties, its most confidential relations, and in the performance of the holiest offices which man can render to man.

As, therefore, with best wishes for your prosperity and happiness, we bid you farewell, may we not ask of you, never to forget your high calling, but ever to acquit yourselves like men.

Art. II.—*Case of Paralysis at St. Marie's Hospital.* Reported by E. P. Christian, M. D., Detroit.

The following case, is in some respects novel, presenting a peculiar form of paralysis; and is interesting as regards the condition manifested, its cause, and the treatment adopted.

Edward Bouchard, aged seventeen, came under the care of Dr. Pitcher, at St. Marie's Hospital, on the 25th of November last; was brought in perfectly helpless, exhibiting a state of complete loss of the power of motion in all the voluntary muscles below the neck, and with almost entire abolition of sensation throughout the same extent. The slightest change of position in his body or limbs being effected only by the aid of an assistant, and without any sensation on his part of the application of the assistant's hand. His surface was persistently cold and dry, appetite moderate, but his stomach would retain only light soups, and in a small quantity at one time; bowels constipated, evacuations occurrring once in five or six days. No difficulty in urinating, complained of no pain or uneasiness, his only suffering consisting in coldness and inability to change his positions.

Gave his previous history as follows: Had been employed during the season in fishing, at Mackinac, and had suffered very much from exposure to wet and cold. Says he had not for weeks slept with dry clothes on. The disturbance commenced with a sensation of numbness at the same time, in both fingers and toes, which gradually extended up the limb and over the body, until he was deprived of both sensation and the power of motion in them. When he entered the Hospital, had been in this condition about one month, and about two months had elapsed since the commencement of the difficulty.

Nov. 26. Was directed to be put on the use of Quinine and Morphine in small doses, repeated daily, to have the limbs painted daily with Tinct. Iodine, the bowels opened as indications advised, with Alt. Pills. The indications being to raise the vital powers, stimulate the capillaries which appeared to be in a torpid condition, and equalize the circulation. This treatment was pursued with slight variations until Feb. 1st, but without satisfactory results. There was a barely perceptible return of sensation, very slight and of slow progress.

Feb. 1. Was ordered the application of friction by the hand over the limbs, to be repeated daily. Under this treatment, the improvement was rapid and unequivocal. After a few repetitions, an agreeable warmth was diffused over the body by the operation, free diaphoresis was excited, and the skin was aroused from its former state of torpidity to new life and action. Sensation was speedily restored with the power of moving the fingers and toes, which was rapidly extended to other joints, and all the functions were restored to their natural and healthy actions, within a month from the commencement of this plan of treatment.

What was the pathological condition here exerting, as the cause of the nervous derangement? We have said that the case was peculiar in the condition manifested; because the condition which was here supposed to exist must be a very unusual course of paralysis, as but little is said of it by authors. In regard to the condition, reviewing the generally recognised divisions, we have here neither general paralysis, which includes total loss of sensibility and motion throughout the system, and which cannot occur without extinction of life, although Tweedie says it is only applied to paralysis of the four extremities, whether other parts be affected or not, and may occur as the result of an injury to the cranial or cervical portions of the spinal cord; or may come on gradually, commencing in the toes and fingers, as in this case, but in this class, occurring mostly in aged persons. Neither have we here a case of hemiplegia, which is for the most part the result of cerebral difficulty, nor of paraplegia, which may be the result of either cerebral or spinal difficulty, in which the lower extremities or the lower half of the body is paralyzed, although, according to Boerhaave and Van Swieten, this may include all below the neck; yet in such cases, there is almost always, if not in all cases, relaxation of the sphincters, as well as paralysis of the voluntary muscles, which did not hold in this case. Nor have we local paralysis, or, according to Marshall Hall, nemal paralysis, which may depend upon a variety of causes, as exposure, injuries, tumors, metallic poisons, &c., but where only a single nerve or a small portion of the body is affected.

Now in regard to the cause. This, indubitably, was the long continued exposure to cold and dampness, which is recognized by all writers as a frequent cause of paralysis. But how operating? By producing a morbid impression upon the nervous centres, as by congestions, inflammations, or some other morbid condition in and about their parts. Was this the mode in this case? Aside from the nervous derangement, there was no indication that could lead us to the supposition of the extreme of cerebral or spinal difficulty. There was manifest peripheral difficulty, and I think, therefore, we may rationally account for the nervous derangement, not necessarily by a morbid condition of, or impression upon the centres, suspending their powers; but in the morbid condition of the nervous extremities.

What authorities, have we to corroborate the opinion, that paralysis may be the result of such a condition? Watson says, "paralysis has been ascribed to some primary morbid condition of the nerves which belong to the spinal cord. That the functions of the efferent or motor nerves may be impaired or even arrested by exposure to cold, and by other injurious influences, is both possible and probable; but a disease or disordered state of the afferent nerves, has been assigned as a cause of palsy. This is less clearly conceivable." If it is not conceivable that a diseased or disordered state of the afferent nerves may be a cause of paralysis, a morbid impression being transmitted to the cord, suspensive of its functions; it is then possible and conceivable that the efferent nerves were here so changed in their condition by the influence of the external causes, as to have been rendered incapable of the proper discharge of their healthy functions. But as the same cause, and in a precisely similar manner, was operating on the extremities of both classes of nerves, it is rational to suppose that both were implicated. In fact, if we admit that paralysis may be the result of a morbid condition of the extremities, and that it was so in this case, we must admit that both classes were implicated to account for both loss of motion and sensation.

Again, Eberle says, "reasoning indeed upon the general nature of palsy, we would be led *a priori* to suppose that everything which is capable of disordering the source of nervous power, might give rise to this affection;" but admits that Dr. Powell, in an interesting paper on the subject of paralysis, has adduced some cases which seem to show that both general and local palsy, sometimes depend upon a morbid condition of the nerves alone, independent of any affection of the encephalic mass." Is it indeed less plausible that the muscular and cutaneous extremities of the nerves may be impaired in their functions, than other parts, as the capillaries and sudoriferous glands?

ART. III.—*On a new mode of removing the Placenta.* By Thomas Schneeder, M. D.

To the Editor of the Peninsular Journal:

Dear Sir,—The following article, which I have been persuaded to send to you for publication, is part of an essay which was read before the Medical Society of Chicago. As I am not yet fully acquainted with your language, having been in this country less than a year, I trust you will excuse its imperfections.

If we fix upon a table with the hand or a weight, a fresh placenta, and seizing it with a pair of wide bladed forceps, either by its margin or at the attachment of the cord, turn them once or twice round, we observe that the bulk of the placenta is diminished, and its strength increased so that we have to use more force to tear it apart.

We find also that we are able to push the placenta through a hole made in a board, by twisting it through which no force could make it pass in any other manner, without laceration.

I think that we may with advantage, make use of these two facts in cases where other means of removing the retained placenta have failed, or where severe hermorrhage requires its immediate removal. For instance, when the placenta is retained by spasm of the uterus, two fingers are to be introduced which seize a portion of the placenta. The forceps are to be applied to this portion, turned once or twice round, and moderate traction used.

Should we not succeed in overcoming the spasm, the two fingers hold the twisted portion of the placenta in its position, and the forceps are applied higher up. Thus the placenta diminished in size, and rounded, dilates the os uteri more equally than the fingers, and its ability to endure traction is much increased.

Should the uterine surface of the placenta present itself, we should, if possible, change its position so as to be able to apply the forceps to the margin. The same process may be used in an hour glass contraction as well as in adherent placenta, naturally without using any traction in this last case.

As the periphery of the adherent placenta by twisting it is slightly moved toward the center, the adhesions will easier yield to the separating hand, and the danger of laceration or inversion is less.

If we had to remove a very fragile placenta, we might surely and successfully have recourse to this twisting; and finally, we must apply this method when the placenta is retained after abortion, other means of removing it having been unsuccessful.

Though I have no certain proof for my idea in regard to the first mentioned cases, I remember a case of abortion where, by this proceeding, I evidently saved a life, which case I will in short relate.

Having been called to a woman that had an abortion in the fourth month, was told by the midwife, that three days previous the abortion had taken place, that the placenta had not been naturally expelled nor had she herself been able to remove it; and that some hours before my arrival a severe flooding had taken place which had reappeared whenever the patient recovered from fainting. The funis was torn off, and the midwife had removed as much of the placenta as she had been able to reach, so that I could only just touch some of the remaining part.

I ordered applications of cold water both internally and externally, and a strong dose of ergotine, and went home for a proper pair of forceps; but the husband came running after me and informed me that I would probably find his wife dead, as the hermorrhage had become worse than ever before.

When I came back, without trying to revive the patient, I immediately introduced my hand and seized with the forceps as much of the placenta as I could reach. For three several times, however, I could only remove small portions, but was at last able, by applying the above mentioned method, to remove the whole.

It is not in slight cases that I would advise this method of twisting the placenta, though even then it might be used successfully; but where danger is urging, various other means having failed, it seems to me a method not only theoretically true, but practically useful.

On the different modes of delivery, I have read Naegele, Siebald, Scantzony, Cazean, Lievee, Ramsbotham, and Churchill, without finding mentioned the twisting of the placenta; therefore I call this idea a new one. Whether it will prove a good one, experience will show.

Chicago, April 20, 1854.

ART. IV.—*The American Medical Association.*

On the second of May, the American Medical Association met at St. Louis, Mo., in Verandah Hall, and in the absence of the venerable President, (Dr. Knight, of Conn.) the meeting was called to order by the first Vice President, Dr. U. Parsons, of R. I. A full delegation was in attendance, some from nearly every State in the Union, but proportionably a larger number were from the young and vigorous Western States.

Letters from the President, regreting his inability to be present, and abounding in expressions of solicitude for the welfare of the Association and the profession, were read. After which the Association was welcomed to the city, in behalf of the profession of St. Louis, by the Chairman of the Committee of Arrangements. Dr. Washington, whose remarks were briefly responded to by the Vice President, Dr. Parsons. After the roll of delegates was called, the Association was announced as organized and ready for business.

Reports of the Committee of Publication and of the Treasurer of the Association, were read and accepted, and a series of resolutions appended to the first report, requiring that each delegate should pay an assessment of three dollars before being entitled to a seat in that body, and that all permanent members shall pay an annual assessment of the same amount, or after being notified by the Treasurer, of their delinquency, should be stricken off the list of permanent members, was subsequently adopted by the Association. Members thus paying are entitled to a volume of the transactions.

A recess of fifteen minutes was then taken to allow the Delegates from each State to appoint one of their number as a member of a Committee for the nomination of officers for the ensuing year.

After the Association was called to order, Dr. D. Brainard, of Chicago, moved a resolution that hereafter, the meetings of the Associations be held alternately at the South, East and West. It was objected that the North was not mentioned, whereupon the mover so modified the resolution as to read the South, the North and West, when by some it was objected that the East was left out—by others that the Middle States were excluded—while the inquiry was made by others whether California was considered as belonging to the West—when on motion, and after some irregular discussion, the resolution was disposed of by being laid upon the table, and the meeting adjourned.

On the re-assembling of the Association in the afternoon, the Vice President, Dr. Parsons, read a valedictory address, referring in appropriate terms to the occasion, to the improvement of the profession in the rich and mighty West, the future seat of empire, and to the distinguished dead of the profession during the past year.

A report of a committee previously appointed to prepare memoirs of the members of the Association who were victims of the Norwalk disaster, was read, stating that the committee had the labor in hand, and asked for further time to complete it in a suitable manner.

A communication was read from the American Medical Society of Paris, returning thanks for the volumes of the transactions of this Association presented to them.

Dr. Gross, of Louisville, Ky., offered a proposition to change the constitution so as to require that the election of President be at the close of each session of the Association, rather than at the beginning, in order to give him time before the active performance of duty to become familiar with Parliamentary rules.

The proposition, according to the constitution, was laid over for one year.

Dr. Gross also moved that hereafter it be considered out of order for the committee of arrangements to provide expensive entertainments for the Association.

After considerable discussion during which it was suggested that wine and tobacco should be excluded from the public entertainment, the resolution was adopted.

The nominating committee presented the names of the following gentlemen as officers of the Association, who were unanimously elected as such—viz:

Dr. C. A. Pope, of St. Louis, President.

VICE PRESIDENTS.

Dr. Fenner, of New Orleans.
Dr. N. S. Davis, of Chicago, Ill.
Dr. Wragg, of Charleston, S. C.
Dr. Green, of Massachusetts.

SECRETARIES.

Dr. LaMoine, of Mo.
Dr. West, of Pa.

TREASURER.

Dr. Condie, of Pennsylvania.

Dr. Palmer, of Chicago, moved that the next meeting of the Association be held in the city of Philadelphia. Carried unanimously.

Dr. Brodie, of Detroit, presented an invitation in behalf of the profession of that city to make Detroit the place of meeting of the Association at its earliest convenience.

Dr. Atlee, of Pa., chairman of a committee appointed to procure a stone for the Washington Monument, reported that he had procured a block of American Marble, and the services of an American artist to execute a very beautiful and appropriate design, the cost of which would be $1000; a moderate proportion of which had been contributed, and asking the members to furnish the remainder.

Dr. Davis, of Chicago, moved that all resolutions should be made in writing and signed by the mover, and also that no member should speak more than fifteen minutes upon any one subject, or more than once until all others had spoken who wished to do so. Carried; when after some other unimportant business, the meeting adjourned.

In the evening entertainments were given by several Government Physicians of St. Louis, and by ex-Mayor Bennett. Sumptuous provisions were made by these gentlemen, and the companies enjoyed themselves in the usual agreeable manner.

SECOND DAY.

The Second Association met this morning at nine o'clock, the President, Dr. Pope, in the chair.

After the reading of the minutes, &c., Dr. Atbee, of Pa., called for the reading of a memorial from the American Medical Society of Paris, wherein it was urged as a means of raising the qualifications of medical practitioners, that a board of examiners for license to practice, be appointed in each State, independent of the Medical Schools, the professors of which have a pecuniary interest in passing all applicants. This subject has been frequently discussed in the Association, and is considered by many as the only mode of preventing the introduction of unworthy and disqualified persons into the rank of the profession.

The memorial was referred to the Committee on Medical Education.

The Association now arrived at the point in its proceedings of the greatest interest in a scientific point of view — viz. the consideration of the Annual Reports of Committees on Professional subjects. Many of the committees were not prepared to report, and those only will be referred to who were.

Dr. J. Cain, of Charleston, S. C.,—on Epidemics of South Carolina, Florida, Georgia and Alabama, read an abstract of his report. The report was referred to the committee of publication.

Dr. W. L. Sutton, of Georgetown, Kentucky, also presented a similar report on the epidemics of Tennessee and Kentucky, which took the same reference.

Dr. George Mendenhall, of Cincinnati, O., read an abstract of a report on the epidemics of Ohio, Indiana and Michigan, which report was disposed of in the same manner.

Dr. M. said he had received a paper from Dr. Pitcher, of Detroit, one of the members of the committee, which would be appended to his in the published transactions.

Dr. Palmer spoke of the plan recently adopted by the State Society of Michigan, for keeping in different parts of the State full and accurate meteorological records, and also records of the state of health, and the prevalence of particular diseases in each locality, which records were to be collected and arranged by a committee for that purpose, and the account transmitted to the proper committee of the Association. He urged upon other States to follow the example, and referred to the immense advantage to truth and science, which would result from such a course being generally adopted.

Dr. Atlee, of Pa., very earnestly and ably urged the importance of the subject, and the necessity of co-operation of all the profession with the committee having these reports in charge.

Dr. R. S. Holmes, of St. Louis, read an extract of a report on Epidemic Erysipelas. Referred for publication.

Dr. E. D. Fenner, of New Orleans, read an extended abstract of a report on the Epidemics of Louisiana, Mississippi, Texas and Arkansas. The report is to embrace an account of the terrible ravages of yellow fever in his district, and will possess much interest. The report will also dwell at some length upon the subject of cholera.

Dr. Linton, of St. Louis, expressed his views upon the pathology of yellow fever. He regarded it as only a more severe form of the usual epidemic fevers of the South, and believed it to be produced by the action of *Southern heat* on *Northern blood.* He thought Northerners might generally avoid attacks by moderation in exercise, in exposure to the sun, in eating, and particularly in drinking. He also expressed doubts as to the existence of miasma from vegetable composition, as a cause of these diseases.

A motion was made that Dr. Linton be requested to write out briefly his views just expressed, to be presented to the committee of publication.

Dr. Ramsey, of Tenn. objected to the motion, unless a counter statement be also entered upon the proceedings. He differed with Dr. Linton as to there being no evidence of a miasma; and stated that the disease prevailed in particular localities, and not in others, where the heat and the condition of the blood might be regarded as similar.

Dr. Palmer said he hoped the motion would prevail, and if any member with other views would come forward and state them as clearly and concisely as had Dr. Linton, he would favor their insertion upon the record. He wished, however, that his position should not be misunderstood.

He did not fully agree with Dr. L's. views. He said he believed that the physiological and pathological conditions referred to by Dr. Linton, acted as *predisposing causes* of these diseases, while a peculiar miasmatic poison was necessary to develope the diseases as we found them.

Dr. N. S. Davis read an abstract of a report on the influence of local circumstances on the origin and prevalence of Typhoid Fever. Report referred to committee of publication.

Dr. Donaldson, of Baltimore, gave notice of a report on the present and prospective value of the Microscope in disease. Same reference.

The report of the Committee on Medical Education was received, and referred for publication.

Dr. Pope, Chairman of Committee on Prize Essays, made a report, awarding a prize to an essay, entitled, "An Essay on a new method of treating Un-united Fractures, and certain deformities of the Osseous System."

On opening a sealed packet accompanying the essay, the author was found to be Prof. Brainard, of Chicago.

Dr. Brainard, by request, gave an abstract of his paper.

Dr. Guthrie offered a resolution, approving of the Secretary of the Treasury's recommendation to Congress to abolish or materially modify the duty upon such crude drugs not producible in this country, as are used in the manufacture of chemicals. He stated that our manufactures were of superior character, and should be encouraged. The resolution passed unanimously.

Dr. Stephen W. Williams, of Ill., through his friend, Dr. Johnson, of St. Louis, called up a resolution, laid over from the meeting last year, asking for a committee to be appointed by this Associatian to procure memorials of the eminent and worthy dead among the physicians of the country.

Dr. W. stated that the profession of medicine contains more learned and distinguished men than any other profession or calling, and that some durable memorial of their lives and actions should be presented to the world. The resolution passed.

Dr. French offered a resolution asking the appointment of a committee to enquire what State or other Societies, represented in this Association were in fellowship with irregular practitioners.

He said there were rumors that men were here representing societies harboring in their bosoms those who professed adhesion to the miserable deception of Homœpathy. He wished to know whether this were possible. Resolution passed.

Dr. Blachford, of Troy, N. Y., introduced the subject of Hydrophobia, stating that, from investigations made, it would seem that the disease was more likely to occur in cold weather than warm, and that the cry of *mad dog* during the *dog days* was founded more in whim than in reason and experience. The subject needed further investigation.

Dr. Palmer moved that Dr. Blachford be appointed chairman of a committee on the subject to report next year. Carried.

Dr. S. M. Smith, of Ohio, moved that a committee on Insanity be appointed. Carried.

It was then announced that at 4 o'clock, P. M., omnibusses and carriages would be in readiness to convey the members to the residence of Col. O'Fallon, some three miles from the city, an invitation having been extended to them to partake of an entertainment.

In the afternoon, but little business was done.

A few unimportant resolutions having passed, Dr. Davis, of Chicago, presented for inspection a sample of solid milk, said to be capable of keeping any length of time, and made some remarks upon the impurity of milk usually found in cities.

The members very generally made a visit to Athlone, the seat of Col. O'Fallon, one of the most beautiful situations which can well be conceived. It is situated upon an eminence overlooking the river, surrounded by beautiful groves and gardens, and manifesting evidence of great wealth and refined taste.

A fine band of music enlivened the occasion, and after a most agreeable entertainment, the members returned to the city by a most beautiful moonlight.

THIRD DAY.

The Association met at 9 o'clock, A. M., the President, Dr. Pope, in the Chair.

After the minutes were read, &c., Dr. McPheters stated that arrangements had been made with the different lines of travel from St. Louis to convey the members home free of charge, all the lines having agreed to the arrangement excepting the New York and Hudson River Railroad Company.

A communication was read tendering the hospitalities of the city of Burlington, Iowa, to those members who return by the Upper Mississippi.

Dr. Atlee offered a resolution that a copy of the constitution of the Association be appended to each volume of the transactions. Carried.

Dr. Gross moved that a committee of one be appointed to enquire into the causes which obstruct the formation and establishment of our National Medical Literature.

The resolution was carried and Dr. Gross appointed as Committee.

A communication from the officers of the Pacific R. R., was read inviting the Association to an excursion upon their road. The invitation was accepted and 10 o'clock the next day, appointed for the purpose.

Dr. J. Berrien Lindsley, offered a resolution which was referred to the committee on Medical Education with instructions to report thereon—

"That this Association earnestly recommend to the Western Schools which still retain the rule of making four year's practice equivalent to one term at College, the abrogation of that rule, holding out a strong temptation to young men to enter upon the practice of Medicine with little or no preparation."

Dr. Paul F. Eves, of Tenn., submitted a resolution that a committee of three be appointed to report at the next meeting of the Association the best means for preventing the introduction of disease by emigrants into our large cities.

On motion of Dr. Beech, of Mich., the resolution was amended by striking out "large cities," and introducing "country," which amendment prevailed and the motion carried.

The Chair appointed Dr. Dickson of Charleston. S. C., Griscom of N. Y., and E. D. Fenner of N. O., said committee.

Dr. Linton, of St. Louis, offered a resolution that in the opinion of this Association quarantine establishments afford no protection to States and cities against the invasion of epidemics, such as Cholera and Yellow Fever.

Dr. Palmer remarked that many, probably a large proportion of the members present had not given the subject such an investigation as would enable them to express definite and positive opinions, while those who had given it most attention and had the largest opportunity of observing, differed in their views. He objected therefore to a vote being taken upon it, and moved a reference to the committee just appointed. Carried.

Dr. Sayre, of N. Y. offered a resolution that the memorial from Drs. Hammer and Murphy of the American Medical Society of Paris, and referred yesterday to the committee on Medical Education, be withdrawn from said committee and laid upon the table.

Dr. S. supported the resolution by some earnest remarks contending that the document reflected unjustly upon the efficiency of the American Professors of Medicine, and implied that a thorough scientific education could not be given in this country. He repudiated the idea and declared it an insult to the profession of the country.

Dr. Atlee, of Pa., remarked that he knew something of the motive of the young men who wrote the document, and was convinced that it was dictated by the best intentions, and without any desire to underrate the members of the profession or of Medical Science in this country.

Dr. Elbert, of Iowa, said the language of the paper and not of the motives of its authors must be considered, and in that view he considered it worthy of condemnation. He thought it should be withdrawn from the committee and laid upon the table, which would be treating it with silent contempt.

Dr. McIlvain, of Ohio, wished the objection to the document more clearly specified. He believed it to have been sent in good faith, and as containing some truth.

Dr. Edgar, of St. Louis, said it could not be denied that there was much looseness on the part of many Medical Schools in this country in admitting incompetent men into the profession. He thought a board of Censors should be appointed in each State outside of the Schools who should determine the qualifications of Students. This was by no means a new idea in this body, and was worthy to be considered.

After further discussion, during which it was insisted that the language of the document intimated that the means of Medical Education in this country was seriously deficient, the motion of Dr. Sayre prevailed.

The nominating committee made the following

REPORT OF THE COMMITTEE OF NOMINATIONS.

The Committee of Nominations, in fulfilling the duty imposed upon them, recommend the continuance of several of the special committees previously created, and the appointment of some new ones. They, therefore, submit the following list of chairmen of special committees, with the subjects to them committed:

Dr. Worthington Hooker, of New Haven, Ct., on epidemics of New England and New York.

Dr. John L. Atlee, of Lancaster, Pa., on epidemics of New Jersey, Pennsylvania, Delaware and Maryland.

Dr. D. J. Cain, of Charleston, S, C., on epidemics of S. Carolina, Florida, Georgia and Alabama.

Dr. W. D. Sutton, of Georgetown, Ky., on epidemics of Tennessee and Kentucky.

Dr. Thomas Beyburn, of St. Louis, Mo., on epidemics of Missouri, Illinois, Iowa and Wisconsin.

Dr. Geo. Mendenhall, of Cincinnati, Ohio, on epidemics of Ohio, Indiana and Michigan.

Dr. E. D. Fenner, of N. Orleans, La., on epidemics of Mississippi, Louisiana, Arkansas and Texas.

Dr. James Jones, of New Orleans, La., on the mutual relations of yellow and and bilious remittent fever.

Dr. D. F. Condie, of Philadelphia, Pa., on the causes of tuberculous disease.

Dr. Joseph Leidy, of Philadelphia, Pa., on diseases of Parasitic origin.

Dr. A. P. Mersill, of Memphis, Tenn., on the physiological peculiarities and diseases of Negroes.

Dr. Jos. N. McDowell, of St. Louis, Mo., on statistics of the operations for the removal of stone in the bladder.

Dr. E. P. Porcher. of Charleston, S. C., on the toxicological and medicinal properties of our cryptogamic plants.

Dr. Daniel Brainard, of Chicago, Ill., on the constitutional and local treatment of carcinoma.

Dr. Geo. Engleman, of St. Louis, Mo., on the influence of geological formations on the character of disease.

Dr. Henry Taylor, of Mt. Clemens, Mich., on dysentery.

Dr. Horace Green, of New York, on the use and effect of applications of Nitrate of Silver to the throat in local or general diseases.

Dr. P. C. Gooch, of Richmond, Va., on the administration of anæsthetic agents, during parturition.

Dr. Chas. Hooker, of New Haven, Ct., on the diet of the sick.

Dr. E. R. Dabney, of Clarksville, Tenn., on certain forms of eruptive fevers prevalent in Middle Tennessee.

Dr. Sanford B. Hunt, of N. Y., on the hygrometrical state of the atmosphere in various localities, and its influence on health.

Dr. Frank H. Hamilton, of Buffalo, N. Y., on the frequency of deformities in fractures.

Dr. M. P. Pallen, of St. Louis, Missouri, on disease of the prostrate gland.

Dr. H. A. Johnson, of Chicago, Ill., on the execretions as an index to the organic changes going on in the system.

Dr. Leroy H. Anderson, of Sumpterville, Ala., on typhoid fever and its complications as it prevails in Alabama.

Dr. W. H. Byford, of Evansville, Ind., on the pathology and treatment of scrofula.

Dr. N. S. Davis, of Chicago, Ill., on the nutritive qualities of Milk, and the influence produced thereon by pregnancy and menstruation in the human female, and by pregnancy in the cow, and also on the question whether there is not some mode by which the nutritive constituents of milk can be preserved in their purity and sweetness, and furnished to the inhabitants of cities in such quantities as to supercede the present defective and often unwholesome method of supply.

Dr. E. B. Haskens, of Clarksville, Tenn., on the microscopical investigations of malignant tumors.

Dr. Geo. K. Srant, of Memphis, Tenn., on the sulphate of quinia as a remedial agent in the treatment of fevers.

Dr. R. R. McIlvain, of Cincinnati, Ohio, on the study of pathology at the bedside.

Dr. E. S. Cooper, of Peoria, Ill., on orthopædic surgery.

Dr. Andrew F. Jeter, of Palmyra, Mo., on the modus operandi of the envenomed secretions of healthy animals.

Dr. Samuel M. Smith, of Columbus, O., on insanity.

Dr. Rene La Roche, of Philadelphia, Pa., on the jaundice of yellow fever in its diagnotistical and prognostical relations.

Dr. Charles Chandler, of Rockport, Missouri, on malignant periodic fevers.

Dr. S. B. Chase, of Portland, Maine, on Typhoid Fever in Maine.

The committee have also nominated the following

STANDING COMMITTEE.

Committee on Plans of Organization for State and County Societies:—

A. B. Palmer, M. D., of Chicago; R. R. McIlvain, M. D., Ohio; D. L. McGugen, M. D., Iowa; E. R. Peaslee, M. D., N. Hampshire; Thos. Lipscomb, M. D. Tennessee.

Committee on Medical Literature:—

Robert J. Breckenridge, M. D., Ky., chairman; A. A. Gould, M. D., Mass.; D. L. McGugen, M. D., Iowa; J. B. Flint, M. D., Ky.; O. M. Langdon, M. D., Ohio.

Committee on Medical Education:—

Wm. H. Anderson, M. D., Ala.; A. Lopez, M. D., do; Andrew Murray, M. D., Mich.; A. Ramsay, M. D., Tenn.; R. D. Ross, M. D.

Committee on Prize Essays:—

Rene La Roche, M. D., Penn.; Isaac Hays, M. D., do; Alfred Stille, M. D., do; J. B. Biddle, M. D., do; G. W. Norris, M. D., do; Joseph Carson, M. D., do; Joseph Leidy, M. D., do.

Committee of Arrangements:—

Isaac Hays, M. D., Penn.; G. Emerson, M. D., do; Wilson Jewell, M. D., do; Alfred Stille, M. D., do; Francis West, M. D., do; Wm. V. Keating, M. D., do.

Committee on Publication:—

Pliny Earle, M. D., N. Y.; D. Francis Condie, M. D., Penn.; E. S. Lemoine, M. D., Mo.; A. March, M. D., of N. Y.; E. H. Davis, M. D., do; C. R. Gilman, M. D., do.

After the reading of the report, Dr. Rayburn moved its adoption, excepting that portion referring to the Committee of Publication, in the following resolution:

Resolved, That the said report be adopted, with the exception of that portion which refers to the committee on publication.

Upon this resolution and the subject growing out of it a lengthy discussion arose, occupying much of the remainder of the day, and eliciting much warmth and eloquence.

Although, perhaps, carried rather too far, and becoming more personal than was quite agreeable at the time, yet it afforded a relief from the drier details of professional subjects and made members better acquainted with each other.

The question involved was whether the majority of the committee on publication should be changed from Philadelphia to New York, the nominating committee favoring that change, which would carry the publication of the proceedings to the latter city.

The Report of the Nominating Committee was ultimately sustained by a large majority.

The friends of Dr. Condie presented his resignation as Treasurer of the Association.

Dr. Isaac Wood, of New York, was appointed in his stead.

A vote of thanks was tendered to Dr. Condie for his faithful services.

Dr. Mussey, of Cincinnati, was appointed a committee on the effects of alcoholic drinks.

Dr. Phelps, of New York, presented an abstract of a long paper upon the connection of medicine and religion in its origin and its progress. The document was referred to a special committee, consisting of Drs. Atlee, of Pa., and March and Sayre, of N. Y.

Dr. Atlee offered a resolution that the Association earnestly recommend the organization of State and County Medical Societies where they do not exist. Carried.

After some other unimportant business, voting of thanks, &c., the Association adjourned *sine die.*

In the evening the delegates met in the Hall of the Mercantile Library to participate in a public entertainment given by the profession of St. Louis, to the Association.

The room was large and beautifully decorated with evergreens, statues, and other objects of taste, and the walls inscribed with suitable mottoes. The tables were bountifully spread, and great efforts were made on the part of the hosts to preserve order and make every circumstance as agreeable as possible. But in view of what has been witnessed on

several   lar occasions, we can but be rejoiced at the passage of a resolution approving of expensive entertainments; and we are assured,
that Philadelphia will set the example of complying with the spirit of
the resolution, and with the privately expressed wishes of a large majority
of the Association.

On the whole, the present session of the Association has been one of
decided interest. The profession throughout the country is becoming
better organized and more united, and the standard of attainments is
becoming higher. The members parted in the best of feeling, and
attachments were formed which will be lasting and afford the highest
pleasure.

SELECTIONS.

From the Western Lancet.

Cold as an Anæsthetic Agent.   By Thos. Wood, M. D.

When we reflect that every person has experienced the numbing effect of cold on the surface of the body, and experienced the complete insensibility to slight injuries done to the skin of the fingers and hand while exposed to a low temperature of the atmosphere, we are surprised that the idea of using cold in surgical operations has been reserved through all past time, to become a discovery of the present age. It is strange, but true, that the investigating mind in search of an undiscovered principle or fact, often looks far beyond its object, into the obscure distance, and hence fails to detect what is near and obvious; like the untrained miner, in search of the secret treasures of the earth, who fruitlessly delves into the chaotic mountain mass, while he treads the undiscovered golden sands beneath his feet, in his daily walks over the plains.

Since the introduction of cold for the purpose of destroying the pain of surgical operations, I have used it quite freely in various cases. In most, it has more than met my expectations, while in some it has entirely failed, or but partially relieved the suffering.

It is not my present purpose to give a detail of the cases in which I have used it, but rather to give the rules gathered from my experience in its use, and indicate the class of cases to which it seems best adapted.

The degree of cold required to destroy the sensibility of a part is but a little above that of the freezing point of water, and it must be obvious to all that this degree of temperature can not be with impunity extended over a large surface of the body, or made to penetrate to a depth much below the surface in any of the more vital regions; hence its use is naturally restricted to the minor and more superficial operations, and can never take the place of chloroform or some of its kindred agents, in operations involving the deep tissues of the body.

To operations upon the surface, such as removing small warts, tumours, and nævii, or other excrescences from the skin, it seems peculiarly adapted; and for destroying the pain in the extraction of diseased or offending nails from the fingers or toes, it is far preferable to chloroform.

First, it is to be preferred for the reason that in its use there is no danger of fatal injury to the constitution, as in chloroform, for its effects are purely local and circumscribed; and, second, because the insensibility is more complete than when ordinarily obtained by chloroform, and is fully equal to the most overwhelming dose. I have repeatedly witnessed the most perfect composure of countenance in my patients, while a nail of the toe or finger was rudely torn, with a strong forceps, from its matrix, without the least exhibition of a sense of pain, or a consciousness of the progress of the operation, except from sight.

It acts well on the skin, where a small portion is to be removed; but in plastic operations I would not use it, as the refrigeration necessary to remove the pain might so destroy the vitality of the flap, that direct union (upon which success in these operations wholly depends,) would not take place.

It has failed in my hands to be of any service in removing hœmorrhoidal tumors, although, according to some of the European surgeons, it has answered well for them in operations on the anus.

In one case I attempted to remove a string of venerial vegetations from around the verge of the rectum, but was unable to get the part sufficiently chilled to even lessen its sensibility, and I was finally obliged to use the chloroform before the operation was completed.

The failure was, doubtless, owing to the rapid supply of heat to the part from the highly vascular organs in its vicinity, and the difficulty of conducting it away rapid enough to reduce the temperature in the tumors to near the freezing point; and this difficulty, in all probability, will ever prevent its successful use in operations on the painful tumors of the anus and rectum.

Cold has also failed to give much relief from the pain of opening paronychia.

While it numbs the surface of the finger, it does not lessen the sensibility toward the bottom of the wound, even when the application is made a considerable time previous to the use of the bistuary.

To chill a part that is to be subjected to an operation, for instance, a finger or toe, it is only necessary to get some pounded ice or snow, and mix it with some common salt, and apply it, taking care to not extend it much beyond the region to be operated on. From three to four minutes will mostly suffice to remove all feeling from the attachments of a toe nail.

It is no matter how rapidly the temperature is reduced, but after the operation, it is very essential that it should be raised cautiously and slowly up to the vital standard again. To effect this object safely, a towel or large cloth should be saturated with cold ice-water, and allowed to remain on the part until reaction is fully established.

From the New York Medical Times,

Case of Croup — Tracheotomy — Successful result. By JAMES W. MINOR, M. D., Surgeon of Brooklyn City Hospital.

C. A.; male; æt. 18 months: was attacked with croup, Tuesday, Dec. 20, 1853. Was promptly and efficiently treated by an intelligent parent, with the remedies usually resorted to, and generally successful in domestic practice. The next (Wednesday) he appeared to be as well as usual, except a little hoarseness and occasional cough, which was scarcely heeded; though from the subsequent development of the disease, they must have been of such a character as would have excited alarm in an educated ear. As night approached, the hoarseness and cough increased rapidly, with all the well-marked characteristics of this formidable disease. The remedies which had previously produced relief were again resorted to; but although they exercised their full specific actions, there was no abatement of the symptoms.

On Thursday evening, Dr. James Crane, of this city, was sent for and found him laboring under all the well-marked symptoms of the disease, viz.: dyspnœa, dry husky voice, and cough, &c. Ordered calomel and antimony every two hours. The antimony had the desired effect, producing free vomiting.

About 3 A. M., Dr. C. was again summoned, but being engaged with another case, Dr. C. R. McClellan was called. He found all the symptoms much aggravated; ordered tincture of sanguinaria in addition to calomel and antimony, but without any visible effect. Was again seen by Dr. C. about 9 A. M., on Friday; at which time the symptoms were so much aggravated as to induce him to request a consultation with Dr. McClellan. The urgency of the case led to the opinion that further medical treatment would be of no avail, and that surgical interference would probably be required.

With this view I was summoned between 9 and 10 A. M. On my arrival, the little sufferer was laboring for breath, with the mouth and nostrils dilated, and muscular apparatus of respiration in the most intense state of action; the face and neck suffused with carbonated blood; the breathing stridulous, and voice husky; in short, presenting all the most pressing indications for speedy surgical interference, or else a rapid termination in death.

This, together with a brief statement of the previous history of the case by Dr. C., induced me fully to concur with them in the opinion that tracheotomy alone could afford a chance for life; and I proceeded to operate with the least possible delay.

The operation was performed in the usual manner, and presented no features worthy of remark, except in the difficulty in cutting through the rings of the trachea, the delay produced by which, with the violent struggles of the child, had nearly caused asphyxia.

At one time we thought the little patient must die; the pulse being scarcely perceptible, and the respirations faint and few; but by keeping him in an upright position, with the shoulders alternately elevated and depressed, and by the administration of brandy and ammonia, the respiration was gradually restored.

Previous to the introduction of ths tube, the posterior surface of the trachea was observed to be of a yellowish white or buff color, and led me to believe that the inflammation had reached that point, though the subsequent course of the case would favor the opinion that it had been confined to the larynx.

The clearing up of the purple hue of the face and the neck, as the fullness and frequency of the inspirations furnished the blood with oxygen, was most striking and satisfactory. A tube was introduced, and retained by tapes around the neck.

I may here mention that the one which was first introduced gave us some trouble, from not having the rim sufficiently broad and long, in consequence of which it could not be kept steady; my own canula was subsequently introduced, which, having such a rim, answered very well.

The calomel and Dover's powders, which had been previously ordered, were continued, and directions left to clear out the tube with a moistened feather from time to time, to prevent the hardened crust of mucus which accumulates and obstructs it under such circumstances.

Saw him again the same evening, and found no material change, except some febrile re-action, but not more than might be expected. Respiration easy and comfortable, slight mucous rales in the bronchial tubes. The extreme fretfulness and irritability of the child prevented a very accurate examination. Continued powders.

Saturday, 24th: child passed a tolerable night; pulse accelerated; cheeks flushed, and some heat of skin.

The mother informed me that about midnight there had been discharged through the wound, *above the tube,* a tough, tenacious "phlegm," after which the air seemed to pass almost entirely *per vias naturales,* the opening in the convexity of the tube allowing it to do so, illustrating the importance of such an arrangement, permitting the returning functions to be gradually and steadily resumed, as the obstruction is removed.

5 P. M. Still some febrile reaction; respiration perfectly easy and a little accelerated; but not more than would be the case with the same vascular disturbance under other circumstances. Inasmuch as the larynx seemed fully competent to perform its functions, and the trachea seemed almost free from disease, I removed the tube, as it was no longer needed, and would merely act as a foreign body. Fearing, however, that if the wound were closed too soon, a subsequent return of obstruction (in larynx) might take place, it was kept moderately dilated.

The same powders were continued Sunday 25th. Still some vascular disturbance, but not more than necessary for the purposes of reparation. Wound perfectly open, permitting a clear view of the posterior lining of the trachea; but, strange to say, scarcely any air escapes from it. Why is this? It is only in coughing that air in any volume escapes. Directed to continue powders.

Monday. 26th. Doing well; brought edges of wound together with adhesive straps; discontinued powders.

From this time the case progressed rapidly to a favorable termination, the wound closing in less than ten days from the time of the operation.

This case is instructive, as presenting the most favorable circumstances for an operation; being one of purely inflammatory croup, and the inflammation confined chiefly to the larynx and upper portion of the trachea.

There was also the advantage arising from very judicious medical treatment in the first instance, and equally judicious selection of the moment for operation. If it had been performed sooner, there would have been the doubt as to whether nature might not have effected a cure; deferred an hour or two, it would most probably have been too late.

The question as to the propriety of this operation has been much discussed within the last few years.

The English authorities of the highest standing, Porter, Stokes, Cheyne, &c., condemning it almost entirely, from the very indifferent success which has attended the operations of the British surgeons. The profession on the other side of the Channel, on the contrary, quite as generally, and with full as great an array of distinguished names, viz.: Trousseau, Bretonneau, Valleix, Velpeau, &c.. advocating it zealously, they having had a large share of success.

I have no means of showing the comparative success in the two countries, but the French statistics show highly favorable results. Of 173 operations previous to 1850 (of which M. Trousseau performed 135), 45 recovered, or 26 per cent.

Since 1850, the per centage of success has been greatly increased, owing, as M. Trousseau thinks, to improved methods of treatment introduced by him, such as the "use of the double canula," abstaining from the introduction of either water or solutions of nitrate of silver, as formerly, and the application of "a large cravat to temper the inspired air,"* "covering the wound with oiled silk to prevent the formation of false membrane." M. Trousseau thinks it important to prevent the formation of false membrane on the surface of the wound. He also objects to blisters, because, he says, false membrane will form upon the surface. Why, even if it forms, it should be so objectionable, he does not say.

By these improvements, 17 cases treated by M. Trousseau, and 36 in the Children's Hospital, of Paris, (53 in all), 19 recovered, or 36½ per cent.

In this country, Dr. Meigs mentions 19 operations, in which only 1 in 5 recovered, or 20 per cent. The exact statistics, however, I think, would show a much more favorable result.

---

* An india-rubber tube, connected with the canula, and passed through a bucket of water kept constantly warm, its end immersed in the vapor which arises from the water in the bucket, would answer a good purpose, both to temper and moisten the inspired air.

I understand that Dr. Ayres, of this city, has had 2 successful cases out of 4, or 50 per cent., and that Dr. Gescheidt, of New York, 2 out of 3, or 66 6-10 per cent., during the last winter. The successful ones were true membranous croup. Dr. Jno. Cochran, of this city, has had 12 cases, of which only 2 recovered, or 16 6-10 per cent.; but we have reason to believe that such a proportion of the severest operations have been successful, as would greatly reduce the per centage of mortality, according to Dr. Meigs.

In view of such success, we should certainly not be justified in refusing our sanction to this operation, both on the score of humanity and of surgical propriety.

Even if the results had been much less successful, I can see no reason why it should not be classed among the legitimate operations of surgery. Even if the recoveries were only 1 per cent., and it could be shown that no other means offered ony prospect of relief, it should be resorted to; for why permit the helpless little sufferers to die the most frightful and agonizing of deaths , when any means of relief remain untried, however small?

It has been objected "that the larynx is not mechanically closed by false membrane," and that "there is sufficient space in all cases for the access of air;" "that it is extremely difficult to say that exudation has taken place;" "that if the false membrane has extended below the incision, it can afford no relief;" "that bronchitis or pneumonia may exist;" "that the operation is a dangerous one;" "that the risk of inflammation is great," &c., which objections might be easily answered *seriatim*, and shown to be untenable as valid objections to the operation; but it is only necessary to refer to the statistical results for a complete vindication of the operation. M. Valleix says that the number of recoveries are "now too numerous to allow any one to think of opposing the operation."

When statistical tables shall show that medication has relieved a larger proportion of desperate cases than the operation, then we shall be justified in adopting the one and rejecting the other. But, so far from having any such countervailing testimony, either in the form of tabular statements or general professional sentiment, we have already a very fair tabular comparison by M. Valleix, in which 17 out of 54 cases of genuine croup, treated non-surgically, were cured, which is about the same result as in tracheotomy, previous to 1850, and less favorable than the operations since that date.

But we should bear in mind that in the one case the disease is taken in its incipient stage, and full time is allowed to bring to bear to all the appliances and means of medication, both externally and internally; while in the other, when every expedient known to the physician has been exhausted, and the case considered hopeless, so far as medical skill can avail, it is handed over to the surgeon, almost in a dying condition, as a sort of forlorn hope; and, even under such unfavorable circumstances, the mortality is shown to be less than when genuine croup is treated medically alone.

With such facts before us, then, it appears to me impossible to come to any other conclusion, than that tracheotomy should be resorted to when all the means which judicious and experienced medical men deem proper have been tried, and before the vital forces nave been impaired from nervous exhaustion and the circulation of imperfectly aerated blood.

From the Western Lancet.

Fistula in Ano, treated by Iodine Injections. By M. BOINET.

At the meeting of the Institute, of August 1st, M. Boinet read a memoir designed to demonstrate the efficacy of injections of iodine in the radical cure of fistulæ in ano, whatever their form, extent, or complications. Seven cases are detailed, which offer examples of almost every variety of fistulæ: complete, blind or incomplete fistulæ, deep fistulæ, with loss of substance of the intestine, and fistulæ in tuberculous subjects. These observations tend to prove that iodine injections may be advantageously employed in all cases of fistula, but especially in those in which the method by incision is dangerous or ineffectual; such, for example, as extend deeply, or occur in phthisicial patients, or depend upon some alteration of the ischium, the coccyx, or the sacrum.

The advantages of iodine injections over the ordinary method, consist in obtaining a cure more easily and in a shorter time, in avoiding pain and the danger of hæmorrhage, and in permitting the patients to continue at their usual avocations. The following are the conclusions of the memoir:

1. Iodine injections properly administered, can cure radically all cases of fistula, whether complete or incomplete, simple or complicated.

2. They cure them more promptly than the method by incision commonly employed, and with less danger.

3. They produce no pain, and are easily practised.

They permit patients to follow their occupations, and relieve them from daily painful dressings.

5. They are applicable to all cases, and especially to those in which incision or excision are dangerous or impossible.

6. They do no harm even if they are ineffectual, and do not prevent the subsequent use of the knife. It is, therefore, rational to employ them before having recourse to a cutting instrument. —*Gazette des Hopitaux,* No. 92.

EDITORIAL AND MISCELLANEOUS.

We here present our readers with the last number of the first volume of the "Peninsular Journal of Medicine."

We are making arrangements to go on with the Second Volume with an increased Editorial corps, and with a full determination to maintain the JOURNAL in a position among the foremost and best. Our arrangements for securing these objects, will be more fully detailed in a future number.

We present our cordial thanks to those who have sustained this new enter—

prise with their subscriptions and with their pens; and we solicit their co-operation for the coming year. By the continued good will and co-operation, of our friends, we trust that the enterprise will go forward with energy.

We would take occasion also to remark, that at the outset of such a work, there is necessarily a pecuniary loss to those who undertake it; and we doubt not that those subscribers who have not yet remitted, will generously bear this fact in mind, and with a hearty good will to the work, speedily enroll themselves among those marked " paid." both for the past and the coming volume. The medical men of Michigan are rapidly organizing and concentrating their forces, and the JOURNAL, which is their organ, should be among the most carefully cherished objects of their attention. To those who are lukewarm on this subject, we commend a perusal of the declarations and the *deeds* of the State Society at their annual meetings.

The prospect of the profession in Michigan for the future, is brighter than it has been for years. Its attitude is more firm and dignified, and its enemies are passing slowly and surely into relative insignificance. In the coming time we have but to do our duty fully and with strength, and we shall see the time when the very *name* of physician will be spoken with kindly reverence, and its desecration will be a blasphemy against joyful homes which have been rescued from desolation.

Obituary.

Died, in Schoolcraft, Kalamazoo Co., on Saturday the 18th of March last, of injuries received by being thrown from his sulky the Monday previous, Joseph Briggs, M.D., aged forty years.

California Journal of Medicine.

We have received a prospectus of a Journal to be issued under the above title at San Francisco, Cal. It is to be edited by Drs. J. B. Phinney and M.B. Angle.

The Georgia Blister and Critic.

This is a monthly Journal, published at Atlanta, Ga., and edited by H. A. Ramsay, M.D. It is a singular production, apparently devoted to medicine, fun, and the defence of the "peculiar institutions of the South." Such a combination of disconnected objects would not be useful in this region; but as we do not know what peculiar circumstances may be present at that place, we cannot say that it would not be, on some accounts, more desirable there. The editor seems to stand firmly in the regular orthodox ranks, so far as we can judge from the one number which has reached us, and his pages present valuable communications. A misunderstanding between him and the Ga. State Medical Society seems to be removed, and everything returning to harmony.

Rodgers on Epidemics and Sanatory Reform.

A pamphlet published in Rochester, N. Y., intended to arouse and instruct the people and authorities of that city in the means and regulations which ought to be adopted to free the streets from filth and guard the inhabitants from disease. The habits of the people, the condition of the markets, streets, sewers, cemeteries, canals, schools, hospitals, quarentine, pest house, &c., are commented on in a very sensible manner.

NEW WORKS:

Vidal on Venereal, and Fuller on Rheumatism.

We have received these finely got up works from the publishers, S. S. & W. Wood, of New York. *Vidal on Venereal* contains a series of colored plates of unusual beauty. We will present our readers with a review of their contents in our next number.

For sale by A. B Wood & Co., Ann Arbor, Mich.

Lightning Source UK Ltd.
Milton Keynes UK
UKHW022213140219
337291UK00006B/485/P